RECENT ADVANCES IN
CLINICAL PATHOLOGY

RECENT ADVANCES IN
CLINICAL
PATHOLOGY

SERIES V

GENERAL EDITOR

S. C. DYKE, D.M.(OXON), F.R.C.P.(LOND.), F.C.PATH.

Department of Pathology, University of Birmingham; Late Pathologist, The
Royal Hospital, Wolverhampton; The General (Sister Dora) Hospital, Walsall

With 169 Illustrations

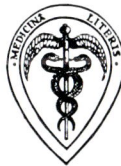

J. & A. CHURCHILL LTD.

104 GLOUCESTER PLACE, LONDON

1968

First Edition	.	.	.	.	.	.	1947
First Edition reprinted	.	.	.	.	.	.	1948
Second Edition	.	.	.	.	.	.	1951
Series III	.	.	.	.	.	.	1960
Series IV	.	.	.	.	.	.	1964
Series V	.	.	.	.	.	.	1968

Standard Book Number
7000·1387·3

*Printed in Great Britain by
T. & A. Constable Ltd., Edinburgh
Printers to the University of Edinburgh*

PREFACE

SINCE the publication of the first volume of this Series in 1947 the whole field of clinical medicine has undergone vast expansion and change; Clinical Pathology consists in the application of the methods of the hospital laboratory to the practice of medicine and its field must expand concurrently with that of the whole of medicine.

One of the effects of this development has been the blurring of the boundaries between what used to be referred to as the different "disciplines" which together constitute the field of pathology in the widest sense. For the sake of convenience this volume continues this division into Sections even though it becomes progressively more unrealistic. Chemical Pathology now plays a basic role in every part of Pathology and no chapter in the present volume fails to make reference to some aspect of it; in many instances particularly in Hæmatology and Histology twenty years ago, these aspects of the subject were not apparent or were only just becoming so; they fell within the sphere of research, but then formed no part of the activities of the pathologist working in a hospital laboratory devoted to immediate clinical problems.

From the beginning a major purpose of the series was to keep the hospital pathologist informed as to the new knowledge continually being accumulated by research workers in every field of science. Even today it is not altogether easy for the hospital pathologist working in a non-teaching hospital to keep himself in touch with all movements and currents of thought in the increasingly swelling flood of new knowledge; at the time of the initiation of the series the hospital pathologist worked largely in isolation; it was the sense of this that led to the formation of the Association of Clinical Pathologists in 1926; with the coming of the Emergency Hospital Service during the Second World War and of the National Health Service in 1948 the number of hospital pathologists in Great Britain greatly increased and thanks to the efforts of the A.C.P., particularly through its Committee on Education, their isolation is now a thing of the past. The first volume of this series was produced under the auspices of the European Association of Clinical Pathologists, which may be regarded as having been the offspring of the A.C.P. and this volume is therefore an emanation of that same parent.

When this series was launched the majority of hospital pathologists were faced with the necessity of dealing as best they could with all and every sort of laboratory investigation required in the practice of medicine; although in Great Britain this has largely ceased to be the case, there remain many parts of the world where a hospital service is still only emergent and where many hospital pathologists still find themselves called upon to deal single-handed with problems in every branch of medical practice; whether working as a member of a team or single-handed, the necessity remains for the clinical pathologist to maintain contact with developments in all fields of clinical medicine, and it has been the aim of the Section Editors to include chapters dealing with the more recent growing-points of their various branches.

The increasing automation of laboratory procedures, more especially in Chemical Pathology, has vastly lightened the work-load of the hospital laboratory; many investigations can now be performed with a speed undreamt of even fifteen years ago when dependance was almost entirely on manual methods. But the introduction of fuller automation and more lately of the computer have brought into the working of the hospital laboratory factors of which it is impossible at this stage in their development to foresee the full effects; it is certain that they will be far-reaching on its whole structure and organization; they can in no way alter its aim and purpose but they may well change the method of approach to their problems of those charged with the direction of the service. When procedures were almost entirely manual it was a prime duty of the pathologist to ensure that the pairs of hands at his disposal were not wastefully employed; it was imperative upon him to keep a watchful eye on the calls upon his department made by his clinical colleagues and even on occasion to remonstrate with them against wasteful and irrelevant demands.

The development of automation bids fair to change this whole outlook; it is becoming increasingly apparent that using multi-channel systems there is a strong case for conducting the full gamut of investigations, particularly on the blood of every patient upon his admission to the wards. From the results it is possible with computer assistance, to construct what have been called "profiles" throwing a flood of light upon many aspects of the work of the laboratory and of the wards. An investigation largely sponsored by the Ministry of Health is now in progress at the Queen Elizabeth Hospital, Birmingham, under the charge of Professor T. P. Whitehead, Director of the Department of Biochemistry of the Hospital; I am indebted to Professor Whitehead for having given me the opportunity of observing the working of this project; one fact which emerges clearly from it is that given multi-channel automation the examination and analysis of several score of specimens of blood for a dozen or more different constituents is less laborious and time-consuming than carrying out only one or two examinations on a few specimens by manual methods. With full automation the future routine will no doubt be the performance of a full range of investigation upon every specimen of blood submitted to the laboratory, even though only one or possibly none of the results may eventually prove relevant to the clinical problem.

Automation first made its appearance in the hospital laboratory in the shape of the Autotechnicon in the division of Histology and until now this has remained the sole automated procedure in this department; the introduction of cybernetics along with automation into Cytology in the shape of devices such as "Cesar" points towards vistas of which it is impossible at this stage to envisage the future prospects.

It is too early yet to form any clear view of the financial aspects of a fully automated laboratory service, but it seems possible that the time will come when one central fully automated and computerised laboratory will deal with much of the laboratory work of many hospitals in its surrounding area.

As General Editor it is a pleasure to me to place on record my gratitude to all those who assisted in the production of this volume; firstly I have to thank the Section Editors who themselves selected the contributors to their various Sections and edited their manuscripts; of these Dr. E. N. Allott remains the only representative along with myself of the editorial staff of the first volume of this series; for this volume I have to welcome three new members on to the editorial staff; on the lamented death of Professor Mary Barber, Professor R. E. O. Williams of St. Mary's Hospital, London, very kindly undertook the Section of Microbiology; Professor G. Wetherley-Mein of St. Thomas's Hospital, London, succeeds Dr. Rosemary Biggs, who found that pressure of other work made it impossible for her to continue to edit the Section of Hæmatology; Dr. A. H. T. Robb-Smith has relinquished the editing of the Section of Histology to Dr. M. S. Dunnill, a member of his own staff at the Radcliffe Infirmary, Oxford; Dr. Robb-Smith was one of the original editorial staff and had continued active upon it throughout all preceding volumes of the series; as General Editor I am deeply grateful to him for support and advice throughout the years.

I have to express my deep regret at the late appearance of this volume; this delay in publication arose from a concatenation of accidents and mishaps lying entirely beyond the control of the editorial staff; as General Editor I have shared to the full in the frustration and annoyance felt by the Section Editors and all contributors, I am deeply indebted to the many authors who, at no little trouble to themselves, brought their contributions up to date during the period of delay; but for their forbearance and co-operation this volume might have ceased to merit the title "Recent"; thanks to them I am happy to believe this not to be the case.

I have to thank Professor R. C. Curran of the Department of Pathology, University of Birmingham, for providing accommodation and assistance without which it would have not been possible for me to have undertaken the preparation of this volume.

S. C. DYKE

Department of Pathology
The Medical School
University of Birmingham

CONTRIBUTORS

D. J. BARTLETT, M.B., B.CHIR., PH.D.
Cytologist, M.R.C. Population Genetics Research Unit, Oxford.

J. R. BATCHELOR, M.D.(CAMB.), M.R.C.S.(ENG.), L.R.C.P.(LOND.)
The East Grinstead Research Trust, Queen Victoria Hospital, East Grinstead, Sussex.

D. BETTY BROWNELL, M.B., CH.B., B.A.O.(DUBL.)
Research Fellow, Neuropathology Department, Radcliffe Infirmary, Oxford.

W. BRUMFITT, M.D., PH.D. M.R.C.P.(LOND.), M.C.PATH.
Consultant Clinical Pathologist, Edgware General Hospital; Senior Lecturer in Bacteriology, St. Mary's Hospital Medical School, London.

I. CHANARIN, M.D.(CAPE TOWN), M.C.PATH.
Reader in Hæmatology and Consultant Hæmatologist, St. Mary's Hospital Medical School, London.

NAOMI DATTA, M.D.(LOND.), M.C.PATH.
Senior Lecturer in Bacteriology, Royal Postgraduate Medical School London; Honorary Consultant Bacteriologist, Hammersmith Hospital, London.

G. C. DE GRUCHY, M.D., B.S., F.R.A.C.P., F.R.C.P.(LOND.)
Professor of Medicine, University of Melbourne, Australia.

J. A. DUDGEON, M.D.(CAMB.), F.C.PATH.
Consultant Microbiologist, The Hospital for Sick Children and Institute of Child Health, Great Ormond Street; Lecturer in Virus Diseases, Institute of Dermatology, University of London.

M. S. DUNNILL, M.D.(BRISTOL), M.R.C.P.(LOND.), M.C.PATH.
Director of Clinical Studies, The University of Oxford; Consultant Pathologist, Radcliffe Infirmary, Oxford.

G. V. FOSTER, M.D., PH.D.
Established Investigator of the American Heart Association; Hon. Lecturer in Chemical Pathology, Royal Post-Graduate Medical School, London.

GEOFFREY FRANGLEN, B.SC.(LOND.)
Lecturer in Chemical Pathology, St. George's Hospital Medical School, London.

A. J. GRIMES, PH.D.
Senior Lecturer in Experimental Hæmatology, Department of Hæmatology, St. Thomas's Hospital Medical School, London.

T. B. HALES, M.B., B.CHIR.(CAMB.), M.C.PATH.
Consultant Chemical Pathologist, Clatterbridge Hospital, Bebington, Cheshire.

R. M. HARDISTY, M.D.(LOND.), M.R.C.P.(LOND.), F.C.PATH.
Consultant Hæmatologist, Hospital for Sick Children, Great Ormond Street, London.

A. V. HOFFBRAND, B.M., B.CH., M.R.C.P.(LOND.)
Lecturer in Hæmatology, Royal Postgraduate Medical School and Hon. Consultant to the Hammersmith Hospital, London.

C. A. HOLMAN, M.B., B.S.(LOND.), M.R.C.P.(LOND.), F.C.PATH.
Consultant Pathologist, Lewisham Group Laboratory.

J. TREVOR HUGHES, M.D.(MANCH.), M.R.C.P.(EDIN.), M.C.PATH.
Consultant Neuropathologist, Radcliffe Infirmary, Oxford.

N. C. HUGHES JONES, D.M.(OXON.), PH.D.(LOND.)
Member, Experimental Hæmatological Research Unit, St. Mary's Hospital, London.

W. J. IRVINE, B.SC.(HNRS.), M.B., B.CH., F.R.C.P.(EDIN.)
Consultant Physician, Royal Infirmary, Edinburgh; Senior Lecturer, Dept. of Therapeutics, University of Edinburgh.

JADWIGA KARNICKI, M.B., CH.B.(WARSAW AND ST. ANDREWS), F.R.C.O.G.
Consultant Obstetrician and Gynæcologist, Lewisham Hospital.

J. C. KELSEY, M.D.(CAMB.), M.C.PATH.
Deputy Director, Public Health Laboratory Service; Administrative Director, Central Public Health Laboratory, London.

J. LIDDELL, M.D.(CAMB.), M.C.PATH.
Consultant Chemical Pathologist, Guy's Hospital, London.

E. J. L. LOWBURY, D.M.(OXON.), F.C.PATH.
Hon. Director, Hospital Infection Research Laboratory, Summerfield Hospital, Birmingham; Bacteriologist, M.R.C. Burns Research Unit, Birmingham Accident Hospital.

N. S. MAIR, M.B., CH.B.(GLAS.), F.C.PATH.
Director, Public Health Laboratory Service, Leicester.

A. A. E. MASSOUD, M.D.(CAIRO), PH.D.(MANCH.), Research Fellow, Department of Virology, and Department of Occupational Health, University of Manchester; Lecturer in Occupational Medicine, Ain Shams University, Cairo.

D. N. MITCHELL, M.D.(LOND.), M.R.C.S.(ENG.)
Member of Medical Staff, Medical Research Council, Tuberculosis Research Unit.

D. L. MOLLIN, B.SC.(WALES), M.B., CH.B., M.R.C.P.(LOND.), F.C.PATH.
Professor of Hæmatology, St. Bartholomew's Hospital Medical School, London.

P. L. MOLLISON, M.D.(CAMB.), F.R.C.P.(LOND.), F.C.PATH., F.R.S.
Professor of Hæmatology, St. Mary's Hospital Medical School, University of London; Director, Dept. of Hæmatology, St. Mary's Hospital.

DELPHINE M. V. PARROTT, PH.D.(GLAS.)
Senior Lecturer, Department of Bacteriology and Immunology, Western Infirmary, Glasgow.

J. PEPYS, M.B., CH.B.(WITS.), M.R.C.P.(LOND.), F.R.C.P.(EDIN.)
Director of Clinical Immunology Research Group, Medical Research Council, London.

A. I. SPRIGGS, D.M.(OXON.), M.R.C.P.(LOND.), M.C.PATH.
Consultant Cytologist, United Oxford Hospitals.

H. STERN, PH.D., M.B., CH.B.(GLAS.), M.C.PATH.
Reader in Virology, University of London; Consultant Virologist, St. George's Hospital, London.

G. TAYLOR, M.D.(MANCH.)
Senior Lecturer in Immunology, Department of Bacteriology, University of Manchester.

G. WALTERS, M.D.(BRISTOL), M.R.C.P.(LOND.), M.C.PATH.
Consultant Pathologist, Wolverhampton Hospital Group.

D. J. WEATHERALL, M.D.(LIVERP.), M.R.C.P.(LOND.)
Senior Lecturer in Haematology, Dept. of Medicine, University of Liverpool; Hon. Cons, Physician (Hæmatology), United Liverpool Hospitals.

ROBERT G. WHITE, D.M.(OXON.), M.R.C.P.(GLAS.)
Gardiner Professor of Bacteriology and Immunology, University of Glasgow.

R. WHITEHEAD, M.D.(LIVERP.), M.C.PATH.
Consultant Pathologist, Radcliffe Infirmary, Oxford.

CONTENTS

SECTION I—MICROBIOLOGY

Editor: R. E. O. WILLIAMS

SECTION II—CHEMICAL PATHOLOGY

Editor: E. N. ALLOTT

SECTION III—HÆMATOLOGY

Editor: G. WETHERLEY-MEIN

SECTION IV—HISTOLOGY

Editor: M. S. DUNNILL

CONTENTS
SECTION V—IMMUNOLOGY

Editor: P. G. H. GELL

SECTION I

MICROBIOLOGY

Section Editor

R. E. O. WILLIAMS

B.Sc., M.D., F.R.C.P., F.C.Path.

Professor of Bacteriology, University of London, and
Dean, St. Mary's Hospital Medical School

Chapter 1

PSEUDOMONAS ÆRUGINOSA

E. J. L. Lowbury

Pseudomonas æruginosa (*pyocyanea*) is an organism of low pathogenicity for healthy subjects, but an important pathogen in patients or tissues with poor resistance. It causes hospital infection of burns, wounds, skin, urinary tract, respiratory tract, ears, eyes and meninges, and has a tendency to invade the bloodstream. In recent years it has attracted more attention and probably caused more illness and death in hospitals than formerly.

There are several reasons for this increased prominence of *Ps. æruginosa*. Unlike *Streptococcus pyogenes* or even, in recent years, *Staphylococcus aureus*, *Ps. æruginosa* has responded poorly to antibiotic therapy. Another factor is the increased number of patients with heightened susceptibility to *Ps. æruginosa*, including those who survive hazards which were formerly a common cause of death, such as fluid loss in severe burns, and those who are treated with immuno-suppressive or steroid drugs. Successful chemotherapy for other pathogens also plays a part by allowing *Ps. æruginosa* to colonize wounds without competition, and certain procedures such as the use of respiratory ventilators and hæmodialysis involve special hazards of contamination.

BACTERIOLOGY

Description and Classification

The blue pigment pyocyanin was described and crystallized (Fordos, 1860) before Gessard (1882) discovered the "bacillus of blue pus". Classical studies on the morphology, cultural characters, pigments and biochemistry of the organism established its position in the genus *Pseudomonas*, of which it became the type species. Members of the genus are commonly distinguished from other Gram-negative bacilli by a positive oxidase reaction (Kovacs, 1956), oxidative metabolism of glucose (Hugh and Leifson, 1953), a positive arginine dihydrolase reaction (Thornley, 1960) and the presence of polar flagella; some species produce characteristic pigments, including the yellow chloroform-insoluble pigment fluorescin, which is produced by almost all strains of *Ps. æruginosa*, and also by *Ps. fluorescens* and *Ps. putida*.

Detailed taxonomic studies of the genus *Pseudomonas* have been reported by Lysenko (1961) and Stanier, Palleroni and Doudoroff (1966), and of the fluorescent pseudomonads, including *Ps. æruginosa*, by Liston, Wiebe and Colwell (1961), Rhodes (1961) and others. Large numbers of tests were made on collections of strains, and quantitative methods, including computer analysis, were used to differentiate species or "clusters", each character being given equal weight. This method of classification, originally proposed by the French biologist Adanson in 1757, has given more precise and stable taxonomies for bacteria than other systems, and it avoids the risk of attaching crucial importance to characters that are likely to be variable (Sneath, 1962). On the basis of such analysis *Ps. æruginosa* has been shown to form a well-defined cluster in the genus *Pseudomonas*. Characters that are shared by most strains of *Ps. æruginosa* are production of the blue chloroform-soluble pigment pyocyanin, reduction of nitrate to nitrogen, production of slime in a chemically defined medium containing potassium gluconate (Haynes, 1951). and growth at 41–43°C; these characters are rare (and pyocyanin production is unknown) in other species of *Pseudomonas*.

Ps. æruginosa is more widely known in Britain as *Ps. pyocyanea*. The pigment of blue pus was called "pyocyanine" by Fordos (1860), and Gessard (1890) called the organism which he had discovered "le microbe pyocyanique". The name *æruginosa* ("rusty", "full of copper rust") is considered to have priority because it was used by Schroeter (1875) for an organism which he believed to exist as the source of a pigment observed in cultures.

Isolation and Identification

Pseudomonas æruginosa is one of the easier pathogens to isolate and identify. When the growth on agar medium and in broth is characteristic in appearance and odour, and when it produces blue-green pigmentation on an appropriate medium, one may reasonably assume that the organism is *Ps. æruginosa*. But pyocyanin is not visible on blood agar and it often does not appear in nutrient broth. Some strains do not produce pyocyanin at all, or produce it only on special media that enhance the production of this pigment (e.g. Wahba and Darrell, 1965). To ensure that *Ps. æruginosa* is not frequently missed, it is useful to include special methods that show characters commonly shared by *Ps. æruginosa* with other pseudomonads (e.g. fluorescin and oxidase production), as well as those which are uncommon or unknown in other species (see above).

The following procedure is convenient for the examination of clinical specimens in which special emphasis is attached to the isolation of *Ps. æruginosa* (see also Appendix). The specimen is inoculated on horse-blood agar, on improved 0·03 per cent cetrimide agar (Brown and Lowbury, 1965) and in a liquid medium (nutrient broth or cooked meat broth); cetrimide agar is useful both in selecting *Ps. æruginosa* from a mixed culture and (because very few other bacteria grow on it at 37°C) in providing a diagnostic character for the species. The improved medium uses King's medium B (King, Ward and Raney, 1954) as the base; this enhances the production of fluorescin (but not of pyocyanin). After overnight incubation at 37°C, the cultures on blood agar and on cetrimide agar are examined by daylight and under ultraviolet irradiation; cultures on cetrimide agar showing no growth or scanty unpigmented growth are examined again after 42–48 hours' incubation. Cultures in liquid medium are subcultured by "spot inoculation" on plates of cetrimide agar (16–25 cultures per plate), which are examined after 18 hours' incubation. Detection of fluorescence is aided by examination in an ultraviolet viewing cabinet (see Fig. 1) which can be used in an undarkened room (Lowbury, Lilly and Wilkins, 1962). Blue-green or yellow fluorescent growth on blood agar indicates the presence of a fluorescent pseudomonad on the plate, but the pigment diffuses readily through agar and is picked up by other types of bacteria (e.g. *Proteus* spp.), which then fluoresce as brightly as the pseudomonad (Hurst and Lowbury, 1952); it therefore cannot be assumed that any fluorescent colony in a mixed culture is a colony of the pseudomonad present.

Fluorescent growth on cetrimide agar at 37°C is almost always *Ps. æruginosa*. For confirmatory tests, the growth is subcultured to blood agar or nutrient agar, and a pure culture is obtained from a colony. This is examined for oxidase and pyocyanin production; tests for oxidative metabolism of glucose, the arginine dihydrolase reaction, slime production in the special medium containing potassium gluconate, growth at 42°C, reduction of nitrate to gas, and growth as red colonies on 1 per cent tetrazolium agar (Selenka, 1958) give further evidence that the organism is *Ps. æruginosa*, and are useful if the strain does not produce pyocyanin.

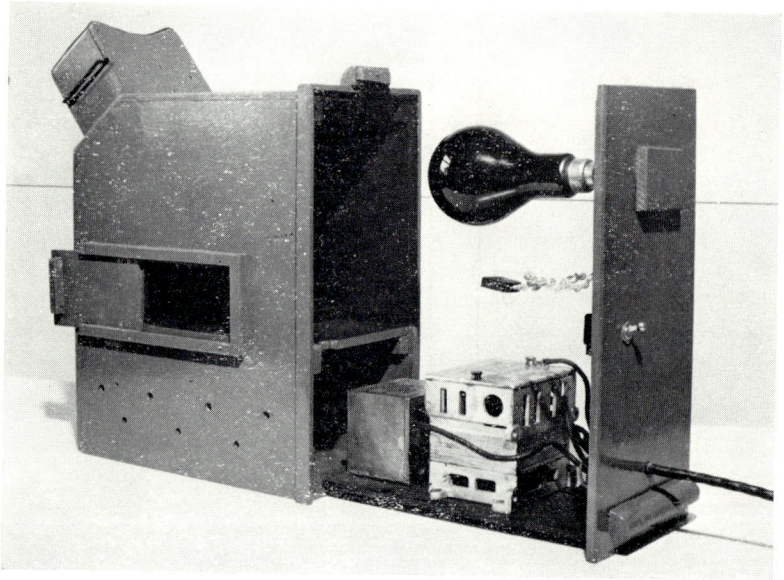

FIG. 1. Cabinet for examination of cultures for fluorescence, with section carrying ultraviolet lamp pulled out from shell. Plate cultures are inserted through the door on the side, and examined through a window projecting from one end of the roof (Lowbury, Lilly and Wilkins, 1962).

Typing Methods

The recognition of a number of different types of *Ps. æruginosa* has been found useful in epidemiological studies. Three methods are available.

Serological Typing. Subdivision of *Ps. æruginosa* into serological types has been studied and developed for many years. Earlier attempts to prepare typing sera were hampered by the use of antigens which did not stimulate good production of O antibodies (e.g. Christie, 1948; Mayr-Harting, 1948; Lowbury and Fox, 1954). In 1957 Habs differentiated *Ps. æruginosa* into 12 serotypes by agglutination with antisera prepared in animals immunized with boiled suspensions. A similar typing scheme was developed by Verder and Evans (1961), and the two systems were recently correlated by Muraschi *et al.* (1966). From these and other studies (Sandvik, 1960; Veron, 1961; Wahba, 1965) a wider range of typing sera has been developed. Most serotypes are found in widely separated parts of the world. Tube or slide agglutination and also precipitin reactions with trichloracetic acid extracts have been successfully used for typing.

Serological typing has been found useful in studies on the sources of hospital infection (e.g. Lowbury and Fox, 1954; Gould and McLeod, 1960; Wahba, 1965; Bassett, Thompson and Page, 1965).

Phage Typing. This method has been studied by Don and van den Ende (1950), Gould and McLeod (1960), Postic and Finland (1961), Graber *et al.* (1962), Sutter, Hurst and Fennel (1965), Shooter *et al.* (1966) and others. It does not result in the definition of distinct types, but gives very numerous pattern reactions which are usually of epidemiological significance. This subdivision is independent of the serological type.

Phage typing has been used successfully in epidemiological studies (e.g. Ayliffe *et al.*, 1965, 1966; Sutter and Hurst, 1966; Phillips, 1966).

Pyocine Typing. Darrell and Wahba (1964) and Gillies and Govan (1966) have developed systems for typing *Ps. æruginosa* by their production of bacteriocines (pyocines), detected by their action on a range of indicator strains. Osman (1965) has recently proposed a different method of typing, in which the strains under investigation are tested for sensitivity to pyocines produced by a range of indicator strains. These methods provide a differentiation of patterns which is only partially independent of serological typing; members of the same serotype have a restricted range of pyocine typing patterns.

Testing for pyocine production has been used with success in epidemiological studies by Wahba (1965), Bassett *et al.* (1965) and others.

By each method a proportion of the strains examined are untypable. In general, the results of serological and pyocine typing have been reproducible and presented no difficulty in interpretation. The interpretation of phage typing, though sometimes easy, often presents great difficulty. On the other hand, while approximately 30 per cent of all typable isolates of *Ps. æruginosa* belong to one serological type (6) and one pyocine type (D), this type can be usefully subdivided into a number of phage types (Asheshov and Parker, personal communication). In two outbreaks studied in Birmingham (Ayliffe *et al.*, 1965, 1966), the strains of *Ps. æruginosa* causing infection could not be distinguished by serological or pyocine typing, but were clearly distinguished by phage typing.

At present it would seem that the combined use of phage typing with one other method gives better differentiation of strains than can be obtained by the use of either method alone.

EPIDEMIOLOGY

Factors that determine how a pathogenic species spreads to cause infection in hospital include its presence in infected patients and in various carrier sites of nurses, patients and others, its viability, and consequent density, in dry and wet environments outside the body, and the presence of susceptible subjects or receptor areas among the patients. A knowledge of these details as they apply in the case of infection with *Ps. æruginosa* helps to explain the peculiar features of its epidemiology and the ways in which it differs from that of *Staphylococcus aureus*.

Ps. æruginosa is carried in the intestinal tract by a small proportion of normal subjects; examination of fæcal specimens or of rectal swabs has shown carrier rates of 11 per cent (Ringen and Drake, 1952), 3 per cent (Lowbury and Fox, 1954), 4 per cent (McLeod, 1958) and 12 per cent (Shooter *et al.*, 1966). Patients in hospital have shown higher carrier rates;

e.g. in the series reported by Shooter *et al.* (1966) 24 per cent of patients carried *Ps. æruginosa* on admission and 38 per cent carried the organism at some time during their stay in hospital. Other sites rarely carry the organisms, but it is found in small numbers, as a contaminant, on the hands of nurses in wards where patients with *Ps. æruginosa* infection are treated (Lowbury and Fox, 1954). The same authors found *Ps. æruginosa* in the upper respiratory tract of some nurses and patients in such an environment, a burns ward.

Like other Gram-negative bacilli, *Ps. æruginosa* is readily killed by drying; though individual strains vary considerably, the great majority of the bacteria die while drying proceeds, and all strains appear to suffer much greater loss than strains of Gram-positive cocci similarly tested (Lowbury and Fox, 1953). Once dry, however, the small residue of living *Ps. æruginosa* survives, as staphylococci do, with little loss for several days if the organisms are protected from light. In fluid environments (e.g. physiological saline) *Ps. æruginosa* survives better than *Staph. aureus* (Pettit, personal communication), and it can multiply in water with minimal nutrient additives. It is also more resistant than most bacteria to certain disinfectants.

Since normal healthy individuals do not suffer from infection with *Ps. æruginosa*, it is (unlike *Staph. aureus*) a hazard almost peculiar to hospitals, and especially in those where "high-risk" patients are treated and where susceptible tissues (e.g. the meninges and the anterior chamber of the eye) are exposed.

There have been many reports in recent years which show the pattern of infection with *Ps. æruginosa* in hospitals. Endemic infections occur where burns provide both a continuing source of cross-infection and a target for fresh infections (Lowbury and Fox, 1954); a similar endemic infection may occur in urological wards (Pyrah *et al.*, 1955). In neurosurgery and ophthalmic surgery (Ayliffe *et al.*, 1965, 1966), infection with *Ps. æruginosa* is occasional and epidemic, arising from the use of contaminated fluids or equipment. Both the endemic and the epidemic situations involve the acquisition of *Ps. æruginosa* from the human or the inanimate environment; it seems likely that self-infection with strains carried in the patient's intestinal canal also occurs in sporadic cases (Shooter *et al.*, 1966).

Contaminated fluids which have or might have caused infection with *Ps. æruginosa* include eye-drops and other ophthalmic solutions (e.g. Thygeson, 1948; Ridley, 1958; Ayliffe *et al.*, 1966); soaps, lotions and certain antiseptics, especially quaternary ammonium compounds, chloroxylenol and chlorhexidine, particularly in bottles with cork closures (Lowbury, 1951); a steroid cream (Noble and Savin, 1966) and lignocaine jelly used for tracheal catheters (Phillips, 1966). Equipment that contains standing water or retains moisture is a common source of contamination with *Ps. æruginosa*, such as air-cooling apparatus (Anderson, 1959), resuscitation equipment for premature infants (Bassett *et al.*, 1965; Rubbo *et al.*, 1966), respirators (Phillips and Spencer, 1965), urine bottles and bedpans (McLeod, 1958) and brushes; in one neurosurgery centre, meningitis was probably acquired through occasional use of a shaving-brush in the pre-operative preparation of the scalp (Ayliffe *et al.*, 1965). The maintenance of high humidity in infant incubators has been associated with a high incidence of infection with *Ps. æruginosa* (Hoffman and Finberg, 1955). Sinks are commonly found contaminated with *Ps. æruginosa*, and may perhaps be a source from which patients become infected. Surgical instruments (e.g. resectoscopes and Bigelow evacuators) have been found to transmit infection when "sterilized" by inadequate disinfectant solution (Moore and Forman, 1966); Rogers (1960) has made similar observations in respect of catheters and other equipment used for removal of tracheal mucus.

As expected, dry reservoirs such as floor dust usually contain very small numbers of *Ps. æruginosa*, and the organism is rarely found in the air; though in some circumstances they may be more numerous and present a hazard. For example, Hurst and Sutter (1966) found that large numbers of *Ps. æruginosa* were present and could survive for weeks in pieces of eschar removed from the floor of a ward occupied by patients with burns. Cellulose wadding used for packing plaster bandages has been incriminated as a source of infection (Sussman and Stevens, 1960), and the removal of dressings from infected burns can cause heavy contamination of air; the use of an air-conditioned dressing station was shown, in a controlled trial, to cause a considerable reduction in the incidence of *Ps. æruginosa* infection of burns (Lowbury, 1954). Although the great majority of *Ps. æruginosa* allowed to dry on the skin die during evaporation of the suspension, the dry hands of nurses attending patients with burns or tracheostomies often carry small or moderate numbers of *Ps. æruginosa*, and may be an important vector of infection.

The resistance of *Ps. æruginosa* to almost all the antibiotics used in hospitals is an important factor by which the organisms gain a selective advantage over others and is enabled to flourish where it is most likely to cause clinical infection. This factor has undoubtedly contributed to the relative and sometimes absolute increase in *Ps. æruginosa* infection in the past 20 years (Yow, 1952; Asay and Koch, 1960).

PATHOGENICITY

Although *Ps. æruginosa* was recognized by earlier workers to be pathogenic in susceptible subjects (see Fraenkel, 1917), it was, until recent times, often dismissed as a harmless saprophyte. The new interest in *Ps. æruginosa* has centred mainly on its tendency to cause septicæmia and death in extensively burned patients (Jackson *et al.*, 1951; Markley *et al.*, 1957; Tumbusch *et al.*, 1961) and in those whose defences are weakened by leukæmia and other malignant disease and by immuno-suppressive treatment (e.g. Forkner *et al.*, 1958; Margaretten *et al.*, 1961).

Strains of *Ps. æruginosa* produce a number of **Toxic Factors**, but there is still uncertainty about their respective rôles in pathogenicity. Liu, Abe and Bates (1961) separated several fractions from the surface of cultures; lethal effects were obtained on intraperitoneal inoculation of mice with extracellular slime and (to a smaller extent) with lecithinase and proteinases; cells washed with acid to remove the slime were non-toxic. The enzymes were found to cause severe local lesions on intradermal injection into rabbits. Pyocyanin caused no toxic effects in these tests, but concentrations of this pigment much lower than those found in infected burns have been found toxic to tissue cultures of human skin (Cruickshank and Lowbury, 1953), and it probably has some part in causing the failure of skin grafts (Jackson *et al.*, 1951). Elastase may have an important rôle in facilitating septicæmic invasion through the walls of blood vessels (Mull and Callahan, 1965), and endotoxins, which have been extracted by Chün-Hsiang *et al.*, (1964), may be important in causing circulatory collapse. Strains of *Ps. æruginosa* vary greatly in their virulence for experimental animals (e.g. Jones *et al.*, 1966), and current studies show some association between virulence of the strain and its production of certain extracellular fractions (Carney and Jones, personal communication).

Characteristic focal, infarct-like lesions have been described in patients with invasive *Ps. æruginosa* infection. They appear as black hæmorrhagic necrotic lesions in burns (see Fig. 5), as ecthymatous foci and ulcerations of unburned skin (see Fig. 2) and in various organs (especially lungs and

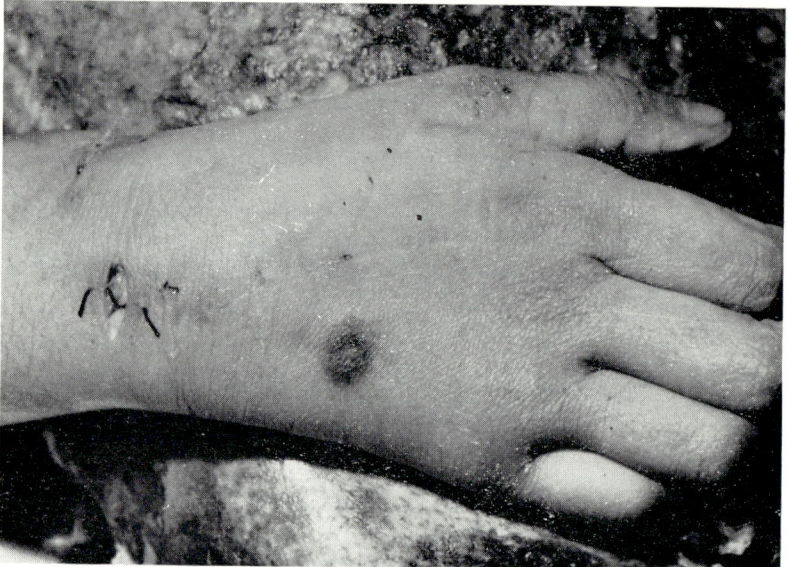

FIG. 2. Focal hæmorrhagic necrotic lesion (ecthyma gangrænosum) in unburned skin of a patient who died with *Ps. æruginosa* septicæmia. (By courtesy of S. Sevitt.)

kidneys) examined at post-mortem (Fraenkel, 1917; Rabin *et al.*, 1961; Sevitt, 1964). Another characteristic feature of invasion by *Ps. æruginosa* is the development of diffuse necrotic and inflammatory lesions in the living tissues subjacent to the colonized slough (burn wound sepsis). In these lesions the walls of blood vessels are densely infiltrated with Gram-negative bacilli (Forkner *et al.*, 1958; Teplitz *et al.*, 1964) (see Figs. 3 and 4). Patients with *Ps. æruginosa* septicæmia commonly have hyperpyrexia and leucocytosis, but sometimes hypothermia and leucopenia, associated with paralytic ileus, hypotension and anuria; this syndrome has been considered to be characteristic of septicæmia with Gram-negative organisms (Tumbusch *et al.*, 1962). These authors have also suggested that the characteristic focal lesion may be a local Schwartzman reaction, and that tissue sensitized by blood-borne organisms may receive a provoking dose of endotoxin released from dead bacterial cells; for this reason they believe that antibiotics (e.g. polymyxin) which kill large numbers of *Ps. æruginosa* may, in some cases, enhance this danger of toxæmia.

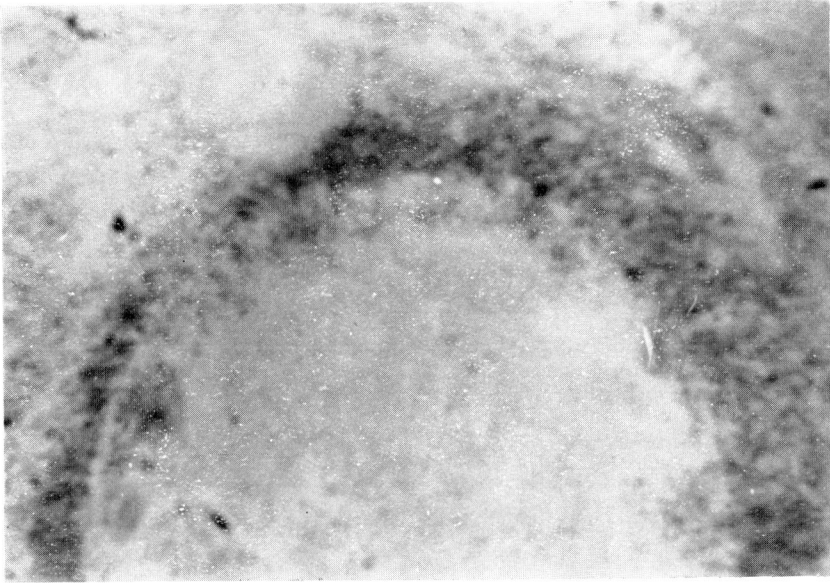

FIG. 3. Vessel in ecthymatous skin lesion infiltrated by Gram-negative rods. The patient died with *Ps. æruginosa* septicæmia. (Gram-Twort, ×900.) (By courtesy of S. Sevitt.)

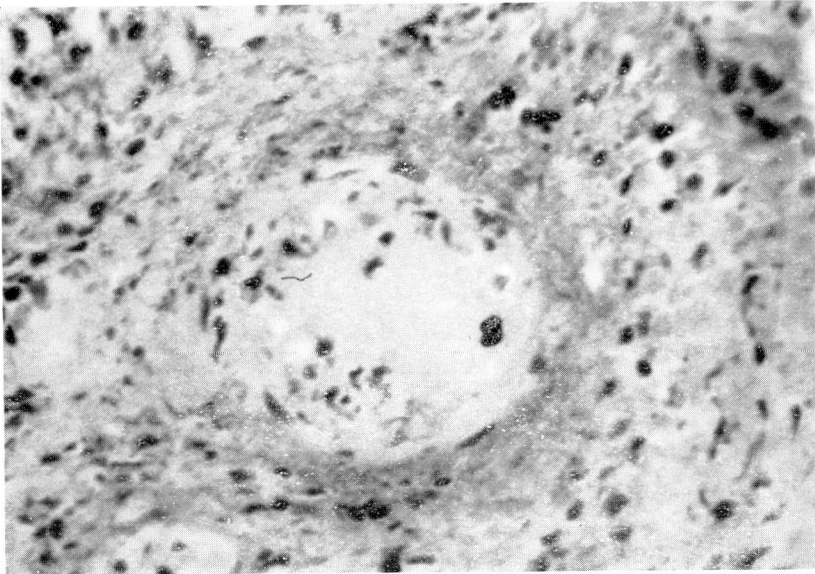

FIG. 4. Small artery in ecthymatous skin lesion infiltrated by Gram-negative rods, from a patient who died with *Ps. æruginosa* septicæmia. (Gram-Twort, ×400.) (By courtesy of S. Sevitt.)

Fortunately most patients whose burns are colonized with *Ps. æruginosa* do not develop invasive infections. The mechanisms that determine invasion involve both a deficiency in the immunity of the host and the production of toxic factors by the bacteria (Liu and Mercer, 1963; Jones and Lowbury, 1965); the conditions for invasion are likely to be present in the more extensively burned patients, possibly associated with increased circulation of steroid hormone (Sevitt, 1955) and with fluctuation in circulating

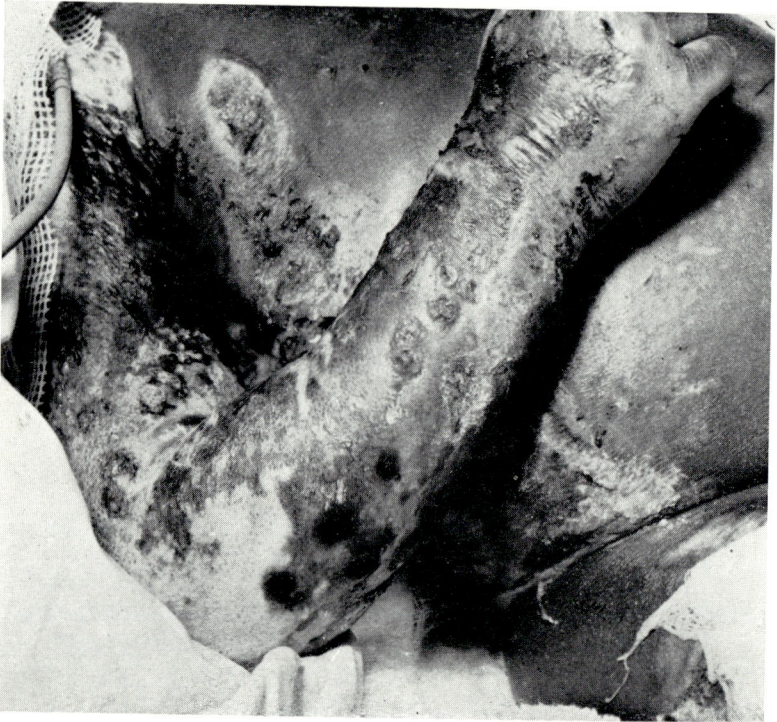

FIG. 5. Black hæmorrhagic necrotic foci in burn of a patient who died with *Ps. æruginosa* septicæmia. (By courtesy of S. Sevitt.)

antibody (Jones and Lowbury, 1963). In chronic bronchitis (Goslings, 1963) and fibrocystic disease of the pancreas, and also in patients with tracheostomies, severe infection of the respiratory tract tends to occur, but invasion of the bloodstream from this source seems to be rare, probably because of adequate levels of circulating antibody (Margaretten *et al.*, 1961).

One of the severest forms of local infection is panophthalmitis, which is likely to occur if *Ps. æruginosa* enters the interior of the eye at operation or through an injury. It has been reported that such an infection may occur and lead to the destruction of the eye of a rabbit into which as few as 50 cells of *Ps. æruginosa* are injected; much larger numbers of *Staph. aureus* were required to produce a similar result (Crompton, 1962).

IMMUNITY

Normal healthy subjects are strongly resistant to invasion by *Ps. æruginosa*. It is usual, too, for the blood of healthy subjects to contain antibody to the organism (Lilley and Bearup, 1928; Gaines and Landy, 1961; Jones and Lowbury, 1965); antibody responses in patients infected with *Ps. æruginosa* have been found (Lilley and Bearup, 1928; Sandiford, 1937; Fox and Lowbury, 1953a; Graber *et al.*, 1961). The importance of such immunity can be judged from the well-known hazard of systemic *Ps. æruginosa* infection in patients treated by whole body irradiation or with immuno-suppressive drugs, and in hypogammaglobulinæmia (Speirs *et al.*, 1963); the susceptibility of tissues and body fluids normally deficient in antibody (cerebrospinal fluid and intra-ocular fluids) is further evidence of the rôle of antibodies in defence.

Gaines and Landy (1961) and Graber *et al.* (1961) found hæmagglutinins to *Ps. æruginosa* lipo-polysaccharide, but no agglutinins to the bacteria, in normal human sera. Bacterial agglutinins were found in patients whose burns were infected with the organism (Graber *et al.*, 1961); mice challenged intraperitoneally with *Ps. æruginosa* were protected by serum from an infected burned patient, but not by normal human serum. Jones and Lowbury (1965) selected sera from two normal subjects, one with an agglutinin titre of 1/110 and one with no detectable agglutinin towards a strain of *Ps. æruginosa*; the former protected burned infected mice against invasive infection with the strain, but the latter gave no protection. These experiments provide evidence of differences in the degree of resistance correlated with agglutination titres. According to Liu and Mercer (1963) it is the antibody to the slime, and not the antibody to the lipopolysaccharide, which is responsible for both protection and agglutination. Some evidence of opsonic activity has been reported (Fox and Lowbury, 1953b), and Liu and Mercer (1963) describe bactericidal effects of antibody, though these may have been non-specific.

High titres of antibody have been found in some burned patients who subsequently died with *Ps. æruginosa* septicæmia (Fox and Lowbury, 1953a). This finding would seem to cast doubt on the protective value of antibody; but it is more probable that the antibody response in these patients came too late to prevent a fatal septicæmia, as in burned, infected mice when prophylactic treatment is delayed for 24 hours or more (Jones and Lowbury, 1966).

While antibodies clearly play an important rôle in protection, the non-specific bactericidins of serum, including the properdin system, though highly active against most strains of *Escherichia coli*, appear to have little or no activity against most strains of *Ps. æruginosa* (Lowbury and Ricketts, 1957).

PROPHYLAXIS

There are, essentially, two ways of protecting patients against *Ps. æruginosa*: (1) by preventing contamination of susceptible tissues, and (2) by preventing invasion. The former includes the whole range of aseptic and antiseptic procedures, and the latter includes immunization and the use of antibiotics.

To prevent post-operative infection in neurosurgery and eye surgery the main emphasis is on aseptic methods, with attention to the special hazards that exist in each situation, by ensuring the sterility of lumbar puncture apparatus, eye-drops, saline solution, and all equipment and materials used at operations, including those required for preparation of the site.

Urinary infection with Gram-negative bacilli, including *Ps. æruginosa*, is a potentially dangerous complication of catheterization, prostatectomy and gynæcological operations; its incidence has been greatly reduced by the combined application of a number of aseptic and antiseptic measures, including closed drainage, disinfection of the urethra, improved disinfection or sterilization of cystoscopes and immobilization of indwelling catheters (Gillespie *et al.*, 1964; Mitchell and Gillespie, 1964).

Infection of burns with *Ps. æruginosa* has been shown, in controlled trials, to be considerably reduced by local prophylactic treatment with polymyxin, and also by dressings such as tulle gras that keep the surface of the burn relatively dry (Jackson *et al.*, 1951; Cason and Lowbury, 1960; Lowbury *et al.*, 1962); the use of a plenum-ventilated room for dressing burns has also led to a significantly reduced incidence of *Ps. æruginosa* in burns. Preliminary results (Cason *et al.*, 1966) suggest that the use of a plastic ventilated isolator, which protects the patients against contact transfer as well as airborne infection, has some value in keeping burns free from *Ps. æruginosa*. More impressive results have recently been obtained with a solution of 0·5 per cent silver nitrate applied in compresses to burns. This method was described by Moyer *et al.* (1965) and studied in a controlled trial on extensively burned patients by Cason *et al.* (1966); in this trial *Ps. æruginosa* appeared in 95 out of 136 (70 per cent) samplings from burns in the control series, treated with penicillin cream, but in only 16 out of 509 samplings (3·1 per cent) from burns treated with silver nitrate compresses; these findings were associated with better clinical results in the patients treated with silver nitrate. A cream containing 0·5 per cent silver nitrate was also found to have a useful prophylactic effect, but less than that of compresses. An alternative method of local prophylaxis against *Ps. æruginosa* which has been favourably reported is the application of a cream containing 10 per cent *p*-amino methyl benzene sulphonamide (Lindberg *et al.*, 1965).

An inner line of defence by antibiotics or antisera against bacteria that break through the outer defences against contamination may be useful in very extensively burned patients, and particularly in those receiving immuno-suppressive treatment. Burned infected mice have been successfully protected against invasive infection with *Ps. æruginosa* by the use of antisera (Millican and Rust, 1960; Jones *et al.*, 1966). Serological protection in actively immunized rabbits, shown by reduction in the skin lesions, has been found when the immunizing and infecting strains were of the same serotype (Fox and Lowbury, 1953b); but cross-reactions occur between some of the serotypes, and a pooled antiserum prepared from six different types gave protection against a range of *Ps. æruginosa* strains, including other types (Jones and Lowbury, 1966). Feller (1966) has found that invasive infection with *Ps. æruginosa* in a burn unit was reduced when patients were given protective treatment with human antiserum prepared in volunteers against one strain.

Systemic prophylaxis by antibiotics has, until recently, had little success. The polymyxins have not prevented death from *Ps. æruginosa* septicæmia, but very large dosages of colistin sulphomethate appeared to have had some prophylactic value in a few patients studied (Jones *et al.*, 1966). Burned infected mice were not protected by such treatment, but successful prophylaxis in mice has been obtained with two new antibiotics, gentamicin and a new penicillin, carbenicillin (Jones and Lowbury, 1967).

CHEMOTHERAPY

Until recently the only antibiotics with some therapeutic value in the treatment of *Ps. æruginosa* infections have been the polymyxins, including colistin. All strains of *Ps. æruginosa* are sensitive *in vitro* to these agents, which are bactericidal. In spite of these potential advantages, however, the polymyxins have been only moderately successful in the treatment of infection with *Ps. æruginosa*. Jawetz (1952), Fekety *et al.* (1962) and others have reported successful results of treatment for urinary infection, but there is a tendency for relapse after treatment when the condition is chronic. Meningitis has been successfully treated with intrathecal injection of polymyxin (Hayes and Yow, 1950; Trapnell, 1954), and good results have been reported in local treatment of external otitis (Farrar, 1954) and wounds (Pulaski *et al.*, 1949); but septicæmia has responded poorly or not at all to the antibiotic (Tumbusch *et al.*, 1961; Kefalides *et al.*, 1964), probably because of inadequate blood levels. Fekety *et al.* (1962) report better results.

In one burned patient with septicæmia, very large dosage of colistin sulphomethate (7 million units daily in a child of 1 year) appeared to remove *Ps. æruginosa* from the bloodstream and even from the burns, but death with meningitis occurred after seven days' treatment; very few organisms were found in the meninges at autopsy. It seemed that the patient had suffered irreparable damage before septicæmia was recognized (Jones *et al.*, 1966). The likelihood of such an outcome makes it seem improbable that any form of chemotherapy would often succeed, and that emphasis should be placed on prophylaxis. Good results in the treatment of septicæmia in burned patients have, however, been reported with gentamicin by Stone *et al.* (1965), and promising results have been obtained in animal studies with carbenicillin (Jones and Lowbury, 1967).

CONCLUSIONS

With the improved control over *Staph. aureus* that has followed the introduction of penicillinase-insensitive penicillins, *Ps. æruginosa* and other Gram-negative bacilli have been found to play a greater rôle, and in some situations have become dominant agents of hospital infection; but there is a prospect of better control over *Ps. æruginosa* by the use of multiple barriers against infection. Further study is needed on the use of isolators, on the value of immunity, active and passive, and on the new antibiotics gentamicin and carbenicillin. Meanwhile there have been real advances in the control of infection in burns by local application of silver nitrate, and in urological surgery by a combination of both aseptic and antiseptic defences.

APPENDIX

The following media and methods are useful in the isolation and recognition of *Ps. æruginosa*:

(1) **Improved Cetrimide Agar** (Brown and Lowbury, 1965). The basal medium is King's medium B: Proteose peptone No. 3 (Difco), 20 g.; New Zealand agar, 15 g.; glycerol, 10 g.; distilled water, 1,000 ml. Adjust to pH 7·2. Autoclave for 15 minutes at 121°C. To 100 ml. of the melted solution add 1 ml. of a 15 per cent solution of K_2HPO_4 (anhydrous) and 1 ml. of a 15 per cent solution of $MgSO_4.7H_2O$, these solutions having been prepared with distilled water and Seitz-filtered. Add a Seitz-filtered solution of 2 per cent cetrimide (B.P.) to the basal medium to give a final concentration of 0·03 per cent.

The medium is selective for *Ps. æruginosa*, which shows brilliant yellow fluorescence in growth after 18 hours' or 42 hours' incubation at 37°C.

(2) **Modified Sierra Medium for Pyocyanin** (Wahba and Darrell, 1965). Bacto peptone 10 g.; NaCl 5 g.; $CaCl_2$ $1H_2O$, 0·2 g.; $MgSO_4$ $7H_2O$, 0·1 g.; agar (Davis), 18·0 g.; water (distilled), to 1,000 ml. Adjust this basal medium to pH 7·4. Add sterile "Tween" 80 to give a final concentration of 1·0 per cent.

Pyocyanin production is shown after 24 hours' incubation of cultures by a deep blue colour which diffuses into the medium.

(3) **Oxidase Test** (Kovacs, 1956). Place two or three drops of fresh 1 per cent tetramethyl *p*-phenylene diamine dihydrochloride solution on Whatman's No. 1 filter paper in a Petri dish. Remove the suspected colony from culture with a platinum loop and rub on to reagent-soaked filter paper in a line 3–6 mm. long. A positive reaction is shown by dark purple colour appearing within 10 seconds. Keep reagent in dark glass-stoppered bottle in the refrigerator and prepare fresh every two weeks.

A positive reaction is given by *Pseudomonas*, *Alkaligenes* and *Aeromonas*, but not by other Gram-negative bacilli.

(4) **Oxidation/Fermentation Test** (Hugh and Leifson, 1953). Use the Difco O/F medium or one containing the following ingredients (per cent w/v): tryptone (Difco), 0·2; NaCl, 0·5; K_2HPO_4, 0·03; agar, 0·3; bromothymol blue, 0·008 (0·8 ml. of a 1 per cent aqueous solution added to 100 ml. of medium); glucose, 1·0. Tube to a depth of about $1\frac{1}{2}$ inches. Sterilize by autoclaving.

Inoculate one loopful of culture into the depth of two tubes; one of the tubes is then covered with a layer of sterile melted petrolatum (Vaseline) to a depth of $\frac{1}{2}$ inch. Examine for colour change after one and three days. Oxidation is shown by colour change in the unsealed tube, fermentation by colour changes in both tubes. Oxidative metabolism is characteristic of the genus *Pseudomonas*.

(5) **Gluconate Oxidation and Slime Production** (Haynes, 1951). Medium (per cent w/v): tryptone, 0·15; yeast extract, 0·10; K_2HPO_4, 0·10; potassium gluconate, 4·0. pH 7·0. Fill into screw-cap bottles and autoclave at 115°C for 10 minutes.

Transfer 1·0 ml. amounts to $6 \times \frac{5}{8}$ in. test tubes. Inoculate two tubes. Incubate and test, after three and seven days, by addition of 1·0 ml. Benedict's reagent (qualitative); mix and heat for 10 minutes in boiling water; cool and examine for colour change and precipitate after five minutes and after standing overnight.

Test for slime production in tube of culture in gluconate medium left standing at room temperature for four days after removal from incubator. Threads of slime can be pulled from the surface with a wire loop, and the presence of slime can be shown by rotating the tube briefly; the contents continue to rotate in the same direction, but then rotate in the reverse direction (a "reverse swirl").

Gluconate oxidation is obtained with cultures of *Ps. æruginosa* and some other Gram-negative bacilli; slime production in the medium is characteristic of *Ps. æruginosa*, and rarely shown by other species of *Pseudomonas* (Brown and Lowbury, 1966).

References

ANDERSON, K. (1959). *Pseudomonas pyocyanea* disseminated from air-cooling apparatus. *Med. J. Aust.*, i, 529.

ASAY, L. D. and KOCH, R. (1960). Pseudomonas infections in infants and children. *New Engl. J. Med.*, 262, 1062.

AYLIFFE, G. A. J., BARRY, D. R., LOWBURY, E. J. L., ROPER-HALL, M. J. and WALKER, W. MARTIN (1966). Post-operative infection with *Pseudomonas æruginosa* in an eye hospital. *Lancet*, i, 1113.

AYLIFFE, G. A. J., LOWBURY, E. J. L., HAMILTON, J. G., SMALL, J. M., ASHESHOV, E. A. and PARKER, M. T. (1965). Hospital infection with *Pseudomonas æruginosa* in neurosurgery. *Lancet*, ii, 365.

BASSETT, D. C. J., THOMPSON, S. A. S. and PAGE, B. (1965). Neonatal infections with *Pseudomonas æruginosa* associated with contaminated resuscitation equipment. *Lancet*, i, 781.

BROWN, V. I. and LOWBURY, E. J. L. (1965). Use of an improved cetrimide agar medium and other culture methods for *Pseudomonas æruginosa*. *J. clin. Path.*, 18, 752.

CASON, J. S., JACKSON, D. M., LOWBURY, E. J. L. and RICKETTS, C. R. (1966). Antiseptic and aseptic prophylaxis for burns: use of silver nitrate and of isolators. *Brit. med. J.*, ii, 1288.

CASON, J. S. and LOWBURY, E. J. L. (1960). Prophylactic chemotherapy for burns: studies on the local and systemic use of combined therapy. *Lancet*, ii, 501.

CHRISTIE, R. (1948). Observations on the biochemical and serological characteristics of *Pseudomonas pyocyanea*. *Aust. J. exp. Biol. med. Sci.*, 26, 425.

CHÜN-HSIANG, L., CHIEN-YIN, H., HSING-MIN, C. and CHÜN, S. (1964). Studies on septicæmia in extensive burns. *Chin. med. J.*, 83, 779.

CROMPTON, D. O. (1962). Ophthalmic prescribing. *Aust. J. Pharm.*, Oct. 30, p. 1020.

CRUICKSHANK, C. N. D. and LOWBURY, E. J. L. (1953). The effect of pyocyanin on human skin cells and leucocytes. *Brit. J. exp. Path.*, 34, 583.

DARRELL, J. H. and WAHBA, A. H. (1964). Pyocine typing of hospital strains of *Pseudomonas pyocyanea*. *J. clin. Path.*, 17, 236.

DON, P. A. and VAN DEN ENDE, M. (1950). A preliminary study of the bacteriophages of *Pseudomonas æruginosa*. *J. Hyg., Camb.*, 48, 196.

FARRAR, D. A. T. (1954). Use of polymyxin B in the external ear. *Brit. med. J.*, ii, 629.

FEKETY, F. R., NORMAN, P. S. and CLUFF, L. E. (1962). The treatment of Gram-negative bacillary infections with colistin. *Ann. intern. Med.*, 57, 214.

FELLER, I. (1966). The use of pseudomonas vaccine and hyperimmune plasma in the treatment of seriously burned patients. In *Research in Burns*, ed. Wallace and Wilkinson, Edinburgh, p. 470.

FORDOS, M. (1860). Recherches sur la matière colorante des suppurations bleues; pyocyanine. *C.R. Acad. Sci.*, 51, 215.

FORKNER, C. E., FREI, C. E., EDGCOMB, J. H. and UTZ, J. P. (1958). Pseudomonas septicæmia: observations on twenty-three cases. *Amer. J. Med.*, 25, 877.

FOX, J. E. and LOWBURY, E. J. L. (1953a). Immunity to *Pseudomonas pyocyanea* in man. *J. Path. Bact.*, 65, 519.

FOX, J. E. and LOWBURY, E. J. L. (1953b). Immunity and antibody to *Pseudomonas pyocyanea* in rabbits. *J. Path. Bact.*, 65, 533.

FRAENKEL, E. (1917). Weitere Untersuchungen über die Menschen-pathogenität des Bacillus pyocyaneus. *Z. Hyg. InfektKr.*, 84, 369.

GAINES, S. and LANDY, M. (1961). Prevalence of antibody to pseudomonas in normal human sera. *J. Bact.*, 69, 628.

GESSARD, C. (1882). Sur le coloration bleue et verte des linges à pansements. *C.R. Acad. Sci.*, 94, 536.

GESSARD, C. (1890). Nouvelles recherches sur le microbe pyocyanique. *Ann. Inst. Pasteur*, 4, 88.

GILLIES, R. R. and GOVAN, J. R. W. (1966). Typing of *Pseudomonas pyocyanea* by pyocine production. *J. Path. Bact.*, 91, 339.

GILLESPIE, W. A., LENNON, G. G., LINTON, K. B. and SLADE, N. (1964). Prevention of urinary infection in gynæcology. *Brit. med. J.*, ii, 423.

GOSLINGS, W. R. O. (1963). Factors affecting the frequency of infection in medical patients. In *Infection in Hospitals* (ed. Williams and Shooter), Blackwell, p. 21.

GOULD, J. C. and McLEOD, J. W. (1960). A study of the use of agglutinating sera and phage lysis in the classification of strains of *Pseudomonas æruginosa*. *J. Path. Bact.*, 79, 295.

GRABER, C. D., CUMMINGS, D., VOGEL, E. H. and TUMBUSCH, W. T. (1961). Measurement of the protective effect of antibody in burned and unburned patients' sera for *Pseudomonas æruginosa* infected mice. *Tex. Rep. Biol. and Med.*, 19, 268.

GRABER, C. D., LATTA, R., VOGEL, E. H. and BRAME, R. (1962). Bacteriophage grouping of *Pseudomonas æruginosa*. *Amer. J. clin. Path.*, **37**, 54.

HABS, I. (1957). Untersuchungen über die O-Antigene von *Pseudomonas æruginosa*. *Z. Hyg. Infektionskr.*, **144**, 218.

HAYES, E. R. and YOW, E. (1950). Meningitis due to *Pseudomonas æruginosa* treated with polymyxin B. *Amer. J. med. Sci.*, **220**, 633.

HAYNES, W. C. (1951). *Pseudomonas æruginosa*—its characterization and identification. *J. gen. Microbiol.*, **5**, 939.

HOFFMAN, M. A. and FINBERG, L. (1955). Pseudomonas infections in infants associated with high-humidity environments. *J. Pediat.*, **46**, 626.

HUGH, R. and LEIFSON, E. (1953). The taxonomic significance of fermentative versus oxidative metabolism of carbohydrates by various gram negative bacteria. *J. Bact.*, **66**, 24.

HURST, L. and LOWBURY, E. J. L. (1952). Transfer of fluorescin from *Pseudomonas pyocyanea* to colonies of other bacteria. *J. clin. Path.*, **5**, 359.

HURST, V. and SUTTER, V. L. (1966). Survival of *Pseudomonas æruginosa* in the hospital environment. *J. infect. Dis.*, **116**, 151.

JACKSON, D. M., LOWBURY, E. J. L. and TOPLEY, E. (1951). *Pseudomonas pyocyanea* in burns: its role as a pathogen and the value of local polymyxin therapy. *Lancet*, **ii**, 137.

JAWETZ, E. (1952). Infections with *Pseudomonas æruginosa* treated with polymyxin B. *Arch. intern. Med.*, **89**, 90.

JONES, R. J., JACKSON, D. M. and LOWBURY, E. J. L. (1966). Antiserum and antibiotic in the prophylaxis of burns against *Pseudomonas æruginosa*. *Brit. J. plast. Surg.*, **19**, 43.

JONES, R. J. and LOWBURY, E. J. L. (1963). Staphylococcal antibodies in burned patients. *Brit. J. exp. Path.*, **44**, 576.

JONES, R. J. and LOWBURY, E. J. L. (1965). Susceptibility of man to *Pseudomonas æruginosa*. *Lancet*, **ii**, 623.

JONES, R. J. and LOWBURY, E. J. L. (1966). Antiserum and antibiotics in the prophylaxis against *Pseudomonas æruginosa*. In *Research in Burns* ed. Wallace and Wilkinson, Edinburgh, p. 474.

JONES, R. J. and LOWBURY, E. J. L. (1967). Prophylaxis and therapy for *Pseudomonas æruginosa* with carbenicillin and with gentamicin. *Brit. med. J.*, **iii**, 79.

KEFALIDES, N. A., ARANA, J. A., BAZAN, A., VELARDE, N. and ROSENTHAL, S. M. (1964). Evaluation of antibiotic prophylaxis and gamma-globulin, plasma, albumin and saline-solution therapy in severe burns. *Ann. Surg.*, **159**, 496.

KING, E. O., WARD, M. K. and RANEY, D. E. (1954). Two simple media for the demonstration of pyocyanin and fluorescin. *J. Lab. clin. Med.*, **44**, 301.

KOVACS, N. (1956). Identification of *Pseudomonas pyocyanea* by the oxidase reaction *Nature, Lond.*, **178**, 703.

LILLEY, A. B. and BEARUP, A. J. (1928). Generalized infections due to *Pseudomonas æruginosa* (Bacillus pyocyaneus) with a study of the characteristics of local strains of organism. *Med. J. Aust.*, **i**, 362.

LINDBERG, R. B., MONCRIEF, J. A., SWITZER, W. E., ORDER, S. E. and MILLS, W. (1965). The successful control of burn wound sepsis. *J. Trauma*, **5**, 601.

LISTON, J., WIEBE, W. and COLWELL, R. R. (1963). Quantitative approach to the study of bacterial species. *J. Bact.*, **85**, 1061.

LIU, P. V., ABE, Y. and BATES, J. L. (1961). The roles of various fractions of *Pseudomonas æruginosa* in its pathogenesis. *J. infect. Dis.*, **108**, 218.

LIU, P. V. and MERCER, C. B. (1963). Growth, toxigenicity and virulence of *Pseudomonas æruginosa*. *J. Hyg., Camb.*, **61**, 485.

LOWBURY, E. J. L. (1951). Contamination of cetrimide and other fluids with *Pseudomonas pyocyanea*. *Brit. J. industr. Med.*, **8**, 22.

LOWBURY, E. J. L. (1954). Air conditioning with filtered air for dressing burns. *Lancet*, **i**, 292.

LOWBURY, E. J. L. and FOX, J. E. (1953). The influence of atmospheric drying on the survival of wound flora. *J. Hyg., Camb.*, **51**, 203.

LOWBURY, E. J. L. and FOX, J. E. (1954). The epidemiology of *Pseudomonas pyocyanea* in a burns unit. *J. Hyg., Camb.*, **52**, 403.

LOWBURY, E. J. L., LILLY, H. A. and WILKINS, M. D. (1962). A cabinet for the detection of fluorescent bacterial cultures. *J. clin. Path.*, **15**, 339.

LOWBURY, E. J. L., MILLER, R. W. S., CASON, J. S. and JACKSON, D. M. (1962). Local prophylactic chemotherapy for burns treated with tulle gras and by the exposure method. *Lancet*, **ii**, 958.

LOWBURY, E. J. L. and RICKETTS, C. R. (1957). Properdin and the defence of burns against infection. *J. Hyg., Camb.*, **55**, 266.

LYSENKO, O. (1961). *Pseudomonas*—an attempt at a general classification. *J. gen. Microbiol.*, **25**, 379.

McLeod, J. W. (1958). The hospital urine bottle and bedpan as reservoirs of infection by *Pseudomonas pyocyanea*. *Lancet*, i, 394.

Margaretten, W., Nakai, H. and Landing, B. H. (1961). Significance of selective vasculitis and the "bone marrow syndrome" in pseudomonas septicæmia. *New Engl. J. Med.*, 265, 773.

Markley, K., Gurmendi, G., Chavez, P. M. and Bazan, A. (1957). Fatal pseudomonas septicæmias in burned patients. *Ann. Surg.*, 145, 175.

Mayr-Harting, A. (1948). Serology of *Pseudomonas pyocyanea*. *J. gen. Microbiol.*, 2, 31.

Millican, R. C. and Rust, J. D. (1960). Efficacy of rabbit pseudomonas antiserum in experimental *Pseudomonas æruginosa* infection. *J. infect. Dis.*, 107, 389.

Mitchell, J. P. and Gillespie, W. A. (1964). Bacteriological complications from the use of urethral instruments: principles of prevention. *J. clin. Path.*, 17, 492.

Moore, B. and Forman, A. (1966). An outbreak of urinary *Pseudomonas æruginosa* infection acquired during urological operations. *Lancet*, ii, 929.

Moyer, C. A., Brentano, L., Gravens, D. L., Margraf, H. W. and Monafo, W. W. (1965). Treatment of large human burns with 0·5 per cent silver nitrate solution. *Arch. Surg.*, 90, 812.

Mull, J. D. and Callahan, W. S. (1965). The role of the elastase of *Pseudomonas æruginosa* in experimental infection. *Exp. Molec. Pathol.*, 4, 567.

Muraschi, T. F., Bolles, D. M., Moczulski, C. and Lindsay, H. (1966). Sero'ogic types of *Pseudomonas æruginosa* based on heat-stable antigens: correlation of Habs' (European) and Verder and Evans' (North American) classifications. *J. infect. Dis.*, 116, 84.

Noble, W. C. and Savin, J. A. (1966). Steroid cream contaminated with *Pseudomonas æruginosa*. *Lancet*, i, 347.

Osman, M. A. M. (1965). Pyocine typing of *Pseudomonas æruginosa*. *J. clin. Path.*, 18, 200.

Phillips, I. (1966). Post-operative respiratory tract infection with *Pseudomonas æruginosa*. *Lancet*, i, 903.

Phillips, I. and Spencer, G. (1965). *Pseudomonas æruginosa* cross infection due to contaminated respiratory apparatus. *Lancet*, ii, 1325.

Postic, B. and Finland, M. (1961). Observations on bacteriophage typing of *Pseudomonas æruginosa*. *J. clin. Invest.*, 40, 2064.

Pulaski, E. J., Baker, H. J., Rosenberg, M. L. and Connell, J. P. (1949). Laboratory and clinical studies of Polymyxin B and E. *J. clin. Invest.*, 28, 1028.

Pyrah, L. N., Goldie, W., Parsons, F. M. and Raper, F. P. (1955). Control of *Pseudomonas pyocyanea* infection in a urological ward. *Lancet*, ii, 314.

Rabin, E. R., Graber, C. D., Vogel, E. H., Finkelstein, R. A. and Tumbusch, W. J. (1961). Fatal Pseudomonas infection in burned patients. *New Engl. J. Med.*, 265, 1225.

Rhodes, M. E. (1961). The characterization of *Pseudomonas fluorescens* with the aid of an electronic computer. *J. gen. Microbiol.*, 25, 331.

Ridley, F. (1958). Sterile drops and lotions in ophthalmic practice. *Brit. J. Ophthal.*, 42, 641.

Ringen, L. M. and Drake, C. H. (1952). A study of the incidence of *Pseudomonas æruginosa* from various natural sources. *J. Bact.*, 64, 841.

Rogers, K. B. (1960). Pseudomonas infections in a children's hospital. *J. appl. Bact.*, 23, 533.

Rubbo, S. D., Gardner, J. F. and Franklin, J. C. (1966). Source of *Pseudomonas æruginosa* infection in premature infants. *J. Hyg., Camb.*, 64, 121.

Sandiford, B. R. (1937). Observations on *Pseudomonas pyocyanea*. *J. Path. Bact.*, 44, 567.

Sandvik, O. (1960). Serological comparison between strains of *Pseudomonas æruginosa* from human and animal sources. *Acta path. microbiol. scand.*, 48, 56.

Schroeter, J. (1875). *Ueber einige durch Bacterien gebildete Pigmente*. Beiträge zur Biologie der Pflanzen (ed. F. Cohn) Heft ii, p. 109.

Selenka, F. (1958). Über die abgrenzung von *Pseudomonas æruginosa* gegen *Pseudomonas fluorescens* und *Pseudomonas putida* auf TTC-Nährböden. *Arch. Hyg., Berl.*, 142, 569.

Sevitt, S. (1955). Splenic eosinopenia and adreno-cortical hyperactivity. *J. Path. Bact.*, 70, 65.

Sevitt, S. (1964). Bacterial invasion after extensive burns. *Acta chirurg. Plast.*, 6, 173.

Shooter, R. A., Walker, K. A., Williams, V., Horgan, G., Parker, M. T., Asheshov, E. and Bullimore, J. (1966). Fæcal carriage of *Pseudomonas æruginosa* in hospital patients: possible spread from patient to patient. *Lancet*, ii, 1331.

Sneath, P. H. A. (1962). The construction of taxonomic groups. In *Microbiol Classification*, ed. Ainsworth and Sneath, Cambridge, p. 289.

Speirs, C. F., Selwyn, S. and Nicholson, D. N. (1963). Hypogammaglobulinæmia presenting as *Pseudomonas* septicæmia. *Lancet*, ii, 710.

Stanier, R. Y., Palleroni, N. J. and Doudoroff, M. (1966). The ærobic pseudomonads: a taxonomic study. *J. gen. Microbiol.*, 43, 159.

STONE, H. H., MARTIN, J. D., HUGER, W. E. and KOLB, L. (1965). Gentamicin sulfate in the treatment of *Pseudomonas* sepsis in burns. *Surg. Gynec. Obstet.*, **120**, 351.

SUSSMAN, M. and STEVENS, J. (1960). *Pseudomonas pyocyanea* wound infection: an outbreak in an orthopædic unit. *Lancet*, **ii**, 734.

SUTTER, V. L. and HURST, V. (1966). Sources of *Pseudomonas æruginosa* infection in burns. *Ann. Surg.*, **163**, 597.

SUTTER, V. L., HURST, V. and FENNELL, J. (1965). A standardised system for phage typing *Pseudomonas æruginosa*. *Health Lab. Sci.*, **2**, 7.

TEPLITZ, C., DAVIS, D., MASON, A. D. and MONCRIEF, J. A. (1964). *Pseudomonas* burn wound sepsis: pathogenesis of experimental pseudomonas burn wound sepsis. *J. Surg. Res.*, **4**, 200.

THORNLEY, M. J. (1960). The differentiation of *Pseudomonas* from other gram-negative bacteria on the basis of arginine metabolism. *J. appl. Bact.*, **23**, 37.

THYGESON, P. (1948). Acute central hypopyon ulcers of cornea. *Calif. Med.*, **69**, 18.

TRAPNELL, D. H. (1954). *Pseudomonas pyocyanea* meningitis successfully treated with polymyxin. *Lancet*, **i**, 759.

TUMBUSCH, W. T., VOGEL, E. H., BUTKIEWICZ, J. V., GRABER, C. D., LARSON, D. L. and MITCHELL, E. T. (1961). Septicæmia in burn injury. *J. Trauma*, **i**, 22.

TUMBUSCH, W. T., VOGEL, E. H., BUTKIEWICZ, C. D., GRABER, C. D., LARSON, D. L., and MITCHELL, E. T. (1962). The rising incidence of Pseudomonas septicæmia following burn injury, in *Research in Burns* (ed. Artz), Philadelphia, p. 235.

VERDER, E. and EVANS, J. (1961). A proposed antigenic scheme for the identification of strains of *Pseudomonas æruginosa*. *J. infect. Dis.*, **109**, 183.

VÉRON, M. (1961). Sur l'agglutination de *Pseudomonas æruginosa*: subdivision des groupes antigeniques 0:2 et 0:5. *Ann. Inst. Pasteur.*, **101**, 456.

YOW, E. M. (1952). Development of proteus and Pseudomonas infections during antibiotic therapy. *J. Amer. med. Ass.*, **149**, 1184.

WAHBA, A. H. (1965). Hospital infection with *Pseudomonas pyocyanea*: an investigation by a combined pyocine and serological typing method. *Brit. med. J.*, **i**, 86.

WAHBA, A. H. and DARRELL, J. H. (1965). The identification of atypical strains of *Pseudomonas æruginosa*. *J. gen. Microbiol.*, **38**, 329

Chapter 2

THE DETECTION AND ASSESSMENT OF
URINARY INFECTION

W. BRUMFITT

IN the last decade there has been an increasing awareness of the potential danger of urinary tract infection. Details of many of the approaches which have been made to the problem will be found in two symposia (Quinn and Kass, 1960; Kass, 1965). Since a number of recent reviews on the general problem of pyelonephritis and urinary tract infection are also available (Kleeman, Hewitt and Guze, 1960; Freedman, 1963; Brumfitt and Percival, 1964), this chapter will be concerned with some particular aspects which are likely to concern the clinical bacteriologist. The need for more widespread screening of populations at risk will be discussed and the various laboratory procedures available for diagnosis of urinary infection evaluated. The use of special techniques for the localization of infection within the urinary tract and the relation of these findings to the outcome of treatment will be dealt with in some detail.

A crucial factor in the understanding of urinary infection was the introduction of quantitative methods which have made it possible to decide when bacteria are actually multiplying in the bladder urine. Rantz and Keefer (1940), when assessing the value of sulphanilamide in the treatment of urinary tract infection, reported that patients with acute pyelonephritis regularly had 100,000 or more organisms per ml. of urine. Further quantitative studies were carried out by Marple (1941) and Harris, Murray, Paine, Kilham and Finland (1947). However, it remained for Kass (1956, 1957, 1960, 1962 a and b) to study systematically the detection and natural history of bacteriuria in various groups of patients. These studies established the value of the "clean-catch" midstream urine for bacteriological investigation and confirmed the diagnostic significance of 100,000 bacteria per ml. of urine. Subsequent studies by Kass and his co-workers suggested the relation of bacteriuria to other conditions such as hypertension and premature birth.

Kass's work was further expanded by Kunin, Deutscher and Paquin (1964), who carried out an important investigation on an apparently healthy population of almost 16,000 schoolchildren and found the prevalence of significant bacteriuria to be 1·2 per cent in schoolgirls but only 0·03 per cent in boys. When 107 of the schoolchildren who were found to have bacteriuria were studied radiologically, caliectasis (calyceal dilation) was demonstrated in 13·7 per cent and ureteric reflux in 18·7 per cent. These findings, together with studies on children who were referred to hospital and found to have urinary infection (Steele, Leadbetter and Crawford, 1963; Smellie, Hodson, Edwards and Normand, 1964; Hodson and Wilson, 1965; Smellie, 1967), indicated that in children uncontrolled infection can lead to progressive renal scar formation and that in some of these patients death from chronic pyelo-nephritis occurred at an early age. Thus, in children at least, there seems to be strong evidence to link asymptomatic bacteriuria and chronic pyelo-nephritis. Kunin *et al.* (1964) also showed that, following treatment, 75 per cent of infections recurred within two years.

Quantitative bacteriological study of the urine provides a method for the detection and hence treatment of urinary infection at an asymptomatic phase. For example, the eradication of asymptomatic bacteriuria in early pregnancy is effective in reducing considerably the later incidence of the serious condition of acute pyelonephritis which, according to Tenney and Little (1958), is the commonest cause of hospital admission during pregnancy.

However, the detection of bacteriuria also allows an approach to be made to the prevention of chronic disease in the community since renal damage resulting from infection is often unrecognized until a relatively late stage of its development. The ideal approach would therefore be to recognize the population at risk and then to detect and eliminate infection at an asymptomatic stage.

Long-term follow-up of patients who have had urinary infection is also important and in a four-year follow-up of patients who had bacteriuria in pregnancy, we found that 69 per cent of those who had failed two or more courses of treatment during pregnancy were still infected and radiological examination revealed abnormalities in 68 per cent. Perhaps even more surprising was the finding that 19 per cent of those who had responded to a single course of chemotherapy were still infected and 23 per cent showed radiological abnormalities (Brumfitt, Leigh and Gruneberg, 1967). These various observations raise the question as to whether underlying renal damage and susceptibility to infection were present before the pregnancy in some of the patients. There is evidence that bacteriuria is as prevalent in non-pregnant women of childbearing age as in pregnant women in the same community. Sleigh, Robertson and Isdale (1964) found that 8 per cent of 397 women attending an infertility clinic in Edinburgh had bacteriuria compared with 6·6 per cent of 1,684 pregnant women. In Jamaica, 4 per cent of adult women studied in a "door-to-door" survey, most of whom were presumably not pregnant, had bacteriuria (Kass, Savage and Santamarina, 1965), whilst the prevalence in pregnant women in the same community was 3·5 per cent (Stuart, Cummins and Chin, 1965). If these findings are repre-sentative of other communities, they suggest that bacteriuria detected during pregnancy has preceded the pregnancy in a substantial proportion of cases.

The evidence that urinary tract infection in children can rapidly progress to chronic pyelonephritis has already been presented and Smellie (1967) found that the detection and effective control of the infection in children resulted in resumption of renal growth even though the scarring had already taken place.

It has already been stressed that many infections are asymptomatic, but it is also important to appreciate that the presence of symptoms is a poor guide to infection. About half of the patients seen in general practice with symptoms suggesting urinary infection prove not to have significant bacteriuria (Mond, Percival, Williams and Brumfitt, 1965) and many authors have pointed out that the symptomatology of urinary tract infection in children may be atypical. Thus the laboratory and pathologist must clearly play a major part in the organization of screening programmes for the detection of urinary tract infection in groups of patients known to be at risk.

Significant Bacteriuria

The term "significant bacteriuria" was introduced to describe the situation where bacteria are actually multiplying in the bladder urine and therefore means that a true urinary infection is present. Under these circumstances the bacterial population will ordinarily exceed 100,000 per ml. of urine. However, bacteria may have entered the urine as contaminants from the container used for collection, from vaginal and faecal contamination, from the peri-urethral area and from the urethra itself. Urethral contaminants in urine rarely exceed 1,000 bacteria per ml., and other forms of contamination can be avoided by the proper preparation of the patient and either prompt processing of the specimen or storage at 4°C. Details of a suitable collection technique for midstream urine specimens and the organization needed for screening large numbers of patients have been described in detail and will not be repeated here (Brumfitt and Percival, 1964; Williams, Leigh, Rosser and Brumfitt, 1965). If careful collection procedures are used, 96 per cent agreement between two positive specimens is obtained in women (Kass, 1962a); in the male (except for the newborn), collection of satisfactory midstream specimens presents no problem provided that proper instructions are given and almost 100 per cent agreement between two specimens is found.

Roberts, Robinson and Beard (1967) have pointed out that antiseptic solutions should not be used for perineal swabbing since small amounts of antiseptic may contaminate the urine and reduce the bacterial count sufficiently to mask the infection.

Special Collection Procedures

Although in the great majority of patients infection can be diagnosed or excluded by well-taken midstream urine specimens, in a few instances equivocal results are obtained even after repeating the test several times. Provided that antibacterial substances are absent from the urine, the explanation may be that the patient has repeatedly contaminated the specimen. Alternatively, there may be a true infection with a reduced bacterial count due to factors such as frequency of micturition, especially if associated with hydration and diuresis (Cox and Hinman, 1961), but exceptional drinking and frequency of micturition is usually necessary to reduce the bacterial concentration below the significant level (O'Grady and Cattell, 1966).

Where midstream specimens repeatedly give equivocal results, the problem can be solved by direct sampling of the bladder urine by a suprapubic puncture (Beard, McCoy, Newton and Clayton, 1965; Stamey, Goven and Palmer, 1965). This procedure is particularly useful in women after vaginal operations and in the early puerperium when contamination from vaginal discharge is difficult to avoid. The use of the urethral catheter is a less satisfactory alternative to suprapubic aspiration because of the danger of introducing infection (Beeson, 1958; Brumfitt, Davies and Rosser, 1961).

Quantitative Estimation of Bacteria

If infection can be defined precisely only by counting the bacteria, it is obviously desirable that this procedure should be carried out routinely. The standard bacteriological technique would involve making tenfold dilutions of the urine followed by surface viable counts, which is expensive

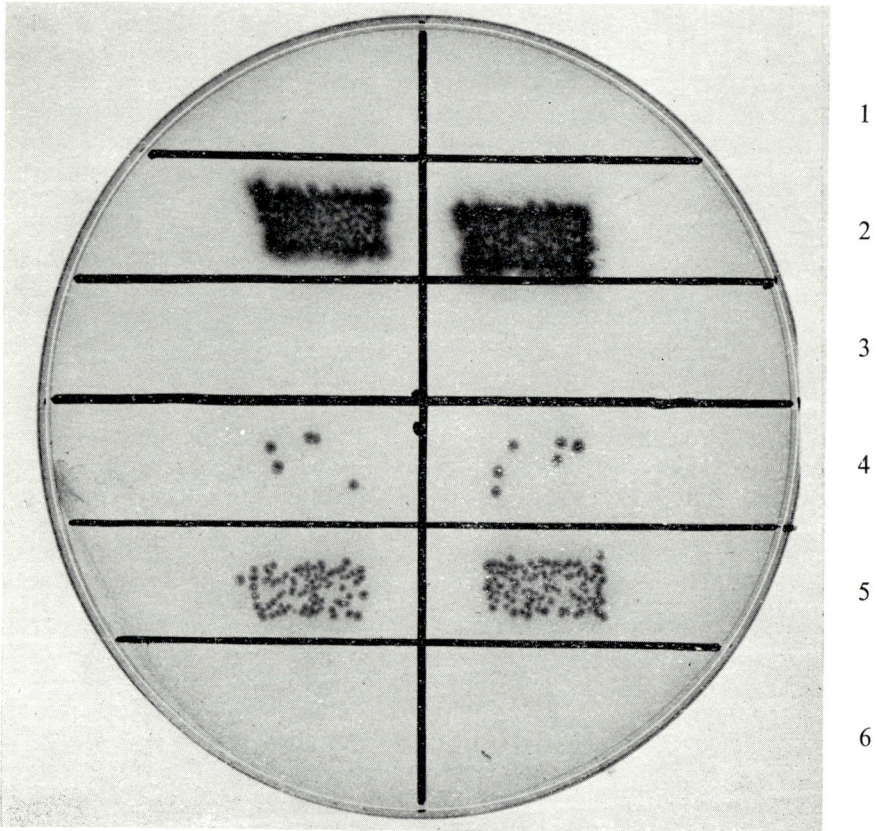

FIG. 1. Results obtained on 6 urines by the filter-paper technique. Duplicate impressions have been made from each specimen and the plates incubated overnight. The results are: urines 1, 3 and 6 not infected; urine 4 equivocal (beween 5 and 24 colonies on the inoculated area) and urines 2 and 5 infected (25 colonies or more).

both in materials and technicians' time, and although, in practice, only two culture plates, one inoculated with 0·1 ml. neat urine and the other with 0·1 ml. of a hundredfold dilution, are needed to distinguish between true infection and contamination, even this is impracticable for routine use on all specimens.

A number of workers have described simpler methods of quantitating bacteria in the urine, and of these the most popular has been based upon the use of a "standard" loop (O'Sullivan, FitzGerald, Meynell and Malins, 1960; McGeachie and Kennedy, 1963; Guttman and Stokes, 1963). However, the standard loop technique requires the use of a whole culture plate for each specimen, the technique of inoculating the plate must be carefully controlled and care must be taken to see that the loop does not become distorted.

We have developed a method which we find both suitable and economical for screening large numbers of urines (Leigh and Williams, 1964; Brumfitt, 1965). It involves dipping a sterilized absorbent filter-paper strip of standard size into the urine and then laying a measured area of the paper on to a well-dried MacConkey agar plate. The number of colonies corresponding to 10^5 bacteria per ml. of urine is determined by comparison with a standard curve. The test can be performed rapidly and uses little material because six to eight urine samples can be examined in duplicate on one culture plate and the results read very quickly (Fig. 1).

In rural clinics and practices, where bacteriological facilities are inaccessible, delay in transport to the laboratory may be unavoidable. For use in such situations transport media have been described which allow quantitatve bacteriology to be carried out on the urine specimens. The transport medium is carried on either a metal or plastic spoon (Mackey and Sandys, 1965, 1966) or coated on an ordinary microscope slide (Guttmann and Naylor, 1967a, 1967b). The spoon or slide is dipped into the urine and then posted to the laboratory in a sealed container where it is incubated. The results given by these two methods compare well with surface viable counts but preparation of the transport material and reading of the results is easier with the slide technique. A problem in interpretation may arise when urinary counts exceed 10^6 per ml., because with undiluted urine confluent growth occurs, and in the absence of individual colonies differentiation between gross contamination and true infection can be difficult.

Chemical Methods for Detecting Infection

It would be ideal if a chemical test could be devised which would detect significant bacteriuria with the same ease and accuracy as the chemical tests for the detection of glucose and protein in urine. A number of chemical tests have been developed, but unfortunately they are less reliable than bacteriological methods. The tri-phenyl tetrazolium chloride (TTC) test and nitrite tests are the best of the chemical procedures available, but both require incubation at 37°C for several hours if accurate results are to be obtained. Both of these tests have been used for screening large numbers of urine specimens (Kincaid-Smith *et al.*, 1964; Sleigh, 1965).

Tri-phenyl Tetrazolium Chloride (TTC) Test. This test depends upon the ability of respiring bacteria to reduce the soluble colourless tri-phenyl tetrazolium chloride to the red insoluble tri-phenyl formazan which is seen as a red precipitate. When 2 ml. of urine are incubated with 0·5 ml. of the reagent for 4 hr. at 37°C a positive result is given by urines containing 100,000 or more bacteria per ml. A number of workers have used the TTC test, and one study showed a 96 per cent correlation with bacterial counts (Simmons and Williams, 1962), but others have found it to be unreliable (Guze and Kalmanson, 1963a; Bulger and Kirby, 1963). Technical reasons for the discrepancy could be failure to maintain an alkaline pH which is essential for the accuracy of the test and variation in the quality of batches of TTC. When reading the test, even slight red colouration of the precipitate must be recorded as positive and such changes may be missed by the inexperienced eye. The presence of red cells in the urine may also cause difficulty.

Nitrite Test. Nitrites are easy to detect chemically and are not found in normal urine. Cruickshank and Moyes (1914) noted that the presence of nitrites in urine was associated with coliform bacilluria, but they found the test for nitrites to be positive in only about half of those patients with infected urine. Sleigh (1965) developed a modification of this test which involved addition of nitrate to the urine followed by incubation of the urine at 37°C for 4 hr. before testing for nitrite. Using this technique, 69 of 71 specimens (97 per cent) with significant bacteriuria were detected. Smith, Thayer, Malta and Utz (1961) had previously added nitrate to the urine specimen and then allowed it to stand at room temperature for 1 hr. before testing for nitrite, but this did not achieve the same high proportion of positive tests as the incubation procedure described by Sleigh.

Urinary White Cell Counts

In studying white cells in the urine it is important to distinguish between leucocytes and tubular cells (Prescott and Brodie, 1964). It is also well known that white cells are unstable under alkaline conditions, and failure to appreciate this leads to errors. Survival of leucocytes under various conditions of pH, osmolality, temperature and time has recently been studied in detail by Triger and Smith (1966).

Three methods of estimation of urinary white cells are available: the white cell excretion rate, the white cell concentration and microscopy of the centrifuged deposit.

White Cell Excretion Rate. The most accurate method of estimating white cells in the urine is to determine the white cell excretion rate, but serious errors will arise if the bladder is not completely emptied, and since the whole urine specimen is needed for the test, contamination is rather likely to occur. An excretion of 400,000 W.B.C. per hour has been suggested as the upper limit of normal by Hutt, Chalmers, MacDonald and de Wardener (1961), but *average* excretion rates for groups of normal subjects are much lower than this (Addis, 1926; Rofe, 1955; Houghton and Pears, 1957), so that an excretion rate below 400,000 per hr. may be abnormal for a particular individual.

White Cell Concentration. The concentration of white cells is easily estimated by counting the number of white cells in a carefully collected midstream urine specimen. Because a midstream specimen is used, vaginal contamination is less of a hazard than when the total volume needs to be collected.

More than 10 white cells per c.mm. is regarded as being abnormal and this concentration is always associated with a white cell excretion of 400,000 per hour or more, regardless of rate of urine flow.

As with the white cell excretion rate, however, it is difficult to determine what concentration of white cells can be regarded as normal, and counts as low as 3 per c.mm. can sometimes be associated with abnormal excretion rates.

Microscopy of Centrifuged Deposit. Many routine laboratories merely examine a centrifuged deposit of urine. Although this is a relatively crude method, a gross excess of white cells is readily detected and the method has the advantage that simultaneous examination for casts and crystals can be undertaken. We centrifuge 7 ml. of urine at 1,500 r.p.m. for 10 min., immediately pour off the supernatant and examine one drop of the deposit under a cover glass. More than one white cell per high-power field indicates an excess of white cells and a count carried out on the uncentrifuged urine in such cases will be greater than 10 per c.mm. Obviously, this method is associated with a number of variables and is unsuitable for the detection of a relatively small increase in white cell excretion.

The Significance of an Increased White Cell Excretion

An increase in white cell excretion results from inflammation within the urinary tract, and is not necessarily the result of infection. Furthermore, its presence gives no indication of the site of the inflammation, and the idea that pyuria is indicative of pyelonephritis (or other renal lesion) is fallacious.

Mond, Percival, Williams and Brumfitt (1965) found that only about half of the female patients seen in general practice with symptoms of urinary infection had a significant bacteriuria but that 47 per cent of the non-infected patients had an excess of white cells in the urine. It was concluded that the symptoms and laboratory findings in these non-infected patients were the result of a urethritis unassociated with urinary infection. The work of Csonka, Williams and Corse (1966) suggests that the ætiology of this syndrome may, in some cases, be infection by T-strains of mycoplasma.

Localization of the Site of Infection within the Urinary Tract

Bacterial invasion of the kidney can be diagnosed with some confidence when infected urine is found in association with the clinical picture of loin pain, loin tenderness and fever. However, it is of importance to know whether involvement of renal tissue has occurred when symptoms are confined to the lower urinary tract, or where there is only asymptomatic bacteriuria. Four methods have been used to detect such involvement: ureteric catheterization, serum antibody titration, estimation of concentrating ability and the detection of enzymes excreted in the urine.

Ureteric Catheterization (Brumfitt, 1965; Stamey, Govan and Palmer, 1965; Fairley, Bond and Adey, 1966). This is the most obvious method but one which is justified only in special circumstances. It has the advantage of allowing distinction to be made between unilateral and bilateral infection which may be of advantage where surgery is contemplated. Strictly speaking, this technique only detects infection of the ureteric urine but in practice this is almost always associated with infection of the renal parenchyma.

Serum Antibody Titration. Antibodies against the O-antigen of Gram-negative bacteria causing infection can be detected in the patient's serum by the hæmagglutination test (Neter, Bertram, Zak, Murdock and Arbesman, 1952) or direct bacterial agglutination (Percival, Brumfitt and de Louvois, 1964). It has also been shown that invasion of the kidney parenchyma is associated with a raised antibody titre (Brumfitt and Percival, 1963; Percival, Brumfitt and de Louvois, 1964; Ehrenkranz and Carter, 1964). Winberg, Andersen, Hanson and Lincoln (1963) also found a rise in antibody titre in children with acute urinary tract infection if the urine-concentrating capacity was also impaired but not in similar children with acute infections and a normal concentrating capacity.

Estimation of Concentrating Ability. Winberg (1959) found that 17 of 22 infants and children with urinary tract infections had impaired concentrating ability, although creatinine clearance and urine acidification were normal. Kaitz (1961) investigated patients with bacteriuria and found subnormal concentrating capacity in 9 of 20 pregnant women with significant bacteriuria, but in none of 30 non-bacteriuric controls. Similar observations have been made by Norden and Tuttle (1965) and Elder and Kass (1965). The concentration test depends upon patient co-operation and Seligman and Hewitt (1965) present data showing how failure of co-operation can lead to an apparently impaired concentration defect when further investigation of the patients after the infusion of vasopressin (pitressin) showed that no defect was present.

Excretion of Enzymes in the Urine. The possibility that renal damage might be detected by the appearance of enzymes that are present in high or relatively high concentration in renal tissues has been studied by a number of workers. Urinary lysozyme, lactic acid dehydrogenase and beta-glucorunidase have all been investigated. Beta-glucuronidase is present in kidney lysosomes and Bank and Bailine (1965) reported that this enzyme appeared in excess in the urine of patients suffering from both acute and chronic pyelonephritis. Roberts, Frampton, Beard and Karim (1967) studied the value of the test for detecting renal damage in pregnancy and in puerperal women. They found that some patients with bacteriuria and abnormal pyelograms had normal levels of beta-glucuronidase whilst a number of control patients without bacteriuria had abnormally high levels. It was concluded that the test was unlikely to be of value in the management of urinary infection.

The Diagnosis of Chronic Pyelonephritis

It cannot be emphasized too strongly that patients with chronic pyelonephritis may have a sterile, protein-free urine, with a normal white cell excretion. Recurrent infections and increased white cell excretion are indicative of active disease and point to the need for investigation of the urinary tract, but are not sufficient evidence to permit a diagnosis of chronic pyelonephritis.

Renal biopsy has proved to be disappointing because of the relatively small sample of tissue together with the patchy nature of the pyelonephritic lesion. Heptinstall (1966) has stressed the importance of examining the whole kidney macroscopically in addition to microscopically and improved radiological techniques have allowed many of these macroscopical changes such as renal size, scarring and calyceal changes to be defined with considerable accuracy (Hodson, 1959; Rosenheim, 1963). The relationship of scars to a dilated deformed calyx has also been emphasized by Smith (1962), who was able to determine whether a scar was due to infection or to arteriosclerosis with a good degree of accuracy.

Another method that has been used to diagnose chronic pyelonephritis is to study the white cell excretion before and after the injection of certain biological substances. These are of some interest and will, therefore, be considered in detail.

White Cell Provocation Tests. Pears and Houghton (1959) reported that following the administration of bacterial cell-wall lipo-polysaccharide (bacterial pyrogen) to 17 patients with chronic pyelonephritis the excretion rate of cells in the urine increased significantly within 30 minutes in all cases. They also noted that in three patients with other forms of chronic renal disease no increase occurred following pyrogen. However, further work by Hutt, Chalmers, MacDonald and de Wardener (1961), Leather, Wills and Gault (1963) and Montgomerie and North (1963) did not entirely confirm these findings since positive tests were found in only about half of the patients with chronic pyelonephritis. Positive tests were also obtained with renal lesions other than chronic pyelonephritis. Hutt *et al.* (1961) also found that the test might be positive in some patients who had suffered from upper urinary tract infection but in whom treatment had made the urine sterile and in whom the white cell excretion had returned to normal. They considered that a significant white cell excretion following administration of pyrogen revealed persisting inflammation and called for further treatment.

Katz, Bourdo and Moore (1962) found that corticosteroids administered parenterally also stimulated the excretion of white cells in pyelonephritic dogs and that in man the test was a useful alternative to the pyrogen test since the unpleasant side effects of pyrogen were avoided (Katz, Velasquez and Bourdo, 1962). I have suggested that lipopolysaccharide and prednisolone act in the same way because the serum corticosteroid levels increase following the administration of lipopolysaccharide (Brumfitt, 1965). However, the recent observation by V. H. T. James (personal communication) that the injection of lipopolysaccharide did not produce a rise in plasma cortisol levels of four normal subjects within 30 min. casts some doubt on this theory since Pears and Houghton (1959) observed that the increase in white cell excretion regularly occurred within 30 min. after the injection of lipo-polysaccharide. N. W. H. Ormonde (personal communication) also noted that of 19 positive tests 17 showed a doubling of white cell excretion within 30 min. of administration of prednisolone.

Our experience with the prednisolone test is based on the study of 50 patients with chronic pyelonephritis. Twenty (40 per cent) gave a positive test, but two patients with chronic glomerulonephritis also gave positive results (Brumfitt and Percival, 1964; Brumfitt, 1965). We confirmed the finding of Hutt *et al.* (1961) that some patients who had recently had successful treatment for urinary tract infections gave positive tests. Of the 26 patients studied, eight (30 per cent) gave a positive test and none of these showed evidence of chronic pyelonephritis. Unlike Hutt *et al.* (1961), we could not find evidence that this indicated persistent renal infection since, although no patient was given further treatment, and urine specimens were examined at regular intervals for the next two years, none showed a relapse of infection due to the same organism.

The reasons for the discrepancies in findings of the various workers mentioned are difficult to explain, for in all cases the patients were studied carefully and the ætiology of the renal lesion established. However, in the present state of our knowledge certain conclusions seem inevitable. First, the white cell stimulation test may be positive in chronic pyelonephritis, but positive results are also found with other forms of chronic renal disease. Second, positive tests occur in patients who do not have chronic pyelo-nephritis but have been recently treated for a urinary tract infection, and third, positive tests may occur with latent lesions in the lower urinary tract.

An investigation by Briggs, Kennedy and Goldberg (1963) showed that white cell excretion was also increased after the injection of iron-sorbitol-citric-acid.

Characterization of Organisms encountered in Bacteriuria

The genus and species of bacteria causing urinary tract infection depend upon many factors including whether infection is acquired in hospital or at home, and whether instrumentation of the urinary tract has been carried out. Infections acquired during antibacterial chemotherapy are likely to be due to resistant bacteria, and when the host defence mechanisms are impaired, organisms which do not commonly invade the urinary tract may infect the urine. However, enterobacteria are by far the most frequent cause of urinary infection. In patients who acquire their infection outside hospital, *E. coli* accounts for more than 80 per cent of uncomplicated cases and *Proteus mirabilis* is found in many of the remainder. *Staph. albus* occasionally causes infection but it is an unusual pathogen, although its presence on the skin makes it a frequent contaminant if specimens are not collected carefully. Details of the distribution and antibiotic sensitivities of organisms commonly found in urinary infections are given by Kass (1955), Finland, Jones and Barnes (1959) and Grossberg, Petersdorf, Curtin and Bennett (1962).

Serotypes of *Escherichia coli* in Urinary Infections. The serological classification of *E. coli* (Kauffman, 1944) has permitted a detailed study of the epidemiology and natural history of urinary tract infection. It is now clear that most *E. coli* infections that cause urinary infections belong to a few of the 147 different O-groups (Ujváry, 1958; Rantz, 1962; Turck and Petersdorf, 1962). The most common varieties are O75, O6, O2, O4 and there has been heated discussion as to whether this means that these organisms are specially pathogenic for the urinary tract or whether they represent the common fæcal strains of *E. coli*. In a study of patients in a domiciliary practice we found that the *E. coli* serotype causing a particular urinary infection frequently predominated in the bowel of the patient. Furthermore, the serotypes in the fæces of healthy people in the community where the infections arose were very similar to those causing the urinary infections and were also those commonly found by other workers (O75, O6, O2, O4, etc.). It is not possible to review the literature on this subject, but at present most workers agree that the serotype of the *E. coli* causing an acute urinary infection is likely to be the same as the predominant *E. coli* serotype in the fæces. However, this does not exclude the possibility that a particular O-serotype may have increased pathogenicity for the urinary tract. Further evidence is needed to resolve this problem.

Use of Serotyping to distinguish between Re-infection and Relapse. Re-infection has obviously occurred when the urine becomes sterile after treatment but later is found to be infected with a different organism, such as *Proteus mirabilis*. However, if the organism is still *E. coli* it is possible that the original infecting strain has persisted or that the urine has become re-infected. A change of serotype is proof that re-infection has occurred and the finding of the same serotype usually indicates relapse, particularly if this serotype is absent from the fæces.

Bacterial "Variants" as a Cause of Persistent Infection

Braude, Siemienski and Jacobs (1961) demonstrated "protoplast" formation in the human urine under conditions of increased tonicity and antimicrobial therapy. Guze and Kalmanson (1963b) produced experimental enterococcal pyelonephritis in the rat and, following apparently successful penicillin treatment, were able to isolate protoplasts from kidney homogenates. In other experimental studies Alderman and Freedman (1963) injected *E. coli* "protoplasts" into the renal medulla of rabbits and some developed pyelonephritis. More recently, Gutman, Turck, Petersdorf and Wedgwood (1965) have isolated "L forms" or "protoplasts" from the urine of 11 of 57 (19 per cent) patients with chronic urinary tract infection and pyelonephritis.

These studies are interesting because they provide a possible explanation for persistent infection in the renal medulla. Further work is desirable in order to define the nature of the "variants" more precisely and particularly to see whether they are really *E. coli* spheroplasts.

Relationship of Bacteriuria to Acute and Chronic Pyelonephritis

Few would dispute the relationship of asymptomatic bacteriuria to severe symptomatic infection such as acute pyelonephritis or Gram-negative bacteræmia. In the experimental animal it has been demonstrated that, if sustained, infection of the kidney can result in chronic pyelonephritis showing histological features very similar to those characteristic of the disease in man. It is also clear that, in the child, uncontrolled urinary tract infection can progress within a decade to renal failure due to chronic pyelo-nephritis. At post-mortem the characteristic macroscopical and microscopical changes are found. Control of infection in the child permits resumption of renal growth and arrest of the scarring process, indicating that active infection causes the lesion, rather than that it is due to a secondary change initiated by the infection.

In the adult, the relationship of bacteriuria to chronic pyelonephritis is less clear since few prospective studies on patients with urinary infection are available. It has been suggested that bacteriuria, which is common in the elderly, is a benign condition as far as progressive renal damage is concerned, but properly designed prospective studies are required to resolve this question.

Pyelonephritis as a Cause of Renal Failure

Although chronic pyelonephritis was described by Wagner in 1882, its importance was not immediately recognized and it is not mentioned by Volhard and Fahr (1914). Over the last two decades, however, the situation has radically changed and nowadays chronic pyelonephritis is regarded by many workers as the commonest cause of renal failure.

However, the diagnosis of chronic pyelonephritis at necropsy is not always easy and several workers have pointed out the difficulties in distinguishing chronic pyelonephritis from chronic interstitial nephritis of non-bacterial origin (Freedman, 1963; Pawlowski, Bloxdorf and Kimmelsteil, 1963; Kimmelsteil, 1966). Also, unless the whole kidney is examined the importance of the histological changes in terms of significant renal damage cannot be assessed. Kimmelsteil and his co-workers have suggested that at post-mortem examination culture of the bladder urine and renal tissue helps to decide whether the chronic interstitial fibrosis is the result of bacterial infection

This approach does not seem valuable since many patients acquire urinary infection during their terminal illness and, in half, bacteria can be demonstrated in the kidney (Brumfitt and Percival, 1963). Pyelonephritis is also common complication of other forms of renal disease, such as glomerulonephritis (Relman, 1963). Furthermore, in the later stages of chronic pyelonephritis the urine may be sterile for prolonged periods of time, and the affected kidney removed from patients with unilateral chronic pyelonephritis is often sterile (Brumfitt and Percival, 1962).

It is no doubt because of these difficulties that the frequency of chronic pyelonephritis found at autopsy by various authors varies so greatly. Similarly, diagnosis of the underlying lesion in kidneys removed at homotransplantation suffers from the diagnostic problems already discussed. Also, although it is true that such kidneys are removed from patients with renal failure, the bias in selection of cases is important. For example, the presence of lower urinary tract disease, often present in chronic pyelonephritis but uncommon in glomerulonephritis, would make patients suffering from the latter condition more likely candidates for transplantation.

Conclusion

During the last decade a large number of studies have shown urinary tract infection to be an important cause of morbidity and mortality in the community. The infection is frequently asymptomatic and persistent and even when treated tends to recur. The relationship of urinary infection to chronic pyelonephritis and renal failure seems clear in children. In adults, prospective studies indicate that persistent bacteriuria is also associated with renal damage, but in the absence of urinary tract abnormalities the factors which determine whether renal damage will occur in the individual patient are less well defined. The value of post-mortem studies in demonstrating the frequency of chronic pyelonephritis is impaired by lack of uniform criteria of diagnosis.

The need for detection, treatment and follow-up of urinary infections in certain groups in the community is obvious. Although less dramatic than chronic dialysis or transplantation, by partially or completely preventing chronic bacterial infections of the kidney and their sequelæ, such detection and treatment provides a more effective and economical approach to the problem. Examination for bacteriuria should not be confined to patients in hospital for it is also widespread in the apparently healthy community and therefore constitutes a major problem in preventive and community medicine.

References

ADDIS, T. (1926). The number of formed elements in the urinary sediment of normal individuals. *J. clin. Invest.*, **2**, 409.

ALDERMAN, M. H. and FREEDMAN, L. R. (1963). Experimental pyelonephritis. X. The direct injection of E. coli protoplasts into the medulla of the rabbit kidney. *Yale J. Biol. Med.*, **36**, 157.

BANK, N. and BAILINE, S. H. (1965). Urinary beta-glucuronidase activity with urinary tract infection. *New Engl. J. Med.*, **272**, 70.

BEARD, R. W., McCOY, D. R., NEWTON, J. R. and CLAYTON, S. G. (1965). Diagnosis of urinary infection by suprapubic bladder puncture. *Lancet*, **ii**, 610.

BEESON, P. B. (1958). The case against the catheter. *Amer. J. Med.*, **24**, 1.

BONDY, P. K. (1966). Therapeutic considerations in diabetes mellitus. In *Controversy in Internal Medicine*, eds. Ingelfinger, Relman and Finland. Saunders, London, p. 499.

BRAUDE, A., SIEMENSKI, J. and JACOBS, I. (1961). Protoplast formation in human urine. *Trans. Ass. Amer. Phycns.*, **74**, 234,

BRIGGS, J. D., KENNEDY, A. C. and GOLDBERG, A. (1963). Urinary white cell excretion after iron-sorbitol-citric acid. *Brit. Med. J.*, **ii**, 352.

BRUMFITT, W. (1965). Urinary cell counts and their value. *J. clin. Path.*, **18**, 550.

BRUMFITT, W., DAVIES, B. I. and ROSSER, E. AP I. (1961). Urethral catheter as a cause of urinary tract infection in pregnancy and puerperium. *Lancet*, **ii**, 1059.

BRUMFITT, W., LEIGH, D. and GRUNEBERG, R. N. (1967). Bacteriuria in pregnancy, with reference to prematurity and long term effects on the mother. In: *Symposium on Pyelonephritis*, Edinburgh 1966. E. & S. Livingstone, p. 20.

BRUMFITT, W. and PERCIVAL, A. (1962). Problems in the ætiology, diagnosis and treatment of pyelonephritis. *Brit. J. clin. Pract.*, **16**, 253.

BRUMFITT, W. and PERCIVAL, A. (1963). Specific antibody response of patients with significant bacteriuria. Proc. 2nd International Congress of Nephrology. Eds. Vostal, J. and Richet, G. *Excerpta med., Amst.*, p. 260.

BRUMFITT, W. and PERCIVAL, A. (1964). Pathogenesis and laboratory diagnosis of non-tuberculous urinary tract infection: a review. *J. clin. Path.*, **17**, 482.

BULGER, R. J. and KIRBY, W. M. M. (1963). Simple tests for significant bacteriuria. *Arch. intern. Med.*, **112**, 742.

COX, C. E. and HINMAN, F. (1961). Experiments with induced bacteriuria, vesical emptying and bacterial growth on the mechanism of bladder defence to infection. *J. Urol.*, **86**, 739.

CRUICKSHANK, J. and MOYES, J. M. (1914). The presence and significance of nitrites in urine. *Brit. med. J.*, **ii**, 712.

CSONKA, G. W., WILLIAMS, R. E. O. and CORSE, J. (1966). T-strain mycoplasma in non-gonococcal urethritis. *Lancet*, **ii**, 1292.

EHRENKRANZ, N. J. and CARTER, M. J. (1964). Immunologic studies in urinary tract infections. *J. Immunol.*, **92**, 798.

ELDER, H. A. and KASS, E. H. (1965). Renal function in bacteriuria of pregnancy. *Progress in Pyelonephritis*, ed. Kass, E. H. Davis, Philadelphia, p. 81.

FAIRLEY, K. F., BOND, A. G. and ADEY, F. D. (1966). The site of infection in pregnancy bacteriuria. *Lancet*, **i**, 939.

FINLAND, M., JONES, W. F. and BARNES, M. W. (1959). Occurrence of serious bacterial infections since introduction of antibacterial agents. *J. Amer. med. Ass.*, **170**, 2188.

FREEDMAN, L. A. (1963). Pyelonephritis and urinary tract infection. In *Diseases of the Kidney*, eds. Strauss, M. B. and Welt, L. G. Churchill, London, p. 469.

GROSSBERG, S. E., PETERSDORF, R. G., CURTIN, J. A. and BENNETT, I. L. (1962). Factors influencing the species and antimicrobial resistance of urinary pathogens. *Amer. J. Med.*, **32**, 44.

GUTMAN, L. T., TURCK, M., PETERSDORF, R. G. and WEDGWOOD, R. J. (1965). Significance of bacterial variants in urine of patients with chronic bacteriuria. *J. clin. Invest.*, **44**, 1945.

GUTTMANN, D. and NAYLOR, G. R. E. (1967). The Dip-Slide, an aid to quantitative urine culture in general practice. *Brit. med. J.*, **3**, 343.

GUTTMANN, D. and STOKES, E. J. (1963). Diagnosis of urinary infection. *Brit. med. J.*, **i**, 1384.

GUZE, L. B. and KALMANSON, G. M. (1963a). Observations on the use of the triphenyl tetrazolium chloride test to determine significant bacteriuria. *Amer. J. med. Sci.*, **246**, 691.

GUZE, L. B. and KALMANSON, G. M. (1963b). Persistence of bacteria in "protoplast" form after apparent cure of pyelonephritis in rats. *Science*, **143**, 1340.

HARRIS, H. W., MURRAY, R., PAINE, T. F., KILHAM, L. and FINLAND, M. (1947). Streptomycin treatment of urinary tract infections—with special reference to the use of alkali. *Amer. J. Med.*, **2**, 229.

HEPTINSTALL, R. H. (1966). *Pathology of the Kidney*. Churchill, London.

HODSON, C. J. (1959). The radiological diagnosis of pyelonephritis. *Proc. R. Soc. Med.*, **52**, 669.

HODSON, C. J. and WILSON, S. (1965). Natural history of chronic pyelonephritic scarring. *Brit. med. J.*, **ii**, 191.

HOUGHTON, B. J. and PEARS, M. A. (1957). Cell excretion in normal urine. *Brit. med. J.*, **i**, 622.

HUTT, M. S. R., CHALMERS, J. A., MACDONALD, J. S. and DE WARDENER, H. E. (1961). Pyelonephritis—Observations on the relation between various diagnostic procedures. *Lancet*, **i**, 351.

KAITZ, A. L. (1961). Urinary concentrating ability in pregnant women with asymptomatic bacteriuria. *J. clin. Invest.*, **40**, 1331.

KASS, E. H. (1955). Chemotherapeutic and antibiotic drugs in the management of infections of the urinary tract. *Amer. J. Med.*, **18**, 764.

KASS, E. H. (1956). Asymptomatic infections of the urinary tract. *Trans. Ass. Amer. Phycns.*, **69**, 56.

KASS, E. H. (1957). Bacteriuria and the diagnosis of infections of the urinary tract. *Arch. intern. Med.*, **100**, 709.

KASS, E. H. (1960). Bacteriuria and pyelonephritis of pregnancy. *Arch. intern. Med.*, **106**, 194.

KASS, E. H. (1962a). Pyelonephritis and bacteriuria. A major problem in preventive medicine. *Ann. intern. Med.*, **56**, 46.

KASS, E. H. (1962b). Prevention of apparently non-infectious disease by detection and treatment of infections of the urinary tract. *J. chron. Dis.*, **15**, 665.

KASS, E. H. (Editor) (1965). *Progress in Pyelonephritis*. Davis, Philadelphia.

KASS, E. H., SAVAGE, W. D. and SANTAMARINA, B. A. G. (1965). The significance of bacteriuria in preventive medicine. In *Progress in Pyelonephritis*, p. 3.

KATZ, Y. J., BOURDO, S. R. and MOORE, R. S. (1962). Effect of pyrogen and adrenal steroids in pyelonephritis. *Lancet*, **i**, 1140.

KATZ, Y. J., VELASQUEZ, A. and BOURDO, S. R. (1962). The prednisolone provocative test for pyelonephritis. *Lancet*, **i**, 1144.

KAUFFMANN, F. (1944). Zur Serologie der coli-grupps. *Acta Path. Microbiol. scand.*, **21**, 20.

KIMMELSTEIL, P. (1966). Asymptomatic bacteriuria a hypothetical concept, should be treated with caution. In *Controversy in Internal Medicine*. Eds. Ingelfinger, F. J., Relman, A. S. and Finland, M. Saunders, London.

KINCAID-SMITH, P., BULLEN, M., MILLS, J., FUSSELL, U., HUSTON, N. and GOON, F. (1964). The reliability of screening tests for bacteriuria in pregnancy. *Lancet*, **ii**, 61.

KLEEMAN, C. R., HEWITT, W. L. and GUZE, L. B. (1960). Pyelonephritis. *Medicine*, **39**, 3.

KUNIN, C. M., DEUTSCHER, R. and PAQUIN, A. (1964). Urinary tract infection in school-children: an epidemiologic, clinical and laboratory study. *Medicine*, **43**, 91.

LEATHER, H. M., WILLS, M. R. and GAULT, H. M. (1963). Bacterial pyrogen in the diagnosis of pyelonephritis. *Brit. med. J.*, **i**, 92.

LEIGH, D. A. and WILLIAMS, J. D. (1964). Methods for the detection of significant bacteriuria in large groups of patients. *J. clin. Path.*, **17**, 498.

MACKEY, J. P. and SANDYS, G. H. (1965). Laboratory diagnosis of infections of the urinary tract in general practice by means of a dip-inoculum transport medium. *Brit. med. J.*, **2**, 1286.

MACKEY, J. P. and SANDYS, G. H. (1966). Diagnosis of urinary infections. *Brit. med. J.*, **1**, 1173.

McGEACHIE, J. and KENNEDY, A. C. (1963). Simplified quantitative methods for bacteriuria and pyuria. *J. clin. Path.*, **16**, 32.

MARPLE, C. D. (1941). The frequency and character of urinary tract infections in an unselected group of women. *Ann. intern. Med.*, **14**, 2220.

MOND, N. C., PERCIVAL, A., WILLIAMS, J. D. and BRUMFITT, W. (1965). Presentation diagnosis and treatment of urinary tract infections in general practice. *Lancet*, **i**, 514.

MONTGOMERIE, J. Z. and NORTH, J. D. (1963). Evaluation of the pyrogen test in chronic pyelonephritis. *Lancet*, **i**, 690.

NAYLOR, G. R. E. and GUTTMANN, D. (1967). The Dip-Slide: a modified dip inoculum transport medium for the laboratory diagnosis of infections of the urinary tract. *J. Hyg., Camb.*, **65**, 367.

NETER, E., BERTRAM, L. F., ZAK, D. A., MURDOCK, M. R. and ARBESMAN, C. E. (1952). Studies on hæmagglutination and hæmolysis by *Escherichia coli* antiserum. *J. exp. Med.*, **96**, 1.

NORDEN, C. W. and TUTTLE, E. P. (1965). Impairment of concentrating ability in pregnant women with asymptomatic bacteriuria. In *Progress in Pyelonephritis*. Ed. Kass, E. H. Davis, Philadelphia, p. 73.

O'GRADY, F. and CATTELL, W. R. (1966). Kinetics of Urinary Tract Infection. *Brit. J. Urol.* **38**, 149.

O'SULLIVAN, D. J., FITZGERALD, M. G., MEYNELL, M. J. and MALINS, J. M. (1960). A simplified method for the quantitative bacterial culture of urine. *J. clin. Path.*, **13**, 527.

PAWLOWSKI, J. M., BLOXDORF, J. W. and KIMMELSTEIL, P. (1963). Chronic pyelonephritis: a morphologic and bacteriologic study. *New Engl. J. Med.*, **268**, 965.

PEARS, M. A. and HOUGHTON, B. J. (1959). Response of infected urinary tract to bacterial pyrogen. *Lancet*, **ii**, 1167.

PERCIVAL, A., BRUMFITT, W., and DE LOUVOIS, J. (1964). Serum antibody levels as an indication of clinically inapparent pyelonephritis. *Lancet*, **ii**, 1027.

PRESCOTT, L. F. and BRODIE, D. E. (1964). A simple differential stain for urinary sediment. *Lancet*, **ii**, 940.

QUINN, E. L. and KASS, E. H. (Editors) (1960). *Biology of Pyelonephritis*. Churchill, London.

RANTZ, L. A. (1962). Serological grouping of *Esch. coli*. Study in urinary tract infection. *Arch. intern. Med.*, **109**, 37.

RANTZ, L. A. and KEEFER, C. S. (1940). Sulfanilamide in treatment of infections of the urinary tract due to bacillus coli. *Arch. intern. Med.*, **65**, 933.

RELMAN, A. S. (1963). Clinical aspects of chronic glomerulonephritis. In *Diseases of the Kidney*. Eds. Strauss, M. B. and Welt, L. G. Churchill, London, p. 320.

ROBERTS, A. P., ROBINSON, R. E. and BEARD, R. W. (1967). Some factors affecting bacterial colony counts in urinary infection. *Brit. med. J.*, **i**, 400.

ROBERTS, A. P., FRAMPTON, J., KARIM, S. M. M. and BEARD, R. W. (1967). Estimation of β glucuronidase activity in urinary infection. *New Engl. J. Med.*, **276**, 1468.

ROFE, P. (1955). The cells of normal human urine. *J. clin. Path.*, **8**, 25.

ROSENHEIM, M. L. (1963). Problems of chronic pyelonephritis. *Brit. med. J.*, **i**, 1433.

SELIGMAN, S. J. and HEWITT, W. L. (1965). Urinary concentration tests on postpartum bacteriuric women. In *Progress in Pyelonephritis*. Ed. Kass. Davis, Philadelphia, p. 558.

SIMMONS, N. A. and WILLIAMS, J. D. (1962). A simple test for significant bacteriuria. *Lancet*, **i**, 1377.

SLEIGH, J. D. (1965). Detection of bacteriuria by a modification of the nitrite test. *Brit. med. J.*, **i**, 765.

SLEIGH, J. D., ROBERTSON, J. G. and ISDALE, M. H. (1964). Asymptomatic bacteriuria in pregnancy. *J. Obstet. Gynæc. Brit. Comm.*, **71**, 74.

SMELLIE, J. M. (1967). Medical aspects of urinary infection in children. *J. Roy. Coll. Phycns.*, **1**, 189.

SMELLIE, J. M., HODSON, C. J., EDWARDS, D. and NORMAND, I. C. S. (1964). Clinical and radiological features of urinary infection in childhood. *Brit. med. J.*, **ii**, 1222.

SMITH, J. F. (1962). The diagnosis of the scars of chronic pyelonephritis. *J. clin. Path.*, **15**, 522.

SMITH, L. G., THAYER, W. R., MALTA, E. M. and UTZ, J. P. (1961). Relationship of the Greiss nitrite test to bacterial counts in the diagnosis of urinary tract infection. *Ann. intern. Med.*, **54**, 66.

STAMEY, T. A., GOVAN, D. E. and PALMER, J. M. (1965). The localisation and treatment of urinary tract infections: the role of bactericidal urine levels as opposed to serum levels. *Medicine*, **44**, 1.

STEELE, R. E., LEADBETTER, G. W. and CRAWFORD, J. D. (1963). Prognosis of childhood urinary tract infection. *New Engl. J. Med.*, **269**, 883.

STUART, K. L., CUMMINS, G. T. M. and CHIN, W. A. (1965). Bacteriuria, prematurity and hypertensive disorders of pregnancy. *Brit. med. J.*, **i**, 554.

TENNEY, B. and LITTLE, A. B. (1958). Obstetrics. *New Engl. J. Med.*, **259**, 625.

TRIGER, D. R. and SMITH, J. W. G. (1966). Survival of urinary leucocytes. *J. clin. Path.*, **19**, 443.

TURCK, M. and PETERSDORF, R. G. (1962). The epidemiology of non-enteric *E. coli* infections prevalence of serologic groups. *J. clin. Invest.*, **41**, 1760.

UJVÁRY, G. (1958). Uber die atiologische Rolle der Escherichia-coli-Gruppe bei extraenteral ulokalisierten Infeltionen; biochemische und serologische untersuchurigen. *Zbl. Bakt. I. Abt. Orig.*, **170**, 394.

VOLHARD, F. and FAHR, TH. (1914). Die Brightsche Nierenkrankheit. Berlin, Springer.

WAGNER, E. (1882). Der Morbus Brightii, Handbuch der Krankheiten des Harnapparates, **8**, 352. Leipzig, F. C. W. Vogel.

WILLIAMS, J. D., LEIGH, D. A., ROSSER, E. AP I. and BRUMFITT, W. (1965). The organisation and results of a screening programme for the detection of bacteriuria of pregnancy. *J. Obstet. Gynæc. Brit. Comm.*, **72**, 327.

WINBERG, J. (1959). Renal function studies in infants and children with acute, non-obstructive urinary tract infections. *Acta pædiat.*, **48**, 577.

WINBERG, J., ANDERSEN, H. J., HANSON, L. A. and LINCOLN, K. (1963). Studies of urinary tract infections in infancy and childhood. I. Antibody response in different types of urinary tract infections caused by coliform bacteria. *Brit. med. J.*, **ii**, 524.

Chapter 3

THE LABORATORY DIAGNOSIS OF INFECTION WITH
PASTEURELLA PSEUDOTUBERCULOSIS

N. S. Mair

HUMAN infection with *Pasteurella pseudotuberculosis* was generally regarded, until a few years ago, as rare. Knapp (1959) could find records of only some 15 authenticated cases between 1910 and 1952. The majority of these were characterized by a severe typhoid-like illness with enlargement of the liver and spleen and an invariably fatal outcome. In 1953 Masshoff and Dölle observed in the mesenteric glands of children suffering from acute mesenteric lymphadenitis certain pathological changes which they described as an "abscess-forming reticulocytic lymphadenitis", probably of viral origin since the changes in the affected glands resembled those found in cat-scratch fever and lymphogranuloma inguinale. In the following year, however, Knapp (1954) and Knapp and Masshoff (1954) investigating similar cases reported the isolation of *P. pseudotuberculosis* from enlarged mesenteric glands in which the histological changes were identical with those described by Masshoff and Dölle. Since then, several hundred cases of *P. pseudotuberculosis* infection have been diagnosed in many countries of Europe, including Great Britain.

Acute mesenteric lymphadenitis due to *P. pseudotuberculosis* occurs mainly in young males between 5 and 15 years of age. The clinical picture is that of acute or subacute appendicitis. Laparotomy reveals in most cases a normal-looking or slightly inflamed appendix. The mesenteric lymph glands, especially those in the ileo-cæcal angle, are inflamed and swollen, and the mesentery frequently shows redness, either diffuse or limited to the region of the affected lymph nodes. Sometimes the terminal ileum and cæcum show gross hyperæmic swelling and œdema which may be mistaken for a malignant tumour or Crohn's disease. Besides the septicæmic and appendiceal forms, infection with *P. pseudotuberculosis* may appear less commonly as an acute enteritis, an acute intussusception or as erythema nodosum occurring in the course of acute mesenteric lymphadenitis.

According to Mollaret (personal communication, 1967) infection with *P. pseudotuberculosis* probably accounts for about 5 per cent of cases of acute mesenteric lymphadenitis in France. In Great Britain, Mair and his colleagues (1960), in a study of 17 consecutive cases of acute mesenteric lymphadenitis, found evidence of infection with *P. pseudotuberculosis* in three cases (18 per cent).

The diagnosis is established by the isolation of the organism from the lymphatic glands, by the demonstration of specific antibodies in the serum, by histological examination of the lymph nodes and by the response to a specific skin-test antigen. In a few cases of septicæmia *P. pseudotuberculosis* has been cultivated from the blood during life, but more often diagnosis has been made at autopsy when the organism has been isolated from the numerous abscesses found in the liver and spleen (Knapp, 1959).

ISOLATION OF *P. PSEUDOTUBERCULOSIS*

From Mesenteric Lymph Glands. The organism is found most frequently in the swollen and congested glands situated in the ileo-cæcal angle. A small node distant from the ileo-cæcal angle, while it may still yield a culture, may be devoid of the characteristic necrotic lesions. There is no record of isolation of *P. pseudotuberculosis* from lymph nodes at sites other than the mesentery.

The gland is ground up in digest broth and loopfuls of the suspension are inoculated on 5 per cent horse-blood agar and into digest broth. Cultures are incubated aerobically and anaerobically at 22°C and 37°C. The lower temperature is to be preferred since *P. pseudotuberculosis* grown at 37°C tends to become "rough" and to lose its motility. As a rule, antigenic analysis is only possible with strains grown at 22°C. In isolated cases growth in primary culture only takes place at 22°C (Mair *et al.*, 1960) or under anaerobic conditions (Knapp, 1960). Growth is visible after 24 hours at 37°C in the form of flat, dry, non-hæmolytic colonies with crenated edges and a dull granular surface. After 24 hours at 22°C small, moist, transparent colonies with entire edge and smooth shining surface are produced. Minute colonies appear on MacConkey's medium after 24 hours at 37°C. In broth, growth is diffuse at 22°C and tends to be more viscous at 37°C.

Attempts to demonstrate the presence of *P. pseudotuberculosis* in smears or impression smears of gland tissue by Gram's method, or by a modified acid-fast technique recommended by Cook (1952) for the recognition of the organism in tissues, have rarely proved successful.

The results of animal inoculation with gland suspension must be viewed with caution. *P. pseudotuberculosis* is often present in the guinea-pig as a latent infection which may become manifest as the result of inoculation. At the same time, strains of *P. pseudotuberculosis* lacking in pathogenicity for guinea-pigs have been isolated from human mesenteric lymph glands. For these reasons guinea-pig inoculation should only be done when attempts to culture the organism have failed.

From the Blood. Apart from the septicæmic form of the disease, the organism has only once been isolated from the blood (Graber and Knapp, 1955). When blood culture is attempted, incubation should continue for at least 10 days before the culture is discarded as negative.

From the Fæces. Up to the present, fæcal culture has been successful in only a small number of cases, probably because a completely satisfactory selective medium for the isolation of *P. pseudotuberculosis* from contaminated material is still lacking. The customary selective media used in the diagnosis of salmonella are not entirely suitable for the routine isolation of *P. pseudo-tuberculosis*. Most promising results have been obtained using tellurite media with or without the addition of antibiotics.

Morris (1958) devised a medium consisting of sheep blood agar containing novobiocin, potassium tellurite, erythromycin and actidione. Paterson and Cook (1963) modified this medium by the addition of nystatin and crystal violet according to the formula: to 200 ml. tryptic digest agar add 10 ml. peptic digest of sheep blood, novobiocin (0·2 per cent) 2·0 ml., erythromycin (0·2 per cent) 0·5 ml., nystatin (50,000 units per ml.) 0·8 ml., and crystal violet (Gurr 548, 0·1 per cent) 0·5 ml. Brzin (1963) claimed equally good results with a medium in which the antibiotics and crystal violet were replaced by potassium tellurite (4–7 ml. of a 1 per cent solution in 100 ml. of medium). Certain selective media, such as that devised by Knisely and his colleagues (1964) for the isolation of *P. pestis*, are equally suitable for *P. pseudotuberculosis*; derived from Morris's medium (with the addition of sodium azide, hæmin and nystatin), this medium is claimed to give results superior to those previously obtained.

A method of enrichment of fæces (or pathological material in general) previous to culture has been described by Paterson and Cook (1963). Based on the fact that *P. pseudotuberculosis* is able to multiply at +4°C, it consists in keeping a 10 per cent suspension of fæces in a solution of phosphate buffer (*p*H 7·6) at +4°C for 28 days. Subcultures are made from the 7th day onwards.

IDENTIFICATION OF *P. PSEUDOTUBERCULOSIS*

Identification of the organism is not difficult. Its motility at 22°C, its ability to grow on MacConkey's medium and to decompose urea and the caseous nodules produced in guinea-pigs after experimental inoculation help to distinguish it from other members of the *Pasteurella* group.

Motility is sometimes difficult to demonstrate in broth cultures. For this reason it has been suggested that human strains are less motile than those of animal origin (Knapp, 1954; Knapp and Masshoff, 1954), while others have even held the view that strains of human origin are invariably non-motile. However, the motility of both human and animal strains can be readily demonstrated by use of a Craigie tube incubated at 18°–20°C. In practice it usually suffices to inoculate at the same time two Craigie tubes, one of which is incubated at 37°C and the other at 18°–20°C.

Just as constant is the presence of urease which produces a rapid colour change in the heavily inoculated urea medium.

To these two major characteristics is added sensitivity of *P. pseudotuberculosis* to certain bacteriophages highly specific for this organism and *P. pestis*. Since the latter presents no problem in Great Britain, the use of

TABLE I

Differential Diagnostic Characteristics of *P. pseudotuberculosis*

	P. pseudo-tuberculosis	*P. pestis*	*Y. entero-colitica*	*P. septica*	*P. hæmo-lytica*
Motility (20°C)	+	—	+	—	—
Motility (37°C)	—	—	—	—	—
Aesculin	+	+	—	—	—
Melibiose	+	—	—	—	—
Rhamnose	+	—	—	—	—
Saccharose	—	—	+	+	+
Salicin	+	+	—	—	—
Urease	+	—	+	—	—
Indole	—	—	—	+	—
β-Galactosidase	+	+	+	—	—
Oxidase	—	—	—	+	+
Ornithine-Decarboxylase	—	—	+	+	—
PST-Phage (lysis)	+	+	—	—	—

bacteriophage constitutes a remarkably specific and practical method of diagnosis. Two tubes of peptone water are inoculated with a culture of *P. pseudotuberculosis*. To one tube is added a drop of bacteriophage suspension and both tubes are incubated at 37°C. After overnight incubation the tube containing the bacteriophage shows complete clearing.

Table I shows the principal diagnostic features which distinguish *P. pseudotuberculosis* from the other members of the *Pasteurella* group.

The determination of the antigenic structure will confirm the identification of the organism and indicate the serological type to which it belongs. Typing is done by a slide agglutination technique using single-factor O-agglutinating antisera prepared from rabbits hyperimmunized with smooth strains of the different serotypes (Table II) boiled for $2\frac{1}{2}$ hours (Mair *et al.*, 1960). One

TABLE II

Antigenic Constitution of *P. pseudotuberculosis* according to Thal (1966)

Type	Subtype	Somatic antigens			Flagellar antigens
		Rough antigen	Type-specific antigen	Subtype-specific antigen	
I	I A	1	2	3	a, c
	I B	1	2	4	a, c
II	II A	1	5	6	a, d
	II B	1	5	7	a, d
III		1	8	...	a
IV	IV A	1	9	11	b
		1	9	11	a, b
	IV B	1	9	12	a, b, d
V		1	10	...	a, e (b)

loopful of serum diluted 1 in 10 is rubbed into one drop of a dense suspension of bacilli in saline. Specific agglutination occurs in 10–30 seconds after mixing. Another drop of bacillary suspension is placed on the slide as a saline control to detect autoagglutination.

SEROLOGICAL TESTS IN DIAGNOSIS

Pasteurella pseudotuberculosis is divided into five serological types each of which is characterized by thermostable strongly type-specific O-antigens and thermolabile H-antigens. The antigenic constitution of the different types is shown in Table II.

Antibodies to *P. pseudotuberculosis* can be demonstrated in the blood during the acute phase of the illness. By means of agglutination tests with live, smooth suspensions of *P. pseudotuberculosis* titres of 1/80 to 1/12,800 have been recorded. The tests are specific only for Types I, III and V. The specificity of the agglutination test for Types II and IV is affected by the antigenic relationships which exist between *P. pseudotuberculosis* Type II and O-factors 4 and 27 of the salmonella B group and between *P. pseudotubercu-*

losis Type IV and O-factors 9 and 46 of the salmonella D group and O-factor 14 of the salmonella H group. In order that a serological diagnosis can be made it is necessary to absorb the patient's serum with the corresponding strain of the B, D or H group; such absorptions are not often necessary since more than 90 per cent of *P. pseudotuberculosis* infections in man are caused by Type I.

Slide-agglutination Test. Stock cultures of the five serotypes of *P. pseudotuberculosis* grown at 22°C on thickly poured tryptose agar plates and kept in the +4°C refrigerator are used for the slide-agglutination test and for preparing suspensions for the Widal test. Since high agglutinin titres are often present during the acute phase of the illness, the slide test, which is carried out with the patient's serum used neat or diluted against the different serotypes, is of value in indicating the causative type. Because of the risk of spontaneous agglutination a positive slide test must be confirmed by tube-agglutination.

Tube-agglutination Test. Antibody can best be demonstrated with living suspensions from agar cultures or with cultures killed by 0·25 per cent phenol or formalin. Heat-killed (100°C) antigen is not agglutinated or only weakly agglutinated by human antisera (Knapp, 1956).

Agglutinating antigen is prepared by growing the organism on tryptose agar at 22°C. After 48 hours the growth is harvested in normal saline, centrifuged, resuspended in saline, agitated with glass beads in a shaker for 20 minutes, and finally diluted to a density equivalent to No. 10 Brown opacity tube. Agglutination tests are carried out in ½-in. wide round-bottom tubes. One drop of the concentrated suspension is added to 1·0 ml. of each serum dilution and to two tubes containing saline and a 1/20 dilution of normal serum which serve as controls to detect spontaneous agglutination. The tubes are incubated for two hours at 37°C, left in the refrigerator overnight, and read two hours after removal next morning. Similar results are obtained using Dreyer's technique and incubating the suspensions for 24 hours at 52°C. The living antigen must be freshly prepared each time, but the antigen killed by phenol or formalin may be used for several months.

A reading of 1/160 or more can usually be regarded as significant. Agglutinins decline rapidly and as a rule disappear within two or three months. According to Knapp (1959), persistence of agglutinins at a high level is a sign of continuing infection in the lymph nodes.

Complement-fixation Test. There is little to be gained by carrying out complement-fixation tests since the titres obtained are always lower than those of agglutination.

Immunofluorescence. Schmidt (1965), comparing the results of agglutination tests with those of immunofluorescence, found that the latter, besides being just as specific, had the advantage of detecting incomplete antibody and providing an answer in 2–3 hours.

HISTOLOGICAL DIAGNOSIS

Macroscopically, the lymph glands are usually considerably enlarged, soft and inflamed. In the fully developed condition small yellow abscesses can be seen on the cut surface.

Microscopically the characteristic lesions consist of a few round or oval abscesses about 1 to 5 in number. Occasionally dissemination of nodular lesions of a miliary character are observed. The abscess appears first as a reticulocytic infiltration usually in the interfollicular zone of the cortex of the lymph gland. Later, the centre of the abscess is occupied by an area of necrosis rich in cellular debris, with some polymorphonuclear leucocytes and a few reticulum cells and histiocytes. The central area of necrosis is surrounded by a zone of reticulum cells arranged in a manner much more haphazard than one sees in sarcoidosis. At the periphery of this zone a few plasma cells and occasionally eosinophils can sometimes be recognized.

These changes, while characteristic, are not specific since similar lesions are also observed in cat-scratch fever and lymphogranuloma inguinale, but their presence in a mesenteric gland should make one suspect *P. pseudotuberculosis* infection.

INTRADERMAL TEST

Preparation of the Allergen. A smooth strain of Type I *P. pseudotuberculosis* is grown on nutrient agar for 48 hours at 37°C. The growth is harvested in normal saline using about 30 ml. saline for the growth in a Roux flask. Five to ten drops of toluene are added to the suspension, which is then kept at 37°C in sealed tubes for three weeks. Once a week the stoppers are removed and 4–5 drops of toluene poured on the cotton-wool in the neck of each tube, which is again sealed. At the end of three weeks the suspensions are centrifuged and the supernatant filtered. The filtrate is heated at 56°C for 1 hour and after being tested for sterility it is diluted 1 in 10 in saline and distributed in ampoules, samples of which are again tested for sterility.

The test is carried out by the injection of 0·05–0·1 ml. of the allergen into the skin of the forearm. To exclude rare early reactions which are regarded as negative, the reading is made at 48 hours. A positive reaction is characterized by the appearance of a slightly raised and indurated, sometimes itching or tender, erythematous zone 1–2 cm. in diameter which takes one to three days to disappear.

This allergen, according to Mollaret (1965), never gives false positive reactions either in healthy subjects or in patients with other diseases including enteric infections. The narrow specificity of the allergen is associated with an absence of type specificity which permits its use whatever the serotype causing the illness. While a positive intradermal test is definite evidence of sensitization to *P. pseudotuberculosis*, like the tuberculin and brucellin reactions, it does not necessarily indicate the presence of active infection since skin sensitivity may persist for at least five to six years. This persistence of skin reactivity fortunately compensates for the brevity of the period during which a serological diagnosis can be made and is of value in providing a retrospective diagnosis.

TAXONOMY OF THE PASTEURELLA GROUP

In view of the close relationship between *P. pestis* and *P. pseudotuberculosis* and the differences between them and other members of the *Pasteurella* group, many workers consider that both species should be placed in a new genus, *Yersinia*, as proposed by Van Loghem (1946). The two organisms would then be designated as *Yersinia pestis* and *Yersinia pseudotuberculosis*. The genus *Pasteurella* would be represented by *P. multocida*, *hæmolytica*, *ureæ* and *pneumotropica*. The bacillus of tularæmia, *P. tularensis*, would be removed from the genus *Pasteurella* to form the genus *Francisella* and be called *Francisella tularensis*.

In the last few years a group of organisms variously described as *P. pseudotubereulosis* Type b (Dickinson and Mocquot, 1961), Pasteurella X (Daniels and Goudzwaard, 1963; Knapp and Thal, 1963), Germ X (Mollaret and Chevalier, 1964) has been recognized as a cause of enteritis and mesenteric lymphadenitis in man (Carlsson, Ryd and Sternby, 1964; Winblad, Nilehn and Sternby, 1966). According to Frederiksen (1964), these organisms possess characteristics sufficiently distinct to separate them from *P. pseudotuberculosis* (Table I), yet resemble *P. pseudotuberculosis* sufficiently to justify their inclusion in the genus *Yersinia* as a separate species: *Yersinia enterocolitica*.

References

BRZIN, B. (1963). Growth of Pasteurella pseudotuberculosis on tellurite media. *Zbl. Bakt. l. Abt. Orig.*, **189**, 543.

CARLSSON, M. G., RYD, H. and STERNBY, N. H. (1964). A case of human infection with *Pasteurella pseudotuberculosis* X. *Acta path. microlobl. scand.*, **62**, 128.

COOK, R. (1952). A method of demonstrating Pasteurella pseudotuberculosis in smears from animal lesions. *J. Path. Bact.*, **64**, 228.

DANIELS, J. J. H. M. and GOUDZWAARD, C. (1963). Enkele stammen van een op Pasteurella pseudotuberculosis gelijkend, niet geidentificeerd species, geisoleerd bij knaagdieren. *T. Diergeneesk.*, **88**, 96.

DICKINSON, A. B. and MOCQUOT, G. (1961). Studies on the bacterial flora of the alimentary tract of pigs. *J. appl. Bact.*, **24**, 252.

FREDERIKSEN, W. (1964). A study of some Yersinia pseudotuberculosis-like bacteria ("Bacterium enterocoliticum" and "Pasteurella X"). *Proc. XIV Scand. Congr. Path. Microbiol.*, Oslo, p. 103.

GRABER, H. and KNAPP, W. (1955). Die abscedierende reticulocytäre Lymphadenitis mesenterialis (Masshoff) als Bestandteil eines enteralen Primärkomplexes und Folge einer Infektion mit Pasteurella pseudotuberculosis. *Frankf. Z. Path.*, **66**, 399.

KNAPP, W. (1954). Pasteurella pseutotuberculosis als Erreger einer mesenterialen Lymphadenitis beim Menschen. *Zbl. Bakt. l. Abt. Orig.*, **161**, 422.

KNAPP, W. (1956). Die Agglutinationsreaktion und ihre Besonderheiten in der Serodiagnostik menschlicher Infektionen mit Pasteurella pseudotuberculosis. *Z. Hyg. InfektKr.*, **143**, 261.

KNAPP, W. (1959). Pasteurella pseutotuberculosis unter besonderer Berucksichtigung ihrer humanmedizinischer Bedeutung. *Ergebn. Mikrobiol.*, **32**, 196.

KNAPP, W. (1960). Die Laboratoriumsdiagnose von Infektionen mit Pasteurella pseudotuberculosis. *Ärzt. Laborat.*, **6**, 197.

KNAPP, W. and MASSHOFF, W. (1954). Zur Aetiologie der abscedierenden reticulocytären Lymphadenitis. *Dtsch. med. Wschr.*, **79**, 1266.

KNAPP, W. and THAL, E. (1963). Untersuchungen über die kulturell-biochemischen, serologischen, tierexperimentellen und immunologischen Eigenschaften einer vorlaufig "Pasturella X" bennanten Bakterienart. *Zbl. Bakt. l. Abt. Orig.*, **190**, 472.

KNISELY, R. F., SWANEY, L. M. and FRIEDLANDER, H. (1964). Selective media for the isolation of Pasteurella pestis. *J. Bact.*, **88**, 491.

LOGHEM, J. J. VAN (1946). La classification du bacille pesteux. *Ann. Inst. Pasteur*, **72**, 975.

MAIR, N. S., MAIR, HÉLÈNE J., STIRK, E. M. and CORSON, J. G. (1960). Three cases of Acute Mesenteric Lymphadenitis due to *Pasteurella pseudotuberculosis*. *J. clin. Path.*, **13**, 432.

MASSHOFF, W. and DÖLLE, W. (1953). Über eine besondere Form der sog. mesenterialen Lymphadenitis: "Die abscedierende reticulocytäre Lymphadenopathie". *Virchows Arch. path. Anat.*, **323**, 664.

MOLLARET, H. H. (1965). Le laboratoire dans le diagnostic d'infection humaine à bacille de Malassez et Vignal. *Gaz. med. Fr.*, **72**, 3457.

MOLLARET, H. H. and CHEVALIER, A. (1964). Contribution à l'étude d'un nouveau groupe de germes prochès du bacille de Mallassez et Vignal. *Ann. Inst. Pasteur*, **107**, 121.

MORRIS, E. J. (1958). Selective media for some "Pasteurella" species. *J. gen. Microbiol.*, **19**, 305.

PATERSON, J. S. and COOK, R. (1963). A method for the recovery of Pasteurella pseudotuberculosis from fæces. *J. Path. Bact.*, **85**, 241,

SCHMIDT, J. (1965). Vergleichende Untersuchungen über den Nachweis von Pasteurella pseudotuberculosis-Antikorpern mit der indirekten fluoreszenzserologischen Methode und der Widalschen Reaktion. *Arch. Hyg., Berlin*, **149**, 154.

THAL, E. (1966). Weitere Untersuchungen über die thermolabilen Antigene der Yersinia pseudotuberculosis (Syn. Pasteurella pseudotuberculosis). *Zbl. Bakt. l. Abt. Orig.*, **200**, 56.

WINBLAD, S., NILEHN, B. and STERNBY, N. H. (1966). *Yersinia enterocolitica* (Pasteurella X) in Human Enteric Infections. *Brit. med. J.*, **2**, 1363.

Chapter 4

ACQUISITION OF ANTIBIOTIC RESISTANCE BY BACTERIA

Naomi Datta

DURING the comparatively few years that have elapsed since the introduction of sulphonamides, pathogenic bacteria have been exposed to an increasing number of different forms of chemotherapeutic and antibiotic attack. They have defended themselves well. Resistant strains have frequently appeared after the introduction of new antibacterial drugs, and although mortality from bacterial infections has dropped precipitously, largely because of the effectiveness of these drugs, bacterial disease is by no means conquered. It presents very different clinical problems from those of the pre-sulphonamide days. Drug-resistance, especially in bacteria causing hospital infections, is now common. This is partly due to the emergence of resistant strains of species formerly drug-sensitive and partly the result of increased incidence of infection with species such as *Pseudomonas æruginosa* (Watt and Okubadejo, 1967) which were always resistant to the most clinically effective drugs.

Antibacterial drugs are the magic bullets sought by Erhlich, lethal to invading micro-organisms and harmless to man. Their targets must be vulnerable areas of the bacterial economy which are not duplicated in mammalian cells. The drugs have been developed empirically because chemical knowledge is inadequate to enable them to be aimed at clearly visualized structures or reactions; but a study of the effects of the drugs has shown that vulnerable areas lie in the synthesis of bacterial cell walls and in the bacterial ribosomes, which are different from those of higher organisms (see Symposium 1966). Bacteria may be resistant to a drug if they lack its specific target, or if a barrier protects the target from the drug, or if the drug is destroyed before it can reach the target.

The means by which previously sensitive bacteria acquire resistance has long been a matter of both practical and theoretical interest. New light has recently been shed on the subject in the case of two important groups of organisms, the staphylococci and the coliform group of Gram-negative bacilli, including salmonellæ and shigellæ.

If sensitive bacteria are exposed to antibacterial drugs in the laboratory, resistant variants can usually, though not always, be obtained. Resistance acquired in this way is often the result of mutation, with selection of those rare clones able to grow in the presence of the drug (Cavalli-Sforza and Lederberg, 1956). In some instances, it is claimed, adaptation to drug resistance occurs without mutation, in which case all the cells in a culture are understood to develop resistance in response to the presence of the drug (Dean, 1960).

Until 1960 it was believed that drug resistance acquired by sensitive bacteria in their natural environment must be of the same nature, that is either mutational or adaptive, although resistant bacteria isolated from natural sources did sometimes differ in various respects from resistant variants selected in the laboratory (Barber, 1947).

An important third method by which sensitive bacteria become resistant is now recognized: that is, by the acquisition of genes governing drug resistance from an outside source. The concept of foreign genetic material entering a living cell, becoming part of the cell and replicating with it, so that descendants of the cell many generations later still display the acquired character, is still novel. But evidence is accumulating to show that bacterial characters, and drug-resistance ones in particular, are frequently acquired in this way.

R FACTORS IN THE ENTEROBACTERIACEÆ

Infectious drug resistance was discovered in Japan in 1959 and is now recognized as a world-wide problem (see Watanabe, 1963; Datta, 1965).

Drug-resistance factors, or R factors, are extrachromosomal genetic elements (episomes or plasmids); they are transmitted directly from one cell to another among the Enterobacteriaceæ by cell contact or conjugation. They carry resistance to antibacterial drugs, frequently multiple resistance to several unrelated drugs. Transfer can take place between Gram-negative bacilli of many genera—all the "coliform" group, including such unrelated species as *Vibrio choloræ*, *Pasteurella pestis*, *Serratia marcescens*, *Proteus* and *Pseudomonas*. Intergeneric transfer has repeatedly been demonstrated in natural circumstances, in the bowel of man and experimental animals (Walton, 1966).

The R factors that were first discovered rendered their host cells resistant simultaneously to four drugs: streptomycin, the tetracyclines, chloramphenicol and the sulphonamides. Since then resistance to kanamycin and neomycin (Lebek, 1963) and to ampicillin and cephaloridine (Anderson and Datta, 1965) has been found to be carried by R factors and it is now not uncommon to isolate bacteria resistant to the whole of this range of drugs, and able to transmit the entire resistance pattern to sensitive bacteria with which they come in contact.

The transmissible element itself, the R factor, cannot be separated from the host bacteria in active form. Culture media from which resistant (R+) bacteria have been removed by filtration or centrifugation will not transmit resistance, the presence of the donor bacteria themselves is required. Foreign DNA has, however, been demonstrated in bacteria carrying R factors. The density of bacterial DNA depends on its guanine-cytosine (G+C) content and is characteristic of the genus from which it is derived (Marmur, Falkow and Mandel, 1963). DNA extracted from bacteria and centrifuged to equilibrium in a cæsium-chloride density gradient normally forms a narrow band at a level determined by its density. If R factors are introduced into bacterial cultures and the DNA extracted and centrifuged in this way, the host DNA forms a band in its normal position and clearly defined minor bands are also seen, presumably representing R-factor DNA. Some R factors appear as a single band with a density indicating a 50 per cent G+C content, which is like chromosomal DNA of *Escherichia*, *Shigella* and *Salmonella*. Other R factors show bands of more than one density (Falkow, Citarella, Wohlhieter and Watanabe, 1966) which suggests that they may have more than one evolutionary origin (Fig. 1).

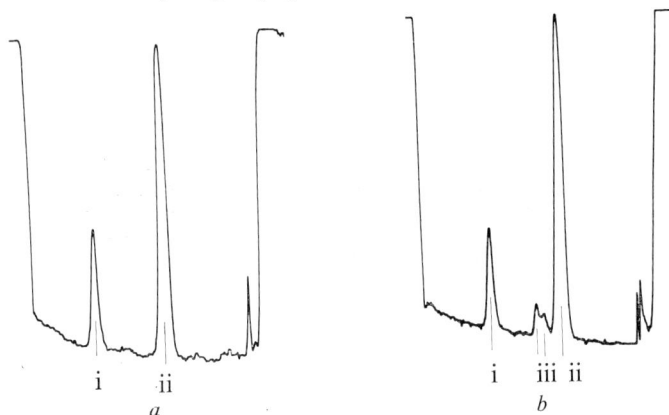

FIG. 1. Microdensitometer tracings of CsCl density gradient photographs. Bands representing DNA appear as peaks identified by roman numerals below.

(*a*) DNA extract of sensitive *Proteus mirabilis*
(i) reference DNA   (ii) Proteus DNA

(*b*) DNA extract of the same *Proteus mirabilis* carrying an R factor.
(i) reference DNA
(ii) Proteus DNA
(iii) R factor DNA.

(From Falkow *et al.*, 1966, *J. mol. Biol.*, 17, 102).

Genes carried by R Factors

R factor DNA carries genes for resistance to specific drugs and also genes determining bacterial conjugation and the ability to transfer DNA. Only a little is known about the changes produced in the host bacteria by the resistance genes. It was believed at first that multiple resistance might be the result of a general impermeability to drugs, but R+ cultures sometimes lost their resistance to one or more of the drugs while retaining transmissible resistance to the others, so evidently each resistance was controlled by a specific determinant (Watanabe, 1963). The great variety of patterns of infectious drug resistance which have since been reported in naturally occurring bacteria also shows that each resistance must be specific, and evidence for production of enzymes determined by R factor genes is accumulating.

Resistance Determinants. *Ampicillin.* Bacteria with R factors conferring ampicillin-resistance synthesize intracellular penicillinases which hydrolyse ampicillin as well as benzyl penicillin and a range of other penicillin- and cephalosporin-derivatives (Datta and Kontomichalou, 1965). The penicillinase production varies both quantitatively and qualitatively according to the R factor which controls it, and those R factors producing a high level of enzyme activity confer resistance to a high concentration (1,000 μg./ml. or more) of ampicillin. One R factor penicillinase has been purified and found to have a lower molecular weight and a wider substrate range than penicillinases from Gram-positive organisms (Datta and Richmond, 1966). Other R factors control the production of what appear to be, on substrate profile studies, a variety of different enzymes (Datta and Kontomichalou, 1965 and unpublished). *E. coli* and salmonellas have slight penicillinase activity without R factors, but none detectable against ampicillin. On "training" by serial passage to ampicillin resistance, either no more enzyme is produced (Datta and Kontomichalou, 1965) or if penicillinase activity is increased, there is still little activity against ampicillin (Smith, 1963).

Tetracycline. Tetracyclines are actively accumulated in large quantities by tetracycline-sensitive cells (Franklin and Godfrey, 1965), but when an R factor conferring tetracycline resistance was introduced into a culture, much less tetracycline was taken up (Izaki and Arima, 1963). Tetracycline impermeability of R+ cultures behaved, in some cases at least, as though an inducible system was involved, since on first exposure to the drug uptake was equal to that by sensitive cells and growth was temporarily inhibited. After two hours' incubation in tetracycline, the R+ cells no longer accumulated the drug, and multiplied normally (Unowsky and Rachmeler, 1966). Thus, active inhibition of a specific transport system by which tetracyclines cross the cell membrane of sensitive bacteria seems to be provided by R factors. The drug is excluded from the cell, but the ribosomes remain sensitive and protein-building by cell-free extracts of R+ or R− bacteria is prevented by tetracycline (Okamoto and Mizuno, 1964; Unowsky and Rachmeler, 1966). In the case of tetracycline, resistance conferred by R factors appears to be of a similar nature to that developed by laboratory "training", that is by selection of colonies able to grow on increasing concentrations of the drug.

Chloramphenicol. Enzyme inactivation of chloramphenicol by extracts of chloramphenicol-resistant R+ cultures has been reported. Inactivation required the presence of acetyl-coenzyme A, and was effected by acetylation of the drug (Okamoto and Suzuki, 1965; Shaw, 1967). The effect was absent from extracts of sensitive cultures and also from extracts of cultures "trained" to resistance. Inactivation of chloramphenicol by R+ but not by "trained" chloramphenicol-resistant *E. coli* or salmonellæ can be demonstrated by Gott's test (Waterworth, 1966). Reduced uptake of radioactive chloramphenicol by an R+ culture has also been found (Unowsky and Rachmeler, 1966).

Streptomycin. Resistance conferred by R factors differs from that attained by one-step chromosomal mutation and is usually expressed at a lower level. Enzyme inactivation of dihydrostreptomycin by R+ cultures has been reported (Okamoto and Suzuki, 1965), but no information was given about inactivation of streptomycin itself. R factor resistance to streptomycin extends to dihydrostreptomycin, so the basis of this resistance needs clarification. Uptake of radioactive streptomycin was reduced by one of two R factors tested (Unowsky and Rachmeler, 1966).

Kanamycin resistance carried by R factors is not linked to streptomycin resistance, but gives resistance to neomycin, framycetin and paramomycin. A kanamycin-inactivating enzyme in R+ cultures has been found, requiring, like the chloramphenicolase, acetyl-coenzyme A (Okamoto and Suzuki, 1965).

Sulphonamide resistance may be the result of a specific change in permeability of R+ cells to the drugs (Yokota and Akiba, 1961).

Colicine Resistance. Colicines are antibiotic substances produced by coliform bacilli and active against closely related bacteria. Enterobacteria in their natural environment must frequently be exposed to colicines, and colicine resistance has been found to be carried by R factors which give, at the same time, resistance to antibiotics used in medicine (Siccardi, 1966).

Conjugation Genes: Transfer Factors. A transmissible R factor comprises drug-resistance determinants linked to genes which promote conjugation. These two kinds of genes are separable and either can exist in the host bacteria in the absence of the other, maintaining its extrachromosomal nature. A culture with episomal drug-resistance genes cannot transfer them unless it also has determinants for conjugation; these have been termed Resistance Transfer Factors (RTF), but because they are not necessarily always linked to drug resistance, they are better referred to as Transfer Factors (Anderson, 1965), or as conjugation factors (Meynell and Datta, 1966).

Resistance and conjugation genes may be separated in the laboratory by phage transduction. Transducing phages can carry genetic material, either chromosomal or extrachromosomal, from one bacterium to another; if R factors are transduced, they enter a fresh host by means of the phage infectivity instead of by their own infective property. Some transducing phages transfer the complete R factor, that is, its whole complement of genes, drug resistances and infectivity, but others normally transduce the R factor piecemeal and resistance determinants transferred by these phages usually lack infectivity. If another conjugation factor, the F (fertility) factor of *E. coli* K12, is introduced into such a culture, it restores the transmissibility of the drug-resistance determinants (Harada, Kameda, Suzuki and Mitsuhashi, 1964). Anderson has found that, in salmonellæ isolated from natural sources, transmissible R factors are common, but so are non-transmissible drug-resistance factors and also transfer factors unlinked to resistance genes. These latter he first recognized by the fact that, like transmissible R factors, they modified the host's sensitivity to the phages used in typing *S. typhimurium*. He was then able to prove their existence by their ability to mobilize, and render infective, naturally occurring, non-transmissible, drug-resistance determinants (Anderson, 1965).

The F factor of *E. coli* K12 is the bacterial conjugation factor which has been most studied and about which most is known (Hayes, 1964). Cells in an F+ culture synthesize a specialized fimbria or pilus, which can be seen in electron micrographs (Crawford and Gesteland, 1964). It is the receptor for F specific phages and is required for conjugation (Brinton, Gemski and Carnahan, 1964). In F+ cultures nearly all the cells carry the F pilus and nearly all conjugate very quickly (within an hour) if mixed with a F— bacterial population. The conjugating function of R factors is not expressed so freely, and in an R+ culture only about one bacterium in 10^3 or 10^4 conjugates and transfers resistance on mixing with an R— population.

The limitation of mating function in R+ cultures is due to a control mechanism, a repressor produced by the factor itself. The repressor is temporarily absent from bacteria newly infected with an R factor and permanently absent from mutants selected for their ability to promote conjugation freely. When repression is lifted, all the cells in a culture can conjugate, and electron microscopy shows that R+ cells which conjugate also have specialized pili. These special structures, associated with conjugation, are called sex pili (Meynell and Lawn, 1967). Those associated with R factors are of at least two kinds, some which resemble the F pili morphologically and in being receptors for F-specific phages, and others which are shorter than F pili and insusceptible to F phage (Meynell and Datta, 1967). Sex pili are tubular, composed probably of protein, and have a diameter of approximately 100 Å. Whether they are the ducts through which DNA is passed from one cell to another is not known; they are certainly closely associated with the mating process. Phages inject their nucleic acid into bacteria through tubular "tails" of similar dimensions (Hayes, 1964) and it seems likely that nucleic acid is actually transmitted through the sex pili (Fig. 2).

A consideration of the properties of conjugation factors shows them to have much in common with bacteriophages: they are infective particles of

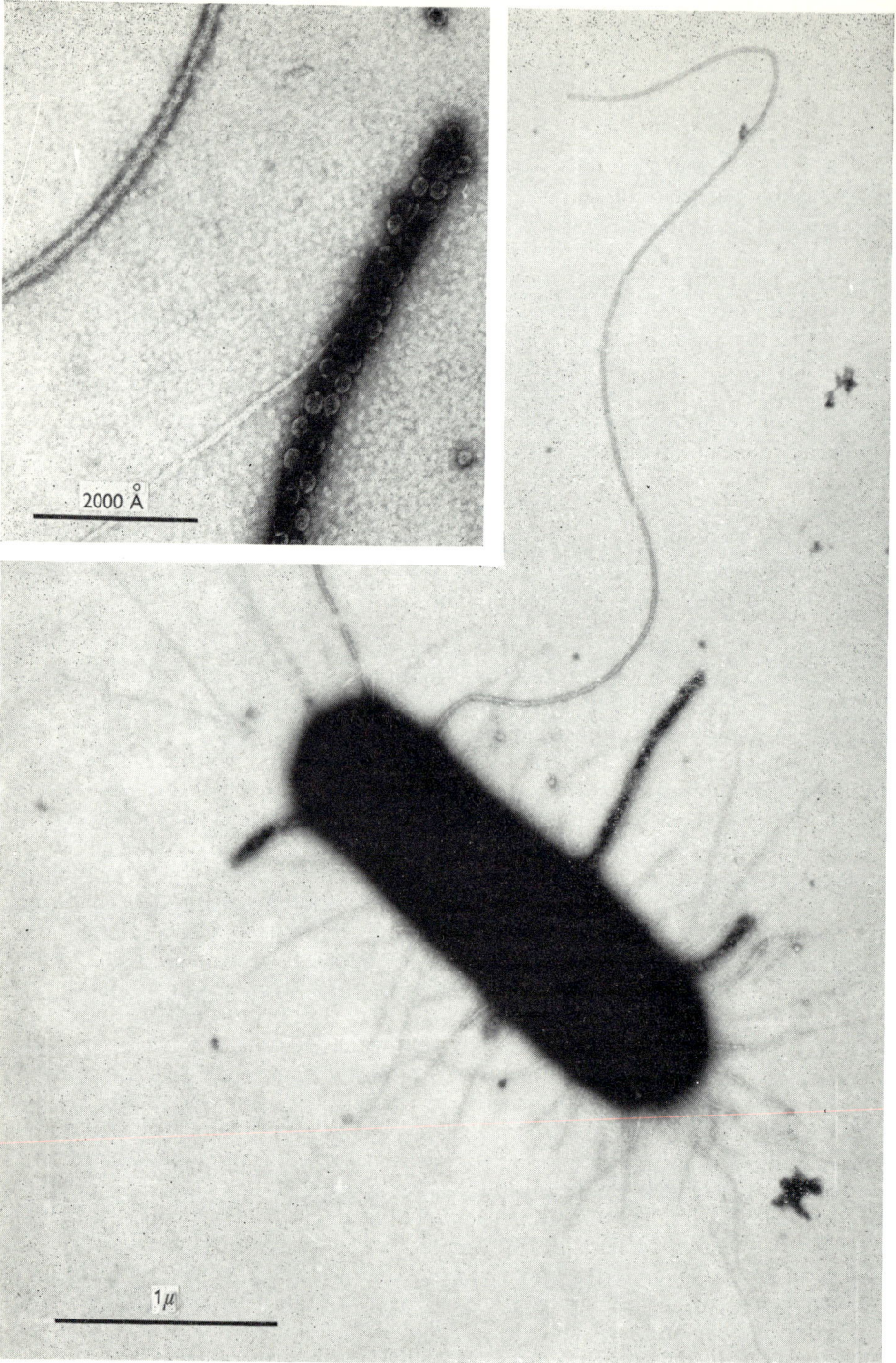

FIG. 2. Electron micrograph of *E. coli* K12 carrying an R factor and mixed with an F-specific phage. Three kinds of appendage can be seen on the bacterium; the sex pili are coated with round phage particles; common pili or fimbriæ have no absorbed particles; flagella can be recognized by their sinuous shape and greater width.

(From Datta, N., Lawn, A. M. and Meynell, E., 1966. *J. gen. Microbiol.*, **45**, 365.)

DNA and although they do not escape from the cell wrapped in a protective protein coat like proper virus particles, they control the synthesis of a protein tube through which they probably reach fresh hosts. They are quite common in enteric bacteria (Meynell and Datta, 1966) and probably play an important part in spreading genetic information through bacterial populations, thus providing a rapid means of adaptation to hostile environments.

The evolutionary origin of the drug-resistance genes with which they are associated in R factors is quite unknown.

Frequency of R Factors. R factors can infect all genera of Gram-negative enteric bacilli and can be found in nature in a wide variety of species. We have some information about their frequency in *Escherichia coli*, salmonellæ and shigellæ. Members of these genera are normally sensitive to all the drugs against which R factors may protect. Resistant variants isolated from natural sources more often than not owe their resistance to R factors, although resistant mutants, particularly to streptomycin, also occur. The incidence of multiple resistance in these species is high and has risen sharply in the last decade. In Japan, multiple-resistance in *Shigella flexneri* was first observed in 1957 and rapidly increased in frequency; by 1964 over 50 per cent of strains isolated were resistant (Watanabe, 1966). *E. coli* with multiple resistance were isolated at the same time as the shigella strains, but their overall incidence was not recorded. In London, *Sh. sonnei* with multiple resistance first appeared towards the end of 1958; there was a general increase in the number of drugs to which *Sh. sonnei* isolates were resistant over the years 1958–65, but the increasing resistance was not an uninterrupted process, and during the period large outbreaks occurred which were caused by drug-sensitive strains. There was even some evidence that sensitive strains were more likely than resistant ones to spread widely in the community (Farrant and Tomlinson, 1966). An increasing frequency of transmissible drug resistance in *Shigella* strains has been observed in the last few years in the United States (Kabins and Cohen, 1966), in Brazil (Trabulsi, S. F., personal communication) and in the Union of South Africa (Watson, 1967).

Multiple drug resistance in salmonellæ has become common during the same period, all over the world. In Holland it increased from 1·6 per cent in 1960 to about 20 per cent in 1965 (Manten, Guinée and Kampelmacher, 1966). It was first observed in England in strains isolated in 1959 (Datta, 1962), but only 2·7 per cent of strains isolated in 1961 were drug-resistant. This proportion had also risen to 20 per cent by 1964 (Anderson, E. S. and Datta, N., unpublished), and has subsequently risen higher still, especially in some phage types associated with bovine infection (Anderson and Lewis, 1965). Drug resistance in salmonellæ causing food poisoning is not of very great clinical importance, but R factors, especially if giving chloramphenicol-resistance, would matter very much in *Salmonella typhi* or *S. paratyphi*. They have been found in *S. paratyphi* (Chabbert and LeMinor, 1966; Anderson and Datta, unpublished) and may already exist in *S. typhi* in India (Murti, Rajyalakshmi and Bhaskaran, 1962) and in Africa (Njoku-Obi and Njoku-Obi, 1965).

Enteropathogenic strains of *E. coli* also very frequently carry R factors giving them multiple drug resistance. The frequency of drug resistance fluctuates from time to time and from place to place. About 50 per cent of strains sent to the Central Public Health Laboratory for serotyping are resistant to one or more antibiotics and in nearly all cases the resistance is transmissible (Smith, 1966; Taylor, J. and Datta, N., unpublished).

Salmonellæ, shigellæ and enteropathogenic types of *E. coli* all give rise to intestinal disease which is likely to be treated with antibacterial drugs. Such treatment inevitably selects resistant strains, so drug resistance would be expected to be commoner in these organisms than in normal intestinal bacteria in healthy people. Little is known of the incidence of R factors in the latter. Smith and Halls (1966), in a small survey, isolated *E. coli* with transmissible drug resistance from 15 of 24 healthy people. Among London preclinical medical students, taken as representing healthy adults without special experience of antibiotics, 3 out of 20 were found to excrete non-pathogenic bacteria with R factors (Datta, N., unpublished). Even in rural areas of Ethiopia, coliform bacteria carrying R factors were detected in a considerable proportion of fæcal specimens collected in the course of a survey of the population (Mann and Gedebou, 1966).

The incidence of R factors in cultures of *E. coli* from urinary infections has been reported as high (over 50 per cent) (Smith and Armour, 1966), and was found to be about 25 per cent in specimens in the diagnostic laboratory of a London Hospital (Pride, R. and Datta, N., in preparation). Here, two frequencies might be expected, with a lower proportion resistant from patients with spontaneous, primary infections than in relapses after therapy or in post-surgical infections; information is not yet available on this point.

Other coliform genera, such as *Klebsiella, Enterobacter, Proteus, Pseudomonas,* frequently carry R factors, but are also almost certainly resistant to certain drugs by virtue of their own chromosomal genes. For example, *Klebsiella* strains almost all synthesize penicillinase and are resistant to ampicillin (Hennessey, T. D., in preparation). Occasional strains are able to transmit ampicillin resistance, by conjugation, to sensitive *E. coli,* but then the donor strain probably had both chromosomal and extrachromosomal genes controlling penicillinase production and only the latter were transferred. Similarly, strains of *Proteus mirabilis* are invariably tetracycline-resistant, presumably as part of their normal genetic make-up, but may sometimes possess, in addition, R-factor genes some of which may confer tetracycline resistance.

Methods of demonstrating Resistance Transfer. When an R + donor culture is mixed in nutrient medium with an R − recipient, some transfer of resistance occurs almost instantly but, because of the repressor mechanism (see p. 47), only a very small proportion of the R + cells conjugate and therefore only a very small proportion of the R − cells receive the factor. If the mixture is incubated for longer (usually overnight), a much higher proportion, sometimes 100 per cent, of the recipient bacteria become resistant, because absence of repressor in the newly infected cells allows free conjugation and the factor spreads rapidly through the R − population. The extent to which this secondary spread occurs depends on the particular R factor and also on the recipient bacteria. *Salmonellæ* often appear to be poor recipients of R factors, perhaps because free spread from newly infected bacteria is less marked than with *E. coli.* Different strains of *E. coli* also vary in their recipient capacity; *E. coli* K12 is a good recipient, F − lines being slightly better than

F+. The use of nutritionally deficient strains provides an extra check on identity to exclude contaminants.

Where a large proportion of the recipient culture receives the R factor after overnight incubation, no special selective medium is required to demonstrate it. For example, a broth culture of a salmonella resistant to tetracycline is mixed with a broth culture of sensitive *E. coli* K_{12}, incubated overnight and the mixture plated by streaking on MacConkey agar containing an appropriate concentration (say 20 μg./ml.) of tetracycline. If lactose-fermenting colonies appear, they are presumably *E. coli* R+ and are purified and identified for confirmation. But lactose-fermenting colonies will only be seen if present in large numbers, since the donor salmonella will grow normally on tetracycline-MacConkey; if spread of resistance through the recipient population has been slight, a more highly selective medium for detecting transfer is needed. For detecting transfer from salmonellæ, shigellæ or other non-lactose-fermenting organisms to *E. coli* "minimal agar", with lactose as sole carbon source and incorporating the appropriate antibiotic, is very satisfactory and allows quantitative experiments to be made. The antibiotic concentration should allow normal growth of the R+ donor but completely inhibit the R− recipient. The minimal agar is made up as follows (modified from Tatum and Lederberg, 1947):

The minimal agar is made up as follows (modified from Tatum and Lederberg, 1947): NH_4Cl 20 g., NH_4NO_3 4, Na_2SO_4 anhydrous 8, K_2HPO_4 12, KH_2PO_4 4, $MgSO_4.7H_2O$ 0·4, Water to 1,000 ml.

Dissolve each salt in cold water in the above order, waiting till each is dissolved before adding the next (a light precipitate will be formed). Filter. Autoclave at 5 lb. for 15 min. No further precipitate should be formed. *p*H 7·2.

Agar: 2 per cent in distilled water.

For use, melt the agar. Mix 3 parts melted agar to 1 part salts solution. Add lactose to a final concentration of 0·2 per cent and appropriate antibiotic. If a nutritionally deficient *E. coli* strain is used as recipient, add also appropriate nutrients to a final concentration of 20 μg./ml.

On minimal lactose medium with added antibiotic, neither resistant non-lactose fermenter nor sensitive *E. coli* will grow, and all colonies should therefore be *E. coli* R+. They should be replated on ordinary media for identification. The number of colonies to develop varies greatly, so it is best to inoculate part of the plate heavily (with say, 0·1, ml. of mixed culture) and streak out from there. If no colonies develop, transfer may yet be detected by centrifuging about 5 ml. of the mixture and spreading the whole deposit on the selective minimal medium. The same minimal medium, with citrate instead of lactose, detects transfer of resistance from *E. coli* to salmonellae. In practice, however, transfer to salmonella strains is often less easy to demonstrate than transfer from one strain of *E. coli* to another.

Another method of selection in transfer experiments is to use a recipient highly resistant to nalidixic acid or streptomycin; the mixed culture is plated on MacConkey agar incorporating the drug to which the recipient is resistant as well as the one for which transfer of resistance is to be looked for. We have found that a non-lactose-fermenting, streptomycin-resistant mutant of *E. coli* K12 is very effective in demonstrating resistance transfer from lactose-fermenting cultures of *E. coli* isolated from clinical material, the only disadvantage being that transfer of streptomycin resistance can only be demonstrated indirectly.

B

RESISTANCE PLASMIDS OF *STAPHYLOCOCCUS AUREUS*

Drug-resistant staphylococci in hospitals pose well-recognized and universal clinical problems. As new antibacterial drugs have been introduced, so strains of *Staphylococcus aureus* resistant to increasing numbers of drugs have become common. It started with penicillin-resistant staphylococci which became endemic in hospitals after the introduction of penicillin into clinical medicine (North and Christie, 1945; Barber, 1947). As other antibiotics were introduced, i.e, streptomycin, chloramphenicol, tetracycline, erythromycin, neomycin, kanamycin, fusidic acid, bacitracin, resistance to them appeared, particularly among strains already resistant to penicillin. The increasing resistance of staphylococci to drugs other than penicillin was interpreted as being the result of natural selection, resistant mutants occurring and replacing the sensitive parent strains, the latter being eliminated by antibiotics in the hospital environment. In the case of penicillin-resistance, however, it was recognized early that mutation to resistance, although it could occur, was not important clinically. Naturally occurring resistant staphylococci owed their resistance to production of penicillinase, while mutants selected in the laboratory by exposing sensitive cultures to penicillin produced no penicillinase, generally grew more slowly than wild strains and apparently lacked virulence. Penicillinase-producing strains had existed before 1940; resistant strains which became common after that date were limited at first to a very few different phage types (Barber and Whitehead, 1949); it appeared that these naturally occurring resistant strains were evolutionary variants selected by the use of penicillin, not mutants of penicillin-sensitive strains occurring during treatment of infected patients.

When penicillin-resistant staphylococci were cultured in the laboratory, it was found that the capacity to produce penicillinase was lost from a proportion of individual cells, sometimes at quite a high rate. For example, cultures of resistant staphylococci, plated in the absence of penicillin, frequently gave between 0·1 per cent and 1 per cent of colonies which were penicillinase-negative, and remained so indefinitely on subculture, even if exposed to penicillin (Barber, 1949). This is a very high frequency for mutation; moreover, if mutation were the explanation, back-mutation to production of penicillinase would be expected to occur. The capacity for penicillinase synthesis can be introduced into penicillinase-negative staphylococci, either naturally occurring, or cocci from which this character has been lost on subculture, by treating them with bacteriophages previously grown in a resistant strain; such penicillinase-positive cultures behave exactly like natural penicillin-resistant strains. Transducing phages are frequently present in staphylococcal isolates and include some of the international typing phages (Ritz and Baldwin, 1961).

Novick (1963) found that penicillin-sensitive staphylococci lacked not only the genes for production of penicillinase protein but also regulatory genes controlling its production. All these genes were transferred together in transduction experiments. This led to the hypothesis (Novick, 1963) that penicillinase genes might be carried on extrachromosomal particles, or plasmids, similar in nature to the R factors of coliform bacilli. Evidence that this is so is as follows: (1) the penicillinase determinant is lost frequently

and irreversibly (Barber, 1949); (2) the penicillinase gene is linked to regulatory and other genes which are transduced with it and lost with it (Novick,
1963; Richmond and John, 1964); (3) the rate of loss is increased by treatment
which does not normally produce mutation, as by growth at 44°C (Fairbrother, Parker and Eaton, 1954) or treatment with acridine dyes (Harmon
and Baldwin, 1964); and (4) the frequency of phage transduction is high, but
is decreased when the transducing phage is irradiated with ultra-violet
(Novick, 1963). (When chromosomal genes are transduced, the frequency
of transfer is lower but is increased by U.V. (Arber, 1960).)

Proof that drug resistance is controlled by extrachromosomal particles
is much more difficult in staphylococci than in coliform organisms, firstly
because the staphylococcal plasmids do not carry genes for conjugation and
resistance transfer, and secondly because hardly anything is known of the
chromosomal genes of *Staph. aureus*, while a great deal is known about the
genetics of *E. coli* (Hayes, 1964).

Other drug resistance, besides penicillinase production, is controlled by
plasmids in staphylococci. Resistance to mercury salts and other heavy
metals is usually linked to genes for penicillinase on plasmids (Moore, 1960;
Richmond and John, 1964) and resistance to erythromycin is occasionally
also so linked (Novick, 1967). Tetracycline resistance, on the evidence already
given for penicillin resistance, can be plasmid-borne, but on a separate
plasmid from the penicillinase ones, since it is transduced or lost independently
(May, Houghton and Perret, 1964; Asheshov, 1966a). On the evidence of a
high rate of loss of several resistance genes together, it seems that resistance
to neomycin and to fusidic acid may also be plasmid-determined. Fusidic acid
resistance may be linked either to a penicillinase plasmid or to a tetracycline-
resistance plasmid (Evans and Waterworth, 1966). The only evidence that
chloramphenicol resistance may be of a similar nature is that naturally
occurring resistant staphylococci inactivate chloramphenicol by acetylation,
like R + *E. coli*, while resistant strains selected from sensitive cultures by
laboratory "training" do not (Suzuki, Okamoto and Kono, 1966); mutation
to production of a new enzyme seems unlikely and the parallel with natural
penicillin resistance is clear.

Simultaneous resistance to neomycin and bacitracin, as well as to
penicillin, mercury salts and tetracycline, is a common feature of a particular
kind of staphylococcus which has become increasingly prevalent in hospitals
since 1960. The genetic basis of the resistance is unknown, but the relationship
of the new strain, which is often of type 84/85, to hospital staphylococci of
type 83A, which preceded it in hospitals, is partly understood and is of great
interest. Changes in phage type are found to be caused by acquisition or loss
of temperate bacteriophages, the new untypable strain is identified as
type 83A, having become lysogenized by a phage which blocks the effect of
the typing phages. However, acquisition of the blocking phage does not
simultaneously render it neomycin and bacitracin resistant; some other
change, possibly mutation but more probably transduction, must be involved
(Parker, 1966).

Penicillinase production, although frequently plasmid-controlled, is not
always so (Asheshov, 1966b), and for other resistances insufficient evidence
of the frequency of their extrachromosomal nature is available. Marked

instability of tetracycline resistance, either at 37° or at 43°–44°C, was found in only a minority (3 out of 50) of strains of *Staph. aureus* (Asheshov, 1966a). Resistance to streptomycin, chloramphenicol, erythromycin, neomycin and bacitracin was relatively stable (May, Houghton and Perret, 1964; Asheshov, 1966a), no loss being observed in several hundred clones. However, this does not preclude the possibility that resistance genes are commonly extra-chromosomal, since the stability of R factors in Gram-negative bacilli is very variable.

As with R factors, the origin of extrachromosomal resistance genes in staphylococci is unknown. It may be that they originated as chromosomal genes in staphylococci and were mobilized by becoming incorporated into bacteriophages, but they may have originated in some quite other organism and might even share a common ancestry with extrachromosomal resistance determinants of Gram-negative bacilli. The means by which they are acquired by sensitive bacteria, however, is different in staphylococci. Gram-negative bacilli carrying R factors cannot transfer their resistance genes to staphylo-cocci, nor is any means known by which staphylococci might transfer resistance to other genera. The probable means by which resistance plasmids are disseminated among staphylococci is phage transduction. Transducing phages are common in staphylococci and transfer of resistance has been demonstrated in experimental animals infected simultaneously with two strains of *Staph. aureus*, one of which carried transducing phage (Novick and Morse, 1967). The phages are limited to staphylococci as hosts, therefore whatever the ultimate origin of the resistance determinants, they are now presumably established in staphylococci. Their integration as chromosomal genes might represent either their origin or the latest stage in their evolution.

METHICILLIN RESISTANCE

The introduction of penicillinase-resistant penicillins, methicillin and cloxacillin, gave medicine an advantage over multiple-resistant *Staph. aureus* which is still maintained after several years. From the first it was considered possible that, as with earlier drugs, resistant strains of staphylococci might emerge and become endemic in hospitals. However, *Staph. aureus* is the only human pathogen in which a high degree of penicillin resistance has developed, and as that has been due to the special circumstances of its having or acquiring penicillinase as a defence, the new resistant penicillins gave grounds for optimism (Chain, 1962). Resistance to methicillin and cloxacillin does occur. Resistant strains were isolated before methicillin was introduced (Jevons, 1961) and have become somewhat commoner since, but they have not spread widely; their distribution is very uneven and does not seem to be closely related to the therapeutic use of methicillin (Parker, 1966).

Resistant strains have peculiar properties. The basis of resistance is not drug destruction; no staphylococcal penicillinase has been found with more than slight hydrolytic activity against methicillin or cloxacillin (Ayliffe and Barber, 1963; Dyke, K., in preparation), and although naturally occurring methicillin-resistant strains are also penicillinase producers, penicillinase-negative variants remain methicillin-resistant (Parker and Jevons, 1964; Seligman, 1966b). The mechanism of resistance seems to be a general, but moderate, tolerance to all penicillins, independent of penicillinase. This tolerance characterizes the whole culture, and is best demonstrated on plates with an increased electrolyte concentration (e.g. 5 per cent NaCl) which, by giving osmotic support to the bacteria, allows the development of normal colonies in the presence of methicillin. Without added electrolytes, resistant strains still grow on medium containing concentrations of drug, sometimes up to 500 μg./ml., on which control strains, whether penicillinase positive or negative, show no growth, but in these circumstances a heavy inoculum is required and the bacteria are affected by the drug, even in quite low concentrations (5 μg./ml.); growth is sparser and less regular than on control plates and the morphology seen in stained films is abnormal (Barber, 1964). Resistant strains also give rise to occasional mutants, able to form single colonies on high concentrations of drug even with normal electrolyte concentrations; they revert, however, when subcultured without drug, to the original lower level of resistance (Sutherland and Rolinson, 1964; Seligman, 1966a).

Resistant strains can cause severe infections (Stewart and Holt, 1963). Whether the highly resistant, but unstable, mutants seen in laboratory experiments contribute to such infection is not certain; indeed it is impossible to assess the efficacy of methicillin or cloxacillin in the treatment of "resistant" infections. In such infections the interest of the patient demands treatment with a drug or drugs to which sensitivity is clearly demonstrable, a drug other than a penicillin, and for this reason it is important for clinical laboratories to recognize methicillin-cloxacillin-resistant staphylococci. Unfortunately, sensitivity tests are even less easy to interpret than with other antibiotics. Although methicillin-resistance, when tested by incorporation of the drug in solid medium, is accompanied by resistance to cloxacillin, resistant strains do not necessarily appear resistant when tested with filter-paper discs impregnated with the latter. If methicillin is used in the disc, the diameter of the zone of inhibition, again, is sometimes only slightly less than with sensitive controls, but resistance is also recognized by the development of colonies within the zone (Garrod and O'Grady, in preparation).

CONCLUSIONS

In this account of some new findings and ideas on acquired drug resistance in bacteria, only a small part of the subject has been covered. It would be wrong to give the impression that selection of resistant mutants is not an important means by which bacteria acquire resistance in nature. Mutants resistant to certain drugs, such as streptomycin, erythromycin, nalidixic acid, are easily isolated in the laboratory and also make their appearance during treatment of infections. Some examples of acquired resistance, such as the tetracycline resistance now common in hæmolytic streptococci and not rare in pneumococci, have not been discussed, for nothing is known of their genetic or biochemical basis.

Understanding of the mechanisms of resistance is necessary for the planning of therapeutic régimes. For instance, the emergence of resistant mutants can be prevented by the use of more than one drug at a time, since simultaneous mutation to two unrelated drugs would be an impossibly rare event. Double or treble chemotherapy for tuberculosis is effective in preventing resistance for this reason. But where bacteria may become infected with several resistance genes simultaneously, double chemotherapy will not be effective in preventing it and may encourage the dissemination of multiple-resistant pathogens. Again, if resistance is acquired from other bacteria, it should only develop in situations where there is a mixed flora, such as the large bowel or in superficial infections, and would not be expected to emerge during the course of a deep tissue infection.

Research into the mode of action of antibiotics and the basis of antibiotic resistance in bacteria is one field where new knowledge of molecular biology has a direct bearing on practical problems of clinical medicine.

References

ANDERSON, E. S. (1965). Origin of transferable drug-resistance factors in the Enterobacteriaceæ. *Brit. med. J.*, **ii**, 1289.

ANDERSON, E. S. and DATTA, N. (1965). Resistance to penicillins and its transfer in Enterobacteriaceæ. *Lancet*, **i**, 407.

ANDERSON, E. S. and LEWIS, M. J. (1965). Drug resistance and its transfer in *Salmonella typhimurium*. *Nature, Lond.*, **206**, 579.

ARBER, W. (1960). Transduction of chromosomal genes and episomes in *Escherichia coli*. *Virology*, **11**, 273.

ASHESHOV, E. (1966a). Loss of antibiotic resistance in *Staphylococcus aureus* resulting from growth at high temperature. *J. gen. Microbiol.*, **42**, 403.

ASHESHOV, E. (1966b). Chromosomal location of the genetic elements controlling penicillinase production in a strain of *Staphylococcus aureus*. *Nature, Lond.*, **210**, 804.

AYLIFFE, G. A. J. and BARBER, M. (1963). Inactivation of benzylpenicillin and methicillin by hospital staphylococci. *Brit. med. J.*, **ii**, 202.

BARBER, M. (1947). Staphylococcal infection due to penicillin-resistant strains. *Brit. med. J.*, **ii**, 863.

BARBER, M. (1949). The incidence of penicillin-sensitive variant colonies in penicillinase-producing strains of *Staphylococcus pyogenes*. *J. gen. Microbiol.*, **3**, 273.

BARBER, M. (1964). Naturally occurring methicillin resistant staphylococci. *J. gen. Microbiol.*, **35**, 183.

BARBER, M. and WHITEHEAD, J. E. M. (1949). Bacteriophage types in penicillin-resistant staphylococcal infection. *Brit. med. J.*, **ii**, 565.

BRINTON, C. C., GEMSKI, P. and CARNAHAN, J. (1964). A new type of bacterial pilus genetically controlled by the fertility factor of *E. coli* K12 and its role in chromosome transfer. *Proc. natn. Acad. Sci., U.S.A.*, **52**, 776.

CAVALLI-SFORZA, L. L. and LEDERBERG, J. (1956). Isolation of preadaptive mutants in bacteria by sib selection. *Genetics*, **41**, 367.

CHABBERT, Y.-A. and LE MINOR, L. (1966). Transmission de la resistance à plusieurs antibiotiques chèz les "Enterobacteriacæ." *Presse med.*, **74**, 2407.

CHAIN, E. B. (1962). Penicillinase-resistant penicillins and the problem of the penicillin-resistant staphylococci. In *Resistance of the Bacteria to the Penicillins*, p. 14. Ciba Foundation Study Group No. 13, Churchill, London.

CRAWFORD, E. M. and GESTELAND, R. F. (1964). The absorption of bacteriophage-R17. *Virology*, **22**, 165.

DATTA, N. (1962). Transmissible drug resistance in an epidemic strain of *Salmonella typhimurium*. *J. Hyg., Camb.*, **60**, 301.

DATTA, N. (1965). Infectious drug resistance. *Brit. med. Bull.*, **21**, 254.

DATTA, N. and KONTOMICHALOU, P. (1965). Penicillinase synthesis controlled by infectious R factors in Enterobacteriaceæ. *Nature, Lond.*, **208**, 239.

DATTA, N. and RICHMOND, M. H. (1966). The purification and properties of a penicillinase whose synthesis is mediated by an R factor in *Escherichia coli*. *Biochem. J.*, **98**, 204.

DEAN, A. C. R. (1960). Chloramphenicol resistance of *Bact. lactis ærogenes* (*Aer. ærogenes*). II. Production of highly resistant strains in non-selective conditions. *Proc. roy. Soc. B.*, **153**, 329.

EVANS, R. J. and WATERWORTH, P. M. (1966). Naturally-occurring fusidic acid resistance in staphylococci and its linkage to other resistances. *J. clin. Path.*, **19**, 555.

FAIRBROTHER, R. W., PARKER, L. and EATON, B. R. (1954). The stability of penicillinase-producing strains of *Staph. aureus*. *J. gen. Microbiol.*, **10**, 309.

FALKOW, S., CITARELLA, R. V., WOHLHIETER, J. A. and WATANABE, T. (1966). The molecular nature of R factors. *J. mol. Biol.*, **17**, 102.

FARRANT, W. N. and TOMLINSON, A. J. H. (1966). Some studies on the epidemiology of Sonne dysentery. Changes in colicine type and antibiotic resistance between 1956 and 1965. *J. Hyg., Camb.*, **64**, 287.

FRANKLIN, T. J. and GODFREY, A. (1965). Resistance of *Escherichia coli* to tetracyclines. *Biochem. J.*, **94**, 54.

GARROD, L. P. and O'GRADY (1968). *Antibiotic and Chemotherapy*. Livingstone, Edinburgh and London (2nd edition).

HARADA, K., KAMEDA, M., SUZUKI, M. D. and MITSUHASHI, S. (1964). Drug resistance of enteric bacteria. III. Acquisition of transferability of nontransmissible R (TC) factor in cooperation with F factor and formation of FR (TC). *J. Bact.*, **88**, 1257.

HARMON, S. A. and BALDWIN, J. N. (1964). Nature of the determinant controlling penicillinase production in *Staphylococcus aureus. J. Bact.*, **87**, 593.

HAYES, W. (1968). *The Genetics of Bacteria and Their Viruses*. 2nd Ed. Blackwell, Oxford.

ISAKI, K. and ARIMA, K. (1963). Disappearance of oxytetracycline accumulation in the cells of multiple drug-resistant *Escherichia coli. Nature, Lond.*, **200**, 384.

JEVONS, M. P. (1961). "Celbenin"-resistant staphylococci. *Brit. med. J.*, **i**, 124.

KABINS, S. A. and COHEN, S. (1966). Resistance-transfer factor in Enterobacteriaceæ. *New Engl. J. Med.*, **275**, 248.

LEBEK, G. (1963). Über die Entstehung mehrfachresistenter Salmonellen. Ein experimenteller Beitrag. *Zbl. Bakt. Abt., l, Orig.*, **188**, 494.

MANN, P. G. and GEDEBOU, M. (1966). Infectious transfer of drug resistance between intestinal bacteria. *Ethiopian med. J.*, **4**, 181.

MANTEN, A., GUINÉE, P. A. M. and KAMPELMACHER, E. H. (1966). Incidence of resistance to tetracycline and chloramphenicol among *Salmonella* bacteria found in the Netherlands in 1963 and 1964. *Zbl. Bakt. l, Abt. Orig.*, **200**, 13.

MARMUR, J., FALKOW, S. and MANDEL, M. (1963). New approaches to bacterial taxonomy. *Ann. rev. Microbiol.*, **17**, 329.

MAY, J. W., HOUGHTON, R. H. and PERRET, C. J. (1964). The effect of growth at elevated temperatures on some heritable properties of *Staphylococcus aureus. J. gen. Microbiol.*, **37**, 157.

MEYNELL, E. and DATTA, N. (1966). The nature and incidence of conjugation factors in *Escherichia coli. Genet. Res. Camb.*, **7**, 141.

MEYNELL, E. and DATTA, N. (1967). Mutant drug resistance factors of high transmissibility. *Nature, Lond.*, **214**, 885,

MEYNELL, G. G. and LAWN, A. M. (1967). Sex pili and common pili in the conjugational transfer of colicin factor Ib by Salmonella typhimurium. *Genet. Res., Camb.*, **9**, 359.

MOORE, B. (1960). A new screen test and selective medium for the rapid detection of epidemic strains of *Staphylococcus aureus. Lancet*, **ii**, 453.

MURTI, B. R., RAJYALAKSHMI, K. and BHASKARAN, L. S. (1962). Resistance of *Salmonella typhi* to chloramphenicol. *J. clin. Path.*, **15**, 544.

NJOKU-OBI, A. N. and NJOKU-OBI, J. C. (1965). Resistance of *Salmonella typhosa* to chloramphenicol. *J. Bact.*, **90**, 552.

NORTH, E. A. and CHRISTIE, R. (1945). Observations on the sensitivity of staphylococci to penicillin. *Med. J. Aust.*, **ii**, 44.

NOVICK, R. P. (1963). Analysis by transduction of mutations affecting penicillinase formation in *Staphylococcus aureus. J. gen. Microbiol.*, **33**, 121.

NOVICK, R. P. (1967). Penicillinase plasmids of *Staphylococcus aureus. Fed. Proc.*, **26**, 29.

NOVICK, R. P. and MORSE, S. I. (1967). *In vivo* transmission of drug resistance factors between strains of *Staphylococcus aureus. J. exp. Med.*, **125**, 45.

OKAMOTO, S. and MIZUNO, D. (1964). Mechanism of chloramphenicol and tetracycline resistance in *Escherichia coli. J. gen. Microbiol.*, **35**, 125.

OKAMOTO, S. and SUZUKI, Y. (1965). Chloramphenicol-, dihydrostreptomycin- and kanamycin-inactivating enzymes from multiple drug-resistant *Escherichia coli* carrying episome "R". *Nature, Lond.*, **208**, 1301.

PARKER, M. T. (1966). Staphylococci endemic in hospitals. *Sci. Basis of Med. ann. Rev.*, p. 157.

PARKER, M. T. and JEVONS, M. P. (1964). A survey of methicillin resistance in *Staphylococcus aureus. Post grad. med. J.*, **40**, Dec. (Suppl.) 170.

RICHMOND, M. H. and JOHN, M. (1964). Cotransduction by a staphylococcal phage of the genes responsible for penicillinase synthesis and resistance to mercury salts. *Nature, Lond.*, **202**, 1360.

RITZ, H. L. and BALDWIN, J. N. (1961). Transduction of capacity to produce staphylococcal penicillinase. *Proc. Soc. exp. Biol., N.Y.*, **107**, 678.

SELIGMAN, S. J. (1966a). Methicillin-resistant staphylococci: genetics of the minority population. *J. gen. Microbiol.*, **42**, 315.

SELIGMAN, S. J. (1966b). Penicillinase-negative variants of methicillin-resistant *Staphylococcus aureus. Nature. Lond.*, **209**, 994.

SHAW, W. V. (1967). The enzymatic acetylation of chloramphenicol by extracts of R factor-resistant *Escherichia coli. J. biol. Chem.*, **242**, 687.

SICCARDI, A. G. (1966). Colicin resistance associated with resistance factors in *Escherichia coli. Genet. Res., Camb.*, **8**, 219.

SMITH, D. H. and ARMOUR, S. E. (1966). Transferable R factors in Enteric bacteria causing infection of the genito urinary tract. *Lancet*, **ii**, 15.

SMITH, H. W. (1966). The incidence of infective drug resistance in strains of *E. coli* isolated from diseased human beings and domestic animals. *J. Hyg., Camb.*, **64**, 465.

SMITH, H. W. and HALLS, S. (1966). Observations on infective drug resistance in Britain. *Brit. med. J.*, **i**, 266.

SMITH, J. T. (1963). Penicillinase and ampicillin resistance in a strain of *Escherichia coli. J. gen. Microbiol.*, **30**, 299.

STEWART, G. T. and HOLT, R. J. (1963). Evolution of natural resistance to the newer penicillins. *Brit. med. J.*, **i**, 308.

SUTHERLAND, R. and ROLINSON, G. N. (1964). Characteristics of methicillin-resistant staphylococci. *J. Bact.*, **87**, 887.

SUZUKI, Y., OKAMOTO, S. and KONO, M. (1966). Basis of chloramphenicol resistance in naturally isolated resistant staphylococci. *J. Bact.*, **92**, 798.

SYMPOSIUM (1966). "Biochemical Studies of Antimicrobial Drugs." Soc. for Gen. Microbiol. Camb. Univ. Press.

TATUM, E. L. and LEDERBERG, J. (1947). Gene recombination in the bacterium *Escherichia coli. J. Bact.*, **53**, 673.

UNOWSKY, J. and RACHMELER, M. (1966). Mechanisms of antibiotic resistance determined by resistance-transfer factors. *J. Bact.*, **92**, 358.

WALTON, J. R. (1966). *In vivo* transfer of infectious drug resistance. *Nature, Lond.*, **211**, 312.

WATANABE, T. (1963). Infective heredity of multiple drug resistance in bacteria. *Bact. rev.*, **27**, 87.

WATANABE, T. (1966). Infectious drug resistance in enteric bacteria. *New Engl. J. Med.*, **275**, 888.

WATERWORTH, P. M. (1966). False resistance to chloramphenicol. *J. med. Lab. Tech.*, **23**, 96.

WATSON, C. E. (1967). Infectious drug resistance in shigellæ in Cape Town. *S. Afr. med. J.* **41**, 728.

WATT, P. J. and OKUBADEJO, O. A. (1967). Changes in incidence and ætiology of bacteræmia arising in hospital practice. *Lancet*, **i**, 210.

YOKOTA, T. and AKIBA, T. (1961). *Igaki to Seibutsugaku (Med. Biol.)* **58**, 151 (in Japanese). Cited by Watanabe (1963).

Chapter 5

RUBELLA

J. A. DUDGEON

IN recent years our concept of rubella as a human pathogen has changed. From being classed as a disease of minor importance, rubella is now recognized as a disease in which severe damage can be caused to the developing fœtus. From being classed as an infectious disease that did not call for research or warrant the development of a vaccine, rubella is now the subject of intensive research towards that end. The reasons for this change can be traced to events of the past 30 years. Prior to this, rubella was accepted as one of the least troublesome of the infectious diseases of childhood and adolescence. The mortality rate was low and complications few in comparison with the more virulent childhood infections, measles, scarlet fever and diphtheria. There is little to suggest from early medical records that the disease seen in the nineteenth century and termed rubella by Veale (1866) a hundred years ago, differed in any significant way from the disease that is seen today. The clinical and epidemiological features recorded by Maton (1815), Veale (1866), Edwards (1890) and many others do not suggest that any significant change has occurred in the disease itself. Fifty years ago Hess (1914) produced experimental evidence that rubella was caused by a virus, but this was not confirmed until 1938, when Hiro and Tasaka (1938) successfully transmitted the disease to children.

Current interest in rubella stems from the important observations made three years later by Norman A. Gregg, an Australian ophthalmologist. Following an extensive epidemic of rubella in Australia in 1940, Gregg (1941) observed a number of congenital malformations of the eye and heart in newborn infants which he attributed to the fact that the mothers had contracted rubella early in pregnancy. Nearly a quarter of a century later another severe rubella epidemic occurred, this time in the United States, and again congenital malformations were encountered in the offspring of women who contracted rubella in pregnancy, as they had been on numerous occasions since Gregg's original observations. But on this occasion many severe and bizarre clinical manifestations were observed in addition to those of the classical rubella syndrome type. Just prior to this epidemic another discovery of the greatest importance had been made. Two groups of investigators working independently—Weller and Neva in Boston (1962) and Parkman, Buescher and Artenstein in Washington (1962)—reported the isolation of rubella virus in cell cultures. The development of laboratory tests soon followed and, when the rubella epidemic occurred two years later, a unique opportunity arose to test them.

The unusual epidemiological behaviour of rubella during the period 1962–65 together with intensive clinical and virological investigations into the disease, its cause and effects have led to the acquisition of a mass of new information on many different aspects of rubella. The pathogenic potentialities of rubella virus are clear and the conditions under which these become manifest are now better understood. From the point of view of human ecology, rubella is clearly a disease of extraordinary interest in which the host-parasite relationship is of special significance.

BIOLOGICAL AND OTHER PROPERTIES OF RUBELLA VIRUS

Isolation of the Causative Virus

Experimental studies in the 1940s pointed to the fact that the virus had a restricted host range. Habel (1942) carried the virus through five consecutive passages on the chorio-allantois of chick embryos. No lesions developed, but material from the fifth passage produced clinical evidence of rubella in rhesus monkeys. Anderson (1949) reported cytopathic changes in monkey kidney cultures inoculated with nasopharyngeal washings, but the findings were not confirmed. What limited information there was available at this time was obtained from experimental studies with monkeys and human volunteers (Hiro and Tasaka, 1938; Habel, 1942; Anderson, 1949; Krugman et al., 1953; Krugman and Ward, 1954).

Isolation was finally achieved independently by Weller and Neva (1962) and by Parkman, Buescher and Artenstein (1962) with cell cultures and techniques found successful in the isolation of the viruses of poliomyelitis, measles and the common cold. Once a means of recognizing the presence of rubella virus (RV) in cultures had been established further detailed studies of the properties of the virus followed. From this it became clear that the host range of rubella was by no means as restricted as was previously thought to be the case.

Cytopathic Effect (CPE) of RV in Cell Cultures. Weller and Neva detected the presence of rubella virus in primary human amnion cultures (PHA) inoculated with urine and blood from patients with clinical rubella (Weller and Neva, 1962). Initially, only a few cells appeared to be affected and cytopathic changes were slow. On primary isolation these took 20 to 60 days to develop, but with virus adapted by passage CPE was evident much earlier. On the twentieth passage CPE was noted by the fourth day with 80 per cent destruction of the cell sheet. In the early stages after inoculation isolated cells appeared refractile, they became rounded and pseudopodia-like projections appeared. Finally, affected cells disintegrated but the cytopathic changes tended to remain focal with many cells remaining unaffected (Weller and Neva, 1965).

Interference by RV in Cell Cultures. Parkman, Buescher and Artenstein (1962) detected rubella virus in primary African Green Monkey kidney culture (AGMK) inoculated with throat washings from cases of rubella. No CPE was detected in the inoculated cultures but they showed resistance to challenge when inoculated with ECHO 11 virus, whereas uninoculated cultures showed typical CPE when challenged. The interference effect of RV was shown to be serially transmissible in AGMK cultures, and the effect was inhibited by rubella antiserum. Since these observations it has been shown that the virus can be cultured in many other types of cell culture.

Some of these are listed in Table I. The presence of virus can be detected either by cytopathic effect or by the interference phenomenon.

TABLE I

Susceptibility of Cell Cultures to Rubella Virus*

Tissue, species and origin of cell culture	Type of cell	Designation	Evidence of virus growth
Human amnion	Primary	PHA	(i) CPE (ii) Interference with Sindbis virus
African green monkey kidney	Primary	AGMK	Interference
Rhesus monkey	Continuous cell line	LLC-MK2	(i) Interference (ii) CPE
Grivet monkey	Continuous cell line	BSC-1	(i) Interference (ii) CPE
Green monkey	Continuous cell line	GMK	CPE
Bovine embryo	Primary		Interference
Human fibroblast	Diploid cell strain	WI-38 WI-26	(i) Interference (ii) Inhibition of growth
Rabbit kidney	Continuous cell line	RK-13	CPE
Rabbit kidney	Primary		CPE
Rabbit cornea†	Continuous cell line	SIRC	CPE

* Details can be found in the report of the Seminar on Measles and Rubella, Paris, June 1964, in *Archiv. fur die Gesamte Virusforschung* (1965), vol. 16.
† Leehøy, J. (1966).

Cytopathology in Cell Cultures

The earliest changes seen by direct microscopy are swelling of cells and loss of cell outline. As infection progresses, cells become rounded and finally fall off the glass. The cytopathic changes in PHA (Weller and Neva, 1962) and RK-13 cultures (McCarthy *et al.*, 1963) tend to remain focal, and even after several days' incubation unaffected cells can still be seen. In stained preparations of PHA, RK-13, LLC-MK2 much the same type of change can be seen. These consist of loss of nuclei, fragmentation and clumping of the nuclear chromatin with the appearance of nuclear and cytoplasmic inclusions. As infection progresses, the amount of cytoplasmic inclusion material increases. Examples of the cytopathic effect of rubella virus in RK-13 cells are shown in Figure 1.

Interference

Interference by RV in AGMK cultures can be demonstrated with many viruses besides ECHO 11 virus. With 100 to 1,000 tissue-culture infective doses of virus (TCID 50) interference has been demonstrated with five strains

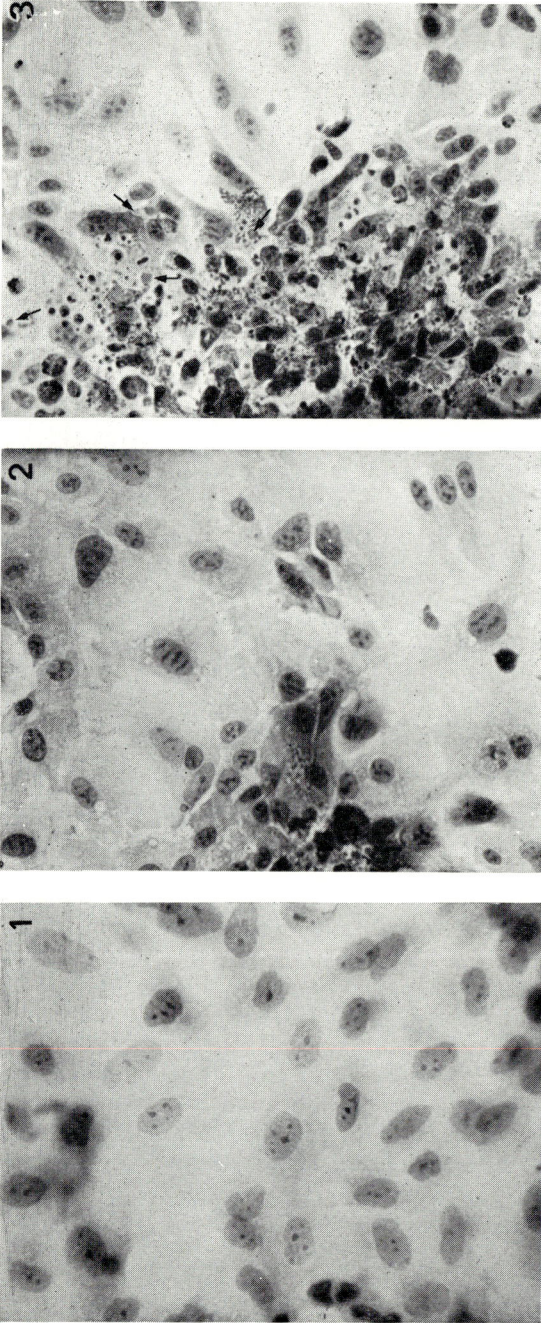

Fig. 1. To illustrate the cytopathic effect of rubella virus in RK-13 cells

1. Uninoculated cells controls.
2. Early focal change at 4 days showing loss of nucleoli in affected cells.
3. CPE at 7 days; cells are grossly distorted with deeply staining nuclei.
   Numerous inclusions and aggregations of granular material in cytoplasm.
   Several inclusions marked with arrow.
        Staining by hemotoxylin and eosin. ×100.

of ECHO virus; polioviruses types 1 and 2; Coxsackie A9 and B1, 3 and 5; para-influenza 2; measles; mumps, and eastern equine encephalitis (EEE) virus. Interference with influenza A could only be demonstrated with a low dose of challenge virus and it was incomplete with herpes simplex virus. None could be detected with five strains of adenovirus (Parkman, 1965).

Antigenic Types

As far as is known, only one antigenic type of rubella virus exists.

Pathogenicity in Animals

RV produces no evidence of infection in guinea-pigs, rabbits, adult or newborn mice or fertile eggs. Ferrets are susceptible to intranasal inoculation. Parkman *et al.* (1965) have shown that rhesus monkeys are susceptible to infection. Inoculated animals usually develop a subclinical infection with viræmia, nasopharyngeal infection and production of antibody. Transplacental infection also occurs.

Particle Size

Filtration studies show that the virus passes through filters of 300 mμ pore diameter but not through 100 mμ filters. Rubella virus appears to be similar in size to para-influenza type 3 (Parkman, 1965), but some evidence has been obtained of a particle size between 50 and 100 mμ (McCarthy *et al.*, 1963).

Nucleic Acid

Rubella virus is not inactivated by treatment with 5-iodo-2, deoxyuridine (IDU). In this respect it resembles RNA viruses such as measles and poliovirus and is unlike DNA viruses such as vaccinia and herpes, which are inhibited by IDU. The growth of RV in tissue culture can be inhibited by amantadine (1-adamantanamine-hydrochloride) which has been shown to have an inhibitory effect on certain of the myxoviruses which are known to be RNA viruses (Cochran and Maassab, 1964).

Effect of Chemicals

Infectivity of RV is completely destroyed by treatment with ethyl ether and chloroform. It is inactivated by 1 : 4000 formalin at 37°C.

Thermal Stability

The virus is stable at −70°C for at least three years. Infectivity is lost at 37°C at the rate of 0·5 log units per hour; at 56°C the rate of loss is 1·5 to 3 log units per hour. The virus is stable at pH ranges from 6·6 to 8·2.

CLINICAL FEATURES

Contrary to general belief, the diagnosis of rubella can be extremely difficult. In the presence of an epidemic in which the diagnosis has been confirmed by laboratory tests a diagnosis of rubella on clinical grounds can usually be made with some confidence, but in sporadic cases this is more difficult. Rubella lacks a pathognonomic sign; lymphadenopathy is an important and fairly constant feature, but is not sufficiently specific for rubella. Unlike measles, marked clinical variation occurs in rubella, and the rash when present may simulate other exanthems, including measles, enterovirus infections, scarlet fever and toxic erythemata. Detailed accounts of the clinical manifestations of rubella can be found in publications by Krugman and Ward (1954, 1964), Krugman (1965) and by Young and Ramsay (1963) in this country. These latter authors found that the main features in 114 cases[1] of rubella admitted to an Infectious Disease Unit in a London hospital and diagnosed on clinical grounds were as follows:

1. Mild prodromal symptoms, usually absent in children, but in adults consisting of a tonsillo-pharyngeal infection (85 per cent) and little or no coryza.
2. Lymphadenopathy was one of the earliest features of rubella; the glands most frequently involved were the cervical, sub-occipital and post-auricular (97 per cent).
3. Suffusion of the eyes with a feeling of "grittiness" (83 per cent).
4. A maculo-papular rash which, as in measles, appears first on the face including the skin around the mouth and behind the ears and then spreads downwards; the rubella rash is usually discrete and seldom blotchy as in measles or as red as in scarlet fever.
5. Occasional petechial lesions on the palate (23 per cent).

Now that laboratory tests are available for the diagnosis of rubella, further data have become available from virologically established cases.

Age of Infection. Rubella is uncommon in infants; in young children it is usually a very mild disease often presenting as a febrile illness with adenopathy but without a rash. In an epidemic of rubella in the Pribilofs in 1963 only 30 per cent of children aged 0–14 years had a rash; in the age-group 15–20 years 90 per cent had a rash (Brody et al., 1965).

Clinical Variation. This is very marked, and particularly so in children. Rubella without a rash occurs in 20–25 per cent of cases, but adenopathy may be found in a proportion of cases on careful palpation. In studying the incidence of rubella in military recruits, Buescher (1965) reported a ratio of 1 : 6·5 of overt to subclinical infections. Horstmann et al. (1965) found a ratio of 1 : 1 in institutionalized children.

The rash usually lasts three days but may last as long as five. The rash may be biphasic and a change from a maculo-papular rash to the bright red blush of scarlet fever may be seen.

Complications are few; arthritis or arthralgia occurs in about 5 per cent of cases. The joints most commonly affected are the hands, wrists, knees and ankles. Encephalitis occurs but is less common than after measles. Mild thrombocytopenia is also sometimes seen. Leucopenia is more commonly encountered in rubella than in measles and enterovirus exanthems.

[1] I am indebted to Dr. S. A. Young and Dr. A. Melvin Ramsay for permission to include their description of these cases. The figures in brackets refer to the incidence of the main clinical feature.

the C-F test is in the diagnosis of recent infections. Preferably both neutralization and C-F tests should be carried out on the same specimens. Several C-F antigens have been described; a cell-associated antigen in AGMK and in RK-13 cells (Sever and Huebner, 1965); and a C-F antigen prepared from a chronically infected

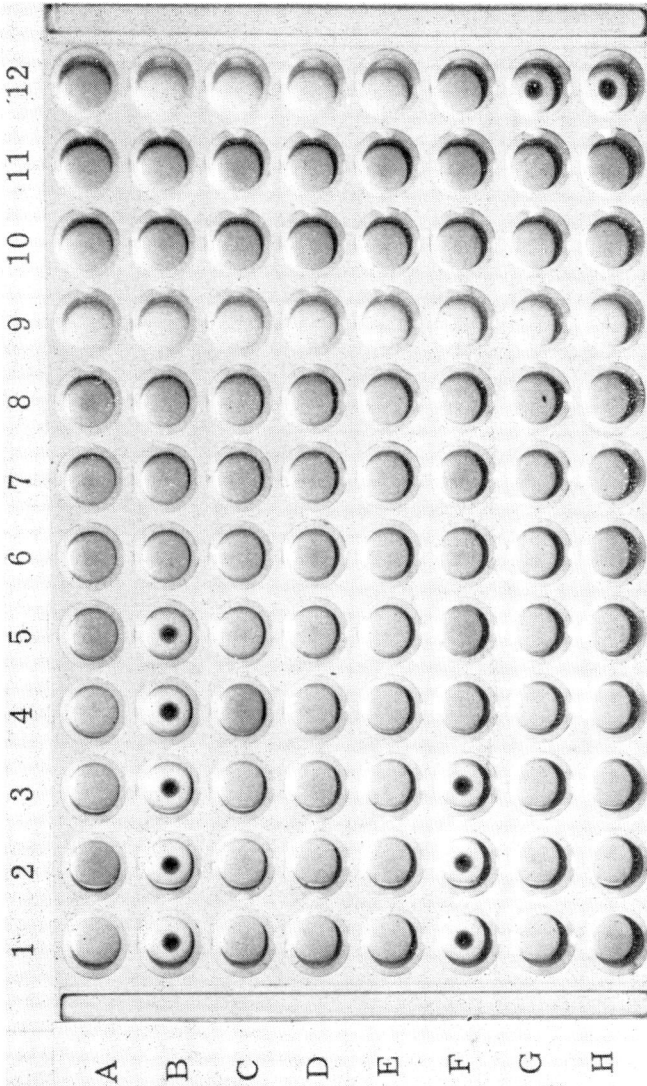

FIG. 6. Complement-Fixation (CF) test for rubella. Micromethod.

Row 1–8 across: serum dilutions 1/4–1/512.
Row 10: serum controls.
Row 11: normal antigen.
Row 12: complement and cell controls.
Rows A–G down: test sera same as in Figure 5. (See Table IV for details.)

line of LLC-MK2 cells (Stern, 1965) and a fluid and cell-phase antigens in BHK-21 cells (Schmidt and Lennette, 1966). The C-F test can be carried out by a micro-technique in Perspex dishes on a Perspex plate. Serial 2-fold dilutions of serum are tested against 4 units of antigen with 2 units of complement. Fixation is allowed to occur overnight after which sensitized red cells are added and the tests read. The end-point is taken as the serum dilution showing 3 to 4 + fixation of complement.

HAI Test. Recently Stewart et al. (1967) have described a hæmagglutinin-inhibition (HAI) test for rubella. The hæmagglutinating antigen (HA) is prepared by growing rubella virus to high titre in BHK-21 cells with serum treated with kaolin to remove non-specific inhibitors. Serial dilutions of serum pretreated with kaolin are made in dextrose-gelatin-veronal buffer; 4 units of HA antigen and an equal volume of a suspension of day-old chick red cells are added to each serum dilution. The titre of the serum is taken as the highest dilution showing complete or almost complete inhibition of hæmagglutination. The HAI test can be carried out in WHO Perspex dishes or by a microtechnique on Takatsy plates. HAI antibody appears to parallel neutralizing antibody in time of appearance and persistence.

Indirect Fluorescent Antibody Technique. Antibodies can also be detected by the indirect method of immunofluorescence with a chronically infected line of monkey

TABLE IV

Row	Patient Number	Age	Days after Rash (R) or Contact (C)	HAI (Plate A) Figure V	CF titre (Plate B) Figure VI	Further details and comments
A	1	20	1 (R)	4	<4	Rubella virus isolated; specific rise in HAI and CF antibodies
B	1	20	24 (R)	>2048	64	
C	2	19/12	2 (R)	<4	<4	No virus isolated; no change in HAI or CF antibody titre
D	2	19/12	27 (R)	<4	<4	
E	3	2	14 (R)	<4	<4	No rubella antibody present
F	4 (Mother of 3 above)	24	4 (C)	16	512	Mother probably immune
G	5	23	7 (C)	<4	<4	No evidence of rubella infection
H	5	23	32 (C)	<4	<4	

kidney cells (LLC-MK2) as antigen (Brown *et al.*, 1965). This method is useful as a screening test and the results correlate with the presence of neutralizing antibody.

The value of virus isolation and serological procedures for rubella can be seen from the results shown in Figures 5 and 6 and Table IV. The two infants had rashes diagnosed clinically as rubella; both were in close contact with women in the early stages of pregnancy.

Diagnosis of Congenital Rubella

The same procedures should be used as outlined above. In addition to nasopharyngeal swabs, urine, and where appropriate, biopsy material from liver and cataractous lens tissue should be examined for presence of virus. Sera should be examined for antibody. Persistence of neutralizing antibody is found in 95 per cent of cases of congenital rubella and complement-fixing antibody in about 70 per cent (Plotkin *et al.*, 1967). C-F antibody declines to a low level at 2 to 3 years of age. High levels of IgM are found in the sera of infants with congenital rubella (Soothill *et al.*, 1966).

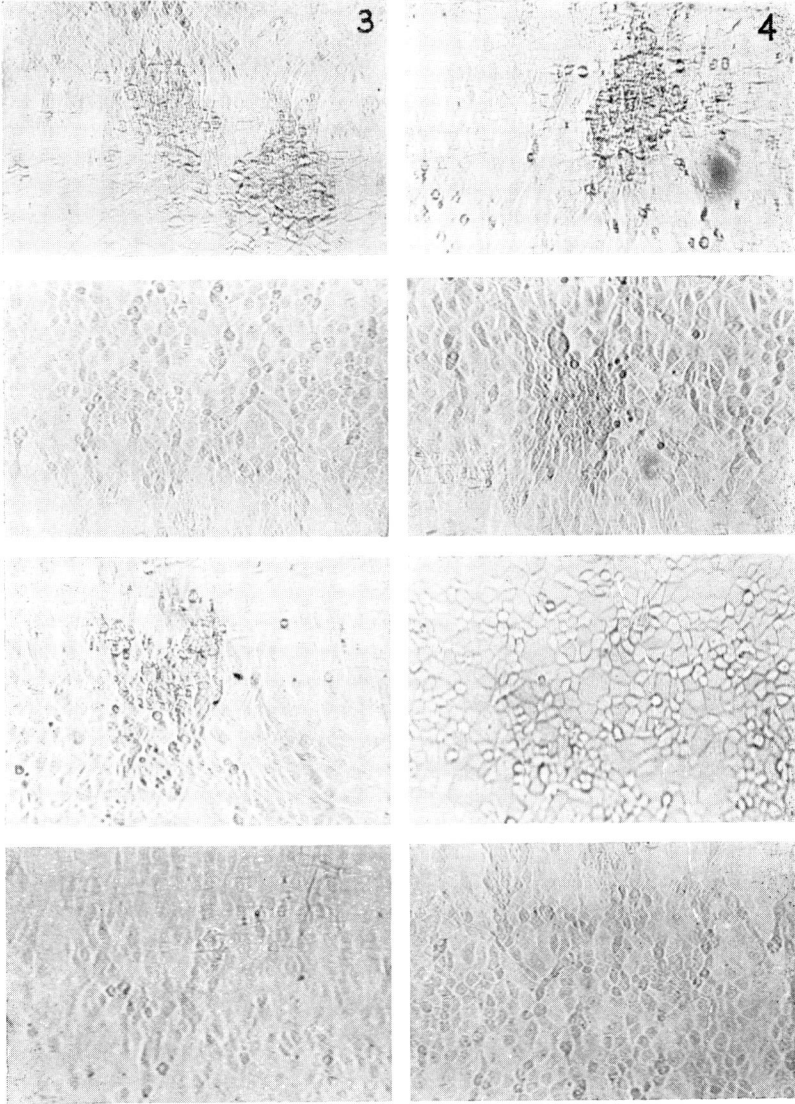

added 10 to 100 IN (interfering doses) of rubella virus in an equal volume. After incubation at 37°C for one hour, 0·1 ml. of the serum-virus mixtures is inoculated into four culture tubes of AGMK cultures which are then incubated at 35°C for five days. After this time half the tubes are challenged with 1,000 to 10,000 TCID 50, ECHO 11 or other challenge virus and the tubes read for evidence of interference or growth of the challenge virus (Buescher, 1964). Cultures showing growth of ECHO 11 virus contain no rubella virus and indicate inhibition by rubella antibody; those showing no cytopathic effect indicate interference from rubella virus and absence of rubella antibody (see Fig. 2). By this method serum neutralizing titres of 4–64 are obtained. Sera without antibody have titres of less than 4.

(ii) *Cytopathic inhibition*. The tests are carried out in RK-13 cells. The preliminary stages of preparation of the serum-virus mixtures are similar to those described above for the interference-inhibition test, except that more consistent results are obtained with uninactivated serum. After incubation at 35°C inoculated cultures are read at three and seven days and the presence of antibody is determined by inhibition of the cytopathic effect of the virus (Dudgeon *et al.*, 1964). Examples of the cytopathic changes seen in a neutralization test are shown in Figure 4.

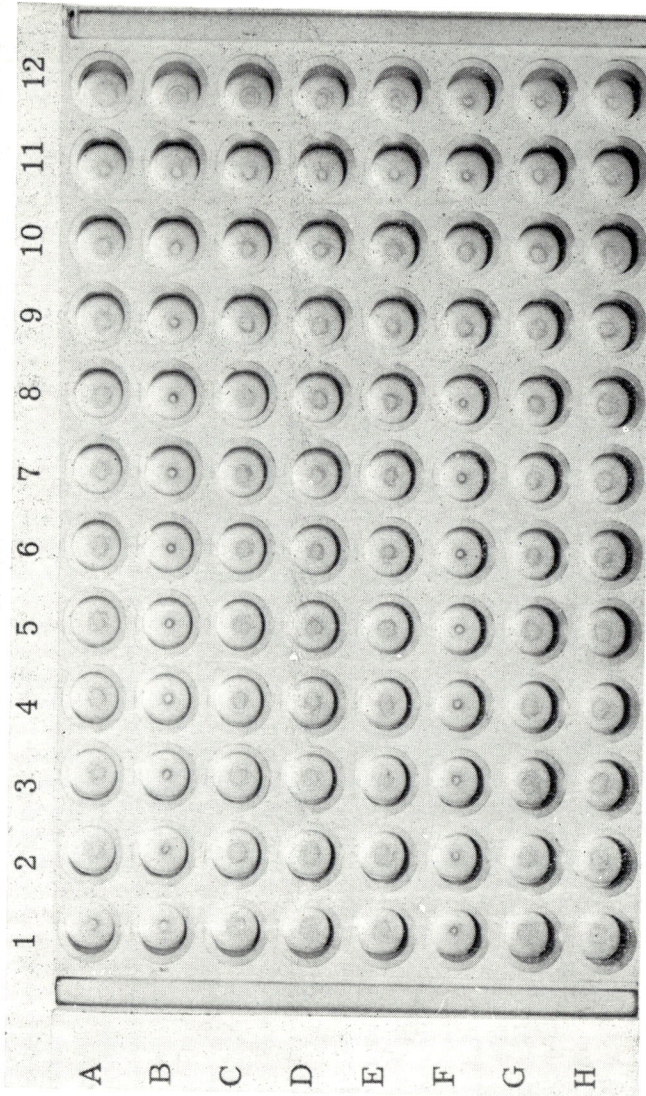

FIG. 5. *Hemagglutination-inhibition (HAI) test for rubella. Micromethod.*
Row 1–10 across: serum dilutions 1/4–1/2048.
Row 11: serum controls.
Row 12 down: virus titrations.
Rows A–H down: test sera. (See Table IV for details.)

Both the interference-inhibition and cytopathic-inhibition methods yield satisfactory and reproducible results provided that an adequate system of controls is included in each test.

Complement-fixing Antibody (C-F) appears a little later than VN antibody, it takes longer to develop and does not persist for as long as neutralizing antibody (Sever and Fabiyi, 1966). It is important therefore not to collect the convalescent sample too early, preferably nearer the 28th than the 21st day. The main value of

Prophylaxis

Passive Immunization. Attempts to prevent rubella with gamma globulin have produced results which vary considerably in their apparent effectiveness (Lundström, 1965). In a study of the effect of gamma globulin in 30,746 pregnant women in Great Britain, it was found that the attack-rate was 1·95 per cent in family contacts and the incidence of congenital defects in infants whose mothers developed rubella despite prophylaxis was 18 per cent. This is close to what would be expected in unprotected women. However, in treated women who did not develop rubella, there was no excess of rubella-type defects (McDonald and Peckham, 1967). At the best, gamma globulin will reduce the clinical attack rate and thereby the risk of fœtal infection.

Active Immunization. Recently Parkman *et al.* (1966) have reported preliminary results with a strain of rubella virus attenuated by passage in monkey kidney cultures. The vaccine strain produced no evidence of pharyngeal infection, viræmia or contact infection in monkeys and an immune response developed. Thirty-four children were vaccinated; none developed any illness, all developed antibody, but virus in low titre was recovered from the throats of a few of them. No contact infection was detected. More recently, reports of other attenuated strains of rubella virus have been recorded (Conference on Virus and Rickettsial Vaccines, 1967).

References

AINGER, L. E., LAWYER, N. G. and FITCH, C. W. (1966). Neonatal rubella myocarditis. *Brit. Heart J.*, **28**, 691.

ANDERSON, S. G. (1949). Experimental rubella in human volunteers. *J. Immunol.*, **62**, 29.

BRODY, J. A., SEVER, J. L., McALISTER, R., SCHIFF, G. M. and CUTTING, R. (1965). Rubella epidemic on St. Paul Island in the Pribilofs. (1963). *J. Amer. med. Ass.*, **191**, 619.

BROWN, G. C., MAASSAB, H. F., VERONELLI, J. A. and FRANCIS, T. (1965). Detection of rubella antibodies in human serum by the indirect fluorescent antibody technique. *Arch. ges. Virusforsch.*, **16**, 459.

BUESCHER, E. L. (1964). "Rubella" in *Diagnostic Procedures for Viral and Rickettsial Diseases*. 3rd edition. Page 737. The American Public Health Association, New York.

BUESCHER, E. L. (1965). Behaviour of rubella virus in adult populations. *Arch. ges. Virusforsch.*, **16**, 470.

BUTLER, N. R., DUDGEON, J. A., HAYES, K., PECKHAM, C. S. and WYBAR, K. (1965). Persistence of rubella antibody in children with and without embryopathy. *Brit. med. J.*, **ii**, 1027.

COCHRAN, K. W. and MAASSAB, H. F. (1964). Inhibition of rubella virus by 1-adamantanamine hydrochloride. *Fed. Proc.*, **23**, 387.

Conference on Viral and Rickettsial Vaccines (1967). Report of a Meeting in Washington, November 1966. (To be published.)

DUDGEON, J. A., BUTLER, N. R. and PLOTKIN, S. A. (1964). Further serological studies on the rubella syndrome. *Brit. med. J.*, **ii**, 165.

DUDGEON, J. A. (1967). Maternal rubella and its effect on the fœtus. *Arch. Dis. Childh.*, **42**, 110.

EDWARDS, W. A. (1890). "Rubella" in *Cyclopædia of the Diseases of Children*, Young & Pentland, London.

FRIEDMANN, I. and WRIGHT, M. I. (1966). Histopathological changes in the fœtal and infantile inner ear caused by maternal rubella. *Brit. med. J.*, **ii**, 20.

GREEN, R. H., BALSAMO, M. R., GILES, J. P., KRUGMAN, S. and MIRICK, G. S. (1964). Rubella: Studies on its ætiology, epidemiology, clinical course and prevention. *Trans. Ass. Amer. Phycns.*, **77**, 118.

GREGG, N. McA. (1941). Congenital cataract following German measles in the mother. *Trans. ophthmal. Soc. Aust.*, **3**, 35.

HABEL, K. (1942). Transmission of rubella to Macacus mulatta monkeys. *Publ. Hlth. Rep. Wash.*, **57**, 1126.

HESS, A. F. (1914). German measles (rubella): An experimental study. *Arch. intern. Med.*, **13**, 913.

HIRO, Y. and TASAKA, S. (1938). Die Röteln sind eine Viruskrankheit. *Mschr. Kinderheilk.*, **76**, 328.

HORSTMANN, D. M., RIORDAN, J. T., OHTAWARA, M. and NIEDERMAN, J. C. (1965). A natural epidemic of rubella in a closed population. *Arch. ges. Virusforsch.*, **16**, 483.

KORONES, S. B., AINGER, L. E., MONIF, G. R. G., ROANE, J., SEVER, J. L. and FUSTE, F. (1965). Congenital rubella: A study of 22 infants. *Amer. J. Dis. Childh.*, **110**, 434.

KRUGMAN, S. (1965). Rubella: clinical and epidemiological aspects. *Arch. ges. Virusforsch.*, **16**, 477.

KRUGMAN, S. and WARD, R. (1954). The rubella problem. *J. Pediat.*, **44**, 489.

KRUGMAN, S. and WARD, R. (1964). "Rubella" in *Infectious Diseases of Childhood*. Mosby.

KRUGMAN, S., WARD, R., JACOBS, K. G. and LAZAR, N. (1953). Studies on rubella immunization: demonstration of rubella without a rash. *J. Amer. med. Ass.*, **151**, 285.

LEERHØY, J. (1966). The influence of different media on cell morphology or rubella virus titre in a rabbit cornea cell line. *Arch. ges. Virusforsch.*, **19**, 210.

LUNDSTRÖM, R. (1962). Rubella during pregnancy. A follow up study of children born after an epidemic of rubella in Sweden in 1951. *Acta paediat.* (supp.) 133.

LUNDSTRÖM, R. (1965). Experimental studies with rubella: evaluation of gamma globulin for prophylaxis. *Arch. ges. Virusforsch.*, **16**, 513.

LUNDSTRÖM, R., SVEDMYR, A., HAGBARD, L. and KAIJSER, K. (1967). Rubella immunity as related to age and history of overt disease. *Acta paediat.*, **56**, 279.

MANSON, M. M., LOGAN, W. P. D. and LØY, R. M. (1960). Rubella and other virus infections during pregnancy. Reports on Public Health No. 101. London, H.M.S.O.

MATON, W. G. (1815). Some account of a rash liable to be mistaken for scarlatina. *Med. Trans. Coll. Phycns. Lond.*, **5**, 149.

McCARTHY, K., TAYLOR-ROBINSON, C. H. and PILLINGER, S. E. (1963). Isolation of rubella virus from cases in Britain. *Lancet*, **ii**, 593.

McDONALD, J. C. (1967). Gamma globulin prophylaxis of rubella. In *Report on the 1st International Conference on Vaccines Against Viral and Rickettsial Diseases in Man.* Scientific publication No. 147, Pan American Health Organization, Washington, D.C. page 371.

MENSER, M. A., DORMAN, D. C., REYE, R. D. K. and REID, R. R. (1966). Renal artery stenosis in the rubella syndrome. *Lancet*, **i**, 790.

NAEYE, R. L. and BLANC, W. (1965). Pathogenesis of congenital rubella. *J. Amer. med. Ass.*, **194**, 1277.

NAGAYAMA, T., UEDA, K., MIENO, K., NUNOE, T., NISHIO, S. and SEVER, J. L. (1966). Frequency of rubella antibody among pregnant women in the Fukwoka district of Japan. *Fukoka Acta. Med.*, **57**, 303.

PARKMAN, P. D. (1965). Biological properties of rubella virus. *Arch. ges. Virusforsch.*, **16**, 401.

PARKMAN, P. D., BUESCHER, E. L. and ARTENSTEIN, M. S. (1962). Recovery of rubella virus from army recruits. *Proc. Soc. Exp. Biol., N.Y.*, **111**, 225.

PARKMAN, P. D., PHILLIPS, P. E. and MEYER, H. M. (1965). Experimental rubella virus infection in pregnant monkeys. *Amer. J. Dis. Childh.*, **110**, 390.

PARKMAN, P. D., MEYER, H. M., KIRSCHSTEIN, R. L. and HOPPS, H. E. (1966). Attenuated rubella virus I. *New Engl. J. Med.*, **275**, 569.

PETERS, E. R., DAVIS, R. L. (1966). Congenital rubella syndrome. *Clin. Paediat.*, **5**, 743.

PITT, D. and KEIR, E. H. (1965). Results of rubella in pregnancy. *Med. J. Aust.*, **ii**, 647, 691, 737.

PLOTKIN, S. A., BOUÉ, A. and BOUÉ, J. G. (1965). The *in vitro* growth of rubella virus in human embryo cells. *Amer. J. Epidem.*, **81**, 71.

PLOTKIN, S. A., COCHRAN, W., LINDQUIST, J. M., COCHRAN, G., SCHAFFER, D. B., SCHEIE, H. G. and FURUKAWA, T. (1967). The congenital rubella syndrome in late infancy. *J. Amer. med. Ass.*, (In the press.)

PLOTKIN, S. A., DUDGEON, J. A. and RAMSAY, A. M. (1963). Laboratory studies on rubella and the rubella syndrome. *Brit. med. J.*, **ii**, 1296.

PLOTKIN, S. A., OSKI, F. A., HARTNETT, E. M., HERVADA, A. R., FRIEDMANN, S. and GOWING, J. (1965). Some recently recognized manifestations of the rubella syndrome. *J. Pediat.*, **67**, 182.

Rubella Symposium (1965). *Amer. J. Dis. Child.*, **110**, 345.

RUDOLPH, A. J., SINGLETON, E. B., ROSENBERG, H. S., SINGER, D. B. and PHILIPPS, C. A. (1965). Osseus manifestations of the congenital rubella syndrome. *Amer. J. Dis. Child.*, **110**, 428.

SCHIFF, G. M., SUTHERLAND, J. M., LIGHT, I. J. and BLOOM, J. E. (1965). Studies on congenital rubella. *Amer. J. Dis. Child.*, **110**, 441.

SCHMIDT, N. J. and LENNETTE, E. H. (1966). Rubella complement-fixing antigens derived from the fluid and cellular phases of BHK-21 cells. *J. Immunol.*, **97**, 815.

Seminar on Measles and Rubella, Paris, June 1964. Proceedings published in *Arch. ges. Virusforsch.* (1965), **16**.

SEVER, J. L., SCHIFF, G. M. and HUEBNER, R. J. (1964). Frequency of rubella antibody among pregnant women and other human and animal populations. *Obstet. and Gynaecol.*, **23**, 153.

SEVER, J. L., FABIYI, A., MCCALLIN, P. F., CHY, P. T., WEISS, W. and GILKESON, M. R. (1965). Rubella antibody among pregnant women in Hawaii. *Amer. J. Obstet. Gynec.*, **92**, 1006.

SEVER, J. L., HUEBNER, R. J., CASTELLANO, G. A., SARMA, B. S., FABIYI, A., SCHIFF, G. M. and CUSUMANO, C. L. (1965). Rubella complement-fixation test. *Science*, **148**, 385.

SEVER, J. L., HUEBNER, R. J., FABIYI, A., MONIF, G. R., CASTELLANO, G., CUSUMANO, C. L., TRAUB, R. G., LEY, A. C., GILKESON, M. R. and ROBERTS, J. M. (1966). Antibody responses in acute and chronic rubella. *Proc. Soc. exp. Biol., N.Y.*, **122**, 513.

SOOTHILL, J. F., HAYES, K. and DUDGEON, J. A. (1966). The immunoglobulins in congenital rubella. *Lancet*, **i**, 1385.

STERN, H. (1965). Rubella virus complement-fixation test. *Nature*, **208**, 200.

STEWART, G. L., PARKMAN, P. D., HOPPS, H. E., DOUGLAS, R. D., HAMILTON, J. P. and MEYER, H. M. (1967). Rubella-virus haemagglutination-inhibition test. *New Engl. J. Med.*, **276**, 554.

THORBURN, M. and MILLER, G. G. (1967). The pathology of congenital rubella in Jamaica. *Arch. Dis. Childh.* (To be published.)

VEALE, H. (1866). History of an epidemic of Rötheln with observations on its pathology. *Edin. Med. J.*, **12**, 404.

WELLER, T. H., ALFORD, C. A. and NEVA, F. A. (1964). Retrospective diagnosis by serologic means of congenitally acquired rubella infections. *New Engl. J. Med.*, **270**, 1039.

WELLER, T. H. and NEVA, F. A. (1962). Propagation in tissue culture of cytopathic agents from patients with rubella-like illness. *Proc. Soc. exp. Biol., N.Y.*, **111**, 215.

WELLER, T. H. and NEVA, F. A. (1965). Biological characteristics of rubella virus as assayed in a human amnion culture system. *Arch. ges. Virusforsch.*, **16**, 393.

YOUNG, S. E. J. and RAMSAY, A. M. (1963). Diagnosis of rubella. *Brit. med. J.*, **ii**, 1295.

Chapter 6

HUMAN CYTOMEGALOVIRUS INFECTIONS

H. STERN

PRIOR to 1956, cytomegalic inclusion disease was believed to be rare and usually fatal. Generally the diagnosis was made at post-mortem by finding "cytomegalic cells" in the tissues. These are very large cells, up to 40 μ in diameter, with a large nucleus containing a single prominent inclusion body. In stained tissue sections the inclusion body is typically separated by a wide unstained halo from the well-defined and thickened nuclear membrane, giving rise to the so-called "owl's eye" appearance (Figs. 1 and 2). Multiple, small, basophilic-staining intracytoplasmic inclusion bodies are also sometimes present. Based on the distribution of cytomegalic cells two forms of disease were recognized: disseminated and localized. Disseminated disease was seen most often in newborn infants, causing symptoms which often closely resembled those of erythroblastosis fœtalis and congenital syphilis. Because most of the cases were diagnosed at post-mortem, the impression arose that the neonatal disease was usually if not always fatal. It accounted for 1–2 per cent of unselected pædiatric autopsies in Boston and St. Louis in the United States, as well as in Finland, Germany and France (Farber and Wolbach, 1932; McCordock and Smith, 1934; Wyatt *et al.*, 1950; Ahvenainen, 1952; Seifert and Oehme, 1957; Fruhling *et al.*, 1960). In other parts of the United States and also in Great Britain it was apparently much less common (Potter, 1957; Crome and France, 1959; Symmers, 1960). It was considered that after 4 years of age disseminated disease was extremely rare and most cases, whether children or adults, occurred as a complication of chronic debilitating disease such as leukæmia and lymphoma which depress the defence mechanisms of the body, especially when steroids and cytotoxic drugs were used in treatment (Wong and Warner, 1962).

The localized form of the disease, on the other hand, was relatively common in young children, occurring as an apparently symptomless infection associated with the formation of cytomegalic cells in the salivary glands. These cells were an incidental finding at post-mortems carried out on children who had died of other causes, and were rarely seen outside the age range 2 months to 5 years. They were described in 10–12 per cent of unselected autopsies on children in Europe and the United States, although in Britain the incidence was only 5 per cent or less (Löwenstein, 1907; Farber and Wolbach, 1932; McCordock and Smith, 1934; Seifert and Oehme, 1957; Baar, 1955; McDonald, personal communication). After early childhood localized disease was also rare, and affected not the salivary glands but the lungs in patients with depressed immunity, or the gastro-intestinal tract around chronic ulcerative and granulomatous lesions (Wong and Warner, 1962).

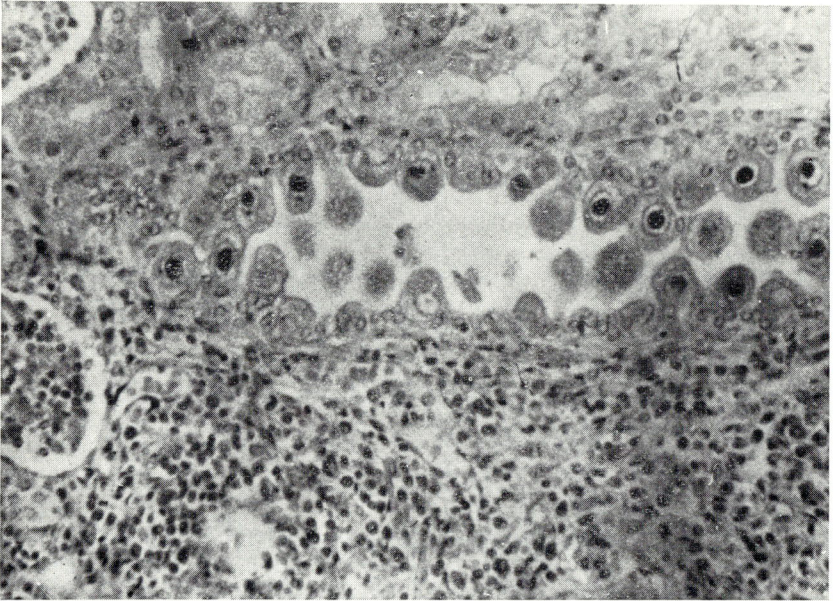

FIG. 1. H. and E. stained section of kidney from a case of neonatal cytomegalic inclusion disease. Note the desquamation of cytomegalic cells into the renal tubule ($\times$ 300).

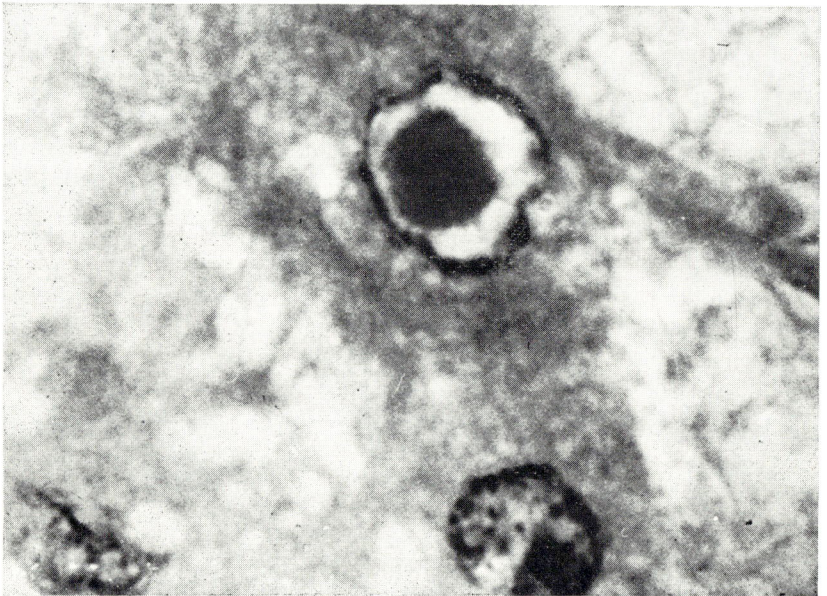

FIG. 2. H. and E. stained section of liver from a case of neonatal cytomegalic inclusion disease showing a typical cytomegalic cell ($\times$ 1500).

The human cytomegalovirus was isolated for the first time in 1956 (Smith, 1956; Rowe *et al.*, 1956; Weller *et al.*, 1957), and it soon became apparent that infection, far from being rare, is widespread in both children and adults and is of considerable clinical importance. Not only is neonatal disease more common than previously suspected but most cases are now known to survive, often with residual damage to the central nervous system. In fact, the cytomegalovirus may prove to be one of the most important causes of microcephalic mental deficiency. Infection in young children appears to be associated with liver damage, and in adults it has recently been shown to be the cause of a type of Paul-Bunnell-negative infectious mononucleosis. Finally, cytomegalic inclusion disease is a common and important hazard of the immuno-suppressive treatments now being used for malignant disease and renal homotransplantation.

PROPERTIES OF THE VIRUS

Cytomegaloviruses are widely distributed among mammalian species, infection being recognized by the presence of "cytomegalic" cells usually in the salivary glands (Andrewes, 1964). Those that have been isolated have proved to be highly species-specific, both *in vivo* and in tissue culture, and antigenically distinct. They are members of the herpesvirus group. The human cytomegalovirus is identical in size and structure with herpes simplex (Fig. 3). It is formed of a deoxyribonucleic acid core with a surrounding icosahedrally shaped capsid, about 110 mμ in diameter and composed of 162 hollow, elongated, polygonal capsomeres, and an outer lipoprotein

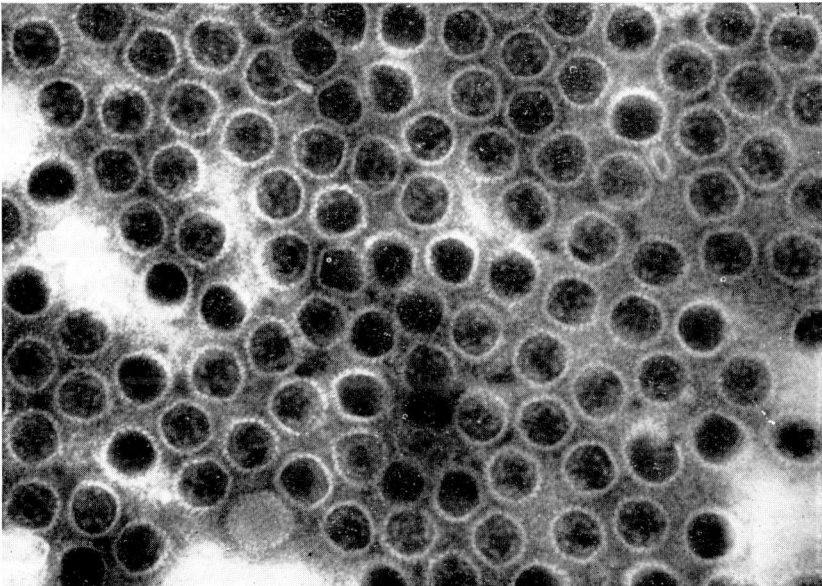

FIG. 3. Electron micrograph of cytomegalovirus capsid formation in the nucleus of an infected tissue culture cell ($\times$ 100,000).

C

envelope (Smith and Rasmussen, 1963; Wright *et al.*, 1964; Crawford and Lee, 1964). The overall diameter is 150–190 mμ. The virus is relatively labile, and specimens for virus isolation should be taken into a suitable transport medium and cultured within a few hours of collection. Freezing is best avoided. In a transport medium containing 10 per cent serum and 25 per cent sorbitol, the virus usually remains infective at 4°C for at least 24 hours.

Replication of the virus takes place in the nucleus of the infected cell with formation of the characteristic intranuclear inclusion body (Luse and Smith, 1958; Stern and Friedmann, 1960; Goodheart *et al.*, 1964). Cytoplasmic inclusions are formed by aggregation of lysosomes around virus particles that have migrated into the cytoplasm (McGavran and Smith, 1965; Ruebner *et al.*, 1965). Although the virus is predominantly epitheliotropic *in vivo*, in tissue culture paradoxically it grows only in human fibroblasts. The cytopathic effect is quite specific, with the development of focal lesions consisting of a few swollen, rounded and irregularly shaped cells which, after staining, can be seen to possess the typical intranuclear inclusion bodies (Figs. 4 and 5). On primary isolation the initial lesions appear usually within five to seven days and then progress slowly over a period of several weeks to involve the greater part of the cell sheet. The bulk of the virus remains cell-associated, but is readily liberated from the infected cells by grinding or sonic disruption.

Different strains of human cytomegalovirus show some degree of antigenic heterogeneity in cross-neutralization tests with human sera (Weller *et al.*, 1960). Antigenic analysis, however, has been handicapped by difficulty in preparing typing antisera in animals, although this has recently been achieved in monkeys (Plummer and Benyesh-Melnick, 1964). As yet it is not certain whether the antigenic differences are sufficiently great to warrant division into distinct serotypes. Fortunately, the human viruses possess common group-specific complement-fixing antigens (Medearis, 1964; Stern and Elek, 1965). This facilitates the identification of fresh isolates and provides a method for routine serological diagnosis.

EPIDEMIOLOGY

Serological surveys have now clearly shown that infection with cyto-megalovirus is common both in children and adults. In London, infection appears to be relatively infrequent in early childhood, since only 6 per cent of children aged 6 months to 5 years have complement-fixing antibodies, but thereafter antibodies become increasingly prevalent to reach maximum frequency by 25–35 years of age (Stern and Elek, 1965; Table I). The bulk of infection occurs, therefore, in schoolchildren and young adults. Very similar findings have been obtained by Hanshaw (1966a) in Rochester, New York, but elsewhere the incidence of infection has often been much higher, especially in pre-school children. Thus, in Washington, D.C., and in Puerto Rico anti-bodies were found in 25–35 per cent of 5-year-old children, and in 70–80 per cent of adults over 35 (Rowe *et al.*, 1956; Mendez-Cashion *et al.*, 1963). In fact, the incidence of infection varies widely among small children of different countries, ranging from 15 per cent in Virginia to as high as 85 per cent in Egypt (Rowe, 1960). Similar results had been obtained in earlier

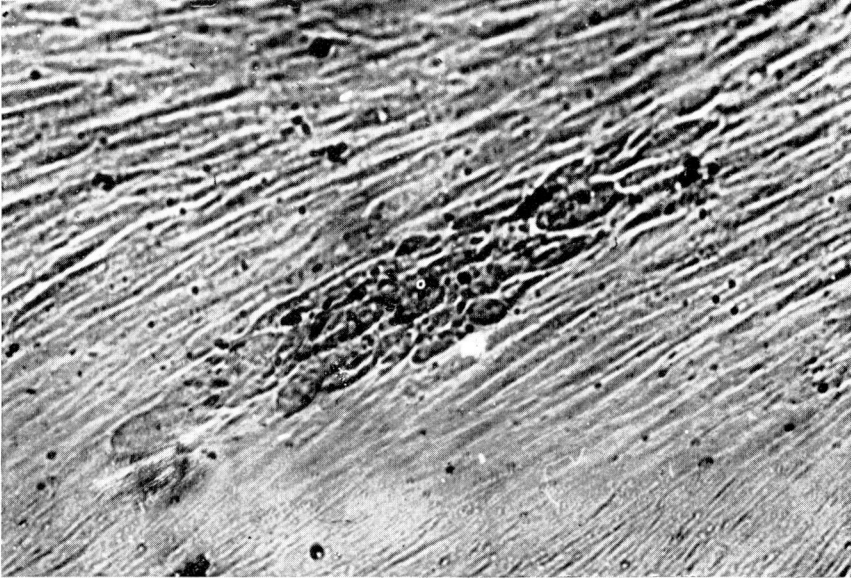

FIG. 4. Cytopathic effect of human cytomegalovirus in human embryonic lung fibroblasts (× 260).

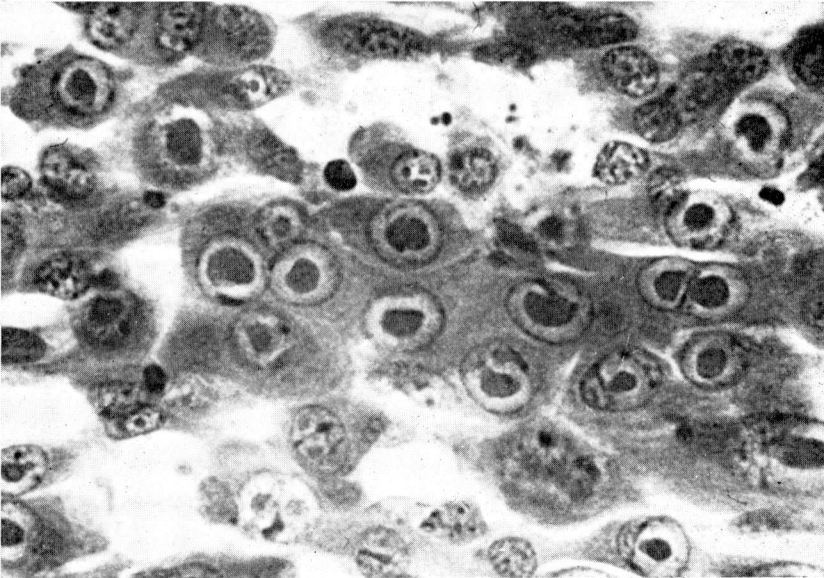

FIG. 5. H. and E. stained monolayer of cytomegalovirus-infected fibroblasts, showing characteristic intranuclear inclusion bodies (× 700).

histological studies which had demonstrated cytomegalic cells in the salivary glands of 5–12 per cent of unselected pædiatric autopsies in Britain, Europe and the United States as compared with 18 and 32 per cent in Venezuela and Indonesia (Farber and Wolbach, 1932; McCordock and Smith, 1934; Prawirohardjo, 1938; Potenza, 1954; Baar, 1955; Seifert and Oehme, 1957). These differences are almost certainly dependent on socio-economic status. As with herpes and poliovirus, improved living standards and hygiene reduce the chances of infection in early childhood, and the first large increase in infection occurs in older children when they come together at school.

The frequency of infection in neonates and in infants under 6 months old cannot be determined by serology because of the high frequency of maternal antibodies. These indicate only infection in the mother at some time in the past, although some of these infections occur during gestation as shown in the United States by Sever *et al.* (1963), who found antibody conversion in

TABLE I

*Incidence in London of Cytomegalovirus
Complement-fixing Antibodies*

Age-groups (years)	No. positive / No. tested	Percentage positive
$<\frac{1}{2}$	3/9	33
$\frac{1}{2}$–4	11/184	6
5–9	15/97	15
10–14	54/257	21
15–24	47/130	36
25–34	62/114	54
35–75	46/85	54

as many as 6 per cent of pregnant women. We isolated virus from 3 per cent of 118 randomly selected and apparently healthy newborn babies in the Maternity Unit of St. George's Hospital, London, and from 10 per cent of unselected admissions to the pædiatric wards in the age-group 2–6 months (Table II). Most of the latter infections were probably acquired post-natally and were benign. Two of the neonatal excreters, on the other hand, subsequently developed symptoms of brain damage, but without typical symptoms of the classical neonatal disease.

Newborn babies who survive intra-uterine infection go on excreting virus in the throat and urine for periods as long as two to three years or more (Weller and Hanshaw, 1962). This is also the case when small children are infected. We collected urine and throat swabs from unselected admissions to two London general hospitals and cultured them for cytomegalovirus; 10 per cent of children between 2 months and 5 years of age were found to be excreting virus (Table II), and some of these children, apparently healthy, are still doing so after two years. On the other hand, although infection is known to be common, from the serological studies, in schoolchildren and adults only a single excreter, aged 6, was detected out of 101 children

5–10 years old, and none was found among the older children and adults. Similar results have been reported elsewhere (Rowe *et al.*, 1958; Benyesh-Melnick *et al.*, 1964b). Why healthy infants and children under 5 or 6 years of age should deal less efficiently with cytomegalovirus infection than their elders is obscure. Prolonged excretion of virus occurs in these children despite high levels of neutralizing antibody in the blood, and the finding of cytomegalic cells in the salivary glands appears to be associated with the carrier state. It cannot yet be entirely excluded, however, that transient excretion of virus occurs in the subclinical infection of older individuals. It would be difficult to detect this in epidemiological surveys in which only single specimens were examined.

When primary infection occurs in adults with immunological defects (Jacox *et al.*, 1964) or undergoing intensive immuno-suppressive therapy for

TABLE II

Excretion of Cytomegalovirus in Unselected
Neonates and Hospital Admissions in London

Age-groups	No. positive / No. tested	Percentage positive
neonates	3/118	3
2–5 months	3/32	10
$\frac{1}{2}$–4 years	10/104	10
5–9 years	1/101	1
10–14 years	0/72	...
15–24 years	0/102	...
25–34 years	0/100	...
35–59 years	0/100	...
60+ years	0/100	...

leukæmia or renal homotransplantation (Duvall *et al.*, 1966; Kanich and Craighead, 1966), they do excrete virus and for prolonged periods. Prolonged virus excretion has also been reported in apparently healthy mothers who had given birth to infants with cytomegalic inclusion disease, and disturbances of steroid metabolism may be a factor here (Medearis, 1964; Frank *et al.*, 1966). Although these women may continue to excrete virus for long periods, even into the early months of the next pregnancy, their antibody is fully protective and there is no evidence for the occurrence of subsequent congenital infections.

Small children who are long-term excreters of virus probably constitute the main reservoir of infection in the community. Spread is presumably mainly respiratory, particularly in view of the frequency of pulmonary lesions in fatal cases of disease (Wong and Warner, 1962). The relatively low incidence of cytomegalovirus antibodies in young children as compared with other virus antibodies, such as those to herpes simplex, suggests that the cytomegalovirus does not spread easily, perhaps because of its lability in the extracellular environment, and that close and prolonged contact may be necessary for effective cross-infection. High infection rates are seen in institutionalized populations and boarding schools and among family contacts (Weller and Hanshaw, 1962; Rowe *et al.*, 1958; Stern and Elek, 1965). Indeed, when one virus excreter is recognized, then almost certainly siblings and other close family contacts under 6 years of age will also be found to be excreting virus (Stern *et al.*, 1963; Stern and Tucker, 1965; Hanshaw *et al.*, 1965).

The continuing high incidence of complement-fixing antibodies in the population beyond 35 years of age suggests, by analogy with herpes simplex, that infection is followed by persistence of the virus in the body in a latent form. However, at present there is no evidence for recurrent reactivations of cytomegalovirus infection in healthy persons, as occurs with herpes simplex, but activation of latent infection has been invoked to explain the occurrence of cytomegalic inclusion disease as a complication of diseases and treatments which depress the defence mechanisms of the body (Nelson and Wyatt, 1959). There is good evidence for this in the frequency with which cytomegalic cells are found in fatal cases of renal homotransplantation; the high incidence of 50 per cent correlates well with the incidence of complement-fixing antibodies in the general population (Hill *et al.*, 1964; Rifkind, 1965; Kanich and Craighead, 1966). Some of these cases are, however, primary exogenous infections, as shown by the development of antibodies during the course of the patient's illness (Rifkind, 1965; Duvall *et al.*, 1966).

CLINICAL FEATURES

Neonatal Diseases

The classical syndrome of neonatal cytomegalic inclusion disease, which follows infection *in utero*, presents at birth or shortly afterwards with jaundice, thrombocytopenic purpura, severe erythroblastic or hæmolytic anæmia, hepatosplenomegaly, pneumonitis and often evidence of neural damage which may be associated with periventricular calcification, microcephaly and choroidoretinitis. About half the cases are premature, and most have a low birth weight. Jaundice, typically of the direct-reacting, regurgitation type, may persist with fluctuating intensity for several months, but the purpura usually clears up fairly quickly. Hepatosplenomegaly is an almost invariable feature and can persist for a year or longer. Choroidoretinitis and periventricular calcification are found in about a quarter of the cases, and the latter is pathognomonic of cytomegalovirus infection. Liver biopsy may be diagnostic by demonstrating the presence of cytomegalic cells, but these can be very scanty or apparently absent even when the virus is readily isolated from the biopsy material; the histological features include nuclear and cellular swelling, focal necrosis, round-cell infiltration and bile stasis. Giant-cell transformation occurs in some cases, and the clinical and histological features may closely conform to Craig and Landing's criteria for a diagnosis of neonatal giant-cell hepatitis (Weller and Hanshaw, 1962; Stulberg *et. al.*, 1966).

The disease is not infrequently fatal, but probably most cases survive. While complete recovery is possible, the majority have residual abnormalities due to brain damage, of which the most important are mental deficiency and microcephaly. These were present in 29 out of 37 surviving cases studied in the United States (Weller and Hanshaw, 1962; Medearis, 1964; Hanshaw,

1966b). Microcephaly may be obvious at birth, but often does not become apparent until after some weeks or even months. Other residual abnormalities are epilepsy, cerebral palsies, hydrocephalus, blindness and deafness.

Occasionally disease does not become manifest until the post-neonatal period, between 1 and 4 months of age or later. There may have been uneventful progress until then, but often there is a history of transient respiratory distress at birth or of failure to thrive. The symptoms are more variable and ill-defined than in the neonate, and are often those of pneumonitis, which resists treatment with antibiotics, or of gastro-intestinal involvement with intractable vomiting and diarrhœa. Hepatosplenomegaly, jaundice and purpuric or maculo-papular rashes may also occur (Smith and Vellios, 1950; Wyatt et. al., 1950; Medearis, 1957; Handshaw, 1966b). It may be difficult in these cases to decide whether the infection is congenital or acquired after birth. Periventricular calcification, when present, is good evidence for long-standing and therefore probably intra-uterine infection. Some cases, however, have underlying debilitating diseases, such as fibrocystic disease of the pancreas, which might have been responsible for converting what would have been an otherwise minor and localized post-natal infection into disseminated disease. Subclinical infections undoubtedly occur in the post-neonatal period. We have isolated cytomegalovirus from three infants, aged 2–5 months, who showed no evidence of cytomegalic inclusion disease (Table II). One of these has thalassæmia major, but, after splenectomy, has made good progress. The other two, aged 2 and 3 months, had been admitted to hospital with a group-A-streptococcal sore throat and chickenpox respectively. They were still excreting virus six months later, but apart from a slightly raised serum alkaline phosphatase in the younger infant they have shown completely normal physical and mental development. Congenital disease presenting in the post-neonatal period is, however, often fatal and survival may be followed as in typical neonatal cases, by mental retardation and microcephaly (Hanshaw, 1966b).

Clinical neonatal disease, as described above, is comparatively uncommon. Virus isolation studies, however, provide direct evidence that fœtal infection is more common than previously suspected, and occurs without the severe symptoms of the classical neonatal syndrome (Stern 1968).

At St. George's Hospital, urine and throat swabs were collected on the day of birth from 118 apparently healthy babies. Three were found to be excreting virus (Table II). One of these developed a scanty petechial rash on the face and head some hours after birth, but this rapidly disappeared and no other abnormalities were found. After 3 months, however, she was recognized to be mentally retarded and microcephalic. The second infant had a normal birth, and the only abnormality was some disturbance of liver function tests which persisted until 6 months of age. At 2 years he is a perfectly healthy child despite continuing virus excretion. We have previously seen a very similar case (Stern and Tucker, 1965). The third infant was also apparently well at birth but at 3 months showed a marked degree of generalised muscular hypotonia which persisted. At 2 years he is obviously retarded both physically and mentally. These less-conspicuous forms of neonatal infection, therefore, may be followed by complete recovery, but also, as in the classical sydrome, by serious damage to the central nervous system.

Cytomegaloviruses are undoubtedly important causes of brain damage in early life, and may prove to be the single most important cause of microcephaly. Hanshaw (1966a), in a retrospective study of non-institutionalized mentally deficient children, demonstrated antibody in 18/41 (44 per cent) children with microcephaly, this proportion being significantly higher than in the mentally deficient cases who were normocephalic (3·9 per cent) or in normal control children of the same age-group. Two of the 18 had experienced transient jaundice or purpura after birth and four had periventricular calcification, but none of them gave a typical history of neonatal cytomegalic inclusion disease. The preliminary results from a comparable study in London have been very similar to those of Hanshaw (Stern, 1965). In view of the fact that entirely symptomless intra-uterine infection has not been recorded (Rowe *et al.*, 1958; Weller and Hanshaw, 1962; Medearis, 1964) virus excretion in the neonate must be looked on with grave suspicion, particularly with regard to subsequent mental development.

True developmental malformations of the central nervous system have also been described following infection of the fœtus early in gestation, namely micropolygyria and porencephaly (Hartmann, 1948; Diezel, 1954; Born, 1955; Verron, 1955; Marie *et al.*, 1957; Wolf and Cowen, 1959; Nelson and Wyatt, 1959; Crome, 1961). Although virus has been isolated from some newborn infants with congenital heart disease and congenital biliary atresia (McAllister *et al.*, 1964; Benyesh-Melnick *et al.*, 1964a; Stern and Tucker, 1965), there is as yet insufficient evidence to incriminate it as a cause of congenital abnormalities outside the nervous system. Nevertheless, the close similarities in the pathogenesis and clinical manifestations with congenital rubella indicate the need for continuing investigation of the teratogenic potentialities of cytomegalovirus infection.

Acquired Cytomegalovirus Infections

Infection with cytomegalovirus outside the neonatal period is probably mostly subclinical. However, two clinical syndromes have now been recognized: liver disease in children and an atypical Paul-Bunnell-negative form of infectious mononucleosis in adults. There is also a suspicion that respiratory symptoms are a further manifestation of primary infection, particularly in view of the frequency of pulmonary involvement when cytomegalovirus infection complicates diseases and therapy which seriously depress immunity. A history of episodes of pneumonia or influenza-like illnesses in early pregnancy has been obtained from women who have given birth to cases of neonatal cytomegalic inclusion disease (Weller and Hanshaw, 1962; Medearis, 1964). Seven out of the 13 children, aged 2 months to 6 years, who were found to be excreting cytomegalovirus (Table II) had been admitted to hospital with respiratory disease; two were diagnosed clinically as croup, and two others with radiological evidence of pneumonitis as whooping-cough. No other bacterial or viral cause was found for their symptoms. Hanshaw (1966b) has also described pneumonitis occasionally resembling whooping-cough in small children excreting cytomegalovirus. However, respiratory illnesses are extremely common, and more evidence is required before cytomegalovirus infection can be firmly linked ætiologically with respiratory disease in otherwise healthy children or adults.

Liver Disease. Primary cytomegalovirus infection in young children is followed by prolonged virus excretion in the throat and urine. Rowe *et al.* (1958) first showed, in Washington, that many of these children, although outwardly well, have such abnormalities as hepatomegaly, splenomegaly, spider angiomata and abnormal liver function tests. Hanshaw *et al.* (1965) isolated cytomegalovirus from the urine of 20 apparently healthy children, aged 2–7 years, during the course of a survey in Rochester, N.Y.; 14 of these had hepatomegaly, five had splenomegaly, two had spider angiomata and 17 of 19 children examined had abnormal liver function tests. We isolated virus from 29 children between 6 months and 8 years of age in surveys in London, and thirteen of twenty tested had abnormal liver function (Stern 1968). These findings indicate that chronic infection in children may be clinically significant, with selective damage to the liver. The children are often without subjective symptoms, but the liver damage can be sufficiently severe to cause manifest illness. Twenty-four children with unexplained liver disease were recently referred to us for virus studies, and cytomegalovirus was isolated from three of them. These, aged 4, 5 and 8 years, had each presented with a febrile illness which in one case was followed by jaundice. On examination they were found to have hepatosplenomegaly and abnormal liver function tests. A four-fold rise in cytomegalovirus antibody was demonstrated during the course of the illness in two of the cases, while a serum specimen taken from the third case a month after onset showed a high complement-fixing antibody titre. Hanshaw *et al.* (1965) also examined 23 children with unexplained hepatomegaly or chronic liver disease and demonstrated virus excretion in nine (39 per cent), a significantly higher proportion than in control healthy children. Liver disease is often of obscure ætiology in children, and cytomegalovirus must now be considered in the differential diagnosis. Most of the above children seemed to recover completely. Some may, however, progress to cirrhosis and die (Hanshaw *et al.*, 1965).

Cytomegalovirus Mononucleosis. This was first described in 1965 by Klemola and Kääriäinen in Finland, and we have since seen nine cases (Anderson and Stern, 1966; Lamb and Stern, 1966; Stern, 1968). The clinical picture is that of a febrile illness of three to six weeks' duration associated with blood changes typical of infectious mononucleosis, namely a relative and absolute lymphocytosis with an abundance of abnormal "glandular fever" cells. The blood changes may be delayed until the second week of illness, but they persist for some weeks. The Paul-Bunnell reaction, however, remains persistently negative. Early symptoms include headache and pains in the neck, back or limbs, and cough is commonly present. Unlike other forms of infectious mononucleosis, exudative pharyngitis is absent and there is usually no lymphadenopathy. Hepatosplenomegaly may or may not occur, but liver function tests have invariably been abnormal. Frank jaundice is probably unusual, but we have seen two such cases. One presented clinically as infectious hepatitis with severe jaundice and liver enlargement, before subsequently developing the typical glandular fever-like blood picture. The other case had had a myocardial infarction. One month after this he became febrile and developed an extensive erythematous eruption, followed, after some days, by jaundice, liver enlargement and the characteristic blood picture Toghill *et al.*, 1697). Other cases have presented with polyneuritis or pericarditis (Ironside and Tobin, 1967; Räsänen and Saikku, 1967). Diagnosis is made by demonstrating a four-fold increase in cytomegalovirus complement-fixing antibody during the course of the illness; peak titres may not be reached until four to six weeks, after onset of symptoms. We have isolated virus from urine and throat in six of the nine cases during convalescence and excretion may continue for three months or more.

Paul-Bunnell-positive and Paul-Bunnell-negative forms of infectious mononucleosis are probably of different ætiology (Belfrage, 1962), and we have failed to show cytomegalovirus infection in over 50 cases of the sero-positive disease. The sero-negative syndrome is certainly of multiple ætiology, now recognized to include toxoplasmosis (Siim, 1951; Beverley and Beattie, 1958), Q fever (Eshchar et al., 1966) and cytomegalovirus infection. Clinically the latter is distinctive in the absence of exudative pharyngitis and lymph-adenopathy, whereas glandular enlargement is characteristic of the toxo-plasmosis and Q-fever illnesses. The age incidence of cytomegalovirus mononucleosis may also be different (Stern, 1968).

We have examined 75 patients diagnosed clinically as Paul-Bunnell-negative infectious mononucleosis; 48 were between the ages of 10 and 29; and the majority of these had enlarged lymph glands and none showed a rising titre of cytomegalovirus antibody. Twenty-seven were aged 30–60, and nine proved to be cases of cyto-megalovirus mononucleosis; eight of them were between 30 and 38 years old and the ninth was 56. The majority of the cases described by Klemola and Kääriäinen (1965) were also in their thirties. How characteristic this age distribution is remains to be seen. The syndrome has, in fact, been described in a 2-year-old girl (Klemola et al., 1966). She developed a prolonged febrile illness with pains and swelling of joints and a widespread red skin rash. There was no tonsillitis or lymphadenopathy, but there was radiological evidence of pneumonitis. The liver was slightly enlarged and liver function tests were abnormal. Two weeks after onset of symptoms typical glandular fever-like changes appeared in the blood with many abnormal mononuclears, which persisted for two weeks. The Paul-Bunnell was persistently negative, but there was a rise in cytomegalovirus antibodies. She recovered after three to four weeks and was well until she contracted measles four months later. This was followed by a recrudescence of the original illness including the blood changes, but this time with marked hepatosplenomegaly and thrombocytopenia. She again recovered, but the hepatosplenomegaly remained for six months and there was prolonged viruria. Liver damage is, of course, a common manifestation of cytomegalovirus infection in small children, but most cases do not seem to develop infectious mononucleosis-like blood changes (Hanshaw et al., 1965; Stern and Tucker, 1965).

The clinical syndrome of atypical, Paul-Bunnell-negative infectious mononucleosis has long been recognized also as a complication of open-heart surgery and other operations requiring massive transfusions of fresh blood (Smith, 1964; Bastin et al., 1965; Reyman, 1966). The incidence of this complication is 3–10 per cent. Some weeks after operation the patient becomes febrile with such symptoms as splenomegaly, hepatomegaly and maculo-papular rashes. He develops the blood picture of infectious mono-nucleosis, and liver function tests are usually abnormal. Some of these cases, at least, are caused by cytomegalovirus, infection probably occurring with the large blood transfusions from multiple donors (Kääriäinen et al., 1966a, b). Such infection may indeed be common, since Kääriäinen and his colleagues could demonstrate the appearance of antibodies in nine out of 21 patients who had no antibody prior to their open-heart operations; eight of these infections, however, were entirely subclinical. This high incidence of transmission of infection indicates the widespread nature of cytomegalovirus infection with active viræmia in the community.

Opportunistic Infections

Prior to 1962 only 54 cases of cytomegalic inclusion disease had been recorded outside early childhood (Wong and Warner, 1962). These occurred mainly as complications of debilitating diseases, such as leukæmia and lymphoma, which seriously depress the defence mechanisms of the body, especially when steroids and other immuno-suppressive drugs were used in treatment. They were diagnosed, usually unexpectedly, at post-mortem or occasionally in biopsy specimens taken for other purposes. Since then, the disease has become relatively common because of the increasing use of intensive immuno-suppressive therapy, and it is now often diagnosed during life by virus isolation. Thus, at the National Institutes of Health in Washington, disseminated cytomegalic inclusion disease was recognized only twice among 394 autopsies on children who had died of leukæmia in the ten years preceding 1962, but in the single following year there were 11 cases among 71 autopsies (Bodey *et al.*, 1965). Others have reported similar findings in fatal cases of childhood leukæmia (Cangir and Sullivan, 1966), while active infection has been demonstrated by virus isolation from throat and urine in as many as a third of adults undergoing treatment with steroids and cytotoxic drugs for leukæmia and Hodgkin's disease (Duvall *et al.*, 1966; Craighead *et al.*, 1967). Patients under immuno-suppressive therapy for renal transplantation are at hazard from opportunistic infections, and pulmonary or disseminated cytomegalic inclusion disease is found in over 50 per cent of those who come to post-mortem (Hill *et al.*, 1964; Rifkind, 1965; Kanich and Craighead, 1966). It seems likely that such therapy causes reactivation of latent infection with resulting dissemination and disease, as is well established for other herpesviruses (Rifkind, 1965; Kanich and Craighead, 1966). Some cases, however, do follow primary exogenous infection, as shown by the development of antibodies during treatment (Rifkind, 1965; Duvall *et al.*, 1966). Primary infections are common in both adults and children, and in patients on immuno-suppressive therapy these otherwise minor or subclinical infections become serious diseases. The incidence of cytomegalovirus excretion in children with leukæmia is no greater than in normal children of the same age, but disseminated disease is more likely to develop (Benyesh-Melnick *et al.*, 1964a).

When disseminated cytomegalic inclusion disease occurs in adults, the commonest sites of lesions are the lungs, adrenals, liver, gastro-intestinal tract, spleen, pancreas and kidneys in that order, while parotid involvement has not been recorded (Wong and Warner, 1962). This contrasts with neonatal cytomegalic inclusion disease in which the kidneys and parotids are almost invariably affected. When the disease is localized it involves usually the lungs or the gastro-intestinal tract. Gastro-intestinal tract disease, unlike either the disseminated or localized pulmonary forms, has been described mostly in patients who have not had underlying reticulo-endothelial disease nor been subjected to intensive immuno-suppressive therapy. The cyto-megalic cells have ordinarily been confined to the stomach or some part of the intestines around chronic ulcerative or granulomatous lesions, such as chronic gastric and duodenal ulcers and ulcerative colitis (Wong and Warner, 1962; Levine *et al.*, 1964). It has been suggested that the cytomegalovirus may be of ætiological significance in these ulcerative lesions, particularly as some cases responded to resection or gamma-globulin treatment (Levine *et al.*, 1964). However, most of the patients were debilitated by prolonged illness and had received some treatment with steroids, so that it is difficult to exclude the possibility of reactivation of latent infection or even primary infection with localization of virus activity at sites of chronic inflammation. A similar explanation could account for the rare reports of finding cytomegalic cells in otherwise healthy persons in localized granulomatous lesions of the orbit, nasal vestibule or anus, in a benign adenolymphoma of the parotid gland and in a cervical biopsy taken because of vaginal discharge (Wong and Warner, 1962; Symmers, 1960; Ross, 1966).

The clinical significance of the complicating cytomegalovirus infection and its influence on the course of the primary disease are still uncertain. In one series of adults who were being treated for leukæmia and Hodgkin's disease no obvious clinical differences were demonstrable between those who were excreting virus and those who were not (Duvall *et al.*, 1966). However, there is often no adequate explanation for episodes of fever, pneumonia, vomiting and diarrhœa, hepatosplenomegaly or hæmorrhagic disorders in treated patients who seem to be in leukæmic remission or who have apparently functioning renal grafts (Rifkind *et al.*, 1964; Rifkind, 1965). The only pathological findings in fatal cases may be an interstitial pneumonia associated with pulmonary or disseminated formation of cytomegalic cells (Hanshaw and Weller, 1961; Hedley-White and Craighead, 1965; Cangir and Sullivan, 1966). Certainly, untoward symptoms in patients with diseases or on therapy known to depress the defence mechanisms of the body should arouse suspicion of opportunistic infection, and indicate the need for extensive virological and bacteriological investigations.

DIAGNOSIS AND TREATMENT

The clinical picture of neonatal cytomegalic inclusion disease may closely resemble other congenital diseases such as rubella, toxoplasmosis or herpesvirus infection, as well as erythroblastosis fœtalis, congenital syphilis, neonatal sepsis and biliary atresia. Moreover, the syndrome may be incomplete, especially when it presents in the post-neonatal period, and congenital cytomegalovirus infection should be included in the differential diagnosis of neonatal or infantile hepatitis, hepatosplenomegaly, purpura, antibiotic-resistant pneumonia, intractable vomiting and diarrhœa or central nervous system disease particularly when associated with microcephaly and mental deficiency. Periventricular calcification, when present, is practically pathognomonic and the diagnosis can also be made by finding desquamated cytomegalic cells in the urine. Urine must be examined fresh as the cells rapidly disintegrate, and since they are usually scanty several specimens should be examined. The critical features are a single large intranuclear inclusion body separated by a clear-cut halo from a well-defined, thickened nuclear membrane (Blanc and Gaetz, 1962; Naib, 1963). However, these cells are demonstrable in only about half of neonatal cases, and they are rarely observed in older patients. The most reliable method of diagnosis is virus isolation from the urine or throat. This is readily accomplished in human embryonic fibroblasts, typical cytopathic effects appearing usually within five to ten days. The earlier in life this is achieved the greater its diagnostic value, since completely benign neonatal infection probably does not occur. In older infants infection may be post-natally acquired and incidental. A high complement-fixing antibody titre in the mother or virus isolation from her will be strong evidence for congenital infection. The absence of antibody in the mother, on the other hand, almost certainly excludes it. The antibody status of the infant is usually of little help in diagnosis. A third or more of newborn babies possess maternal antibodies which are indicative only of infection in the mother at some time in the past, while some infected infants do not start to make complement-fixing antibodies until after 3–6 months. Neutralizing antibody is almost always present early in congenitally infected infants, but the neutralization test for cytomegalovirus antibody is unsatisfactory for routine diagnosis on account of antigenic strain differences which may require the use of the patient's own virus after adaptation to tissue culture.

Cytomegalovirus infection should also be suspected in older children who have unexplained hepatomegaly, splenomegaly or liver disease. The complement-fixation test is probably most useful in the age-group 6 months to 6 or 7 years of age. The possession of complement-fixing antibody then almost invariably means active infection with excretion of virus. Nevertheless, virus isolation should also be attempted, if possible, in these cases as antibody formation is sometimes delayed for several weeks or months after onset of illness and virus excretion (Stern and Tucker, 1965; Stern, unpublished). A liver biopsy may show the presence of cytomegalic cells and confirm the diagnosis. However, since these are often scanty or even absent, some of the biopsy material should be kept for virus culture, which is a more sensitive indicator of infection (Weller and Hanshaw, 1962; Stern et al., 1963; Kanich and Craighead, 1966; Duvall et al., 1966). After early childhood the possession of complement-fixing antibody means only past infection. It is necessary to look for a rising titre of antibody during the course of illness, as in cytomegalovirus mononucleosis, or for virus excretion. The latter is rare in healthy children over 6 or 7 years old and in healthy adults and may signify disease, especially in patients on immuno-suppressive therapy or with immunological defects.

There is no specific therapy. Steroids have been used in the neonatal disease and some of these cases have recovered completely (Birdsong et al., 1956; van Gelderen, 1959; Lelong et al., 1960; Elliot and Elliot, 1962; Gear et al., 1962). However, survival is now known to occur without treatment, so that the value of steroid therapy in this disease is doubtful. Marked clinical improvement has been reported following repeated injections of pooled gamma-globulin in adults with severe cytomegalovirus infections, and further investigation of this form of treatment is indicated (Levine et al., 1964; Jacox et al., 1964).

Appendix

Further evidence of the importance of cytomegalovirus infection in the ætiology of mental deficiency was obtained from the recent study of 360 mentally retarded children in London (Stern and Elek, unpublished). These were aged 6 months to

6 years and were all living at home with their families. 11 per cent of them were found to possess cytomegalovirus complement-fixing antibodies, as compared with 6 per cent of 154 normal control children of the same ages who were examined at the same time (Table III). When the mentally retarded children were analysed according to various associated abnormalities, including epilepsy, cerebral palsy, microcephaly and hydrocephaly, the proportion of microcephalics with antibodies was found to be significantly high. These results support the findings of Hanshaw (1966) in the United States.

TABLE III

Incidence of cytomegalovirus CF antibody in non-hospitalised mentally retarded children

Main associated feature	No. of cases	+ve CF test	% +ve
Epilepsy	48	6	12·5
Cerebral palsy	39	2	5
Microcephaly	54	11	20
Hydrocephaly	25	2	8
None	194	20	10
Total	360	41	11

microcephalics $\quad$ 11/54 $\quad \left. \right\}$ $0·05 > P > 0·02$.
non-microcephalics 30/306

References

AHVENAINEN, E. K. (1952). Inclusion disease or generalised salivary gland virus infection Report of 5 cases. *Acta path. microbiol. scand.* (suppl.), **93**, 159.
ANDERSON, J. P. and STERN, H. (1966). Cytomegalovirus as a possible cause of a disease resembling infectious mononucleosis. *Brit. med. J.*, **1**, 672.
ANDREWES, C. (1964). *Viruses of Vertebrates*, London, Baillière, Tindall and Cox, p. 236.
BAAR, H. S. (1955). Interstitial plasmacellular pneumonia due to Pneumocystis carinii. *J. clin. Path.*, **8**, 19.
BASTIN, R., LAPRESLE, C. and DUFRENE, F. (1965). Syndrome fébrile avec réaction sanguine mononucléosique après chirurgie thoracique. *Presse Méd.*, **73**, 63.
BELFRAGE, S. (1962). Infectious mononucleosis. An epidemiological and clinical study. *Acta med. scand.*, **171**, 531.
BENYESH-MELNICK, M., DESSY, S. I. and FERNBACH, D. J. (1964a). Cytomegaloviruria in children with acute leukaemia and in other children. *Proc. Soc. exp. Biol., N.Y.*, **117**, 624.
BENYESH-MELNICK, M., ROSENBERG, H. S. and WATSON, B. (1964b). Viruses in cell cultures of kidneys of children with congenital heart malformations and other diseases. *Proc. Soc. exp. Biol., N.Y.*, **117**, 452.
BEVERLEY, J. K. A. and BEATTIE, C. P. (1958). Glandular toxoplasmosis. A survey of 30 cases. *Lancet*, **ii**, 379.
BIRDSONG, M., SMITH, D. E., MITCHELL, F. N. and COREY, J. H. (1956). Generalised cytomegalic inclusion disease in newborn infants. *J. Amer. med. Ass.*, **162**, 1305.
BLANC, W. A. and GAETZ, R. (1962). Simplified millipore filter technique for cytologic diagnosis of cytomegalic inclusion disease in examination of urine. *Pediatrics*, **29**, 51.
BODEY, G. P., WERTLAKE, P. T., DOUGLAS, G. and LEVIN, R. H. (1965). Cytomegalic inclusion disease in patients with acute leukemia. *Ann. intern. Med.*, **62**, 899.
BORN, E. (1955). Über fruhkindliche Hirnschädigung bei der Cytomegalie und ihre Abgrenzung gegenüber der Toxoplasmose. *Arch. Psychiat. Nervenkr.*, **193**, 557.
CANGIR, A. and SULLIVAN, M. P. (1966). The occurrence of cytomegalovirus infections in childhood leukemia. *J. Amer. med. Ass.*, **195**, 616.
CRAIGHEAD, J. E., HANSHAW, J. B. and CARPENTER, C. B. (1967). Cytomegalovirus infection after renal allotransplantation. *J. Amer. med. Ass.*, **201**, 725.
CRAWFORD, L. V. and LEE, A. J. (1964). The nucleic acid of human cytomegalovirus. *Virology*, **23**, 105.
CROME, L. (1961). Cytomegalic inclusion body disease. *Wld. Neurol.*, **2**, 447.

CROME, L. and FRANCE, N. E. (1959). Microgyria and cytomegalic inclusion disease in infancy. *J. clin. Path.*, **12**, 427.

DIEZEL, P. B. (1954). Mikrogyrie infolge cerebraler Speicheldrüsenvirusinfektion im Rahmen generalisierten Cytomegalie bei einem Saügling. Virchows *Arch. path. Anat.*, **325**, 109.

DUVALL, C. P., CASAZZA, A. R., GRIMLEY, P. M., CARBONE, P. P. and ROWE, W. P. (1966). Recovery of cytomegalovirus from adults with neoplastic disease. *Ann. intern. Med.*, **64**, 531.

ELLIOT, G. B. and ELLIOT, K. A. (1962). Observations on cerebral cytomegalic inclusion disease of the fœtus and newborn. *Arch. Dis. Childh.*, **37**, 34.

ESHCHAR, J., WARON, M. and ALKAN, W. J. (1966). Syndromes of Q fever. *J. Amer. med. Ass.*, **195**, 390.

FARBER, S. and WOLBACH, S. B. (1932). Intranuclear and cytoplasmic inclusions ("protozoan-like bodies") in salivary glands and other organs of infants. *Amer. J. Path.*, **8**, 123.

FRANK, D. J., DE VAUX, W. D., PERKINS, J. R. and PERRIN, E. V. (1966). Fetal ascites and cytomegalic inclusion disease. *Amer. J. Dis. Childh.*, **112**, 604.

FRUHLING, L., KORN, R., PORTE, A. and FRANCFORT, C. (1960). La Maladie à inclusions cytomégaliques. *Ann. Anat. path. med.-chir.*, **5**, 153.

GEAR, J., LE ROUX, A. F., KESSEL, I. and SICHEL, R. (1962). Generalised cytomegalic inclusion disease. A review and a report of the isolation of virus from cases occurring in Johannesburg. *S. Afr. med. J.*, **36**, 8.

GELDEREN, H. H. VAN (1959). Successfully treated case of cytomegalic disease in a newborn infant. *Acta pædiat. (Uppsala)*, **48**, 169.

GOODHEART, C. R., MCALLISTER, R. M. and FILBERT, J. E. (1964). Human cytomegalovirus. DNA synthesis and migration in infected cells studied autoradiographically. *Virology.* **23**, 603.

HANSHAW, J. B. (1966a). Cytomegalovirus complement-fixing antibody in microcephaly. *New Engl. J. Med.*, **275**, 476.

HANSHAW, J. B. (1966b). Congenital and acquired cytomegalovirus infection. *Pediat. Clin. N. Amer.*, **13**, 279.

HANSHAW, J. B., BETTS, R. F., SIMON, G. and BOYNTON, R. C. (1965). Acquired cytomegalovirus infection. Associated with hepatomegaly and abnormal liver function tests. *New Engl. J. Med.*, **272**, 602.

HANSHAW, J. B. and WELLER, T. H. (1961). Urinary excretion of cytomegaloviruses by children with generalized neoplastic disease. *J. Pediat.*, **58**, 305.

HARTMANN, G. (1948). Über die "protozoenartigen Zellen" in den Organen Neugeborener. *Klin. Med. (Wien)* 3, **281**, 344.

HEDLEY-WHYTE, E. T. and CRAIGHEAD, J. E. (1965). Generalized cytomegalic inclusion disease after renal homotransplantation. *New Engl. J. Med.*, **272**, 473.

HILL, R. B., ROWLANDS, D. T. and RIFKIND, D. (1964). Infectious pulmonary disease in patients receiving immunosuppressive therapy for organ transplantation. *New Engl. J. Med.*, **271**, 1021.

IRONSIDE, A. G. and TOBIN, J. O'H. (1967). Cytomegalovirus infection in the adult. *Lancet*, **ii**, 615.

JACOX, R. F., MONGAN, E. S., HANSHAW, J. B. and LEDDY, J. P. (1964). Hypogammaglobulinemia with thymoma and probable pulmonary infection with cytomegalovirus. *New Engl. J. Med.*, **271**, 1091.

KÄÄRIÄINEN, L., KLEMOLA, E. and PALOHEIMO, J. (1966a). Rise of cytomegalovirus antibodies in an infectious-mononucleosis-like syndrome after transfusion. *Brit. med. J.*, **i**, 1270.

KÄÄRIÄINEN, L., PALOHEIMO, J., KLEMOLA, E., MÄKELÄ, T. and KOIVUNIEMI, A. (1966b). Cytomegalovirus-mononucleosis. Isolation of the virus and demonstration of subclinical infections after fresh blood transfusion in connection with open-heart surgery. *Ann. Med. exp. Biol. Fenn.*, **44**, 297.

KANICH, R. E. and CRAIGHEAD, J. E. (1966). Cytomegalovirus infection and cytomegalic inclusion disease in renal homotransplant recipients. *Amer. J. Med.*, **40**, 874.

KLEMOLA, E. and KÄÄRIÄINEN, L. (1965). Cytomegalovirus as a possible cause of a disease resembling infectious mononucleosis. *Brit. med. J.*, **ii**, 1099.

KLEMOLA, E., SALMI, I., KÄÄRIÄINEN, L. and KOIVUNIEMI, A. (1966). Hepatosplenomegaly after "cytomegalovirus mononucleosis" in a child. *Ann. Pædiat. Fenn.*, **12**, 39.

LAMB, S. G. and STERN, H. (1966). Cytomegalovirus mononucleosis with jaundice as presenting sign. *Lancet*, **ii**, 1003.

LELONG, M., LEPAGE, F., LE-TAN-VINH, TOURNIER, P. and CHANY, C. (1960). Le virus de la maladie des inclusions cytomégaliques. *Arch. franç. Pédiat.*, **17**, 437.

LEVINE, R. S., WARNER, N. E. and JOHNSON, C. F. (1964). Cytomegalic inclusion disease in the gastro-intestinal tract of adults. *Ann. Surg.*, **159**, 37.

LÖWENSTEIN, C. (1907). Über protozoenartige Gebilde in den Organen von Kindern. *Zbl. allg. Path. path. Anat.*, **18**, 513.
LUSE, S. A. and SMITH, M. G. (1958). Electron microscopy of salivary gland viruses. *J. exp. Med.*, **107**, 623.
MCALLISTER, R. M., WRIGHT, H. T. and TASEM, W. M. (1964). Cytomegalic inclusion disease in newborn twins. *J. Pediat.*, **64**, 278.
MCCORDOCK, H. A. and SMITH, M. G. (1934). Intranuclear inclusions: incidence and possible significance in whooping-cough and a variety of other conditions. *Amer. J. Dis. Child.*, **47**, 771.
MCGAVRAN, M. H. and SMITH, M. G. (1965). Ultrastructural, cytochemical, and microchemical observations on cytomegalovirus (salivary gland virus) infection of human cells in tissue cultures. *Exp. mol. Path.*, **4**, 1.
MARIE, J., SÉE, G., GRÜNER, J., HÉBERT, S., GENNES, J. L. and FOUQUET, J. DE (1957). Manifestations cérébrales de la maladie des inclusions cytomégaliques. *Sem. hop., Paris*, **33**, 248.
MEDEARIS, D. N. (1957). Cytomegalic inclusion disease: an analysis of the clinical features based on the literature and six additional cases. *Pediatrics*, **19**, 467.
MEDEARIS, D. N. (1964). Observations concerning human cytomegalovirus infection and disease. *Johns Hopk. Hosp. Bull.*, **114**, 181.
MENDEZ-CASHION, D., VALCARCEL, M. I., ARELLANO, R. R. DE and ROWE, W. P. (1963). Salivary gland virus antibodies in Puerto Rico. *Bol. Asoc. méd. P. Rico*, **55**, 447.
NAIB, Z. N. (1963). Cytologic diagnosis of cytomegalic inclusion-body disease. *Amer. J. Dis. Childh.*, **105**, 153.
NELSON, J. S. and WYATT, J. P. (1959). Salivary gland virus disease. *Medicine (Baltimore)*, **38**, 223.
PLUMMER, G. and BENYESH-MELNICK, M. (1964). A plaque reduction neutralisation test for human cytomegalovirus. *Proc. Soc. exp. Biol., N.Y.*, **117**, 145.
POTENZA, L. (1954). Cytomegaly ("protozoa-like cells") in South American children. *Amer. J. clin. Path. (suppl.)*: Program of the International Congress of Clinical Pathology, Washington, D.C., **24**, 43.
POTTER, E. L. (1957). Placental transmission of viruses. With especial reference to the intra-uterine origin of cytomegalic inclusion body disease. *Amer. J. Obstet. Gynec.*, **74**, 505.
PRAWIROHARDJO, S. (1938). Een onderzoek naar het voorkomen van zoogenaamde protozoaire cellen in de organen van kinderen te Batavia. *Ned. T. Geneesk.*, **52**, 6218.
RÄSÄNEN, V. and SAIKKU, P. (1967). Cytomegalovirus hepatitis. *Lancet*, **ii**, 772.
REYMAN, T. A. (1966). Postperfusion syndrome. *Amer. Heart J.*, **72**, 116.
RIFKIND, D. (1965). Cytomegalovirus infection after renal transplantation. *Arch. intern. Med.*, **116**, 554.
RIFKIND, D., MARCHIORO, T. L., WADDELL, W. R. and STARZL, T. E. (1964). Infectious diseases associated with renal homotransplantation. *J. Amer. med. Ass.*, **189**, 397.
ROSS, L. (1966). Incidental finding of cytomegalovirus inclusions in cervical glands. *Amer. J. Obstet. Gynec.*, **95**. 956.
ROWE, W. P. (1960). Adenovirus and salivary gland virus infections in children. In *Viral Infections in Infancy and Childhood*, edit. By H. M. Rose, P. B. Hoeber, Inc., New York, p. 205.
ROWE W. P., HARTLEY, J. W., CRAMBLETT, H. G. and MASTROTA, F. M. (1958). Detection of human salivary gland virus in mouth and urine of children. *Amer. J. Hyg.*, **67**,57.
ROWE, W. P., HARTLEY, J. W., WATERMAN, S., TURNER, H. C. and HUEBNER, R. J. (1956). Cytopathogenic agent resembling human salivary gland virus recovered from tissue cultures of human adenoids. *Proc. Soc. exp. Biol., N.Y.*, **92**, 418.
RUEBNER, B. H., HIRANO, T., SLUSSER, R. J. and MEDEARIS, D. N. (1965). Human cytomegalovirus infection. Electron microscopic and histochemical changes in cultures of human fibroblasts. *Amer. J. Path.*, **46**, 477.
SEIFERT, G. and OEHME, J. (1957). *Pathologie und Klinik der Cytomegalie*, Leipzig: Georg Thieme.
SEVER, J. L., HUEBNER, R. J., CASTELLANO, G. A. and BELL, J. A (1963) Serologic diagnosis "en masse" with multiple antigens. *Amer. Rev. Resp. Dis.*, **88** (suppl.), 342.
SIIM, J. C. (1951). Acquired toxoplasmosis. *J. Amer. med. Ass.*, **147**, 1641.
SMITH, D. R. (1964). A syndrome resembling infectious mononucleosis after open-heart surgery. *Brit. med. J.*, **i**, 945.
SMITH, K. O., and RASMUSSEN, L. (1963). Morphology of cytomegalovirus (salivary gland virus). *J. Bact.*, **85**, 1319.
SMITH, M. G. (1956). Propagation in tissue cultures of cytopathogenic virus from human salivary gland virus (SGV) disease. *Proc. Soc. exp. Biol., N.Y.*, **92**, 424.
SMITH, M. G. and VELLIOS, F. (1950). Inclusion disease or generalized salivary gland virus infection. *Arch. Path.*, **50**, 86?

STERN, H. (1965). Human cytomegalovirus infection. *Proc. roy. Soc. Med.*, **58**, 346.

STERN, H. (1968). Isolation of cytomegalovirus and clinical manifestations of infection at different ages. *Brit. med. J.* (In press.)

STERN, H. and ELEK, S. D. (1965). The incidence of infection with cytomegalovirus in a normal population. A serological study in Greater London. *J. Hyg. Camb.*, **63**, 79.

STERN, H. and FRIEDMANN, I. (1960). Intranuclear formation of cytomegalic inclusion disease virus. *Nature*, **188**, 768.

STERN, H., LAMBERT, H. P and SHAKESPEARE, W. G. (1963). Isolation of cytomegalovirus in an infant with an angiosarcoma. *Arch. Dis. Childh.*, **38**, 626.

STERN, H. and TUCKER, S. M. (1965). Cytomegalovirus infection in the newborn and in early childhood. Three atypical cases. *Lancet*, **ii**, 1268.

STULBERG, C. S., ZUELZER, W. W., PAGE, R. H., TAYLOR, P. E. and Brough, A. J. (1966). Cytomegalovirus infections with reference to isolations from lymph nodes and blood. *Proc. Soc. exp. Biol., N.Y.*, **123**, 976.

SYMMERS, W. ST. C. (1960). Generalized cytomegalic inclusion-body disease associated with Pneumocystis pneumonia in adults. *J. clin. Path.*, **13**, 1.

TOGHILL, P. J., BAILEY, M. E., WILLIAMS, R., ZEEGEN, R. and BOWN, R. (1967). Cytomegalovirus nepatitis in the adult. *Lancet*, **i**, 1351.

VERRON, G. (1955). Klinische Beiträge zur generalisierten Cytomegalie. Einschlubkörperchenkrankheit Speicheldrüsen-Viruskrankung. *Ann. pædiat.* (*Basel*), **185**, 293.

WELLER, T. H. and HANSHAW, J. B. (1962). Virologic and clinical observations of cytomegalic inclusion disease. *New Engl. J. Med.*, **266**, 1233.

WELLER, T. H., HANSHAW, J. B. and SCOTT, D. E. (1960). Serologic differentiation of viruses responsible for cytomegalic inclusion disease. *Virology*, **12**, 130.

WELLER, T. H., MACAULEY, J. C., CRAIG, J. M. and WIRTH, P. (1957). Isolation of intranuclear inclusion producing agents from infants with illnesses resembling cytomegalic inclusion disease. *Proc. Soc. exp. Biol., N.Y.*, **94**, 4.

WOLF, A. and COWEN D. (1959). Perinatal infections of the central nervous system. *J. Neuropath. exp. Neurol.*, **18**. 191.

WONG, T. and WARNER, N. E. (1962). Cytomegalic inclusion disease in adults. *Arch. Path.*, **74**, 403.

WRIGHT, H. T., GOODHEART, C. R. and LIELAUSIS, A. (1964). Human cytomegalovirus. Morphology by negative staining. *Virology*, **23**, 419.

WYATT, J. P., SEXTON, J., LEE, R. S. and PINKERTON, H. (1950). Generalized cytomegalic inclusion disease. *J. Pediat.*, **36**, 271.

Chapter 7

STERILIZATION, DISINFECTION AND THE PATHOLOGIST

J. C. KELSEY

IN the last edition of the Recent Advances Series the chapter on sterilization was almost entirely concerned with discussing the various methods then available, the advantages and disadvantages of each and methods of testing their efficacy. This article will be more concerned with the use of disinfectants within the hospital, but an attempt will also be made to bring up to date the information previously given on methods of sterilization and to report experience with these methods in the last few years, especially with regard to the sterilization of heat-sensitive materials. There will also be a brief discussion of commercially available pre-sterilized devices for surgical and medical use and of the sterility of some pharmaceutical preparations.

STERILIZATION TECHNIQUES

Of the methods of sterilization available to hospitals the use of dry heat, either as hot-air fan-ovens or as conveyor ovens, has changed little and continues to be simple and reliable for those materials that can withstand this treatment.

High-vacuum steam sterilizers for porous loads have been actively developed, and the value of steam injection, in the form of either a continuous bleed or intermittent pulses, during the evacuation phase as opposed to merely drawing a high pre-vacuum, has been amply confirmed. Devices are now fitted routinely which continuously monitor the partial pressure of air in the sterilizer chamber and do not allow the cycle to proceed if an unacceptable amount of air is present. A new British Standards specification 3970 : 1966 has been published and Part 1 deals with high-vacuum sterilizers for porous loads. This specification includes an air-sampling device and also defines functional performance tests. The value of the Bowie-Dick test for day-to-day use has been amply confirmed. There is still room for improvement in the general reliability of this type of equipment and the need for regular routine maintenance must be emphasized.

Sterilizers that are loaded and unloaded automatically are being installed in some large Central Sterile Supply Departments now being organized along factory lines.

Sterilizers for bottled fluids are described in Part 2 of BS 3970. This requires provision to be made for indicating the temperature from within one or more bottles identical with those comprising the load so that the effectiveness of the sterilizing cycle may be checked. There is also a requirement that the door cannot be opened until the temperature of the bottles is below 80°C, thus minimizing the danger of explosion from premature removal.

Sterilizers for unwrapped instruments and utensils are covered by Part 3 of BS 3970, and Part 4 describes sterilizers of small size, powered by electricity, for treating unwrapped instruments in clinics and surgeries where mains steam is not available. When instruments are to be sterilized wrapped, either individually, in sets, or ready laid out as in the Edinburgh trolley-top system (Bowie, Gillingham, Campbell and Gordon, 1963), high-vacuum sterilizers will be required.

Ionizing Radiation. The use of this for sterilizing heat-sensitive materials is continually expanding, especially for commercially available disposable items. A sterilization service has been made available to hospitals by the United Kingdom Atomic Energy Authority. Cartons containing small items can be sent to the Authority's laboratory for irradiation and are returned within a week (*Lancet,* 1964.)

Ethylene oxide continues to be used commercially and in certain large hospitals for special purposes. Beeby and Whitehouse (1965) described the preparation and use of a bacteriological test object, and Cunliffe (1966), in reporting experience with several commercially available ethylene oxide sterilizers, emphasized the importance of regular bacteriological monitoring if such a process is to be used with confidence. Weymes (1966) limits the use of ethylene oxide sterilizers to certain hospitals "licensed" as being able to supply the necessary supervision. A method has been described for using ethylene oxide in laboratory apparatus when the items to be sterilized are small and the procedure can be carried out and controlled by a competent bacteriologist (Kelsey, 1967).

Sub-atmospheric Steam. Further development has taken place in the use of this either by itself for disinfection or with formaldehyde for sterilization (Alder, Brown and Gillespie, 1966). Many items have now been treated without damage and it is being suggested not only for fabrics and plastic devices but also for wrapped endoscopes and electrical apparatus.

The sterilization of heat-sensitive materials still presents certain problems to the hospital pathologist although many items that used to cause trouble are now available either as disposables or made of heat-resistant plastic. None of the methods available is entirely satisfactory, and care must be exercised in deciding which to use, depending on the amount of supervision that will be available, the extent to which a slight risk of contamination may be accepted, and such operational considerations as the centralization of the more sophisticated sterilization techniques.

When neither pasteurization, low-temperature steam with formaldehyde nor ethylene oxide are available, resource may have to be made to liquid chemical agents. Of these, buffered glutaraldehyde is the most promising, although it is expensive and the material to be sterilized must be scrupulously clean (Rubbo and Gardner, 1965; Ross, 1966). The use of traditional formaldehyde cabinets, which were condemned by Nordgren as long ago as 1939, cannot be countenanced although they are still to be seen in some hospitals. As Blandy (1965) has pointed out, they, and the gum-elastic catheters for which they were largely used, belong in the museum.

The capabilities and limitations of the various methods available for sterilizing medical and surgical equipment have now largely been defined. What remains is to determine how, where and by whom each method may best be used. No item of equipment which may need to be used in a sterile condition should be designed, offered for sale or purchased without a clear understanding of how sterilization may be achieved.

Sterile Water for use in Operating Rooms

This is still best supplied in bottles sterilized by autoclaving. The large amounts of water required for some operating procedures may be provided by the use of several bottles connected together. If for any reason this is not practicable, alternatives are filters or ultraviolet water-processing apparatus. Both these methods have certain disadvantages and bottles are to be preferred wherever possible (Ministry of Health, 1966).

THE CHOICE OF DISINFECTANTS FOR USE IN HOSPITALS

From time to time the hospital pathologist is called upon to advise about a disinfectant policy or about the purchase and use of individual disinfectant agents. In an attempt to help those who are forced to undertake this unenviable task, a committee of the Public Health Laboratory Service was set up and charged in particular with inquiring into the current uses for disinfectants, the categories into which these could be divided, and what tests were proper for the evaluation of particular agents proposed for these different uses. The following discussion on the use of disinfectants in hospitals will draw very substantially from this Committee's report (1965). The results of a questionnaire sent to a number of hospitals showed quite clearly that in most hospitals no coherent policy existed and many disinfectants were used at many strengths and often for quite unsuitable purposes. More hopefully it was also clear that some few hospitals had already succeeded in devising a simple if empirical policy whereby the number of disinfectants and their concentrations were substantially reduced, with the consequent saving of confusion, trouble and expense.

The current uses of liquid disinfectants are often unsuitable or unnecessary. Liquid disinfectants are frequently used in situations where sterilization is required and for which only an adequate heat treatment (or, in the case of disposables, irradiation or ethylene oxide) could be regarded as satisfactory. Such disinfectants as pine fluids, which are known to have a narrow antimicrobial spectrum and to be inactivated by organic matter, are commonly used and it is by no means universally appreciated that many of the more sophisticated agents, such as the quaternary ammonium compounds, can be effectively neutralized by hard water or soap. Expensive and toxic chemicals, such as pure phenol, are used when other cheaper and safer phenolics would be equally effective. When the uses of disinfectants are examined critically it becomes apparent that many are being used as part of a general cleaning programme with the general object of reducing the hazards of cross-infection in the absence of any evidence that such disinfectants make a substantial contribution. Finegold, Sweeney, Gaylor, Brady and Miller (1962) found that floors washed with detergent alone were microbially no cleaner when disinfectants were used. Vesley and Michaelsen (1964) found that adding disinfectants to floor-cleaning solutions neither improved the reduction in bacterial flora immediately after cleaning, nor did it affect the rate at which the floor counts were subsequently increased. Ayliffe, Collins and Lowbury (1966) did find a slightly greater reduction in floor counts after using disinfectants than after soap and water alone, but they too found that recontamination was rapid. It is probable that microbes on such vertical surfaces as walls are held there by strong electrostatic forces and if not removed by ordinary cleaning are likely to stay there and not make any significant contribution to the airborne contamination, though they could be rubbed off on to the clothing of passers by. Terminal disinfection of wards and cubicles is rapidly going out of fashion and is recommended only very sparingly by such authorities as Williams, Blowers, Garrod and Shooter (1966) and the American Public Health Association (1965), whose handbook *Control of Communicable Diseases* is accepted by the health authorities in Great Britain. Smallpox is a special case and is dealt with in the relevant official memorandum (Ministry of Health, 1964). It is hard to escape the conclusion that the only contribution made by many disinfectants used for general cleaning purposes is their smell.

However, there will probably always remain situations in which a disinfectant is necessary, particularly to render safe for subsequent handling objects which are known to be contaminated or are liable to contamination. Such uses can be divided as follows:

Ordinary general disinfection, for example the handling of contaminated instruments, vessels that have contained excreta, dirty floors or floor-mops (where these must still be used), calls for a broad-spectrum disinfectant that will not be readily inactivated by organic matter but which need not act particularly rapidly. In this application the substantial reduction of microbial flora in the liquid phase is important because of the danger of spread of bacteria through spillage or the generation of aerosols, but it is not essential that the innermost recesses of solid masses of contaminated material should be free from bacteria. For disinfecting clean surfaces such as trolley tops, ward furniture or kitchen tables, a broad spectrum is still necessary, resistance to organic matter is less important, but relative rapidity in action is desirable. For disinfecting the skin of hands and operation sites it is necessary to deal both with transient organisms, which are usually removed by simple mechanical washing, and resident organisms, notably staphylococci, which live within the skin and are harder to dislodge. It is against these that those agents (such as hexachlorophane) which when regularly used impart to the skin a continuing antibacterial property are particularly valuable.

The Public Health Laboratory Service Committee, having drawn attention to the need for rationalizing a disinfectant policy and to some of the broad principles involved, was unable to give detailed or specific advice about the actual choice of disinfectant fluids. This was largely because of the lack of satisfactory tests for evaluating disinfectants. The halogens, and in particular hypochlorites, were recommended for the disinfection of clean surfaces and it was suggested that the selection should be made from the approved list of such agents, with or without added detergents, maintained by the Ministry of Agriculture, Fisheries and Food. Where appropriate, alcohol in the form of industrial methylated spirit or isopropanol at a concentration of 70 per cent was advised.

General disinfection against heavy contamination or where much organic matter may be present; phenolic disinfectants are thought to be most suitable and tentative recommendations were made for black or white fluids conforming to BS 2462 and use-dilutions derived from their Chick-Martin coefficient. It was recognized that a number of clear soluble fluids of the lysol type were very suitable in that they had a wide antibacterial spectrum, were relatively insensitive to organic matter and relatively non-toxic. Unfortunately the Chick-Martin test cannot be relied upon to distinguish these fluids from unsuitable substitutes (Kelsey, 1965). Various other tests have been proposed, such as the capacity test of Kelsey, Beeby and Whitehouse (1965) and its modification (Dodd and Kelsey, 1966). In the U.S.A. the disinfectant tests of the Association of Official Agricultural Chemists are commonly used (AOAC, 1960). The German Society for Hygiene and

TABLE

Some Disinfectants currently available* in Britain, together with the Range of Use-dilutions appropriate to Hospitals

Disinfectant	Description	Use-dilution %
Dettol Reckitt & Sons Ltd., Hull	Chloroxylenols with terpineol	5–†
Hycolin William Pearson Ltd., Hull (distributed by Stayne Laboratories, High Wycombe)	Balanced combination of synthetic phenols	0·5–1·5
Izal Izal Ltd. (Newton Chambers & Co. Ltd.), Sheffield	White fluid to BS 2642 WD or WF (an emulsion of coal-tar acids)	0·5–1·0
Portex D.C.R. Portland Plastics Ltd., Hythe, Kent	Dipenidam	0·25–2·0
Printol	A clear soluble disinfectant with a phenolic base	1·25–3·0
Printol D Printar Industries Ltd., Brettenham House, Lancaster Place, Strand, London, W.C.2	A clear soluble disinfectant with a phenolic base, incorporating a detergent system	0·75–2·5
Resiguard Nicholas Laboratories Ltd., Slough	Picloxydine diglutonate, combined with benzalkonium chloride and incorporating a detergent system	0·625–2·5
Savlon HC Imperial Chemical Industries, Macclesfield	Chlorhexidine combined with cetrimide	0·5–2·5
Stericol Izal Ltd. (Newton Chambers & Co. Ltd.), Sheffield	A clear soluble disinfectant with a phenolic base, incorporating a detergent system	0·1–2·0
Sudol Printar Industries Ltd.	A clear soluble disinfectant of the lysol type	0·5–1·0

* This information relates to the situation in October 1967. By the time this chapter is published other disinfectants will almost certainly have been developed.
† Not suitable for use in heavily contaminated situations.

Microbiology (Kliewe *et al.*, 1958) has proposed a set of tests which are widely used on the Continent of Europe.

At present no really satisfactory test structure has been devised, but work on the subject continues. In Britain at least the user must rely either on the reputation of the disinfectant manufacturer or on tests made by himself or by some other worker in whom he has confidence. In the absence of any more official advice the tentative use-dilutions given in the table for some disinfectants of various types available in Britain, based on work done in this laboratory, may be of interest. The lower value is the one that is probably adequate when there is little organic matter present, when contamination is light, and when dilutions are freshly made up in clean containers; the higher value should deal with all but the worst conditions of use (or abuse).

The information given in the Table refers only to antibacterial activity. Other factors will need to be taken into account, including the stability and toxicity of the use-dilutions and the degree of detergency desired. Guidance about these matters and about the precise use-dilutions appropriate to particular situations may be sought in the literature issued by manufacturers, most of whom also operate an advisory service.

When a disinfectant and use-dilution have been selected it is still necessary to ensure that it is used correctly. Kelsey and Maurer (1966) described a simple in-use test for checking the liquid phase of practical sterilization situations and showed that the validity of a use-dilution depends on such practical matters as the accuracy with which the dilution is made up, the cleaning of both the objects to be disinfected and the vessels in which they were stored or used, and the frequency with which the solutions are changed. It is strongly recommended that disinfectant users should carry out some in-use tests routinely both to confirm their choice of agent and dilution and to check that these are being used correctly. The value of in-use tests for the disinfection of surfaces is harder to interpret as it may be impossible to distinguish between disinfection and cleaning. Any assessment based on bacterial counts on surfaces must be regarded as an assessment of the procedures used for environmental hygiene as a whole.

The P.H.L.S. Committee were unable to make any recommendations of their own about skin disinfection and referred their readers to the work of Lowbury and his co-workers (1960a, b, 1963, 1964a, b). This recommended for operation sites a single application of chlorhexidine (0·5 per cent), iodine (1 per cent) or laurolinium (5 per cent) in 70 per cent industrial methylated spirit. Alternatively, repeated washing with hexachlorophane liquid soap or polyvidone iodine should be followed by pre-operative treatment with alcoholic chlorhexidine. For injection or vene-puncture they recommended aqueous or alcoholic solutions of chlorhexidine or laurolinium, and for hands repeated washing with liquid soap or cream containing hexachlorophane (3 per cent) or regular rinsing with aqueous chlorhexidine.

For information about particular disinfectants the P.H.L.S. report should be consulted or, if greater detail is required, such textbooks as that of Sykes (1965) or Rubbo and Gardner (1965). Here it will suffice to point out that pine fluids and similar preparations containing chlorxylenol should not be accepted at their face value without an assurance that they have been tested by a reputable method and shown to be effective. The quaternary ammonium compounds are useful in the food and dairy industry, but their relative inactivity against Gram-negative organisms and their inactivation by hard

Another matter about which the pathologist is sometimes asked to advise is the sterility of pharmaceutical products. In particular, the serious eye infections reported from Birmingham and associated with contaminated eye-lotions have focused attention on this type of product (Ayliffe, Barry *et al.*, 1966). Here again little purpose is served by attempting to carry out sterility tests on individual products, especially in laboratories not skilled in these techniques. The Supplement (1966) to the *British Pharmacopœia Codex* (1963) contains a monograph on eye preparations and gives detailed instructions for their preparation and use. The best safeguard against the hazards of unsterile eye preparations is to insist that only those prepared in accordance with some such standard are used, even if this involves additional expense either in purchase from reputable commercial sources or in providing the hospital pharmacist with adequate facilities. In Britain, the staff of the Pharmaceutical Society's laboratory are always prepared to give advice about the sterilization of particular pharmaceutical preparations; in the U.S.A. the U.S. Public Health Service will advise; energy is better expended in seeking and implementing such specialist advice than in unskilled sterility testing.

CONCLUSION

The voluminous literature on the subject of sterilization and disinfection is evidence of the number of workers who have taken the trouble to report their experiments or their experience. However, this mass of reported information must be sifted, appraised and translated into practical policies, programmes and procedures. Much of this operation must usually be undertaken by the clinical pathologist, whether as volunteer or conscript. His rôle was clearly defined in the report of a symposium held by the Association of Clinical Pathologists as follows:

"The fundamental responsibility of the pathologist in sterilization and disinfection was to advise on what methods were appropriate for carrying out these processes in particular situations, to suggest what controls or tests were necessary, and to demand evidence at short intervals that his advice was being carried out" (*Lancet*, 1965).

Pathologists in Britain could be saved much time, energy and frustration if the broad outlines of policy and programme were to be agreed at Group or Regional level so that the individual pathologist, who has many other tasks to perform, need only be concerned with the local implementation of the agreed measures.

References

ALDER, V. G., BROWN, A. M. and GILLESPIE, W. A. (1966). Disinfection of heat-sensitive material by low-temperature steam and formaldehyde. *J. clin. Path.*, **19**, 83.

American Public Health Association (1965). Control of communicable diseases in man. 10th ed. New York. (Obtainable from H.M.S.O.)

ARMSTRONG, J. A. and FROELICH, E. J. (1964). Inactivation of viruses by benzalkonium chloride. *J. Appl. Microbiol.*, **12**, 132.

Association of Official Agricultural Chemists (1965). *Official Methods of Analysis.* 10th ed. Washington, D.C.

AYLIFFE, G. A. J., BARRY, D. R., LOWBURY, E. J. L., ROPER-HALL, M. J. and WALKER, W. M. (1966). Postoperative infection with *Pseudomonas æruginosa* in an eye hospital. *Lancet*, **i**, 1113.

AYLIFFE, G. A. J., COLLINS, B. J. and LOWBURY, E. J. L. (1966). Cleaning and disinfection of hospital floors. *Brit. med. J.*, **ii**, 442.

AYLIFFE, G. A. J., LOWBURY, E. J. L., HAMILTON, J. G., SMALL, J. M., ASHESHOV, E. A. and PARKER, M. T. (1965). Hospital infection with *Pseudomonas æruginosa* in neurosurgery. *Lancet*, **ii**, 365.

BEEBY, MELANIE M. and WHITEHOUSE, C. E. (1965). A bacterial spore test piece for the control of ethylene oxide sterilization. *J. appl. Bact.*, **28**, 349.

BLANDY, J. P. (1965). Catheterization. *Brit. med. J.*, **ii**, 1531.

BOWIE, J. H., GILLINGHAM, F. J., CAMPBELL, I. D. and GORDON, A. R. (1963). Hospital sterile supplies: Edinburgh pre-set tray system. *Brit. med. J.*, **ii**, 1322.

British Standards Institution (1966). Specification for Steam Sterilizers. Part 1: Sterilizers for porous loads. Part 2: Sterilizers for bottled fluids. BS 3970: 1966. [Part 3: Sterilizers for unwrapped instruments and utensils. Part 4: Sterilizers of small size for unwrapped instruments for use in clinics and surgeries. In course of preparation.]

BRYCE, D. M. (1956). Tests for the sterility of pharmaceutical preparations. The design and interpretation of sterility tests. *J. Pharm. Pharmacol.*, **8**, 561.

CUNLIFFE, A. C. (1966). Ethylene oxide sterilisation. *Brit. Hosp. J. Soc. Serv. Rev.*, **66**, 1162

DODD, A. H. and KELSEY, J. C. (1966). A capacity use-dilution test for disinfectants. A statistical note. *Mon. Bull. Minist. Hlth Lab. Serv.*, **25**, 232.

FINEGOLD, S. M., SWEENEY, E. E., GAYLOR, D. W., BRADY, DORIS and MILLER, L. G. (1962). Hospital Floor Decontamination: Controlled Blind Studies in Evaluation of Germicides. *Antimicrobial Agents & Chemotherapy*, p. 250.

KELSEY, J. C. (1961). Acceptable standards for surgical methods. *Recent Developments in the Sterilization of Surgical Materials*. Symposium, p. 203. London: The Pharmaceutical Press.

KELSEY, J. C. (1965). Disinfectants for use in hospitals. *Brit. med. J.*, **ii**, 592 (corr.).

KELSEY, J. C. (1967). The use of gaseous antimicrobial agents with special reference to ethylene oxide. *J. appl. Bact.*, **30**, 92.

KELSEY, J. C., BEEBY, MALENIE M. and WHITEHOUSE, C. E. (1965). A capacity use-dilution test for disinfectants. *Mon. Bull. Minist. Hlth Lab. Serv.*, **24**, 152.

KELSEY, J. C. and MAURER, ISOBEL M. (1966). An in-use test for hospital disinfectants. *Mon. Bull. Minist. Hlth Lab. Serv.*, **25**, 180.

KLEIN, M. and DEFOREST, A. (1963). The inactivation of viruses by germicides. *Chem. Spec. Mfrs Ass. Proc. Midyear Mtg.*, **49**, 116.

KLIEWE, H., HEICKEN, K., SCHMIDT, B. H., WAGENER, K., WÜSTENBERG, J., OSTERTAG, H., GRUN, L., LAMMERS, TH. and MÜLHENS, K. (editors) (1958). Richtlinien für die Prüfung chemischer Disinfektionsmittel. *Zbl. Bakt. l Abl. Orig.*, **173**, 307.

Lancet (1964). A radiation sterilization service to hospitals (Annotation), **i**, 372.

Lancet (1965). Sterilization, disinfection and the pathologist (Annotation), **ii**, 780.

LOWBURY, E. J. L. and LILLY, H. A. (1960a). Disinfection of the hands of surgeons and nurses. *Brit. med. J.*, **i**, 1445.

LOWBURY, E. J. L., LILLY, H. A. and BULL, J. P. (1960b). Disinfection of the skin of operation sites. *Brit. med. J.*, **ii**, 1039.

LOWBURY, E. J. L., LILLY, H. A. and BULL, J. P. (1963). Disinfection of hands: Removal of resident bacteria. *Brit. med. J.*, **i**, 1251.

LOWBURY, E. J. L., LILLY, H. A. and BULL, J. P. (1964a). Disinfection of hands: Removal of transient organisms. *Brit. med. J.*, **ii**, 230.

LOWBURY, E. J. L., LILLY, H. A. and BULL, J. P. (1964b). Methods for disinfection of hands and operation sites. *Brit. med. J.*, **ii**, 531.

Ministry of Health and Scottish Home and Health Department (1964). *Memorandum on the Control of Outbreaks of Smallpox*. London: H.M.S.O.

Ministry of Health: Medical Supplies Working Party Sterilization Group (1966). Provision of Topical Fluids for Surgical Operations. *Lancet*, **i**, 705.

NORDGREN, G. (1939). Investigations on the sterilization efficacy of gaseous formaldehyde. *Acta path. microbiol. scand.*, Suppl. No. 40.

PROOM, H. (1962). Sterility test regulations and the manufacturer. *Proc. Int. Conf. Bio. Standardisation*, p. 169.

Public Health Laboratory Service: Committee on the Testing and Evaluation of Disinfectants (1965). Use of Disinfectants in Hospitals. *Brit. med. J.*, **i**, 408.

ROGERS, K. B. (1966). Observations on bedpan washers and sterilizers. Abstr. CXIII. *Meet. Path. Soc. G.B.*, London.

ROSS, P. W. (1966). A new disinfectant. *J. clin. Path.*, **19**, 318.

RUBBO, S. D. and GARDNER, JOAN S. (1965). *A Review of Sterilization and Disinfection*, pp. 141, 244. London: Lloyd-Luke.

Supplement (1966) to British Pharmacopœia Codex 1964, p. 77. London: The Pharmaceutical Press.

SYKES, G. (1965). *Disinfection and Sterilization*. 2nd ed. London: Spon.

VESLEY, D. and MICHAELSEN, G. S. (1964). Application of a surface sampling technic to the evaluation of bacteriological effectiveness of certain hospital housekeeping procedures. *Hlth Lab. Sci.*, **i**, 107.

WEYMES, C. (1966). Sterilisation with ethylene oxide at sub-atmospheric pressure. *Brit. Hosp. J. Soc. Serv. Rev.*, **66**, 1745.

WILLIAMS, R. E. O., BLOWERS, R., GARROD, L. P. and SHOOTER, R. A. (1966). *Hospital Infection*, 2nd ed. London: Lloyd-Luke.

SECTION II

CHEMICAL PATHOLOGY

Section Editor

E. N. ALLOTT

D.M.(Oxon), F.R.C.P., F.R.I.C.

Formerly Group Pathologist, Lewisham Hospital, London

Chapter 8

PRACTICAL ASPECTS OF MICROCHEMICAL TECHNIQUES

J. Liddell and T. B. Hales

The technique of measuring the concentration of chemicals in small samples is variously known as microchemistry or ultramicrochemistry. Wilkinson (1960) has defined the former as methods requiring 0·1–0·5 ml., and the latter as methods requiring less than 0·05 ml. (50 microlitres) of sample (1,000 μl.=1 ml.). In this article we define microchemistry as a collection of techniques which allows the concentration of several chemical substances to be estimated in one sample of capillary blood. 0·4 ml. of whole blood can be easily collected from a skin puncture (many experienced operators can readily obtain 1 ml. samples from small babies), and microchemical techniques should use less than 50 μl. of plasma. Convenient volumes usually vary between 5 and 30 μl. There is no advantage for clinical purposes in trying to use smaller samples.

The main clinical use for these techniques is in the investigation and treatment of babies and small children, especially when frequent repeated estimations are required, but they are sometimes of value with adult patients when repeated venipuncture is difficult as in severely burned adults.

The minimum volume of plasma which can be used is controlled by the limitations of the available commercial apparatus. We have therefore listed the essential commercial equipment with which we are familiar and describe its advantages and limitations. This practical information is often difficult to obtain, and is essential when starting these techniques. The exclusion of any item from this article should not be taken as criticism; it simply means that we have not had personal experience of the equipment. References to other equipment are given in the paper by Clayton and Jenkins (1966).

In our experience about 70 per cent of pædiatric chemistry requests are for urea, sodium, potassium, bicarbonate and glucose. These estimations can all be performed on capillary samples with only a small amount of specialized equipment. Such a limited service can be of great value in a hospital with a few children's beds.

Some methods that we have found reliable are listed in Table I and the details are given in Appendix A. These are given to illustrate the basic principles, and as suggestions for those starting a similar service. It is not claimed that they are necessarily the best methods. Variations in local conditions will often make other methods more suitable.

APPARATUS

Tubes and Containers. The prime requirements for this equipment in a microchemistry laboratory are that it should be of a convenient size and scrupulously clean. Washing of glassware is of supreme importance in a microchemical unit.

Whenever possible, we use disposable plastic containers of a variety of sizes. Plastic materials have non-wettable properties desirable in microchemistry, and drops of liquid will remain as discrete globules on their surface. This greatly improves the handling, and reduces evaporation. For larger volumes the disposable containers used in the collection of venous blood are valuable. Stoppered polyethylene tubes of 0·4 ml. capacity are available and are useful for collecting capillary blood samples as well as for chemical estimations. It is easy to fill these tubes nearly to the brim with capillary blood, the stopper then seals the specimen and prevents losses of carbon dioxide.

TABLE I

Summary of Microchemical Techniques

Estimation	Technique	Total sample volume	Final volume
		μl.	ml.
Sodium	Flame photometry⎫		
Potassium	Flame photometry⎭	20	2·0
Bicarbonate	Natelson microgasometer	30	…
Urea	Urease/indopenhol blue	5	5·1
	Chaney and Marbach (1962)*		
Glucose	Kingsley and Getchell (1960)*	40	4·02
	Glucose oxidase		
Calcium	Radin and Gramza (1964)*	30	3·03
Bilirubin	Nosslin (1960)*	30	0·265
Total protein	Biuret	5	0·205
Alkaline phosphatase	Kind and King (1954)*	20	0·36
Inorganic phosphate	Gomori (1942)*	20	0·14
Thymol flocculation	MacLagan (1944)*	30	1·83
Salicylates	Trinder (1954)*	50	0·25
Cholesterol	Searcy and Bergquist (1960)	40	7·0

* Modification of original method.

Pipettes. There are three types of micropipette in common use:

A glass pipette with a capillary tube of uniform bore, calibrated to contain the volume. The Sahli pipette, used for hæmoglobin estimations, and 0·1 and 0·2 ml. graduated shell-back pipettes are common examples.

These pipettes suffer from a number of defects. They require careful washing out in order to include the film of sample adhering to the glass walls. This makes them susceptible to individual variations in technique and limits their use to dilution of the sample in a relatively large volume of reagent. Slight variations in the relationship of the meniscus to the calibration mark may produce considerable errors in the delivered volume. When filled by the conventional method of mouth suction, the sample meniscus is first taken beyond the calibration point and then the excess fluid is slowly drained. This leaves a thin film of sample above the calibration mark which is frequently

D

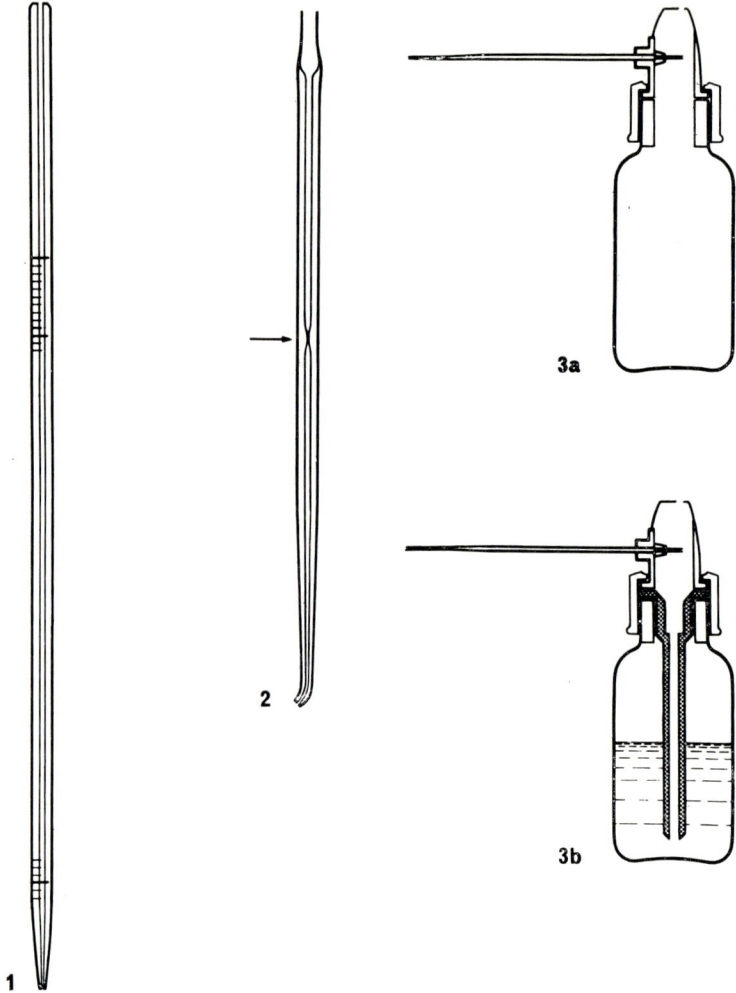

FIG. 1. The three basic types of micropipette:
  1. A 0·1 ml. graduated pipette calibrated to contain.
  2. The Lang-Levy glass constriction pipette.
  3. The Sanz polyethylene overflow pipette when (a) used to deliver plasma samples, (b) as modified for mutliple deliveries of the reagent contained within the bottle.

Operat n of the Sanz pipette in function A:
  1. Hold the polyethylene bottle between the opposed thumb and fingers, leaving the forefinger free to rest lightly on the top of the plastic dome.
  2. Insert the pepette tip below the surface of the sample.
  3. Gently squeeze the bottle.
  4. Occlude the hole on the top of the dome with the forefinger.
  5. Gently release the finger pressure so that sample slowly fills the pipette and one drop overflows from the inner end of the pipette.
  6. Stop the suction by lifting the forefinger.
  7. Remove the pipette from the sample and carefully wipe the tip.
  8. Insert the pipette into the test tube so that the tip touches the wall of the tube just above any fluid level.

[Continued at foot of next page

and variably included in the delivered volume during the washing procedure. This error can be considerably reduced by a modification proposed by Wilkinson (1960). The mouth end of the pipette is connected to a 1 ml. syringe with a short length of tubing, and the syringe is used to aspirate the sample. It is possible then to fill the pipette precisely without overfilling at any stage. This procedure is accurate but time-consuming.

A second type is the *glass constriction pipette*. The Lang-Levy pipette is a frequently used member of this class: the fluid is aspirated beyond the constriction point and allowed to drain to this point before the pipette is carefully wiped. The pipette tip is then inserted into the test-tube and the pipette tapped to start the fluid draining. After gravity drainage is complete, the remainder of the sample is gently blown out into the test-tube. The pipette is not rinsed out with diluent. Like all glass pipettes calibrated to deliver, the Lang-Levy pipette can retain a variable proportion of sample adherent to the wall of the tube. It can give precise results only if the pipette is scrupulously clean. Careful washing is required between each pipetting operation, particularly when protein-containing fluids such as plasma are used.

The "Overflow" Type. Excess fluid aspirated into the pipette is trapped in a large container and cannot be included with the delivered volume. Earlier examples were made of glass, but more recently Sanz (1957) has developed a polyethylene pipette. Because polyethylene is "non-wettable", only a minute amount of fluid remains adherent to the walls after delivery. This improves the reproducibility and also allows successive pipetting of different samples without intervening washing. The pipettes can be cleaned by immersing overnight in a pepsin/HCl mixture or a detergent such as Alconox or Decon 75.

These three types of micropipette are illustrated in the figure, the subscript of which explains the operation of the Sanz pipette. A disadvantage of polyethylene pipettes is that they cannot be used for many organic solvents. The Sanz pipette is marketed commercially by Beckman-Spinco Ltd., in sizes ranging between 5 and 250 microlitres.

There are two points of general importance about the use of micropipettes. The accuracy of such pipettes is always suspect, although their reproducibility is good. For instance, the delivered volume of a series of commercially produced 20 μl. Sanz pipettes tested by us, ranged between 18·9 and 19·6 μl. Since their reproducibility is good, then compensation for this inaccuracy can always be made by incorporating in every estimation a standard which has been put through the entire procedure using the same pipette both for this

---

9. Occlude the dome hole with the forefinger and gently squeeze the bottle so that the pipette contents are slowly delivered. Slight withdrawal of the pipette tip during the last part of the delivery will avoid the blowing of an air bubble into the drop of delivered sample and thus reduce spattering.

Function B:
1. Hold the pipette in the same way.
2. Gently squeeze the bottle so that the reagent rises above the inner end of the pipette.
3. Occlude the hole with the forefinger and continue the gentle pressure so that the reagent is forced along the pipette and one drop is extruded from the outer end to hang on the tip.
4. Lift the forefinger, release pressure on the bottle and wipe the pipette tip with tissue.
5. Deliver the reagent by manœuvres 8 and 9 above.

standard and all the samples. The use of calibration curves or standards introduced halfway through the technical procedure is never permissible in microchemistry.

The second practical point is that it is much better to become thoroughly expert in the use of one, or at the most two, types of pipette and to use them for all estimations. We routinely use the Sanz polyethylene pipette which we have found to be simple and reliable. The reproducibility of these pipettes is good with a coefficient of variation of about 0·5 per cent. In the few instances where organic solvents are required we use Lang-Levy pipettes.

Burettes. Volumetric techniques dominated the early days of micro-chemistry. They have now been largely superseded by the development of modern photoelectric colorimeters requiring only small sample volumes. Where microtitration is still necessary, there are two basic types of micro-burette, both having a titrant volume of the order of 10 μl., with a precision better than 1 per cent.

(1) The *capillary burette*, in which the titrant is expelled by an immiscible liquid, usually mercury, in a capillary tube of very uniform bore. The move-ment of liquid is usually controlled by a screw-operated plunger, and the volume of fluid expelled is a known function of the displacement of the liquid interface along the capillary tube. The disadvantages of this type of apparatus are that it is usually bulky, often temperature sensitive and may give contamination of the titrant by the mercury.

(2) The *displacement burette*, in which the fluid is directly displaced by a plunger of extremely uniform diameter the movement of which is operated and measured by a micrometer screw. Alternatively, the delivered volume may be measured by a dial micrometer often with a zero setting device.

A few general principles apply to titration with any type of microburette. The burette tip should always dip beneath the surface of the liquid in the reaction vessel. This removes errors due to drop formation and the spread of a thin film of liquid up the outside of the burette tip. The tip is preferably made of a non-wettable material with a fine exit hole. This reduces the creep of the titrated fluid up the inside of the burette. The solution being titrated should be constantly mixed during the titration. This is often accomplished by a vibrating rod dipping into the liquid close to the burette tip. It is preferable that the speed of this should be adjustable in order to avoid both undermixing and overvigorous vibration producing splashing. The end-point may be easier to read if the concentration of reagents is higher than that in conventional methods: the error produced by difficulty in reading the end-point is often greater than the volumetric error of the burette. The titration is best performed in a small container making the depth of the liquid approximately the same as the diameter. This not only makes the end-point easier to read but also reduces errors such as the absorption of atmospheric carbon dioxide in acid-base titrations.

Automatic Dilutors. A number of electrically operated machines for the automatic measuring and dilution of small samples (10–200 μl.) are available. We have experience of one of these (made by Hook and Tucker Ltd.) which is both reliable and robust. Their main use in clinical chemistry is probably the pre-dilution of samples before estimation on the Auto-Analyzer.

Colorimeters and Spectrophotometers. The majority of clinical chemistry techniques are now colorimetric, and the volume of the cuvette is the critical factor determining the original size of the sample. Most colorimeters and spectrophotometers require about 3 ml. of solution with a light path of 1 cm. Many published methods which have a final fluid volume greater than this can be easily scaled down so that a smaller sample is adequate. Much can be done using micro-cells, usually of 0·5 ml. capacity, with ordinary colorimeters and spectrophotometers. Particular care must be given to the cleanliness of the optical surfaces, the same cell must be used for standard and test solution and the cuvette filled with a pasteur pipette without scratching the optical surfaces or introducing air bubbles. Polyethylene-tipped pipettes lessen the risk of damaging the light-transmitting surfaces. Care must be taken to ensure that the optical alignment is precise. The danger that part of the light is transmitted through the side wall of the cell and not through the liquid whose optical density is being measured can be avoided by frequently checking that the optical density of a solution in the micro-cell is identical with that of the same solution in a normal cell at the same wavelength. These precautions make the use of micro-cells in normal spectrophotometers rather time-consuming and not suitable for junior staff and we confine their use to more specialized investigations which require a reading in the ultraviolet, since special microchemical instruments are usually limited to the visible region of the spectrum.

The Gilford 300 spectrophotometer will take volumes down to 500 $\mu l.$ and has a 10 mm. light-path. It has an automatic sampling device, a digital presentation of the absorption, and a wavelength range between 340 mμ and 700 mμ. It is possible to calibrate the instrument with a standard so that a direct reading of the concentration of the unknown solution is displayed instead of optical density. The volume of sample required is still too large for some microchemical methods, and for these a special instrument with a very small cuvette is required, such as the Spinco colorimeter made by Beckman.

The Beckman-Spinco colorimeter is a specially designed instrument limited to the visible range, with a volume requirement of 100 $\mu l.$ Its performance has been critically examined by O'Brien, Ibbott and Pinfield (1961) and by Clayton and Jenkins (1966). The latter authors find it necessary to make duplicate readings in order that errors due to trapped air bubbles, incomplete filling of the cuvette and "sticking" of the galvanometer can be detected. Both reviewers comment on the large amount of drift in the zero reading of the instrument. We have not found these difficulties of great importance. We tested one Beckman-Spinco colorimeter which has been in routine use for over six months without an overhaul. The optical density of the standard solution was read 21 times while the zero readings were checked in between each standard with distilled water. The coefficient of variation of the standard readings was 0·9 per cent. The zero drift between successive water readings was nil on 13 out of the 21 readings, 0·001 on five, and 0·002 on three occasions. We fill the machine by using a 100 $\mu l.$ Sanz pipette: this ensures that an adequate volume is inserted and reduces the risk of trapped air bubbles. The effective light path of this machine appeared to be 6 mm.

Flame Photometers. The majority of flame photometers in routine use are sufficiently sensitive. Sodium and potassium are measured with the one plasma dilution, usually 1 : 100. The aspiration rate of these machines can be reduced by lowering the air pressure; and we find that 20 μl. of plasma is sufficient for both a sodium and a potassium estimation.

Gasometers. The Natelson microgasometer is an accurate reliable machine which is simple and quick to use. It is essentially a combination of syringe-pipette and gasometer and requires 30 μl. of sample. We regard it as the best machine for the determination of total carbon dioxide content of plasma, for use in any laboratory using manual techniques. The commonest source of error is the use of improperly stored reagents which are not CO_2 free. The loss of CO_2 in the sample is reduced if capped polyethylene tubes are used for blood collecting and the sample taken directly into the gasometer as soon as centrifugation is complete.

Balances. An ordinary laboratory balance is adequate for making up reagents and standards.

Commercial Systems. Two commercial "systems" are available which provide the chemical pathologist with a do-it-yourself microchemistry kit. We have experience of only one of these, that made by Beckman-Spinco Ltd., and have found it valuable.

The equipment consists of the following:

(1) The prism colorimeter already referred to.

(2) A centrifuge designed to take 20 polyethylene test-tubes of 0·4 ml. capacity. This is a robust machine with a single speed of about 15,000 r.p.m. which is fitted with a timing control. The high speed is useful when separating the plasma in blood samples previously collected in these tubes.

(3) A microtitrator of the displacement type with a dial micrometer and a zero setting device. The fluid to be titrated is placed in disposable polystyrene cups which are held in a rotatable plastic mount. This is a good piece of equipment technically, but we have found the methods for which it was intended (chloride and calcium) to be of limited value.

(4) A mixing device consisting of a rubber cone mounted on an electrically rotated shaft. Such a device is essential in mixing small volumes.

(5) Disposable test-tubes and titration cups.

(6) A selection of Sanz pipettes and plastic containers so that one container will hold all the pipettes required for each estimation.

Acid-Base Measurements. Estimations of blood pH, P_{CO_2} and standard bicarbonate are of great value in pædiatrics particularly during the neonatal period.

We know of two types of apparatus for measuring these and have personal experience of one. The more usual is that designed by Astrup and made by Radiometer Ltd. Measurements of blood pH are made at three different P_{CO_2} levels, and the parameters of clinical importance are calculated from these readings. It is an expensive precision instrument and needs careful experienced supervision.

A newer machine is the blood gas analyser marketed by P. K. Morgan Ltd. This gives a direct measurement of blood pH and blood P_{CO_2} using two different electrodes sensitive to hydrogen ion and carbon-dioxide respectively. It has the advantage of appearing simpler to use and of giving a direct reading of P_{CO_2}. We have little personal experience of this equipment.

There are several different ways of reporting these results. We like to include in the report the hydrogen ion concentration in nano-Equivalent/litre and also both the respiratory and non-respiratory deviation from the normal expressed in the same units. (1 nano-equivalent $= 10^{-6}$ milli equivalents.) This system was described by Whitehead (1965); and its advantages are sometimes not fully appreciated. It permits a direct comparison of the magnitude of the respiratory and non-respiratory components in an acid-base disturbance.

Staff and Space

In our experience microchemical techniques are learnt surprisingly quickly by a competent technician or biochemist. The pipetting techniques can be learnt in a few hours; technicians can do routine work under supervision after about two weeks, and can be considered fully fledged members of the unit after one month. The optimum period for one person to work in a microchemical unit is about six months. A shorter period is uneconomic and a longer period results in boredom and a drop in efficiency.

Microchemical methods are not more time-consuming than other techniques. They do however require concentration to produce accurate results. Careless pipetting, for instance, will produce gross errors. The work load should therefore be such that the technicians do have a few minutes between estimations to relax.

The amount of space required for such a unit within an ordinary laboratory is small, as much of the equipment such as a balance or flame photometer is already standard. The specialized apparatus is small in size; and little room is required for storage of reagents. At Guy's Hospital the unit, which serves 120 children's beds, is staffed by two biochemists and has 24 ft. of laboratory bench. However, smaller laboratories serving only a few pædiatric beds could manage with only about 8 ft. of bench. The work can be done in the middle of an open laboratory, although a side room is preferable.

COLLECTION OF SPECIMENS

The use of capillary blood for analysis has obvious advantages in pædiatrics. The fact that the capillary blood has a composition which approximates closely to that of arterial blood, means that a well-taken capillary sample is preferred to venous blood for investigations such as blood pH.

The collection of satisfactory specimens is not difficult; but the technique requires a certain amount of training and constant practice. Hospital medical staff are commonly inexperienced in this type of collection, which should, therefore, be undertaken by trained laboratory staff. We employ one or two older women with no previous experience of laboratory work as blood collectors on a part-time basis. Such people soon learn how to collect good unhæmolysed samples of capillary blood, and are willing to do this work indefinitely as the frequent contact with children, parents and nurses gives interest.

It has been found convenient to collect specimens directly into disposable stoppered polyethylene test-tubes of 0·4 ml. capacity. The thick rim of these tubes obstructs the flow of blood, so they are modified by cutting off one segment of the rim with a pair of scissors. The thin section of the wall so produced can be applied to the drop of blood.

Heparin is used as an anticoagulant for all specimens except those for plasma glucose. One drop (about 15 μl.) of a 0·5 per cent solution of lithium heparin is placed in each tube using a syringe fitted with a No. 17 needle. The tubes are then dried in an oven at 50°C. Samples for plasma glucose are collected in tubes containing a strip of impregnated filter paper. For this purpose Whatman No. 1 filter paper is soaked in a solution containing 5 g. of potassium oxalate and 3 g. of sodium fluoride per 100 ml. The paper is then dried and cut into strips measuring 30 × 4 mm.

Capillary blood may be obtained from the heel, fingers, toes or ear lobes, the choice being determined to some extent by the age of the patient. It is most important that the skin over the selected part be warm. A satisfactory capillary specimen will never be obtained from a cold site; and it is sometimes necessary to warm the selected area by wrapping it in cotton-wool soaked with warm (but not hot) water for a few minutes. A free flow of capillary blood will then be obtained when the skin is pierced.

The first drop of blood is collected on to the lip of the polythene tube, which is then tapped or flicked until the drop reaches the bottom of the tube. Subsequent drops flow down the wall without difficulty. When the tube is almost full, it is capped, and the small bubble of air will assist in mixing the blood with the dried heparin.

The main factors which give rise to hæmolysis are: contamination with the cleansing fluid, excessive squeezing during collection, and scraping up the blood with the tube. Ether is the most convenient cleansing agent as it produces skin hyperæmia and leaves a clean, dry surface. It should not be used in infant incubators. If another fluid is used, it must be completely removed by a second, dry, sterile swab before the skin is punctured. The skin should be bunched up when it is being stabbed; then the flow of blood is initiated by exerting lateral pressure away from the wound by the thumbs. A gentle milking action is permissible as long as the blood flows freely, but if the flow slows down further squeezing is useless: it will only close the wound. Lateral pressure should then be exerted again, and the flow will usually recommence. It is useful to apply a thin smear of Vaseline over the puncture site before the first drop of blood appears. This makes the drop more stable; and the blood can be collected drop by drop. Any attempt to scoop up blood running over the skin will result in hæmolysis.

In practice we have found that, in routine collection, about 7 per cent of specimens show naked-eye evidence of hæmolysis. However, with sufficient care and patience a satisfactory sample can be obtained even in the most difficult cases.

PRINCIPLES OF MICROCHEMICAL METHODS

There are a few basic principles which need to be considered when choosing a microchemical technique. An advantage of these methods is that only small amounts of reagents are required, and when these are expensive microchemical methods are desirable even if large samples can be relatively easily obtained. The estimation of galactose-1-phosphate uridyl transferase is an example where the price of chemicals is an important factor.

Certain methods are not satisfactory when scaled down because surface effects and the creeping of fluids along container surfaces interfere. Extraction procedures should be avoided. Organic solvents are often not suitable, either because of volatility or because plastic containers with their valuable non-wetting properties cannot be used. Filtration involves unacceptable losses and is replaced by centrifugation. Methods involving precipitation occasion-ally give variable results, and where possible it is better not to precipitate plasma proteins.

After these points have been considered there remain two ways in which results can be obtained from small plasma samples. The first is to use an extremely sensitive method so that standard equipment can be used. For instance, methods are available for determination of urea and glucose which permit the optical density of a final volume of over 3 ml. to be measured in a conventional colorimeter, using a sample volume of a few microlitres. Flame photometry is another method where careful attention to detail will allow the measurement of sodium and potassium in small plasma samples by a normal instrument. The alternative approach is to scale down a standard method so that a plasma volume of less than 50 μl. will produce a solution of more than 100 μl. for the final colorimetry.

We prefer to use sensitive methods wherever possible despite the temporary disadvantages of their unfamiliarity. They allow the smaller laboratory to offer a reasonably comprehensive service with little extra capital expenditure. Even when specialized equipment is available it is reassuring to know that the rare but inevitable failure in this equipment will not produce a catastrophic breakdown in the service. It is technically simple to estimate urea, sodium, potassium, glucose and calcium with ordinary facilities so that the most frequent and urgent estimations can be maintained.

With many estimations, however, it is necessary to use methods of normal sensitivity and special apparatus. It is then often best to scale down a method of known reliability that is already in routine use in that laboratory rather than turn to a new and unfamiliar technique. This has the advantages that separate standards and reagents will not be required for the microchemical version, and that the pathologist is already aware of the potential fallacies and failures of the method. When doing this it is important to ensure that a standard is always used, and that it is treated in exactly the same way as the plasma samples. For instance, some methods involve protein precipitation and use standards which bypass this step. These must be modified.

PRACTICAL SUGGESTIONS

Pædiatricians sometimes feel, perhaps with justification, that their needs are often neglected in a busy routine laboratory. Some children's diseases are virtually unknown in adults and conditions such as galactosæmia and phenylketonuria require time-consuming methods to establish a reliable diagnosis. These conditions are of great biochemical interest and the pathologist who interests himself in the necessary techniques will find them a fascinating problem. Nevertheless, the main need is for ordinary routine investigations to be performed on small samples. Table II shows the investigations done by the microchemical unit at the Children's Hospital, Sheffield, during 1965 and 1966.

Both pædiatricians and pathologists often fail to realize how much can be done to modify existing techniques without any extra expense in apparatus or staff. With colorimetric methods, for instance, the plasma volume required can often be halved by ensuring that the final volume available for colorimetry is not greatly in excess of the minimum required. When choosing a new colorimeter, the cuvette volume should always be an important consideration.

TABLE II

An Analysis of Microchemical Estimations performed at the Children's Hospital, Sheffield

Estimation	1965	1966
Sodium	2,708	4,142
Potassium	2,736	4,228
Bicarbonate	2,676	4,012
Urea	3,211	4,568
Glucose	1,045	...
Calcium	358	471
Bilirubin	302	423
Total protein	252	334
Alkaline phosphatase	160	249
Inorganic phosphate	120	146
Thymol flocculation	86	153
Salicylates	88	158
Cholesterol	40	83

In 1966 the glucose estimations were performed on an Auto-Analyzer in another Sheffield Hospital. The figures are therefore not included.

It can be seen that sodium, potassium, bicarbonate, urea and glucose comprise 90 per cent of the investigations.

Now that the Natelson microgasometer is available there can surely be no justification for any laboratory to buy an older type of gasometer.

But in order to provide a useful selection of estimations on capillary blood some extra equipment and methods will be required. This problem will be faced by two different types of laboratory.

In the small unit serving 10–20 pædiatric beds in a general hospital, little extra expense is involved. Table II shows that urea, electrolytes and glucose are requested far more frequently than any other investigation. These estimations can easily be performed on capillary blood samples. Calcium and cholesterol can also be estimated with conventional apparatus.

A few micropipettes, preferably of the Sanz type, should be purchased. Sodium and potassium can be estimated on 20 μl. of plasma using the sort of flame photometer that is already available in most routine laboratories.

The urea and glucose estimations do not require any specialized apparatus. The bicarbonate estimation will need a Natelson microgasometer which can then be used for all estimations of total CO_2 if this is not already done on automated equipment. It is important to remember that the normal range on capillary samples (about 17–24 mEq./l.) is lower than that for venous blood. This is mainly due to the lower CO_2 content of capillary blood, but also to inevitable losses during the collection process.

Chloride cannot be easily estimated without specialized apparatus. This investigation is of limited clinical value, and patients with electrolyte disturbances can be managed on the basis of the sodium, potassium and bicarbonate estimations.

In a larger unit the purchase of extra equipment and the employment of specially trained staff is justified. The newcomer to this field will probably decide to purchase one of the commercial equipment systems. These systems sometimes include a microtitrator, but this could probably be omitted. We have been disappointed in the titrimetric methods (chloride and calcium) which are frequently required in a clinical laboratory. The end-points are difficult to read and marked errors occur with hæmolysed samples.

Microchemistry, like all branches of chemical pathology, has developed rapidly in the last ten years. At the moment the situation appears relatively stable and satisfactory. It is difficult to forecast future technical developments in any subject. But we suspect that automated methods will soon be available on the microlitre scale. It is already possible to estimate glucose on about 40 μl. of whole blood using an Auto-Analyzer. In one of our laboratories the Auto-Analyzer method for urea, sodium, potassium, chloride and bicarbonate has been modified for a total sample volume of 100 μl. (Michael, C. and Michelin, M. J., unpublished). The method has been in routine use on all electrolyte samples, both adult and paediatric, for over three months.

APPENDIX A

EXAMPLES OF MICROCHEMICAL METHODS

SODIUM AND POTASSIUM
(20 μl. plasma)

These ions are measured, using a single dilution, on an EEL flame photometer. The aspiration rate of the machine is reduced by using an air pressure of 6 lb./sq. in. The linearity of the instrument is improved by adjusting the range of the zero control (a knurled knob, held by a clamp on the inner end of the zero control rod is held firmly while the external knob of this control is forcibly rotated).

Reagents

(1) Three pre-diluted standards are prepared from stock solutions of sodium chloride and potassium chloride:

(a) Sodium 1·00 mEq./l. Potassium 0·020 mEq./l.
(b) Sodium 1·40 mEq./l. Potassium 0·060 mEq./l.
(c) Sodium 1·80 mEq./l. Potassium 0·100 mEq./l.

(2) Working standard (Sodium 140 mEq./l., Potassium 4·0 mEq./l.)

Method. Into a 5 ml. disposable polyethylene container, pipette 20 μl. of plasma, add 2·0 ml. of deionized water and mix. The working standard is treated similarly.

The sample and standard dilutions are read on the flame photometer which has been set with the prediluted standards, the known standard being used to calculate the results.

TOTAL CO₂ CONTENT
(30 μl. plasma)

Reagents

(1) N-*Lactic Acid.* 90 ml. of 85 per cent lactic acid is made up to 1 litre with water.
(2) 3N-*Sodium Hydroxide.* 12 g. NaOH are dissolved in 100 ml. water.
(3) *CO₂ Standard* (22·3 mM./l.). 2·382 g. of sodium carbonate, previously dried at 100°C, is dissolved in one litre and covered with mineral oil.
(4) *Anti-foam Reagent* (Scientific Industries).

Method. The estimation is performed with the Natelson microgasometer (previously described in the "Apparatus" section) using the manufacturer's method. The normal range for capillary blood in infants is 17–24 mM/l.

UREA
(5 μl. plasma)

A modification of the method described by Chaney and Marbach (1962), which depends on the formation of indophenol blue from the ammonia liberated by urease.

Reagents

(1) *Urease Solution.* 25 mg. urease (Sigma type IV) in 60 ml. of 1 per cent E.D.T.A. adjusted to *p*H 6·5. Store in small aliquots at −20°C.
(2) *Urea Standard.* 100 mg. of vacuum-dried urea is dissolved in 100 ml. of water and a little toluene is added as a preservative: stable for one month at 4°C.
(3) "*Solution 1*". 5 g. phenol and 25 mg. sodium nitroprusside are dissolved in 100 ml. of water. Store at 4°C in a brown container.
(4) "*Solution 2*". 32·5 ml. of N-sodium hydroxide plus 3 ml. of N-sodium hypochlorite are made up to 100 ml. with water. Store at 4°C. Deionized water is used throughout.

Method. Into a 5 ml. plastic tube, pipette 5 μl. of plasma and 100 μl. of urease solution: mix and incubate for 5 minutes at 37°C.

Then add 0·5 ml. of solution 1 and 0·5 ml. of solution 2: mix and incubate for a further 10 minutes.

Finally add 4 ml. of deionized water, and read at 630 mμ or with the appropriate filter.

Blank. A blank using water instead of plasma is also put up and treated the same way.

Standard. 5 μl. of the standard urea solution is treated similarly.

Calculation. The blank is subtracted from the test and standard solutions, and the calculation is made in the usual way.

GLUCOSE
(40 μl. plasma)

This can be performed on the Auto-Analyzer by a modified glucose oxidase method, using 40 μl. of whole blood. The manual method is a modification of that of Kingsley and Getchell (1960).

Reagents

(1) *Peroxidase buffer.* Dissolve 5 mg. peroxidase (Sigma) in 125 ml. 0·1 M-KH₂PO₂, adjust to *p*H 7·0 with 0·1 N-NaOH and dilute to 500 ml. with water. Store at −20°C in 20 ml. aliquots.
(2) *o-Dianisidine.* 1 g. per cent in methanol, stored at 4°C.
(3) *Glucose oxidase.* Fermcozyme 653 AM (Hughes and Hughes).
(4) 50 *per cent Sulphuric Acid* (50 per cent in water v/v).

(5) *Standard Glucose Solutions.* Dissolve 1 g. glucose in 100 ml. of 0·25 per cent benzoic acid for the stock solution. The *working standard* (100 mg./100 ml.) is made by diluting the stock solution one in ten with 0·25 per cent benzoic acid.

(6) *Working Solutions* (prepare fresh daily):

"*Solution A*"	20 ml. peroxidase buffer
	0·2 ml. *o*-dianisidine
	40 μl. glucose oxidase
"*Solution B*"	20 ml. peroxidase buffer
	0·2 ml. *o*-dianisidine

Method. Into 5 ml. disposable plastic containers pipette 20 μl. of plasma and 3 ml. of Solution A. Mix and incubate at 37°C for exactly 15 minutes.

Then add 1 ml. of 50 per cent sulphuric acid, and mix and read at 527 mμ or with the appropriate filter in a colorimeter.

Standard. 20 μl. of the working glucose standard is treated in the same way.

Blanks. A blank is prepared for each plasma and for the standard by substituting Solution B for Solution A in the above procedure.

Calculation. The relevant blank values are subtracted from the standard and plasma readings and the calculation is made in the usual way.

CALCIUM
(30 μl. plasma)

Calcium and magnesium can be estimated with an Atomic Absorption apparatus. For laboratories without this facility, calcium is conveniently estimated by a modification of the method of Radin and Gramza (1964). This method requires a spectrophotometer, and depends on the decrease in optical density of the dye Eriochrome Blue produced by calcium at a wavelength of 620 mμ. Magnesium does not interfere at the alkaline *p*H used.

Reagents

(1) *Eriochrome Blue Solution.* 532·7 mg. of dye is dissolved in 1 litre of water acidified with 0·7 ml. of N-HCl. (Stable at room temperature.)

(2) 5N-*Potassium Hydroxide.*

(3) *Stock Calcium Solution.* 625 mg. of dried Analar calcium carbonate are dissolved in 50 ml. of water plus 12·5 ml. N-HCl, and the volume made up to 250 ml. with water: for use this is diluted 1 in 10 ($\equiv$ 10 mg. /100 ml.).

(4) *Alkaline Dye Solution* (prepare fresh and use within one hour): 10 ml. Eriochrome Blue Solution is added to 80 ml. water, and then 10 ml. 5N-KOH is added. Deionized water is used throughout.

Method. Readings are made in the spectrophotometer at 620 mμ using a 3 ml. cuvette. 2·5 ml. of the alkaline dye solution plus 1·5 ml. of deionized water is used to zero the instrument.

Into a second 3 ml. cuvette, pipette exactly 3 ml. of alkaline dye solution and read the optical density (Reading 1). Then add 30 μl. of standard calcium solution (10 mg./100 ml.) mix and read again (Reading 2).

The cuvette must then be washed out with water, rinsed with alkaline dye solution and drained well. A further 3 ml. of alkaline dye is pipetted into the cuvette and Reading 3 is taken. After adding 30 μl. of plasma and mixing, take Reading 4. Readings are best performed in duplicate.

Calculation

$$\text{Plasma calcium} = \frac{\text{Reading 3--4}}{\text{Reading 1--2}} \times 10 \text{ mg./100 ml.}$$

The calculation assumes that plasma diluted 1/100 with 0·5 N-KOH has a negligible optical density. This is true even in the presence of jaundice or hæmolysis. However, lipæmic sera (e.g. in the nephrotic syndrome) do have a significant absorption at 620 mμ and a correction must be made: 30 μl. of plasma are added to 3 ml. of

0·5 N-KOH and the increase in O.D. is determined (Reading 5). The calculation then becomes:

$$\text{plasma calcium} = \frac{(\text{Reading } 3\text{–}4) + 5}{\text{Reading } 1\text{–}2} \times 10 \text{ mg./100 ml.}$$

BILIRUBIN
(30 μl. plasma)

This is a modification of the method of Nosslin (1960), which gives a more accurate value for direct reacting bilirubin than other methods of which we are aware.

Reagents

(1) *Diazo Solution I.* 5·0 g. of sulphanilic acid are dissolved in distilled water containing 15 ml. concentrated hydrochloric acid and made up to 1 litre.

(2) *Diazo Solution II.* Sodium nitrite 0·5 g./100 ml.

(3) *Diazo Reagent.* 10 ml. of diazo I solution is added to 0·25 ml. of diazo solution II. It must be prepared freshly.

(4) *Caffeine Reagent.* 50 g. of caffeine, 75 g. of sodium benzoate and 125 g. of sodium acetate are dissolved in one litre of distilled water.

(5) *Alkaline Tartrate.* Fehling's Solution II. 100 g. of sodium hydroxide and 350 g. of sodium potassium tartrate per litre of distilled water.

(6) *4 per cent Ascorbic Acid.* Approximately 200 mg. of ascorbic acid are dissolved in 5 ml. of distilled water. Prepare fresh daily.

(7) *Standard Bilirubin.* 10 mg. of bilirubin are dissolved in 100 ml. of 5 per cent bovine albumin.

Method. Polyethylene tubes are used for the total, direct and blank reactions. The precise order in which reagents are added is important.

Total. Place in tube 40 μl. distilled water, 10 μl. plasma, 100 μl. caffeine reagent and 30 μl. of diazo reagent. Exactly 10 minutes later add 5 μl. ascorbic acid and 80 μl. alkaline tartrate.

Direct, Place in tube 40 μl. distilled water, 10 μl. plasma, and 30 μl. diazo reagent. Exactly 10 minutes later add 5 μl. ascorbic acid, 100 μl. caffeine reagent an 80 μl. alkaline tartrate.

Blank. Place in tube 40 μl. distilled water, 10 μl. plasma, 5 μl. ascorbic acid, 30 μl. diazo reagent, 100 μl. caffeine reagent and 80 μl. alkaline tartrate.

The total and direct solutions are read at 600 mμ. after setting the instrument to zero absorbance with the blank solution.

Standard. The total and blank reactions are performed in a similar manner.

Calculation. Both the total and the direct-reacting bilirubin values are calculated from the optical density of the standard in the total reaction.

TOTAL PROTEIN
(5 μl. plasma)

This is a modified biuret method. The addition of sodium sulphite has been found to be unnecessary.

Reagents

(1) *Biuret Reagent.* Dissolve 0·15 g. of copper sulphate pentahydrate and 0·60 g. of sodium potassium tarrtate in about 50 ml. of 2·5 N-NaOH (carbonate free); and make up to 100 ml. with distilled water. Store in a dark bottle at 4°C.

(2) *Standard Protein Solution.* A bovine albumin solution of approximately 10 g./100 ml. is prepared; the precise value is determined by a Kjeldahl method.

Method. Into a 0·4 ml. polyethylene test-tube, pipette 0·2 ml. of biuret reagent. Add 5 μl. of plasma, mix, and allow to stand for about 30 minutes. Read at 540 mμ.

Standard and *Blank.* 5 μl. of standard protein solution and water, respectively, are treated in the same way.

Calculation. The blank is subtracted from the test and standard solutions, and the calculation made in the usual way.

ALKALINE PHOSPHATASE
(20 μl. plasma)

The method of Kind and King (1954) has been scaled down and modified.

Reagents

(1) *Reagent I.* 0·128 g. of disodium phenyl phosphate dihydrate, 0·318 g. anhydrous sodium carbonate, 0·168 g. anhydrous sodium bicarbonate and 0·120 g. of 4-aminophenazone are dissolved in 100 ml. of distilled water. Pipette in 0·3 ml. amounts into the polyethylene micro test-tubes and store in the deep freeze. (These are stable for about a month.) Fresh reagent is prepared when the blank has an O.D. greater than 0·10.

(2) *Reagent II.* 4·8 g. of potassium ferricyanide are dissolved in 100 ml. of distilled water. Store at 4°C.

(3) *Standard Phenol Solution.* A stock solution is made by dissolving 100 mg. phenol in 100 ml. 0·1 N-hydrochloric acid. This is diluted 1:4 with water for the working standard (25 mg./100 ml.).

Method. Sufficient tubes containing Reagent I are thawed and warmed to 37°C in a water-bath. 10 μl. of plasma are added, successive tests being staggered by 30 seconds. 50 μl. of Reagent II is added to each tube after it has stood exactly 15 minutes. After mixing, the absorption is read in a microspectrophotometer at 510 mμ. If the O.D. is greater than 1·0, the test should be repeated on 5 μl. of plasma.

Standard. To 0·3 ml. of Reagent I add 10 μl. of the working phenol standard and 50 μl. of Reagent II, mix, and read as above.

Blanks. For the tests, to 0·3 ml. of Reagent I add 50 μl. of Reagent II followed by 10 μl. of plasma. Mix well, and read immediately as above. For the standard blank, the standard solution is replaced by 10 μl. of water.

Calculation.

$$\text{Plasma alkaline phosphatase} = \frac{\text{Test} - \text{Test Blank}}{\text{Std.} - \text{Std. Blank}} \times 25 \text{ King units.}$$

APPENDIX B

COMMERCIAL APPARATUS

This appendix lists a few firms who supply specialized microchemical apparatus. References to other equipment is given in the paper by Clayton and Jenkins (1966).

BECKMAN INSTRUMENTS LTD., Glenrothes, Fife
Sanz pipettes, polyethylene and polypropylene test-tubes of 0·4 ml. and 0·5 ml. capacity. Also supply the Spinco colorimeter, centrifuge, burette and mixer, either as a complete unit or as individual items.

FISON'S SCIENTIFIC APPARATUS LTD., Bishop Meadow Road, Loughborough, Leicestershire
Supply the Natelson microgasometer.

HOOK AND TUCKER LTD., 301 Brixton Road, London, S.W.9
Makers of an automatic dilutor.

V. A. Howe Ltd., 46 Pembridge Road, London, W.11
    Agents for the Astrup apparatus made by Radiometer, Copenhagen.

P. K. Morgan, Ltd., 10 Manor Road, Chatham, Kent
    Blood gas analyser for blood pH and P_{co_2}.

Wright Scientific Ltd., 7 Cardigan Road, London, N.W.6
    Agents for the Gilford spectrophotometer.

Addendum

Since this article was written a further commercial system has been introduced. This is the Eppendorf microlitre system, marketed in this country by V. A. Howe and Co., Ltd., 46 Pembridge Road, London, W.11.

The basis of the system is a new type of pipette. A plunger, used to aspirate and eject reagents and samples, is operated by a push button on the top of the pipette. The fluid dispensed is contained within a disposable polypropylene tip. The sizes available are 5, 10, 20, 50, 100, 200, 500 and 1000 microlitres. The pipette is simple to use although rather expensive.

Other items available are polypropylene test tubes, reagent flasks, rotary shaker, mixer and centrifuge.

References

Chaney, A. L. and Marbach, E. P. (1962. *Clin. Chem.*, **8** 130.
Gomori, G. (1942). *J. lab. clin. Med.*, **27,** 955.
Kind, P. R. N. and King, E. J. (1954). *J. clin. Path.*, **7,** 322
Kingsley, G. R. and Getchell, G. (1960). *Clin. Chem.*, **6,** 466.
Maclagan, N. F. (1944). *Brit. J. exp. Path.* **25,** 234.
Nosslin, B. (1960). *Scandinav. J. clin. lab. Invest.*, **12,** Supp. 49.
O'Brien, D., Ibbott, F, and Pinfield, A. (1961). *Clin. Chem.* **7,** 521.
Radin, N. and Gramza, A. L. (1964). *Clin. Chem.*, **10,** 704.
Searcy, R. L. and Bergouist, L. M. (1960). *Clin. Chim. Acta.*, **5,** 192.
Trinder, P. (1954). *Biochem. J.*, **57,** 301.
Whitehead, T. P. (1965). *Lancet*, **ii,** 1015.

Books and Review Articles:

Clayton, B. E. and Jenkins, P. (1966). Micromethods and micro apparatus for chemical pathology with special reference to paediatrics. *J. clin. Path.*, **19,** 293.
O'Brien, D. and Ibbott, F. A. (1962). *Laboratory Manual of Paediatric Micro- and Ultra-micro-Biochemical Techniques*, 3rd Edit. New York: Harper and Row.
Reinouts van Haga, P., and Wael, J De, (1961). Ultramicro methods. *Adv. clin. Chem.*, **4,** 321.
Sanz, M. C. (1957). Ultramicro methods and standardisation of equipment. *Clin. Chem.* **3.** 406.
Wilkinson, R. H. (1960). *Chemical Micromethods in Clinical Medicine*. Springfield, Illinois: Charles C. Thomas.

Chapter 9

MAGNESIUM METABOLISM

G. V. FOSTER

DURING the past decade, two outstanding developments have accelerated progress in magnesium research. First, the radioactive isotope of magnesium, ^{28}Mg, has become commercially available. Although its relatively short half-life of 21·3 hours and its high cost restrict its general use, ^{28}Mg has already proved an invaluable aid in the study of kinetic problems. Second, the application of flame spectrophotometry to the determination of magnesium has provided an assay technique with a sensitivity hitherto impossible to achieve by other means. Its simplicity of operation has eliminated the tedium of former methods.

Biochemistry. Magnesium is essential for life. It is present as an intracellular ion in all living tissues. Although our knowledge of this metal has grown in recent years, few general conclusions can be made regarding its biochemical function. Its influence on a wide spectrum of enzyme reactions precludes assigning it a single primary rôle in body processes. The importance of magnesium in many of these reactions is difficult to assess. In some, other metal ions may substitute for magnesium. In others, its required presence can be demonstrated only *in vitro*. Unquestionably it plays a rôle in many of the energy storing and releasing reactions involved in oxidative phosphorylation. Indirectly, therefore, it affects all anabolic and catabolic reactions involving carbohydrate, fat and protein. In addition, it is an essential co-factor for some peptidases, ribonucleases and glycolylic and cocarboxylation reactions. Other enzyme systems influenced by magnesium have been reviewed by Wacker and Vallee (1964) and Walser (1967).

The diversity of reactions affected, as well as their widespread distribution in nature, reflect magnesium's evolutionary significance. Basic life processes evolved in a magnesium environment in pre-Cambrian seas. Subsequent internalization of these important biochemical reactions within cell walls followed. By preserving the inorganic milieu, the evolution of terrestial forms of life was made possible.

Pharmacology. The pharmacological properties of magnesium are threefold. It depresses nerve conduction, impairs vascular tone and cardiac function and accentuates the action of posterior pituitary hormones on the uterus.

Magnesium is both a central and a peripheral nervous system depressant. Magnesium sulphate causes a curare-like muscular paralysis in laboratory animals. In larger doses it produces general anæsthesia. The peripheral effect is due to a decreased liberation of acetylcholine at the neuromuscular junction and sympathetic ganglion. It may be antagonized by an excess, or accentuated by a diminution, of calcium.

The cardiovascular effects of the ion include both an influence on the muscular tone of blood vessels and on the conduction of electrical impulses by the myocardium. As the magnesium concentration in the blood is raised, hypotension is the first sign to develop. At higher levels the transmission of electrical impulses is impaired. Both the PT and QRS intervals of the electrocardiogram are increased, as is the height of the T wave. At still higher levels the heart stops in diastole. Intravenous administration of magnesium salts can reverse ventricular arrhythmias due to digitalis intoxication. In this condition a reciprocal interrelationship between calcium and magnesium is found. High concentration of calcium in the blood predisposes to ventricular arrhythmias due to digitalis poisoning.

Finally, magnesium potentiates or confers an oxytocic effect to the posterior pituitary hormones. In *in vitro* experiments even vasopressin can cause contraction of uterine muscle strips when magnesium is present in the suspending medium.

To recapitulate, magnesium affects nerve transmission, muscular contraction and a wide range of important enzyme reactions. These classical biochemical and pharmacological effects were originally demonstrated in acute experiments. The magnesium concentrations under which the results were observed varied greatly from physiological conditions. Of far greater clinical importance are the changes produced by small but chronic aberrations in magnesium balance. The quantitative study of magnesium imbalance has only recently been made possible by more exacting methods of assay.

DETERMINATION OF MAGNESIUM

Flame Spectrophotometry. Estimation of magnesium may be done by either *emission* or *absorption* flame spectrophotometry. These techniques and their application to assays of blood, urine and tissue have been fully described by MacIntyre and his co-workers (Alcock, MacIntyre and Radde, 1960; MacIntyre, 1961; Alcock and MacIntyre, 1966).

Emission flame spectrophotometry entails the spraying of diluted fluid in a hot oxygen-acetylene flame and comparing the emission of excited atoms at 285·2 mμ with standard solutions of magnesium. In addition to a hot flame, a monochromator of very high resolution is needed.

In contradistinction to emission flame spectrophotometry, absorption flame spectrophotometry measures unexcited atoms in the flame (Willis, 1960; Dawson and Heaton, 1961; MacIntyre, 1961). A beam of monochromatic light of the same wavelength is passed through the flame and changes in the light absorbed are measured.

Both methods have the great advantage of being applicable to other heavy metal ions. Theoretically, emission flame spectrophotometry offers greater precision for determining calcium and absorption flame spectrophotometry offers greater precision for magnesium. Recent improvements in many commercial instruments, however, now permit near equal sensitivity for assay of either ion.

Chemical Methods. In general, chemical determinations lack the specificity of flame spectrophotometry. Unless automated, they require considerably more time to carry out. All have the advantage of requiring no specialized instruments other than a colorimeter or fluorometer.

Magnesium may be estimated after removal of calcium as oxalate by precipitation with ammonium phosphate and subsequent assay for phosphate in the residue.

The latter determination may be made by a number of methods (Alcock and MacIntyre, 1966). The technique has been extensively used and modifications are numerous.

A number of colorimetric procedures are available. These include reactions with Titan Yellow, estimation of magnesium as magnesium-8-hydroxyquinoline, titration of magnesium-dye complex with ethyl-diamine tetra-acetate and colour reactions with Erichrome Black T and various azo dyes. Of all the colorimetric methods currently used, the fluorometric method of Hill (1962) appears most promising. However, unless expense is the final determinant, flame spectrophotometry is to be preferred over all other methods.

DISTRIBUTION OF MAGNESIUM IN THE BODY

Magnesium is the fourth most abundant cation in man. It is exceeded in amount only by calcium, sodium and potassium. Of the 2,400 mEq. in the body, approximately two-thirds occur in bone, 1 per cent in extracellular fluid and the remainder in soft tissue (Table I). Despite this disproportionately low concentration of magnesium in plasma, its level is rigorously maintained within the narrow limits of 1·5 to 1·8 mEq./l.

TABLE I

Distribution of Magnesium in Man

(From Aikawa (1964), *reproduced with permission of the U.S. Atomic Energy Commission.*)

Tissue	Concentration mEq./kg. wet weight	Magnesium content, mEq.	Percentage of total
Bone	300	1,500	63
Muscle	12	470	19
Soft tissues	10–15	400	17
Extracellular fluid	2	30	1
Total	—	2,400	100

These compartments must not be thought of as static reservoirs. In healthy man, 15 per cent of the total body magnesium is exchangeable (Avioli, Lynch and Bastomsky, 1963; Avioli and Berman, 1966). Kinetic studies suggest wide variation in the percentage of exchangeable magnesium in different tissues. Muscle, for example, contains 20 per cent exchangeable magnesium, bone only 2 per cent. As might be expected, the percentage proportions can be greatly altered by disease. Hyperthyroidism markedly increases the amount of exchangeable magnesium. Conversely, the reverse is found when thyroid function is suppressed. In Paget's disease, exchangeable bone magnesium can be increased as much as two- or threefold.

Blood. Like calcium, magnesium is partly bound to protein. Under conditions of physiological pH, roughly one-third is protein-bound. The remainder is ionic (Prasad, Flink and McCollister, 1961). The factors which influence this partition are largely obscure. Thyroid hormone, parathyroid hormone, venous stasis, pH and changes in red cell and blood vessel permeability have been claimed to alter the proportion of bound to free cation. Whang and Wagner (1966) have studied the effect of venous occlusion in the forearm. They found that, concomitant with the fall in blood pH, serum magnesium rose, as did the hæmatocrit. The degree of acidosis was felt to be insufficient to explain the change, whereas the increase in red blood cell size could. Loss of water from serum either into red cells, due to pH changes, or into soft tissue, due to increased hydrostatic pressure in the capillaries, results in increased serum concentrations. Under these conditions, magnesium bound to protein is concentrated relative to other freely diffusible components. This is an important clinical consideration. For meaningful determinations, prolonged venous occlusion must be avoided.

Cerebrospinal Fluid. The concentration of magnesium in cerebrospinal fluid is half again as high as in plasma (Pallis, MacIntyre and Anstall, 1965). The observation is of great interest, since it proves that spinal fluid cannot be an ultra-filtrate of plasma.

FACTORS AFFECTING MAGNESIUM METABOLISM

In occidental countries, the average daily intake in man is 250–300 mg. Much of this is obtained from green vegetables, where magnesium is found in the porphyrin group of chlorophyll. No definitive experimental studies have been carried out to determine the minimal daily requirement for man, although the figure 250 mg. has been widely quoted. In comparison to oriental diets, which provide 6–10 mg./kg./day, occidental diets average less than 5 mg./kg. Seelig (1964), in a comprehensive review of the literature on magnesium balance studies, concludes that daily intakes below 6 mg./kg. predispose to negative balance. Failure to retain magnesium under these conditions is more prevalent in men than women. Since western diets can be relatively deficient in magnesium, subclinical deficiency may be more common than is generally recognized.

Absorption

Roughly one-third of the dietary magnesium is absorbed: the remainder is passively excreted in the fæces. Balance is maintained by further loss in urine, sweat and gastric and mammary secretions. The factors which influence these processes are summarized in Figure 1.

Absorption takes place primarily in the small bowel. It begins within an hour after ingestion and continues at a steady rate for 2–8 hours, by which time 80 per cent of the total absorption has taken place. Studies in the rat by Ross (1962) and Hendrix and his collaborators (1963) suggest that the rate increases from proximal duodenum to distal ileum. In man, fairly uniform absorption has been demonstrated throughout the small intestine (Graham, Caesar and Burgen, 1960).

Unlike calcium absorption, which is markedly influenced by vitamin D, no one factor plays a controlling rôle for magnesium. The following sub-sections on factors affecting magnesium metabolism are outlined in somewhat greater detail than in most general reviews for two reasons. First, these areas have recently been intensively investigated. Second, they are important to the chemical pathologist and clinician interested in metabolic balance studies.

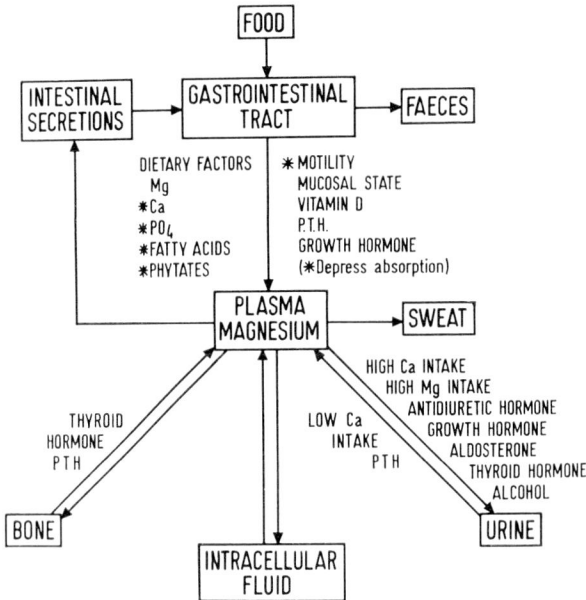

Fɪɢ. 1.—Factors which influence the absorption and excretion of magnesium.

(1) *Size of Magnesium Load.* Graham, Caesar and Burgen (1960), using isotopic magnesium, have studied the effects of varying diets in patients. Absorption was doubled when the normal dietary magnesium requirement was doubled, and halved when a diet low in the cation was fed. The findings suggest that absorption is influenced by the load but that the relationship is not linear. The results are unaffected by depletion or repletion of magnesium over short periods.

(2) *Dietary Calcium.* Alcock and MacIntyre (1960, 1962) have advanced the hypothesis that calcium and magnesium are absorbed by a common transport mechanism from the intestinal tract. Without question, magnesium absorption is increased in calcium deficiency and decreased in the presence of excess calcium. The converse with respect to calcium with varying magnesium diets is likewise true. The interrelationship is not surprising since calcium is found subjacent to magnesium in the same group of the Periodic Table. The hypothesis of a common absorptive mechanism has only been confirmed in animals (Schachter and Rosen, 1959; Alcock and MacIntyre, 1962; Care and Van't Klooster, 1965). Whether or not a similar mechanism exists in man has not yet been shown (Heaton, Hodgkins and Rose, 1964).

(3) *Motility and Mucosal State.* Increased fæcal losses occur in patients with malabsorption syndrome (MacIntyre, Hanna, Booth and Read, 1961; Booth, MacIntyre and Mollin, 1964).

(4) *Vitamin D.* Studies in rats suggest that vitamin D exerts an effect on magnesium absorption similar to that which it exerts on calcium (Hanna, 1961). Animals treated with large doses excrete 60 per cent less magnesium than controls. The effect may be due to an increased uptake of magnesium by the body tissues as shown by Wallach and his collaborators in dogs (Wallach, Bellavia, Schorr and Gamponia, 1966). A similar effect has yet to be demonstrated in man.

(5) *Parathyroid Hormone.* MacIntyre and his associates (MacIntyre, Matthews and Robinson, 1966) have studied the effect of parathyroid hormone in para-thyroidectomized rats. They have convincingly shown that the hormone increases absorption of magnesium throughout the intestine. Their results support the clinical observations of Heaton and Pyrah (1963), who noted in five out of six patients that fæcal magnesium increased following the removal of a parathyroid adenoma.

Presumably the hyperfunctioning parathyroids in these cases were responsible for increased absorption of the cation prior to operation.

(6) *Growth Hormone.* Metabolic balance studies have been carried out in patients either receiving exogenous hormone or with excessive endogenous secretion due to acromegaly (Hanna, Harrison, MacIntyre and Fraser, 1960). The effects of growth hormone resembled those of vitamin D. In all the cases studied, an increase in magnesium absorption was demonstrated.

(7) *Other Factors.* In addition to the above, brief mention should be made of other substances which also affect magnesium absorption. Absorption is increased by high protein intake and neomycin. Fatty acids, phytates and excess phosphate decrease absorption. Like calcium, these combine with magnesium to form insoluble and unabsorbable compounds. Gastro-intestinal handling of the ion is little affected by pH.

Excretion

Magnesium is lost in fæces, sweat and urine.

Fæcal Loss. The loss via the gastro-intestinal tract is variable, depending primarily upon dietary factors. Using ^{28}Mg, Aikawa (1964) found that between 60 and 80 per cent of orally administered magnesium could be accounted for in the fæces. When the isotope was given intravenously, only 1·8 per cent could be recovered. Presumably this latter loss occurred in unabsorbed saliva and pancreatic and gastric secretions. Of these, saliva contains the greatest concentration of magnesium. Between 0·25 and 0·50 mEq. of total magnesium is returned to the gastro-intestinal tract daily by this secretion alone. This should be borne in mind by physicians treating patients requiring prolonged gastric suction.

Sweat Loss. Sweat loss is currently receiving considerable attention by many investigators interested in calcium balance. Unfortunately little information on magnesium losses in sweat is presently available. Seelig (1964), extrapolating data from other sources, has estimated that 0·75 mEq. of magnesium are lost daily on a normal diet. Increased losses can be assumed to occur under circumstances which promote increased perspiration. The effect of environmental temperature has been studied (Consolazio, Matoush, Nelson, Harding and Canham, 1963). As might be anticipated, magnesium losses in perspiration increased at elevated temperatures. The data suggests that there is increased renal and intestinal conservation of magnesium under these conditions. These points are mentioned only to remind the clinician that seasonal variations in excretion and conservation can be anticipated unless environmental temperatures are reasonably controlled.

In lower animals a relationship exists between plasma magnesium levels and body temperature. Magnesium lowers body temperature in dogs. Conversely, in a number of hibernating animals magnesium levels rise during hibernation. The ion may act by depressing the central nervous system. Lowering body temperature in some non-hibernating species produces a similar effect on magnesium. In man this interrelationship between temperature and magnesium has not been shown.

Urinary Loss. Absorption of magnesium from the gastro-intestinal tract and excretion in sweat are poorly controlled processes. Regulation of magnesium balance is principally dependent upon renal handling of the ion. This is substantiated by the direct relationship of dietary intake to its appearance in the urine (Heaton and Parsons, 1961; Barnes, Cope and Harrison, 1958). Most likely excess ionic magnesium in the blood is passed in the urine when the limit of renal tubular resorption is exceeded. Although a Tm has yet to be shown in man, it exists in laboratory animals (Averill and Heaton, 1966).

In the adult on a normal diet, 3–17 mEq. magnesium are excreted daily by the kidney. Diffusible magnesium is filtered by the glomerulus and reabsorbed by the tubules. Whether tubular secretion occurs in man is not known. It occurs in aglomerular fish (Berglund and Forster, 1958), rat (Averill and Heaton, 1966) and dog in the distal tubule (Ginn, Smith, Hammarsten and Snyder, 1959). Most of the factors affecting renal handling of magnesium are poorly understood. The following are known:

(1) *Calcium Intake*. Increased excretion is promoted by increased dietary intake of calcium. Samiy and his colleagues (1960) and Alcock and MacIntyre (1962) have proposed a common transport system in the renal tubule for both ions. If their hypothesis is valid, the absorptive mechanism is saturated by an excess of calcium which reduces tubular reabsorption of magnesium.

(2) *Parathyroid Hormone*. Administration of pure parathyroid hormone diminishes excretion in the rat (MacIntyre, Boss and Troughton, 1963). Its effect in man is less obvious. Urinary excretion of magnesium in patients following removal of parathyroid adenomas did not appreciably alter in five of six patients studied by Heaton and Pyrah (1963).

(3) *Antidiuretic Hormone*. Nielsen (1964) has shown that either lysine or arginine vasopressin increases the rate of both magnesium and calcium excretion in normal subjects. The clinical finding by Hellman and his colleagues (1962) in a patient with porphyria and signs of excessive secretion of antidiuretic hormone supports this observation. During an attack of this disease, signs of magnesium deficiency developed which were readily alleviated by parenteral magnesium. Although the mechanism for the increased urinary excretion is not understood, the finding that both calcium and magnesium are affected further suggests that divalent cations are handled by a similar pathway.

(4) *Growth Hormone*. As well as producing increased gastro-intestinal absorption, growth hormone increases the urinary excretion of magnesium (Hanna, Harrison, MacIntyre and Fraser, 1960). In addition to the above effects, it increases plasma calcium and lowers plasma magnesium and plasma citrate in acromegalic patients. Hanna and his colleagues (1960) have pointed out that, since vitamin D causes similar results, a common biochemical process may exist for both substances.

(5) *Aldosterone*. Conclusive evidence has been presented by Horton and Biglieri (1962) that this hormone increases urinary excretion. Urinary output was measured in four patients with primary aldosteronism. All had values above normal control subjects on comparable diets. Spironolactone given to two patients produced an immediate fall. Stimulation of aldosterone secretion by intravenous infusion of saline markedly increased urinary output of magnesium in those patients with tumours. The observations were confirmed in a bilaterally adrenalectomized patient who was given exogenous hormone. A similar increase in urinary excretion occurred. In all the studies a concurrent increase in potassium excretion was associated with magnesium diuresis.

(6) *Thyroid Hormone*. Urinary excretion of magnesium is 80 per cent

greater in the hyperthyroid patient and 30 per cent less in the hypothyroid patient than in control subjects (Dimich, Rizek, Wallach and Siler, 1966). The changes are explainable by alteration in bone turnover of magnesium. The possible interrelationship between this ion and thyroid hormone has been extensively studied by many workers. Several have suggested that thyroid hormone production or effect might be modified by magnesium. Deficiency of the ion produces thyroid enlargement in the rat (Corradino and Parker, 1962). Conversely, exogenously administered magnesium reduces the weight loss produced in this animal by excessive doses of hormone. The inter-relationship may also exist in man. Goitre has not been reported in mag-nesium deficiency and moderate doses of magnesium have had no obvious effect on hyperthyroidism (Wiswell, 1961). However, large doses have ameliorated clinical and laboratory manifestations of hyperthyroidism and reduced the size of non-toxic goitres in a few patients (Neguib, 1963).

(7) *Alcohol Ingestion.* Oral ingestion of as little as 1 ml. of 95 per cent alcohol per kg. increases urinary magnesium excretion two- to fourfold (McCollister, Flink and Lewis, 1963). Output is unrelated to the changes in urine volume. Undoubtedly the increased excretion partially accounts for the magnesium deficiency in alcoholics with delirium tremens (Flink, Stutzman, Anderson, Konig and Fraser, 1954; Nielsen, 1963).

To recapitulate, of the dietary and hormonal factors which affect urinary excretion of magnesium, all promote output with the exception of parathyroid hormone. The mechanisms by which these alterations are brought about are still poorly understood. Parenthetically, special caution must be taken in assessing the results of all acute studies. McCollister and his colleagues (1963) have shown in normal subjects on controlled diets and fluid intake that progressively more magnesium is excreted in the urine during the course of the day. Late afternoon output exceeds morning output by approximately 10 per cent.

PLASMA MAGNESIUM IN DISEASE

High Plasma Magnesium. Raised values have been reported in uncontrolled diabetes, adrenocortical insufficiency, hypothyroidism, advanced renal failure and acute renal faliure. In these disease states the elevated blood magnesium values do not constitute a management problem and respond to appropriate therapy.

Low Plasma Magnesium. The pathological conditions which may cause abnormally low serum magnesium values are listed in Table II. Besides

TABLE II

Conditions in which Low Serum Magnesium is found

Condition	Reference
Malabsorption syndrome	MacIntyre, I., Hanna, S., Booth, C. C. and Read, A. E. (1961). *Clin. Sci.* **20**, 297. Back, E. H., Montgomery, R. D. and Ward, E. E. (1962). *Arch. Dis. Childh.* **37**, 106. Booth, C. C., MacIntyre, I. and Mollin, D. L. (1964). *Quart. J. Med.* **33**, 401.

TABLE II—*Continued*

Conditions in which Low Serum Magnesium is found—*Continued*

Condition	Reference
Infantile protein malnutrition (Kwashiorkor)	Montgomery, R. D. (1960). *Lancet*, **2**, 74. Montgomery, R. D. (1960). *Lancet*, **2**, 264. Pretorius, P. J., Wehmeyer, A. S. and Theron, J. J. (1963). *Amer. J. clin. Nutr.* **13**, 331.
Prolonged gastric suction	Kellaway, G. and Ewen, K. (1962). *N.Z. med. J.* **61**, 137.
Post-parathyroidectomy	Harmon, M. (1956). *Amer. J. Dis. Child.* **91**, 313. Agna, J. W. and Goldsmith, R. E. (1958). *New Engl. J. Med.* **258**, 222. Potts, J. T., Roberts, B., Ravdin, I. S. and Johnston, C. G. (1958). *Amer. J. med. Sci.* **235**, 206. Hanna, S., North, K. A. K., MacIntyre, I. and Fraser, R. (1961). *Brit. med. J.* **2**, 1253. Walser, M. (1962). *J. clin. Invest.* **41**, 1454.
Hyperthyroidism	Wallach, S., Cahill, L. N., Rogan, F. H. and Jones, H. L. (1962). *J. Lab. clin. Med.* **59**, 195.
Primary aldosteronism	Mader, I. J. and Iseri, L. T. (1955). *Amer. J. Med..* **19**, 976. Milne, M. D., Muehrcke, R. C. and Aird, I. (1957). *Quart. J. Med.* **26**, 317. Horton, R. and Biglieri, E. G. (1962). *J. clin. Endocr.* **22**, 1187.
Renal disease	Smith, W. O. and Hammarsten, J. F. (1958). *Arch. intern. Med.* **102**, 5.
Pyelonephritic renal insufficiency	Nielsen, B. (1962). *Dan. med. Bull.* **9**, 235.
Portal cirrhosis	Stutzman, F. L. and Amatuzio, D. S. (1953). *J. Lab. clin. Med.* **41**, 215.
Prolonged use of diuretics	Smith, W. O., Hammarsten, J. F. and Eliel, L. P. (1960). *J. Amer. med. Ass.* **174**, 77.
Porphyria associated with excessive antidiuretic hormone secretion	Nielsen, B. and Thorn, N. A. (1965). *Amer. J. Med.* **38**, 345.
Chronic alcoholism	Flink, E. B., Stutzman, F. L., Anderson, A. R., Konig, T. and Fraser, R. (1954). *J. Lab. clin. Med.* **43**, 169. McCollister, R. J., Flink, E. B. and Doe, R. P. (1960). *J. Lab. clin. Med.* **55**, 98. Heaton, F. W., Pyrah, L. N., Beresford, C. C., Bryson, R. W. and Martin, D. F. (1962). *Lancet*, **2**, 802.
Delirium tremens	Flink, E. B., Stutzman, F. L., Anderson, A. R., Konig, T. and Fraser, R. (1954). *J. Lab. clin. Med.* **43**, 169. Suter, C. and Klingman, W. O. (1955). *Neurology*, **5**, 691.
Excessive lactation	Greenwald, J. H., Dubin, A. and Cardon, L. (1963). *Amer. J. Med.* **35**, 854.
Hypercalcæmia of malignancy	Eliel, L. P., Smith, W. O. and Thomsen, C. (1960). *J. Oklahoma med. Ass.* **53**, 359.
Osteolytic bone disease	Smith, W. O. and Eliel, L. P. (1956). *Clin. Res. Proc.* **4**, 245.

TABLE II—*Continued*

Conditions in which Low Serum Magnesium is found—*Continued*

Condition	Reference
Renal tubular acidosis	Hanna, S. (1961). *J. clin. Path.* **14**, 410.
Malacic bone disease	Hammarsten, J. F. and Smith, W. O. (1957). *New Engl. J. Med.* **256**, 897.
Recovery phase of diabetic acidosis	Martin, H. E. and Wertman, M. (1947). *J. clin. Invest.* **26**, 217.
Acute pancreatitis	Edmondson, H. A., Berne, C. J., Homann, R. E. and Wertman, M. (1952). *Amer. J. Med.* **12**, 34.
Bronchial asthma	Haury, V. G. (1940). *J. Lab. clin. Med.* **26**, 340.
Pregnancy at term and newborn infants	Wallach, S., Cahill, L. N., Rogan, F. H. and Jones, H. L. (1962). *J. Lab. clin. Med.* **59**, 195.
Familial hereditary hypomagnesæmia	Welt, L. G. (1964). *Yale J. Biol. Med.* **36**, 325.
	Freeman, R. M. and Pearson, E. (1966). *Amer. J. Med.* **41**, 645.

these, hypomagnesæmia has also been reported in idiopathic epilepsy and eclampsia. The findings, however, have been disputed. In general terms, depressed magnesium blood levels are usually found in debilitated patients with chronic disease, suggesting that normal blood values are successfully maintained until reserve stores of the ion are severely depleted.

Hypomagnesæmia can usually be attributed to one of three causes: (*a*) deficient intake or absorption, (*b*) endocrinopathies or (*c*) chronic alcoholism.

Deficient Intake or Absorption. Magnesium deficiency should always be suspected in patients with malabsorption syndrome. Low serum magnesium is found in approximately 30 per cent of patients (Booth, Hanna, Babouris and MacIntyre, 1963). Of these, roughly one-third require replacement therapy. Low values have been reported in cases with idiopathic steatorrhœa, resection of small bowel and ulcerative colitis. Deficiencies could be equally common in any condition with chronic diarrhœa, rapid transit of food through the small intestine or disease interfering with absorption.

Inadequate intake occurs in kwashiorkor, chronic emesis and conditions requiring prolonged gastric suction or intravenous alimentation with insufficient magnesium replacement. Previously healthy subjects more readily withstand magnesium deprivation than do cachectic patients. Deficiency is rarely encountered post-operatively unless there has previously been an underlying disease promoting negative balance.

Endocrinopathies. A number of investigators have reported falls in plasma magnesium following removal of a parathyroid adenoma (Potts and Roberts, 1958; Hanna, North, MacIntyre and Fraser, 1961; Heaton and Pyrah, 1963). Acute hypomagnesæmia is most marked in patients with pre-existing magnesium depletion, bone disease or excessive vomiting. Increased bone uptake following surgery accounts for the changes seen. The falls observed are frequently of sufficient magnitude to require treatment. All patients with parathyroid adenomata should be studied post-operatively for changes in plasma magnesium. If proper analytical facilities are not available, prophylactic magnesium should be given intravenously.

Roughly one-third of patients with hyperthyroidism have hypomagnesæmia. Conversely, hypermagnesæmia occurs in a similar percentage of patients with hypothyroidism. The plasma levels reflect changes in excretion of the cation produced by the hormone. Hypersecretion of thyroid hormone increases the interchangeable body pool of magnesium (Dimich, Rizek, Wallach and Siler, 1966) and turnover rate. Under these conditions aberrations in excretion have a magnified effect on total body stores. The changes in magnesium handling produced by thyroid dysfunction are readily corrected by therapy directed to the underlying cause.

Primary hyperaldosteronism is a relatively rare disease. Hypomagnesæmia occurs in approximately half the patients and may be responsible for some of the neurological manifestations. Magnesium depletion is more commonly associated with secondary hyperaldosteronism. This condition may arise as a complication of renal insufficiency, cirrhosis or congestive heart failure. The cause of depletion is frequently difficult to attribute entirely to the disease. Characteristically œdema is present and renal loss of magnesium may be augmented by prolonged treatment with diuretics.

Mention has been previously made that antidiuretic hormone increases urinary magnesium excretion. A hypersecreting tumour for this hormone has yet to be reported. An increase in hormonal levels has been occasionally found in association with porphyria. Nielsen and Thorn (1965) have described hypomagnesæmia in this condition. Whether the low values reported are due to a direct effect of the hormone or reflect overhydration or rebound secondary hyperaldosteronism has yet to be shown.

Chronic Alcoholism. Magnesium balance in chronic alcoholics may be markedly negative (McCollister, Flink and Doe, 1960), and serum values are often low in patients with delirium tremens. The neurological symptoms, associated with this latter complication, may be related to the deficiency. The causes of negative magnesium balance are varied and frequently multiple. Prominent factors are insufficient dietary intake coupled with increased urinary excretion immediately following drinking. Even in severe depletion, 1–3 mEq. is excreted daily. In addition, liver damage may play a part. Nielsen (1963) has noted the relationship of serum magnesium levels to SGOT levels. In patients recovering from acute alcoholic episodes, serum transaminase levels fall as depressed blood levels return to normal.

Other Causes. Depletion of magnesium stores can occur during excessive lactation where both calcium and magnesium are lost in the mammary secretion. Low serum values are occasionally found associated with hypercalcæmia of malignancy and osteolytic bone disease. In these conditions hypercalcæmia presumably interferes with tubular reabsorption of magnesium on a competitive basis. This mechanism may also be important in renal acidosis and renal acidosis associated with osteomalacia where secondary hyperparathyroidism may occur. Magnesium deficiency is further augmented by distal tubular insufficiency which results in a decreased ability to form ammonia. As a consequence cations are excreted, resulting in further depletion of the body's store of magnesium.

Serum magnesium may be low in acute pancreatitis. Like calcium, magnesium in this condition is frequently precipitated with fat as a soap, Hypomagnesæmia with acute bronchial asthma has been reported to occur in 50 per cent of acute episodes (Haury, 1940). The cause is uncertain although some relation may exist between the eosinophilia found in allergic conditions and the eosinophilia produced by magnesium deficiency in animals (Hungerford and Karson, 1960). Low levels are occasionally found in pregnancy at term. Presumably they can be accounted for by the demands of the fœtus and by hæmodilution secondary to body fluid retention. Low serum values likewise occur in the newborn, reflecting maternal conditions.

Finally, mention should be made that a familial form of hypomagnesæmia may exist. Several probable cases have been described (Gitelman, Graham and Welt, 1966; Freeman and Pearson, 1966). In some, the defect is associated with hypokalæmia and alkalosis.

MAGNESIUM DEFICIENCY

In man, overt magnesium deficiency rarely occurs as an isolated entity. Only in cattle is a naturally occurring disease found. Two types have been described. One form is found in calves raised on unsupplemented whole milk. The other is an endemic disease called "grass staggers" or "grass tetany" which occurs in animals pastured in fields heavily fertilized with inorganic nitrates. This latter condition is thought to be due to the high ammonia content of the diet. Absorption is presumably impaired by the formation of insoluble ammonium magnesium phosphate at alkaline pH. The symptoms in both conditions are similar: restlessness and convulsions, frequently followed by death. Symptoms do not develop until serum magnesium values fall to one-half or one-third of normal levels. Phosphate and calcium concentrations remain unchanged.

Experimental Studies in Animals. Most of what we know of magnesium deficiency has been learned from studies in young, rapidly growing animals subjected to specific dietary restriction. Although symptoms of deficiency vary slightly between species, hyper-irritability and convulsions are always produced. Symptom producing dietary deprivation is always associated with hypomagnesæmia. The bone reserve may lose up to one-third of its magnesium content. In addition, the soft tissue is depleted of magnesium (MacIntyre and Davidsson, 1958).

Extensive investigations have been carried out in the rat. In animals fed a deficient diet, hyperæmia of the ears is always an early sign. This usually appears after about two weeks and subsequently fades. Many of the animals develop alopecia with inflamed skin lesions, and diarrhœa is common. Growth is retarded. The epiphysial cartilages of the posterior head of the tibia have a widened hyper-trophied zone and a narrow proliferating zone (Bernick and Hungerford, 1965). Staining reactions of metaphyseal trabeculæ and the incisal dentine suggest an interference in calcification of cartilage, bone and dentine. Using adult rats, Martindale and Heaton (1964) observed that, although the animals lose weight, the growth of the femur continues at a normal rate until the final stage of deficiency. Changes in plasma magnesium concentrations correspond to net loss of magnesium from bone. Both fall rapidly at first and then more slowly. The results suggest that the skeleton is the principal reservoir of mobile magnesium. When this reserve is depleted, magnesium is lost from the soft tissues, especially skeletal muscle (MacIntyre and Davidsson, 1958; Whang and Welt, 1963).

Eosinophilia and hypercalcæmia develop. The significance of the eosinophilia is not readily apparent. Hungerford and Karson (1960) have reported blood counts significantly higher than those following adrenalectomy. The increase is not dependent upon the integrity of the adrenals, since magnesium deficiency still produces an increase in their absence.

An inverse relationship between plasma calcium and magnesium exists in experimental depletion in the rat. Hypercalcæmia occurs as plasma magnesium levels fall. Consequently, extensive, though variable, calcification of the heart, kidney, liver, cerebellum and skeletal muscles results. Two types of renal lesions have been described: an intratubular deposition of calcium phosphate and a degenerative lesion due to intensive intracellular changes. Primary intratubular calcific deposits have been reported in the proximal convoluted tubule (Ko, Fellers and Craig, 1962) and the broad ascending limb of Henle's loop (Welt, 1964). These sites have high concentrations of calcium and relatively alkaline pH which favour precipitation of calcium salts. Adjacent epithelial changes are thought to occur secondarily to the basic lesion. Primary degenerative lesions have also been noted in the distal segment of the proximal tubule (Hess, MacIntyre, Alcock and Pearse, 1959). Changes occur during the first few days of magnesium deficiency and are characterized by mitochondrial swelling followed later by the appearance of lipid droplets. In older lesions mitochondrial enzymes were decreased in the damaged areas. These lesions subsequently undergo intracellular calcification and necrosis. Changes also occur in the cardiac mitochondria (Heggtveit, Herman and Mishra, 1964). The ultrastructural abnormalities include mitochondrial swelling and vacuolization and fragmentation of the myofibrils. Calcification of damaged mitochondria begins on the cristæ, slowly increasing until the entire mitochondrion is calcified. Aberrations in the appearance of the mucous and goblet cells of the colon and degenerative changes may also occur (Ko, Fellers and Craig, 1962).

Finally, convulsions themselves produce changes in plasma electrolytes (Martindale and Heaton, 1964). Within minutes following a seizure, plasma magnesium, calcium and phosphate rise. Liberation of these ions from bone is the most likely explanation.

Deficiency in Man

The effects of experimentally induced prolonged magnesium depletion have only been reported in two patients (Shils, 1964). Both were fed magnesium deficient synthetic diets: one for 274 days and the other for 414 days. Plasma magnesiums fell slowly over several months to approximately one-third to one-quarter pre-diet control levels and thereafter remained unchanged. The symptoms and signs observed, predominantly in one patient, included personality changes, gastro-intestinal disturbances, gross tremors, fasciculations, abnormal electromyographia and hyporeflexia in the presence of positive Trousseau and Chvostek signs. Despite adequate calcium and potassium intake, hypocalcæmia and hypokalæmia developed in both patients. Following magnesium repletion, serum calcium returned to normal, serum potassium rose and symptoms and signs reverted to normal. Since these findings could in part be explained by hypocalcæmia itself, the observations of Hanna and his associates (Hanna, Harrison, MacIntyre and Fraser, 1960) are pertinent. These investigators studied three hypomagnesæmic patients made normocalcæmic by calcium repletion or vitamin D.

The signs and symptoms they attribute to hypomagnesæmia in uncomplicated magnesium deficiency are: depression, irritability, vertigo, ataxia, dysarthria, tremor, epileptiform convulsions, and muscular weakness. There may be positive Chvostek sign with or without a concomitant Trousseau's sign, a low-voltage electrocardiogram and electroencephalographic changes suggesting a focal cerebral lesion.

In addition, other signs and symptoms may be present. Some may be non-specific. Somnolence, nausea, vomiting, abdominal pain, aggressiveness, paranoid delusions, fasciculations, hyperreflexia, and lowered threshold to galvanic stimulation have been reported in the presence of hypocalcæmia. Some investigators claim that true tetany with carpopedal spasm occurs (Vallee, Wacker and Ulmer, 1960) but this has been questioned.

Diagnosis and Treatment. Magnesium deficiency should be suspect in all patients with conditions known to be associated with hypomagnesæmia. The diagnosis is seldom suggested by symptoms. These are most always of secondary importance to those of the primary underlying disease. Confirmation is made by demonstration of low blood levels of the metal.

In patients with mild to moderate hypomagnesæmia, oral replacement with magnesium chloride, using 0·25–0·50 mEq./kg. daily, will usually suffice until normal magnesium levels are restored. Supplementation up to 4 mEq./kg./day in divided doses may be required in chronic refractory malabsorption. When severe depletion from any cause is present, intravenous therapy should be initially instituted to reduce the likelihood of possible fatal seizures and renal damage. MacIntyre (1967) has proposed that 2 mEq./kg. should be given over a four-hour period when original levels are 0·8 mEq./l. or less.

ACKNOWLEDGEMENT

This work was done during the tenure of an established investigatorship of the American Heart Association.

REFERENCES

AIKAWA, J. K. (1964). In *Dynamic Clinical Studies with Radioisotopes*, p.565, *ed.* by R. M. Kniseley, W. N. Tauxe and E. B. Anderson. U.S. Atomic Energy Commission.
ALCOCK, N. W. and MacINTYRE, I. (1960). *Biochem. J.*, **76**, 19P.
ALCOCK, N. W. and MacINTYRE, I. (1962). *Clin. Sci.*, **22**, 185.
ALCOCK, N.W. and MacINTYRE, I. (1966). *Meth. biochem. Anal.*, **14**, 1.
ALCOCK, N. W., MacINTYRE, I. and RADDE, I. (1960). *J. clin. Path.*, **13**, 506.
AVERILL, C. M. and HEATON, F. W. (1966). *Clin. Sci.*, **31**, 353.
AVIOLI, L. V. and BERMAN, M. (1966). *J. appl. Physiol.*, **21**, 1688.
AVIOLI, L. V., LYNCH, T. and BASTOMSKY, C. (1963). *Clin. Res.*, **11**, 40.
BARNES, B. A., COPE, O. and HARRISON, T. (1958). *J. clin. Invest.*, **37**, 430.
BERGLUND, F. and FORSTER, R. P. (1958). *J. gen. Physiol.*, **41**, 429.
BERNICK, S., and HUNGERFORD, G. F. (1965). *J. dent. Res.*, **44**, 1317.
BOOTH, C. C., HANNA, S., BABOURIS, N. and MacINTYRE, I. (1963). *Brit. med. J.*, **2**, 141.
BOOTH, C. C., MacINTYRE, I. and MOLLIN, D. L. (1964). *Quart. J. Med.*, **33**, 401.
CARE, A. D. and VAN'T KLOOSTER, A. Th. (1965). *J. Physiol. (Lond.)*, **177**, 174.
CONSOLAZIO, C. F., MATOUSH, L. O., NELSON, R. A., HARDING, R. S. and CANHAM, J. E. (1963). *J. Nutr.*, **79**, 407.
CORRADINO, R. A. and PARKER, H. E. (1962). *J. Nutr.*, **77**, 455.
DAWSON, J. B. and HEATON, F. W. (1961). *Biochem. J.*, **80**, 99
DIMICH, A., RIZEK, J. E., WALLACH, S. and SILER, W. (1966). *J. clin. Endocr.*, **26**, 1081.
FLINK, E. B., STUTZMAN, F. L., ANDERSON, A. R., KONIG, T. and FRASER, R. (1954). *J. Lab. clin. Med.*, **43**, 169.
FREEMAN, R. M. and PEARSON, E. (1966). *Amer. J. Med.*, **41**, 645.
GINN, H. E., SMITH, W. O., HAMMARSTEN, J. F. and SNYDER, D. (1959). *Proc. Soc. exp. Biol. (N.Y.)*, **101**, 691.
GITELMAN, H. J., GRAHAM, J. B. and WELT, L. G. (1966). *Trans. Ass. Amer. Phycns.* **79**, 221.
GRAHAM, L. A., CAESAR, J. J. and BURGEN, A. S. V. (1960). *Metabolism.* **9**, 646.
HANNA, S. (1961). *Metabolism*, **10**, 735.
HANNA, S., HARRISON, M., MacINTYRE, I. and FRASER, R. (1960). *Lancet*, ii, 172.

HANNA, S., NORTH, K.A.K., MACINTYRE, I. and FRASER, R. (1961). *Brit. med. J.*, **2**, 1253.
HAURY, V. G. (1940). *J. Lab. clin. Med.*, **26**, 340.
HEATON, F. W., HODGKINSON, A. and ROSE, G. A. (1964). *Clin. Sci.*, **27**, 31.
HEATON, F. W. and PARSONS, F. M. (1961). *Clin. Sci.*, **21**, 273.
HEATON, F. W. and PYRAH, L. N. (1963). *Clin. Sci.*, **25**, 475.
HEGGTVEIT, H. A., HERMAN, L. and MISHRA, R. K. (1964). *Amer. J. Path.*, **45**, 757.
HELLMAN, E. S., TSCHUDY, D. P. and BAKTTER, F. C. (1962). *Amer. J. Med.*, **32**, 734.
HENDRIX, J. Z., ALCOCK, N. W. and ARCHIBALD, R. M. (1963), *Clin. Chem.*, **9**, 734
HESS, R., MACINTYRE, I., ALCOCK, N. and PEARSE, A. G. E. (1959). *Brit. J. exp. Path.*, **40**, 80.
HILL, J. B. (1962). *Ann. N.Y. Acad. Sci.*, **102**, 108.
HORTON, R. and BIGLIERI, E. G. (1962). *J. clin. Endocr.*, **22**, 1187.
HUNGERFORD, G. F. and KARSON, E. F. (1960). *Blood*, **16**. 1642.
KO, K. W., FELLERS, F. X. and CRAIG, J. M. (1962). *Lab. Invest.*, **11**, 294.
MCCOLLISTER, R. J., FLINK, E. B. and DOE, R. P. (1960). *J. Lab. clin. Med.*, **55**, 98.
MCCOLLISTER, R. J., FLINK, E. B. and LEWIS, M. D. (1963). *Amer. J. clin. Nutr.*, **12**. 415.
MACINTYRE, I. (1961). *Advanc. clin. Chem.*. **4**, 1.
MACINTYRE, I. (1967). *Advanc. intern. Med.*, **13**, 143.
MACINTYRE, I., BOSS, S. and TROUGHTON, V. A. (1963). *Nature (Lond.)*, **198**, 1058.
MACINTYRE, I. and DAVIDSSON, D. (1958). *Biochem. J.*, **69**, 6P.
MACINTYRE, I., HANNA, S., BOOTH, C. C. and READ, A. E. (1961). *Clin. Sci.*, **20**, 297.
MACINTYRE, I., MATTHEWS, E. W. and ROBINSON, C. J. (1966). *J. Physiol. (Lond.)*, **184**, 83P.
MARTINDALE, L. and HEATON, W. F. (1964). *Biochem. J.*, **92**, 119.
NEGUIB, M. A. (1963). *Lancet*, **i**, 1405.
NIELSEN, B. (1964). *Acta endocr. (Kbh.)*, **45**, 151.
NIELSEN, B. and THORN, N. A. (1965). *Amer. J. Med.*, **38**, 345.
NIELSEN, J. (1963). *Dan. med. Bull.*, **10**, 225.
PALLIS, C., MACINTYRE, I. and ANSTALL, H. (1965). *J. clin. Path.*, **18**, 762.
POTTS, J. T. and ROBERTS, B. (1958). *Amer. J. med. Sci.*, **235**, 206.
PRASAD, A. S., FLINK, E. B. and MACCOLLISTER, R. (1961). *J. Lab. clin. Med.*, **58**, 531.
ROSS, D. B. (1962). *J. Physiol. (Lond.)*, **160**, 417.
SAMIY, A. H. E., BROWN, J. L., GLOBUS, D. L., KESSLER, R. H. and THOMPSON, D. D. (1960). *Amer. J. Physiol.*, **198**, 599.
SCHACHTER, D. and ROSEN, S. M. (1959). *Amer. J. Physiol.*, **196**, 357.
SEELIG, M. S. (1964). *Amer. J. clin. Nutr.*, **14**, 342.
SHILS, M. E. (1964). *Amer. J. clin. Nutr.*, **15**, 133.
VALLEE, B. L., WACKER, W. E. C. and ULMER, D. D. (1960). *New Engl. J. Med.*, **262**, 155.
WACKER, W. E. C. and VALLEE, B. L. (1964). In *Mineral Metabolism*, Vol. IIA, p. 483, Ed. by C. L. COMAR and F. BRONNER. New York: Academic Press.
WALLACH, S., BELLAVIA, J. V., SCHORR, J. and GAMPONIA, P. J. (1966). *Endocrinology*, **79**, 773.
WALSER, M. (1967). *Ergebn. Physiol.*, **59**, 185.
WELT, L. G. (1964). *Yale J. Biol. Med.*, **36**, 325.
WHANG, R. and WAGNER, R. (1966). *Metabolism*, **15**, 608.
WHANG, R. and WELT, L. G. (1963). *J. clin. Invest.*, **42**, 305.
WILLIS, J. B. (1960). *Spectrochim. Acta*, **16**, 273.
WISWELL, J. G. (1961). *J. clin. Endocr.*, **21**, 31.

Chapter 10

THIN LAYER CHROMATOGRAPHY

Geoffrey Franglen

Thin layer chromatography (TLC) is similar in many ways to the more widely used paper chromatography. In both cases the material under analysis is applied as a small spot or streak to the surface of the separation medium, and chromatographic separation is effected by the passage of suitable solvents through this. In paper chromatography, as is well known, the separation medium is carefully selected filter paper; in TLC it is a powder, such as silica gel or cellulose, which has been spread as a thin, even, adhesive layer on the surface of a sheet of glass or plastic. In both types of chromatography the position of the separated components is usually revealed by treatment of the chromatogram with reagents which convert them into coloured derivatives.

The advantages of TLC over conventional paper chromatography are many. Usually the speed of separation is significantly increased, and, for example, the common amino acids can be analyzed in less than six hours on a two-dimensional chromatogram. In spite of this speed, resolution of the components is as good as, and in some cases considerably better than, those obtained on paper. Sensitivity is greatly increased, and there is the additional advantage that, with some of the separation media used in this technique, it is possible to use corrosive detecting reagents which are unsuitable for normal chromatography, since they destroy paper. In some cases separation by TLC depends, like paper chromatography, on the partition of components between the moving organic phase of the system (the developing solvent) and the stationary watery phase held within the matrix of the medium. It has been more common, however, with this technique to effect separation using the absorptive properties of the separation medium, thus permitting the analysis of mixtures difficult to resolve by partition methods. In contrast to paper, it is easy with TLC to set up a reversed phase system, i.e. the support holds an organic solvent within its matrix whilst the chromatogram is developed with either another organic mixture or one containing water. Such systems permit the easy resolution of hydrophobic compounds such as lipids.

The disadvantages of TLC are primarily mechanical. The powder in which separation takes place has first to be made into a slurry with water or some other solution, and this has to be spread as a very thin and even layer on the supporting glass plate. Many forms of apparatus are available commercially to enable this spreading to be done efficiently and accurately, but, in general, these are rather too expensive to warrant expenditure by a laboratory where only a few chromatograms are likely to be run. In such cases commercially prepared plates are useful. It is also possible to spread plates quite adequately by simple techniques one of which is described in

E 147

this article. Another difficulty may be found in recording or preserving the chromatogram. In spite of various additives to increase the adhesion of the powder to the plate, the dried thin layer chromatogram is usually fragile. It can be fixed by spraying on a plastic coating available commercially as an aerosol, but, in most cases, it is probably sufficient to make a careful drawing or a photograph as a record.

The techniques and applications of TLC in clinical pathology have expanded considerably during the past few years and will probably continue to do so for some time. It is not possible, therefore, at this stage to lay down definitive methods for any particular type of analysis and this article makes no attempt to do so. Instead, general principles of technique are discussed and illustrated by applications of particular interest to the pathologist. It is hoped that the reader will be able to adapt the techniques described to the particular circumstances of his laboratory and to feel free to add such useful innovations as they appear in the literature. A very useful and comprehensive review on TLC has been written by Stahl (1965). Many papers on the technique also appear regularly in the *Journal of Chromatography*, though often the methods described there have to be modified before being applied to the problems of chemical pathology.

General Description of TLC

The separation medium, supplied as a fine, dry powder, is made into a smooth slurry or suspension with water or some other liquid. The materials which have been used most commonly in the TLC of chemical pathology have been silica gel, cellulose powder and superfine "Sephadex" gel. The slurry is spread over a glass or plastic plate as an even layer, generally with a thickness of 100–1,000 μ (0·1–1·0 mm.). This is usually allowed to dry in the open air, and, in some cases, is then "activated" by heating in an oven at a high temperature, followed by cooling in a desiccator. The substance to be analysed is applied in the form of a solution to the surface of the layer. For simple analysis it is usual to make this application as a spot not greater than 2 mm. in diameter, but, for preparative work it is more common to lay the material down in the form of a line. Since it is particularly important that the surface of the layer should not be touched, the application is often effected with the aid of a template to site the spot accurately and to prevent contamination of the plate. The plate is subjected to chromatographic development, usually by ascending solvent flow. When the run is finished, the plate is dried and is sprayed with the detecting reagent; in the case of separations made on "Sephadex" gels, the material is printed on to a piece of filter paper which is stained separately. It is not possible to use the dipping techniques common in paper chromatography, since such procedures break up the fine layer of powder. With two-dimensional analyses, the techniques used are similar to those of paper chromatography, the plate being carefully dried at the end of the first run and then being developed at right angles to this with the second solvent. It is also possible to effect separations by zone electrophoresis. For this, the dry plate has to be evenly sprayed with a suitable buffer before being inserted into the electrophoresis tank. For low voltage work, the simple horizontal tanks supplied for paper or cellulose acetate electrophoresis are suitable, connections from the electrode chambers to the plate being made through filter-paper wicks. High-voltage electrophoresis is possible but is difficult, since particular care has to be taken to cool the plate evenly if the run is to be satisfactory.

MATERIALS APPARATUS AND TECHNIQUES

Separation Media. The separation medium is usually supplied as a fine, dry powder with a particle size of the order of 10 μ, either in a plain form or with various additives. Thus, phosphors, such as fluorescein, may be incorporated to facilitate the detection of material absorbent under ultraviolet light. Again, the less adhesive media may include binders, such as gypsum, to fix the layer to the plate; alternatively, a small amount of soluble starch solution may be added just before use.

The dry powder is made into a slurry by mixing a known weight with a measured amount of water or buffer. All other preparations for spreading the plates should be made before mixing the slurry; this is particularly important when using media containing binders which begin to set after only a few minutes. The slurry must be very smooth if a homogeneous layer is to be obtained, and should be mixed by mechanical stirring rather than by hand. Air bubbles should not be entrapped in the suspension, and, if this does happen, they should be removed by partially evacuating the mixing flask for a moment or two with a water pump.

The manufacturers can now supply many different materials in a form suitable for making separation layers, the more important of these are noted below.

Silica gel is particularly useful for the separation of materials by adsorption chromatography and of acidic compounds.

Aluminium oxide (alumina), in contrast, is more useful for the separation of alkaline compounds.

Kieselguhr does not usually have any significant adsorptive properties and is generally used for separations by partition chromatography. It is thus more useful for the resolution of amphoteric and hydrophilic compounds, such as sugars.

Cellulose powder is particularly useful to the chemical pathologist, since separations on this material often resemble those obtained with paper chromatography, and methods developed for the latter technique can frequently be adapted to TLC with the advantages of increased speed and sensitivity. Some of these adaptations, however, are not completely satisfactory, and, for example, the separation of urinary indoles at present is better by paper chromatography than by TLC on cellulose layers. When a binder is not incorporated in the cellulose powder, more homogeneous layers are obtained when the mixture of powder and water is allowed to stand for about ten minutes before completing the mixing.

Ion-exchange powders have not been extensively used in the TLC of chemical pathology so far. They include powders prepared from the common ion-exchange resins and from the modified celluloses such as DEAE, ECTEOLA, as well as the carboxymethylated, acetylated and phosphate forms. Layers made from such materials can usually only be partially dried before use, and great care has to be taken over drying at the end of the analysis, since they crack very easily.

Superfine "Sephadex" gels have been developed by the firm of "Pharmacia" for the TLC separation of materials by gel filtration. Of the varieties available, the most useful to the chemical pathologist probably is the G-200 grade which permits the resolution of serum proteins in terms of their molecular weights. The dry powder has to be soaked for a considerable time before use to allow it to swell as completely as possible, and, as an example, the G-200 gel should be soaked for at least three days for satisfactory runs.

Plates. The plates supplied for laboratory use are usually of glass with standard sizes of 20×5 cm. (quarter plate), 20×10 cm. (half plate) and 20×20 cm. (whole plate), the last size being used for two-dimensional analyses, as well as for multiple one-dimensional analyses. For preparative work, plates of 40 cm. or even 1 meter have been used, thus permitting the separation of milligram amounts of material in a single run. Since the solvent flow in most analyses rarely exceeds 15 cm., there is little point in using plates greater than 20 cm. in width, and, in fact, many separations have been effected over a much smaller distance, e.g. certain classes of lipids may be adequately separated on thin layer plates made from microscope slides. Good-quality window glass may be used for plates and for the standard sizes, should be about 3 mm. thick. As explained below, with some types of spreader the thickness of the glass has to be constant from plate to plate to within 0·1 mm.

The plates must be scrupulously clean and dry before being spread with the separation layer. They should be soaked for about half an hour in a laboratory detergent, such as "Hemosol", and rinsed completely free of this with distilled or de-ionized water. After draining they should be swabbed with acetone, using a good grade of cotton-wool, and thereafter they should be handled only by the edges. It is appropriate to note at this point that consistently good, unequivocal analyses can be obtained by TLC only by a constant attention to detail and cleanness. The amounts of materials being separated are usually of the order of micrograms or even nanograms, and the contamination of amino acids or lipids from a single fingerprint can completely invalidate an analysis. After use, the plates can be washed free of the separation layer and used again.

Some manufacturers supply plates spread with a wide variety of separation layers ready for immediate use or after activation by heating. Usually these are made on a fairly rigid plastic sheet rather than on glass, and may be cut to size with a pair of scissors. In some cases the layer is sufficiently firmly bound to the plastic support to allow storage of the finished chromatogram in a book. Although these plates are distinctly more expensive than ones made in the laboratory they are beautifully uniform and are very convenient when the number of analyses is small. In the author's experience, these plates tend to run rather more slowly than the corresponding ones made in the laboratory.

Spreading Apparatus. This consists of two parts, a *spreader* which holds the prepared slurry and coats it on to the plates, and a *jig* which holds the glass plates securely in line and provides a guiding edge for the spreader (Fig. 1). The spreader may be made of plastic when only watery slurries are used, but for general use it is better when made from metal, preferably stainless steel. Essentially it consists of a rectangular box to hold the slurry; at the bottom of one of its longer sides is a slot of predetermined width through which the slurry can pass to form an even layer on the plate as the spreader is moved over it. In some types of spreader the size of this slot can be varied and its width has to be set initially, usually by means of feeler gauges. Others provide slots of fixed width, usually 100, 250, 500 and 1,000 μ. Whilst the first type can give a wide variety of slot widths, the author has not found this to be a particular advantage. For most analytical work a slot width of about 250 μ is usually suitable. The spreader must always be washed immediately after use; the slurry must not be allowed to dry in it. Great care must also be taken to avoid scratching the bottom, since this may produce uneven spreading.

There are two main types of jig for holding the glass plates. The simplest consists of a flat-bed on which the plates are butt-ended in line against a raised straight edge which acts as a guide for the spreader. Whilst this is extremely simple in design, it has the disadvantage that the thickness of the glass plates must be identical to within 0·1 mm., otherwise the passage of the spreader cannot be uniform, and chips of glass may be sheared off the edges of the plates. It is necessary therefore, with this type of jig, to use plates made from specially selected glass. This disadvantage is overcome in the second type of jig in which the plates are pressed up against two parallel bars which retain them along opposite edges. The necessary pressure can be exerted mechanically or by inflating a rubber bag beneath the plates. In this way the upper surface of each plate is brought to lie in the same plane, irrespective of their different thicknesses.

A uniform separation layer is essential for good TLC, and the operator will find that a little careful practice in spreading plates leads to a considerable

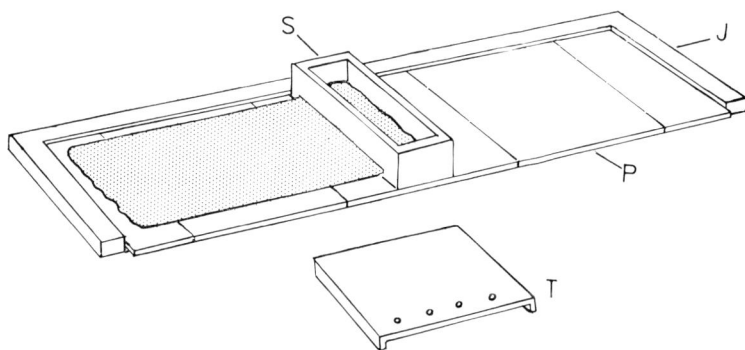

FIG. 1. Simple plate spreading apparatus and template. S, spreader; J, jig; P, plates; T, template.

saving of time later on. It is usually quite easy to see when a plate has been correctly spread; the surface is uniform and free of ripples and no striations can be seen in the layer when the plate is held up to the light. Irrespective of the particular apparatus in use, the spreading of plates follows the same general routine. The correct number and size of clean, dry and greaseless plates are lined up in the jig with an extra quarter plate at each end. These end plates are necessary, since the starting and stopping of the spreader's movement results in the appearance of a ripple in the layer. The spreader with the appropriate slot width is first run over the plates to check that they are correctly aligned before being placed in its starting position on the "run-on" end plate. The correct volume of slurry is prepared, degassed if necessary and then poured gently into the spreader. This is immediately drawn across the plates in a smooth, light movement which does not stop until the spreader is fully on the "run-off" end plate. The spreader should be drawn towards the operator with the slot facing away from him; for most slurries a rate of spreader movement of about 5–10 cm/second is suitable.

It is possible to spread adequate plates with the minimum of equipment, following the technique described by Baron and Economidis (1963). The clean plate is laid on a flat, level surface and is fixed in position by taping strips of ordinary adhesive plaster along the lengths of opposite edges. About 0·5 cm. should lap on to each side of the glass plate, the rest on to the bench surface. A strip of "Sellotape" is stuck over each length of the plaster, thus smoothing its slightly uneven surface. About 15 ml. of slurry is poured over the whole length of the far end of the plate. A half-plate, held at an angle of about 30° and resting on the side strips is pulled smoothly towards the near end, spreading the slurry rather like an enormous blood film. With practice, this technique will give an even layer about 250 μ thick.

Other methods for spreading plates are described in the literature. In one, a thin slurry is prepared and is poured on to the plate resting horizontally on the bottom of a trough. The separation layer is allowed to settle on to the plate and the excess liquid is carefully drawn off. Another way is to spray the slurry on to the plate with a high-pressure air-brush. Whilst they have particular applications, it is difficult with both these methods to obtain even layers.

After spreading, the plates are left undisturbed for up to half an hour, during which time the layer will set or dry sufficiently so that the plates can be moved without being spoilt. It is convenient at this stage to transfer them to a stacking plate holder in which they can be air dried overnight or be heated in an oven for activation. Various forms of plate holders are supplied by most manufacturers of TLC apparatus.

Since the separation layer is usually irregular in thickness at the outside edges of the spread, this should be removed before using the plate by scraping it away with a razor blade, leaving a clear strip about half a centimetre wide down each edge. In some forms of TLC the layer is divided up into separate lanes by scribing lines across it with a broad needle and blowing away the loosened powder. Such lanes need not be rectangular, and, with urinary sugar analyses, Rink and Hermann showed that improved results were obtained with wedge-shaped lanes (see Stahl, 1965). This technique of being able to isolate parts of a chromatogram with a scribed line is particularly useful in two-dimensional analysis. Quite often the solvent of the first run deposits material on the front which then acts as a local restriction to the solvent flow of the second run, thus distorting the chromatogram. By scribing a straight line across the plate just behind the front, this dirty area can be isolated so that the second solvent can run evenly through the rest of the plate. Similarly, a line can be scribed across the plate at the level where it is desired to stop the run in those cases where the length of the run is important.

Application of the Sample. In TLC separation occurs almost immediately with the flow of the solvent through the spot of sample on the plate. There is little point, therefore, in applying the sample a long way up the chromatogram, and it can be safely spotted on about 1·5 cm. from the bottom edge or, for two-dimensional runs, in a bottom corner, 1·5 cm. from adjacent edges. When multiple spots are being run, these may be placed 1·0–1·5 cm. apart, the distance depending on their size.

The position of application may be marked with a sharp, hard pencil or gently with a dissecting needle when the separation layer has a binder incorporated in it. On the whole, however, it is better not to mark the surface, but to use a template to site the spot (Fig. 1). These templates cover a whole plate without touching the separation layer and have locating holes for the pipette. The level of the line of spots on the chromatogram can be marked by making nicks in the outside edges of the layer if desired.

The sample is applied to the separation layer with a micropipette or with a micrometer syringe. It must be remembered that the applied volumes are small, loads of 1 μl. are usual in one-dimensional TLC, and practice may be needed in working with these amounts. For the best results, the spots must be kept as compact as possible, not more than 2–3 mm. in diameter. The sample should be applied slowly, and must not be allowed to flood on to the layer, as it is only too easy to wash out a hole in the chromatogram.

For some forms of quantitation and for preparative work, the sample is applied as a line. It is common in such cases to apply the material in the form of closely set spots. Better runs, however, are obtained if the sample can be gently sprayed on to the layer as a line 0·25–1·00 mm. thick by an apparatus such as that designed by Professor Stahl (1965).

Tanks. These are of glass and must have a really efficient air-tight lid. Paper chromatographic tanks and converted museum jars can be used, but they should not be too big; optimum conditions are usually obtained when the plates just fit the tank. The plates tend to slide about on the floor of plain tanks; this can be prevented by laying a sheet of thick filter paper on the bottom. A pressed tank with a flat bottom is distinctly more convenient to use than the more usual moulded type in which the bottom is bowed. In the former, the plates sit squarely, less solvent is needed and the front migrates at right angles to the edges of the plates. The Shandon Scientific Company makes excellent tanks for TLC.

The need for equilibration of the tank atmosphere with the solvent vapour before starting the run varies with the system of analysis. With some, e.g. separation of amino acids on cellulose powder layers, equilibration is deleterious, and the solvent should be poured into the tank and the loaded plates inserted immediately afterwards. In others, equilibration is essential and the solvent should be kept in the tank for some time before opening the lid briefly to admit the plates. With some solvent systems it may even be necessary to line the larger sides of the tank with sheets of thick filter paper, and to pour solvent over this to increase the area of evaporation. For consistent runs, especially with the more volatile solvents, it is always worth while providing a constant area of evaporation by including the same number of layered plates in the tank, whether they are loaded with sample or not.

Most separations are conducted at room temperature, and the tanks may be sited in the open laboratory. It is important, nevertheless, that the ambient conditions around the tank should be reasonably constant during the period of the run. Tanks should not be placed in direct sunlight nor in a draught. A simple although unsightly way of ensuring constant conditions around a tank is to put an ordinary cardboard box over it.

Solvents. Solvents must always be freshly prepared, since changes can occur on prolonged standing. Reagent grade materials should be used. Great care must be taken in making up the mixtures, since small alterations in composition can materially alter the analysis; this effect is distinctly more noticeable with TLC than with paper chromatography. The amount of solvent poured into the tank should be just enough to cover the separation layer to a depth of 0·5 cm.

Detection and Quantitation. When the solvent has reached the required distance in the layer, the plate is lifted out of the tank and excess solvent is blotted off its lower edge with a piece of filter paper. It is then dried, either with a gentle flow of warm air from a hair drier or in an oven. Large changes in temperature should be avoided in the early stages of drying, especially with watery solvents since this can produce cracks in the layer. With analyses which require a high temperature of drying, it is usually best to allow the plates to dry partially at room temperature before placing them in the oven. Drying must be sufficient to remove all traces of solvent; this is particularly important when the plate is to be subjected to another solvent, as in two-dimensional chromatography, or if it is to be treated with a locating reagent.

Coloured material can obviously be found by simple inspection. Many other compounds can be detected by their fluorescence or absorbence under ultraviolet light of the appropriate wavelength. When the material is absorbent, and thus appears as a dark spot on the plate under ultraviolet light, sensitivity can usually be increased considerably by employing a separation layer which incorporates a phosphor, e.g. DNP—amino acids can be detected down to levels of 5–10 mμg. (nanograms) on a plate of phosphor impregnated silica gel. Moreover, it should not be forgotten that many compounds may be converted to derivatives visible under ultraviolet light after treatment with suitable reagents; such methods often have considerable sensitivity. Almost all lipids, to give an example, may be recognized after spraying the plate with an ethanolic 0·2 per cent w/v solution of 2,7-dichlorofluorescein; they then appear as light-green fluorescent spots under ultraviolet light of 270 mμ. The position of spots located in this way may be recorded by scribing their outline on the plate with a fine point.

Detection of colourless compounds is commonly effected by treatment of the plate with reagents which convert the material to a coloured derivative. Many of the methods developed for paper chromatography can be used with little or no modification (see Smith, 1962). The reagent has to be sprayed evenly on to the plate without flooding it. The spray itself should be of glass and, where possible, should be supplied with air pressure from a pump or an air cylinder; mouth pressure is too irregular for good spraying. Since the inhaling of most of these reagents is not conducive to health and in some cases is frankly dangerous, it is wise to insist that this operation be done with *both the plate and the spray* inside an efficient fume cupboard. The plate should be held nearly vertically, and, if some illumination can safely be provided behind it, this helps to show whether the spraying is even.

Storage. Since it is inconvenient to store thin layer chromatograms, results have to be recorded by some means. The outline and position of the spots can be drawn on a piece of tracing paper carefully placed on the layer. The layer itself may be preserved by spraying on a plastic coating, such as the Merck "Neatan"; when this sets, the layer, embedded in the plastic, may be stripped from the glass and then be stored in a book. The most satisfactory way is to make a photograph of the chromatogram, using fine-grain film and a suitable filter to enhance the contrast between the spots and the layer. The ubiquitous 35-mm. camera is not the best instrument for this work, since the negative needs enlargement and the amount of film loaded in the camera is usually too long for convenience. A good copying apparatus can be made from an old quarter- or half-plate camera with double or triple extension, as supplied by Brunnings in London or Hayhurst in Manchester for about £15. The size of the negative from such a camera is sufficiently large for a simple contact print to be useful. Even more convenient is the "Polaroid" camera adapted for laboratory use. In this instrument the photograph is developed and printed as the film is drawn from the camera after exposure. The running costs are high, but it should be remembered that they replace all the expense and time of the normal developing and printing procedures.

Quantitation. The most accurate form of quantitation involves scraping that area of the separation layer containing the component off the plate into a flask. The component may then be eluted from the support and measured by any suitable means, e.g. absorptiometry, biological activity, direct chemical analysis or measurement of radioactivity.

It is also possible to use the various techniques of densitometry employed in paper chromatography and thus estimate the concentration of the coloured derivative directly on the plate. Since the reaction of most detecting reagents is not rectilinearly proportional to the concentration of the component being located, it is essential that standards should be run on the same plate, and that their concentrations should closely straddle that of the test; with all such methods, extrapolation is dangerous. The simplest method of this kind is to make a direct visual comparison between the unknown and adjacent standards. Both the test material and the standards should have been applied as spots with the same diameter. With care, accuracy can be about ± 25 per cent. It can, however, be increased considerably if the spots are scanned with a reflectance densitometer, e.g. the Joyce-Loebl "Chromoscan". With such an instrument, estimation may be made by integrating the peaks obtained from the test and standard spots rather in the manner of quantitating an electrophoresis strip. Greater accuracy is obtained when the spots are scanned over their whole area with a small circular aperture to find the maximum density (the "peak density" method). In general, the logarithm of the concentration is rectilinearly proportional to the maximum density of the spots, i.e. to the height of the peaks on the scan. Such a method has an accuracy of about ± 2 per cent. It must be emphasized, however, that accuracy of this level can only be obtained when the spots are initially of the same diameter and when the concentrations of the standards straddle that of the test. Since the area of the separated spots in TLC is generally small, estimation by measuring spot areas is usually not sufficiently accurate to be useful.

SUPPLIERS

The following firms in Great Britain can supply apparatus or materials or both for TLC:

Aimer Products Ltd., 56–58 Rochester Place, London, N.W.1. *Apparatus.*
Camlab (Glass) Ltd., Milton Road, Cambridge. *Desaga apparatus, Merck chemicals.*
Pharmacia (GB) Ltd., Paramount House, 75 Uxbridge Road, London, W.5. *Superfine "Sephadex" gels.*
Quickfit and Quartz Ltd., Stone, Staffs. *Apparatus.*
H. Reeve Angel & Co., Ltd., 9 Bridewell Place, London, E.C.4. *"Whatman" TLC powders.*
Shandon Scientific Co., Ltd., 65 Pound Lane, London, N.W.10. *Apparatus.*

SELECTED APPLICATIONS OF THIN LAYER CHROMATOGRAPHY

These methods have been chosen as illustrating the wide variety of techniques which are useful in TLC. The layer thicknesses given are those used by the original authors. It should be noted, however, that, in most cases, good results can be obtained on a layer with a standard thickness of 250 μ or on those spread by the simple technique of Baron and Economidis (1963).

Forminino-glutamic (FIGLU) and Urocanic Acids in Urine
(Roberts and Mohamed, 1965)

Plate Size. 20 × 20 cm. One-dimensional run.
Separation Layer. Cellulose powder MN-300 G (Camlab).
Slurry. Cellulose powder, 15 g., in water, 70 ml., and ethanol, 10 ml., for five whole plates.
Layer Thickness. 200 μ.
Activation. Plates are heated at 105°C for 30 minutes and either stored in a desiccator or reactivated just before use by heating at 105°C for 10 minutes.

Method. The patient should be given L-histidine, 15 g., in tepid water, 300 ml. The urine is collected for eight hours thereafter. It may be preserved with N-HCl, 5 ml., and a few crystals of thymol, and an aliquot stored at −20°C until analysis may be undertaken.

Undesalted urine, 5 μl., is applied in 1 μl. aliquots as a spot 1·5 cm. from the lower edge to duplicate plates.

For semi-quantitation, three 2·5 μl. samples of the following are applied:

"*Control*" *Urine.* Normal urine to which has been added glutamic acid, 50 mg./100 ml.

"*Low*" *Standard.* Normal urine to which has been added glutamic acid, 50 mg./100 ml., FIGLU, 10 mg./100 ml., and urocanic acid, 5 mg./100 ml.

"*High*" *Standard.* Normal urine to which has been added glutamic acid, 50 mg./100 ml., FIGLU, 40 mg./100 ml., and urocanic acid, 20 mg./100 ml.

The volume of each standard should be applied to the plates in 1 μl. aliquots.
Solvent. n-butanol : glacial acetic acid : water 114 : 38 : 60 by vol.
The running distance is 12–13 cm. past the origin; this takes about 2½ hours.

Detection. One plate is dried for 25 minutes in a fan operated oven at 50°C or in a stream of warm air from a hair-drier. It is then placed for one hour in a closed tank containing a breaker of fresh, concentrated ammonia solution to convert the FIGLU to glutamic acid. The excess ammonia is blown off the plate by a stream of warm air for 15 minutes. The other plate acts as a control and is left untreated, being simply allowed to dry in an ammonia-free atmosphere.

FIGLU is detected as a ninhydrin positive spot by spraying the lower half of the plate with a solution of ninhydrin, 0·2 g. and pyridine, 2 drops, in 100 ml. acetone. The density of the spots is maximal after one hour at room temperature and may be preserved by spraying with 0·25 M-nickel sulphate. FIGLU is present when a ninhydrin-positive substance is present in position R_f 0·4–0·5 on the ammonia-treated plate but is absent on the control plate. Glutamic acid runs a little slower than, but clearly separated from, FIGLU.

Urocanic acid is detected by spraying the top half of the plate with the Pauly reagent. This is made as follows: to a solution of sulphanilic acid, 0·9 g., in concentrated HCl, 9 ml., and water, 90 ml., is added one volume of sodium nitrite, 5 per cent w/v, in water. Both these solutions should be cool with a temperature not greater than 15°C. To this mixture is carefully added 2 volumes of anhydrous sodium carbonate, 10 per cent w/v, in water. Urocanic acid appears as a brownish spot in position R_f approximately 0·7.

FIGLU and urocanic acids appearing in the test urines are roughly quantitated by visual comparison with the standard urines; the spots may also be scanned on a reflectance densitometer. The accuracy of such an estimation is about ±20 per cent.

3-Methoxy-4-Hydroxy-D-Mandelic Acid (VMA) in Urine
(O'Neal, Traubert and Meites, 1966)

Plate Size. 20 × 20 cm. Two-dimensional run.
Separation Layer. Cellulose powder MN-300 G (Camlab).
Slurry. Cellulose powder, 15 g., in water, 110 ml., for two whole plates.
Layer Thickness. 500 μ.
Activation. After air drying for 15 minutes, plates are heated at 110°C for 10 minutes.

Method. A 24-hour urine collection is made, using 6 N-HCl, 10 ml., as preservative. Whilst, in contrast to other methods, this technique permits the complete isolation of VMA from contaminants, the chromatogram is clearer and less

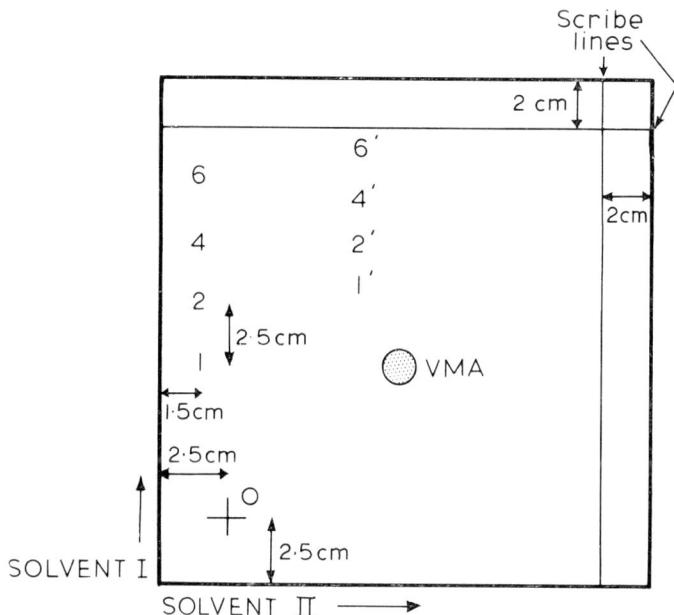

Fig. 2. Layout of 20×20 cm. plate for VMA analysis O, origin; 1, 2, 4, 6, application sites for standards; 1′, 2′, 4′, 6′, sites of standards after chromatography; VMA, site of test VMA after chromatography.

confusing to the novice if the usual dietary restrictions for this estimation are imposed on the patient immediately before and during the urine collection. A volume of urine containing 1·2 mg. creatinine is taken and made up to 5·5 ml. with distilled water. 6N-HCl, 0·5 ml., is added and mixed. Solid NaCl, about 3 g., is added and mixed. Ethyl acetate (reagent grade), 30 ml. is added and the mixture is shaken for 5 minutes, and then centrifuged for 5 minutes in a stoppered tube. 25 ml. of the ethyl acetate layer is removed into a small flask and carefully evaporated to dryness; the residue contains the VMA from that volume of urine containing 1 mg. creatinine. The dry residue is dissolved in ethanol, 1 ml., and 25 μl. is applied to one plate, and 100 μl. to another in a corner 2·5 cm. from each edge.

VMA standards containing 0·02 μg./μl. and 0·04 μg./μl. are made up in ethyl acetate. Apply to each plate 5 μl. of the weaker standard and 5, 10 and 15 μl. of the stronger along a line above the sample as shown in Figure 2; these standards are equivalent to 0·1, 0·2, 0·4 and 0·6 μg. of VMA, respectively.

Lines are scribed across the plate 2 cm. from the top edges for each solvent run.

Solvents. 1st—Isopropanol : concentrated ammonia solution : water 80 : 2 : 18 by vol.

2nd—Benzene : propionic acid : water 100 : 70 : 10 by vol.
Mix the acid and the water together before adding the benzene.

The tank must be fully saturated with solvent vapour and should be lined with filter paper soaked in the solvent. After the first run dry the plates at 110°C for 20 minutes. Before the second run place the plates in the tank for one hour with the lining papers soaked in the second solvent. It is necessary to stand the plates on microscope slides on the bottom of the tank, so that they do not pick up any solvent draining from the lining papers during equilibration.

The running distance for both runs is 15·5 cm. past the origin. This takes about three hours for the first solvent and about 45 minutes for the second.

Detection. The plates are partially dried in a fume cupboard for 15 minutes and then at 110°C for 15 minutes more, and then sprayed with freshly prepared diazotized p-nitroaniline. This is made as follows: p-nitroaniline, 0·15 g., is dissolved in concentrated HCl, 4·5 ml., and water, 95 ml. Just before use, 0·2 vols of 5 per cent w/v aqueous sodium nitrite are added to 10 volumes of this solution and then with care 10 volumes of 10 per cent w/v anhydrous sodium carbonate in water. The test VMA appears as a purple spot near the middle of the plate (see Fig. 2). Other spots, blue, purple or pink, may appear elsewhere on the plate, depending largely on the diet of the subject.

The concentration of VMA is obtained by visual comparison of the test result with the standards to the nearest 0·05 μg. From this the μg. VMA excreted per mg. creatinine is calculated. This method has an accuracy of about $\pm$10 per cent.

This method has a particular advantage in that contaminants due to diet do not overlap the VMA spot and thus lead to an erroneously high estimate. This is in contrast to one-dimensional chromatographic and direct spectrophotometric methods.

Tissue Lipids
(*Strich*, 1965; *Liadsyk and Woolf*, 1967)

Plate Size. 5 × 7·5 cm. One-dimensional run with double development.

Separation Layer. Silica gel G (Camlab).

Slurry. Silica gel, 5·5 g., in water, 12 ml., for 11 plates.

Layer Thickness. 100 μ.

Activation. Plates are heated at 80°C for 30 minutes and then cooled at room temperature.

Method. Unfixed tissue is cut into a block about 1 cm. wide and 2–3 mm. thick This is "snap-frozen" and cut into 40-μ sections. A single section is mounted on the *unspread* plate along a line 1 cm. from the bottom edge. The plate is then spread with the slurry.

Solvents. 1st—Petroleum ether (40°–60°C) : diethyl ether : glacial acetic acid 80 : 20 : 1 by vol.

2nd—Chloroform : methanol : water 65 : 25 : 4 by vol.

The first solvent resolves cholesterol, cholesterol esters, triglycerides and free fatty acids into separate classes (see Fig. 3). The plate is dried and rerun in the same dimension with the second solvent to separate the phospholipids (see Fig. 3). The running distance is over the full-length of the plate, 7·5 cm., and takes about 5–6 minutes for the first solvent, and about 8–10 minutes for the second.

Detection. 1. The plate is placed for 10 minutes in a closed jar containing iodine crystals. The spots are not permanent, but this technique is useful for ascertaining the separation after the first solvent.

2. The plate is sprayed with phosphomolybdic acid, 10 per cent w/v, in ethanol and heated at 80°C for 10 minutes. The lipids appear as blue bands on a yellow background.

3. Lipids may also be detected by destructive charring with a dehydrating acid (Jones, Bowyer, Gresham and Howard, 1966). The plate is placed for 2 minutes in a closed tank containing a little sulphuryl chloride (SO_2Cl_2). It is removed

quickly and held over a steaming water bath for 30 seconds, thus converting the sulphuryl chloride in the layer to a mixture of sulphuric and hydrochloric acids. The chromatogram is then placed on a hot plate thermostatically controlled at 200°C. The lipids are charred in a few seconds.

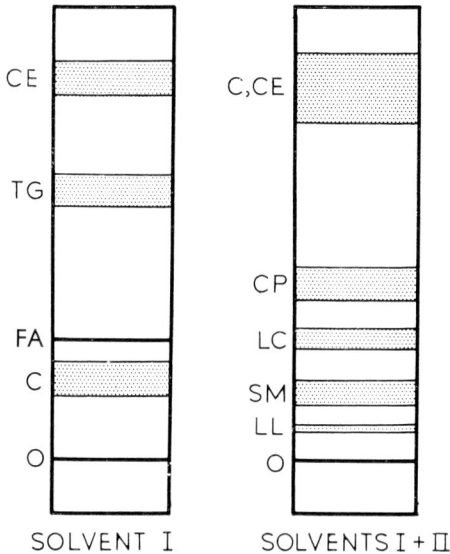

FIG. 3. Distribution of lipids. O, origin; C, cholesterol; CE, cholesterol esters; TG, triglycerides; FA, free fatty acids; CP, cephalin: LC, lecithin; SM, sphingomyelin; LL, lysolecithin. Note that the phospholipids remain at the origin in the first solvent.

Amino Acids in Plasma and Urine
(*Jones and Heathcote*, 1966)

Plate Size. 20 × 20 cm. Two-dimensional run.
Separation Layer. Cellulose power MN-300 (Camlab).
Slurry. Cellulose powder, 15 g., in water, 70 ml., and ethanol, 10 ml., for five plates.
Layer Thickness. 300 μ.
Activation. Air dry at room temperature overnight.

Method. Plasma samples should be deproteinized and desalted by any suitable means. The author finds the following method convenient. Plasma, 0·5 ml., is mixed with saturated picric acid in water, 3 ml., and stood at room temperature for 15 minutes. The mixture is centrifuged and the supernatant carefully drawn off. The precipitate is broken up with a glass rod and washed with more saturated picric acid solution, 2 ml. The mixture is again centrifuged and the supernatant pooled with the first. This extract is desalted by passing it through a small ion-exchange column of either "Dowex" 50 × 8 or "Zeo-Karb" 225, both in the acid phase. The column is washed free of picric acid with a little distilled water, after which the amino acids are eluted from it with 4N-ammonia solution. The eluate is collected and dried, and the residue of amino acids is dissolved in 10 per cent v/v isopropanol in water, 0·5 ml., for application to the plate.

Urine samples may be applied directly, but superior results are obtained when they are desalted before application. It should be noted that, in general, salt causes even more distortion on a thin layer plate than it does on a paper chromatogram.

The sample is applied in a lower corner, 1·5 cm. from each edge. The volume of a single application should be 1 μl. or less. For optimum results the amount of each amino acid applied should be around 0·05 μM. Good results are obtained with a volume of plasma extract equivalent to 10 μl. of the original sample, or with that volume of desalted urine containing 6 μg. of creatinine. The application should be made in aliquots of 1 μl.

Solvents. 1st—Isopropanol : formic acid : water 40 : 2 : 10 by vol.

2nd—*tert*-Butanol : methyl-ethyl ketone : concentrated ammonia solution : water 50 : 30 : 10 : 10 by vol.

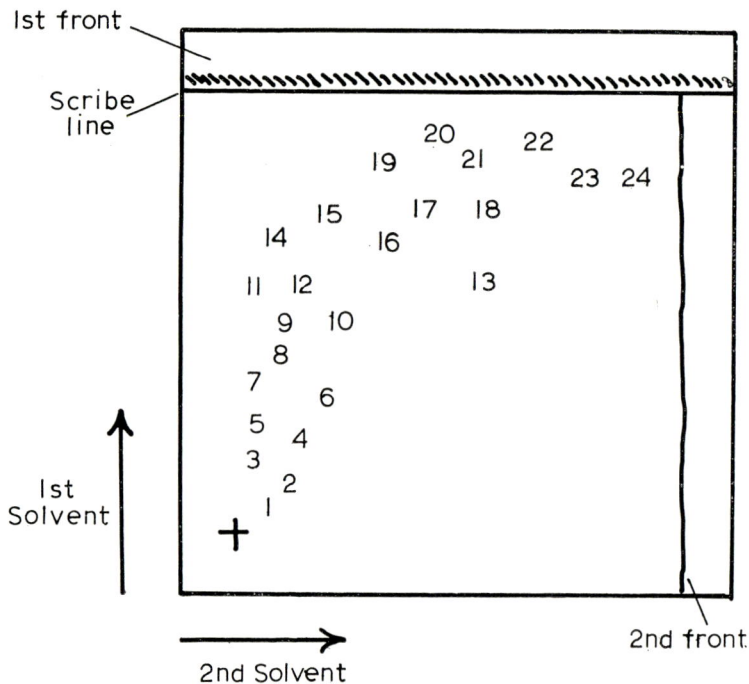

Fig. 4.—Distribution of amino acids, 1, cysteine; 2, cysteic acid; 3, ornithine; 4, histidine; 5, lysine; 6, taurine; 7, arginine; 8, glutamine; 9, glycine; 10, serine; 11, aspartic acid; 12, hydroxyproline; 13, threonine; 14, glutamic acid; 15, α-alanine; 16, proline; 17, tyrosine; 18, tryptophane; 19, β-amino-butyric acid; 20, valine; 21, methionine; 22, phenylalanine; 23, *iso*leucine; 24, leucine.

The first solvent usually deposits yellow material along the front. This should be isolated by scribing a line across the chromatogram just behind the front before running the second solvent. With both solvents it is necessary to place the plate in the tank immediately after adding the solvent so that the tank atmosphere is not saturated with vapour prior to development. The running distance for both solvents is 12–13 cm. past the origin. This takes about 3 hours for the first solvent and about $2\frac{1}{2}$ hours for the second.

Detection. The plate is dried in a stream of warm air from a hair drier until no smell of solvent is detectable. It is then sprayed with ninhydrin (Ninhydrin 0·3 g., glacial acetic acid, 20 ml., collidine, 5 ml., in ethanol to 100 ml.) and heated in a stream of warm air.

Twenty-three common amino acids may be unambiguously separated by this method, and also leucine from isoleucine (see Fig. 4).

Serum Proteins
(*Morris*, 1964)

Plate Size. 20 × 10 cm. or 20 × 20 cm. One-dimensional run.
Separation Layer. Superfine "Sephadex" G-200 (Pharmacia).
Slurry. "Sephadex", 1 g., in buffer, 25 ml., of composition 0·1 M-TRIS, 0·2 M-NaCl, *p*H 8·0. Soak for 3–5 days.
Layer Thickness. 500 μ.
Equilibration. Place the plate immediately after spreading in a flat tank at an angle of about 30° to the horizontal. Supply buffer solution of the above composition to the top edge of the plate from a reservoir through a filter-paper wick overlapping the layer by about 0·5 cm. Lap another filter-paper wick on the bottom edge to allow even drainage of the buffer off the plate. Allow the buffer to flow through the plate in the closed tank overnight before loading with sample.

Method. Apply to the wet plate the sample of serum, 2 μl., at a position 1·5 cm. from the *upper* edge. Apply as a marker 1 per cent w/v Blue Dextran 2000 (Pharmacia), 2 μl.

Allow TRIS-buffer of the above composition, to flow until the Dextran marker has moved about 15 cm. from the origin. This takes about six hours.

Detection. Soak a piece of "Whatman's" filter paper, No. 3 MM, the size of the plate, in the buffer and blot it lightly and evenly. Lift the plate out of the tank and place it on a level surface. Lay the wet filter paper on the separation layer, being careful not to trap air bubbles under it. Heat the plate and the filter paper at 100°C for 30 minutes. Stain the filter paper with any dyeing system used for paper electrophoresis of proteins, e.g. 10 minutes in 1 per cent w/v Ponceau S in 5 per cent w/v aqueous trichloracetic acid, followed by washing in dilute acetic acid.

Serum proteins will be divided into three components by this technique, according to their molecular size. The fastest moving component is largely macroglobulins, the slowest albumin and transferrin, whilst the middle component is mostly γ-globulins. This method enables sera giving similar paraprotein patterns by electrophoresis to be classified either as macroglobulinæmic or as myeloma-like.

References

BARON, D. N. and ECONOMIDIS, J. (1963). *J. clin. Path.*, **16**, 484.
JONES, D., BOWYER, D. E., GRESHAM, G. A. and HOWARD, A. N. (1966). *J. Chromatog.*, **24**, 226.
JONES, K. and HEATHCOTE, J. G. (1966). *J. Chromatog.*, **24**, 106.
LIADSKY, C. and WOOLF, N. (1967). *J. Atherscler. Res.*, **7**, 718.
MORRIS, C. J. O. R. (1964). *J. Chromatog.*, **16**, 167.
O'NEAL, J. P., TRAUBERT, J. W. and MEITES, S. (1966). *Clin. Chem.*, **12**, 441.
ROBERTS, M, and MOHAMED, S. D. (1965). *J. clin. Path.*, **18**, 214.
SMITH, I., Ed. (1962). *Chromatographic and Electrophoretic Techniques*, London: Heinemann Medical Books.
STAHL, E., Ed. (1965). *Thin Layer Chromatography*. Berlin: Springer-Verlag.
STRICH, S. J. (1965). *J. Physiol.*, **178**, 3P.

SECTION III

HÆMATOLOGY

Section Editor

G. WETHERLEY-MEIN
M.D.(Cantab.), M.R.C.P.(Lond.)
Professor of Hæmatology, St. Thomas's Hospital Medical School, London

Chapter 11

PLATELET FUNCTION

R. M. HARDISTY

THE RÔLE OF PLATELETS IN HÆMOSTASIS AND THROMBOSIS

PLATELETS have long been recognized as playing an essential part in the arrest of hæmorrhage at sites of vascular injury, and in intravascular thrombus formation. From the observation that thrombocytopenia is typically associated with widespread spontaneous capillary hæmorrhages, it must also be inferred that platelets are essential for the maintenance of the normal impermeability of capillary endothelium to red cells, though the mechanism of this function of platelets continues to defy explanation.

The Hæmostatic Process

Within seconds of injury, platelets begin to clump in and around the cut end of a vessel, adhering to the vessel wall and surrounding tissues to form a hæmostatic plug. At first friable, the plug soon becomes firmer in structure, leading within minutes to the final arrest of bleeding. Fibrin formation, in which platelet constituents also play a part, has meanwhile begun in the immediate vicinity and provides further resistance to the outflow of blood, though the bulk of the hæmostatic plug is composed of tightly packed platelets. Local vasoconstriction also plays a part in reducing the outflow of blood and is mediated in part by the action of vasoconstrictor substances, chiefly 5-hydroxytryptamine (5 HT, serotonin), released from the platelets during their aggregation. Finally, the fibrin clot retracts, and this phenomenon which serves to increase the compactness and tensile strength of the clot, is also mediated by a platelet constituent, the contractile protein thrombosthenin. Platelets thus not only form the main bulk of the hæmostatic plug, but contribute in various other ways to its efficacy.

Much additional light has been shed in recent years on the interrelationships of these hæmostatic functions of platelets. The main stimulus for the renewed activity in this field derives from the demonstration by the Norwegian workers (Hellem, 1960; Gaarder *et al.*, 1961) that an active principle from red cells, subsequently identified as adenosine diphosphate (ADP), greatly increases the adhesiveness of platelets to foreign surfaces such as glass and also brings about the aggregation of platelets, one to another, when added to platelet-rich plasma *in vitro*. Born (1956a, b) had already shown that platelets contain high concentrations of adenosine triphosphate (ATP), which is broken down to ADP during clotting; it has subsequently been demonstrated that both connective-tissue extracts (Hovig, 1963) and thrombin (Käser-Glanzmann and Lüscher, 1962) release sufficient ADP from platelets themselves to bring about their aggregation. Platelet aggregation in turn

makes phospholipid (platelet factor 3) available for the acceleration of
thrombin formation (Hardisty and Hutton, 1966), and thrombin, besides
converting fibrinogen to fibrin, releases 5 HT and other active principles
from the platelets and also consolidates the plug, making the platelet
aggregate irreversible (Grette, 1962; Spaet and Zucker, 1964).

There is evidence that the exposure of blood constituents to connective
tissue at the site of injury acts as a trigger mechanism for the hæmostatic
process in three distinct ways: exposed collagen causes adhesion and subsequent aggregation of platelets and also activates the intrinsic plasma clotting
system through its action on factor XII (Niewiarowski et al., 1965); and
factor X is simultaneously activated by a tissue factor in the presence of
factor VII. An attempt has been made in Figure 1 to indicate some of these
interrelationships, and to illustrate the central rôle of the platelets in the
hæmostatic mechanism.

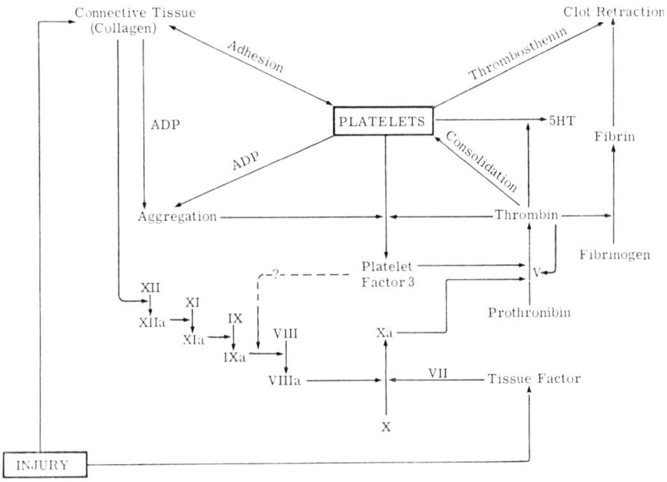

FIG. 1. The rôle of platelets in hæmostasis.

Thrombus Formation

Since the original observations of Bizzozero (1882), it has been realized
that the granular masses which form at the site of non-penetrating injuries to
mammalian arteries are composed of platelets, which adhere to the injured
vessel wall. Examination of sections of such white thrombi by light and
electron microscopy shows that their structure is closely similar to that of
hæmostatic plugs: both are composed of tightly packed masses of platelets
with little or no fibrin between them (French et al., 1964). The rate of growth
and embolization of white thrombi are essentially unaffected by agents which
influence blood coagulation (Honour and Ross Russell, 1962), but are
stimulated by the application of ADP or ATP to the site of injury (Honour
and Mitchell, 1964) and diminished by inhibitors of platelet aggregation,
such as adenosine (Born et al., 1964). From these and other studies it would
appear that thrombus formation represents a sequence of events closely

similar to those involved in the formation of a hæmostatic plug, but occurring within the lumen of a vessel. Just as more diffuse fibrin formation may subsequently occur in the stagnant blood behind a hæmostatic plug so, in certain hæmodynamic conditions, and particularly on the venous side, may red thrombus, composed of red cells enmeshed in a fibrin network, form around the compact white thrombus adherent to the vessel wall.

It would seem, then, that platelet aggregation, and subsequent changes involving consolidation of the platelet mass and local fibrin formation, are common to both hæmostatic plugs and thrombi. The problem of naturally occurring thrombosis in man centres on the question: what sets this chain of events in motion within the uninjured vessel? Does a thrombotic tendency reflect an abnormality of vessel walls, so that normal platelets are exposed to collagen or other tissues to which they adhere, with consequent liberation of ADP resulting in aggregation? May it reflect abnormal patterns of blood flow at certain sites? Or may it be entirely attributable to an inherent abnormality of the constituents of the blood, and in particular to an increased tendency of the platelets to adhere to the vascular wall or to aggregate together? It is in the attempt to answer this last important question that most tests of platelet behaviour are carried out today, though at the other end of the scale they have provided more clear-cut information about the pathogenesis of a small group of rare bleeding disorders.

INVESTIGATION OF PLATELET FUNCTION

The following discussion is concerned with the principles underlying some of the methods currently used for the investigation of platelet function, and particularly their relationship, so far as it is understood, to the rôles of platelets in hæmostasis and thrombosis. The value and limitations of the methods in the study of bleeding and thrombotic disorders are indicated, but technical details are not given; for these the reader is referred to the original descriptions cited.

Adhesion to Connective Tissue

This, the first activity of platelets after injury to a vessel, has been studied by applying platelet-rich plasma (PRP) to mildly traumatized mesentery of the rabbit or rat, and observing the adhesion and subsequent aggregation and morphological changes of the platelets microscopically (Hugues, 1962; Spaet and Zucker, 1964). The method, which is essentially an experimental one, does not lend itself to quantitative assessment of the relative "adhesiveness" of platelets of different subjects to collagen, nor is there any evidence that a bleeding disorder or a thrombotic tendency may be due to an abnormality of the affinity of platelets for connective tissue. This property of platelets, unlike aggregation, does not require the presence of calcium or ADP and is normal in thrombasthenia. Adhesion to collagen results in the liberation of ADP from the platelets, and this in turn leads to their aggregation or cohesion, one to another—a property which can be examined quantitatively *in vitro* in response to connective tissue fragments as well as to other aggregating agents (see below). Figures 2 and 3 illustrate respectively the adhesion of platelets to collagen fibres, and their aggregation.

Borchgrevink (1960) devised a method for measuring platelet adhesiveness *in vivo*, based on the difference between the platelet counts in venous blood and in blood issuing from a standard cut on the forearm. In a series of normal

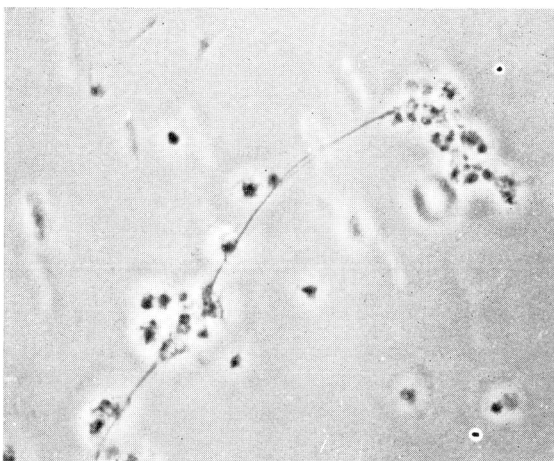

FIG. 2.   Adhesion of platelets to a collagen fibre *in vitro*. Subsequent aggregation was inhibited by the addition of adenosine to the platelet-rich plasma. Phase contrast, ×1120.

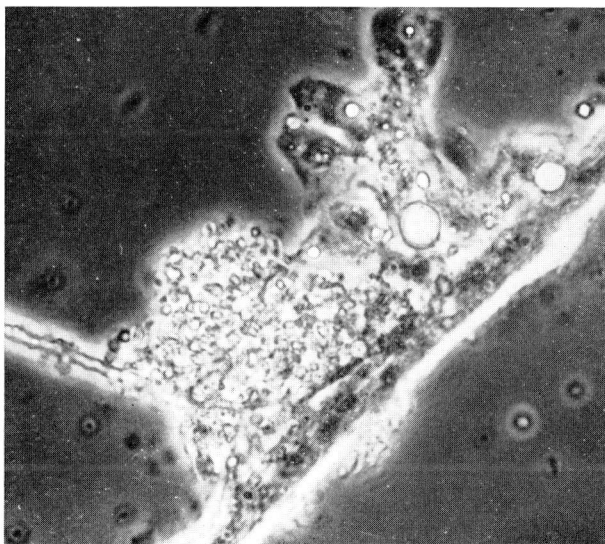

FIG. 3.—Aggregation (cohesion) of platelets at the site of adhesion to collagen fibres in traumatized rat mesentery. Phase contrast, ×1120.

subjects, he found the mean platelet count of the forearm blood to be 37 ± 7.5 per cent lower than the venous platelet count, and suggested that this difference represented the proportion of platelets retained in the wound in the course of hæmostatic plug formation. While this method provides a useful adjunct to the bleeding time in the experimental study of hæmorrhagic disorders, it certainly is not purely a measurement of adhesion of platelets to connective tissue but also reflects their subsequent aggregation. This is borne out by Borchgrevink's own observation of greatly diminished "*in-vivo* adhesiveness" in a patient with thrombasthenia. He has also obtained low results in a variety of conditions associated with long bleeding times, including von Willebrand's disease and macroglobulinæmia (Borchgrevink, 1961), and it is probable that the test has no more specific significance than that of the bleeding time itself. Muckle (1964) has observed abnormalities in this test in a number of patients with hereditary hæmorrhagic telangiectasia, and Castaldi *et al.* (1966) have made similar observations in uræmic patients

Aggregation

When aggregating agents, such as ADP, are added to PRP in a stirred system, the resulting platelet aggregation results in a progressive decrease in optical density of the mixture (Fig. 4). This forms the basis of the turbidi-

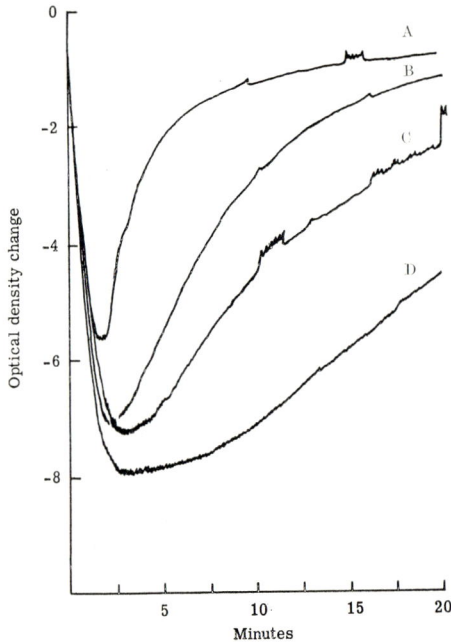

FIG. 4. Optical density changes during aggregation and subsequent disaggregation of platelets in platelet-rich plasma. ADP was added at zero time to give the following final concentrations: A. 0·5 μM; B, 1·0 μM; C, 2·0 μM; D, 20 μM.

metric method of Born (1962) and O'Brien (1962) for the quantitative study of platelet aggregation; full details of the method, and an analysis of the effects of controllable variables, are given by Born and Cross (1963). This method has proved of great value in the investigation of the mode of action of various aggregating and disaggregating agents, the rôle of calcium ions and plasma co-factors in the aggregation process, and interrelationships between aggregation and other platelet functions. It was designed as a research procedure, in which the effect of varying individual conditions could be studied while keeping the remainder of the system constant, and not primarily as a clinical test. Quite wide variation may be noted in the response pattern of platelets to aggregating agents in this system, not only between patients but from day to day in the same individual; much of this variation is due to uncontrollable differences in parameters not directly related to the platelets themselves (Harrison, Emmons and Mitchell 1967). For example, differences in venous hæmatocrit and ESR will affect the yield of platelets in PRP, and perhaps also the aggregating characteristics of the sample studied: there is evidence to suggest that small amounts of ADP released from the red cells during preparation of PRP may cause aggregation of some platelets which then sediment with the red cells, leaving a relatively less responsive population of platelets in the supernatant plasma. The number of leucocytes present in the PRP will also influence the result (Harrison, Emmons and Mitchell, 1966), as they inactivate ADP and so produce reversal of ADP aggregation, while having no effect on aggregation produced by noradrenaline. Finally, various plasma constituents contribute to the total optical density of PRP, so that no constant relationship holds good between the degree of platelet aggregation and either the relative or the absolute change in optical density.

For reasons such as these, the clinical applications of this method are limited, and great caution must be exercised in interpreting differences in behaviour between samples of PRP in this system. Nevertheless, certain wide deviations from the normal pattern may be recognized. Thus in thrombasthenia, there is a complete failure of the platelets to aggregate in response to any stimulus, whether ADP, noradrenaline, 5 H.T, collagen or thrombin (Hardisty et al., 1964; Zucker, 1964); this defect is so gross that it can easily be detected by simply shaking PRP with one-half volume of 100 μM ADP for about a minute, and observing by the naked eye; failure to aggregate is pathognomonic of thrombasthenia. In afibrinogenæmia, platelet aggregation by ADP can be shown by the turbidimetric method to be defective and to be corrected by the addition of fibrinogen; aggregation by collagen and thrombin occurs normally (Hardisty and Hutton, 1966; Inceman et al., 1966).

Macmillan (1966) has shown that platelet aggregation in response to ADP, like that brought about by adrenaline, occurs in two phases in most normal subjects, the second phase being due in each case to the action of ADP released from the platelets themselves. Hardisty and Hutton (1967) have studied a number of patients with mild bleeding symptoms and long bleeding times, in whom no second-phase aggregation occurred, apparently because of a defect of platelet ADP release; these patients' platelets also showed little or no aggregation in response to collagen suspensions. Similar observations have been made in other patients by Hirsh et al. (1967), O'Brien (1967) and Caen et al. (1968), and it appears that the increased bleeding time observed after aspirin ingestion is the result of a similar defect of platelet aggregation, caused by inhibition of ADP release (Weiss and Aledort, 1967). Castaldi *et al.* (1966) have observed a defect of platelet aggregation in a number of uræmic patients. No abnormality of aggregation by ADP or collagen has been found in von Willebrand's disease.

There is no direct evidence that a tendency to thrombosis is ever due to an increased responsiveness of platelets to a given concentration of ADP or of other aggregating agents. This is one possible explanation of some of the findings obtained with glass adhesiveness tests (see below), but for the reasons given above, the investigation of platelet aggregation in PRP is not likely to be helpful in the differentiation of such patients from normal.

Adhesiveness to Glass

Wright (1941, 1942) was the first to study the "adhesiveness" of platelets to glass as an index of a thrombotic tendency. She measured the percentage of platelets which disappeared from whole blood rotated in a standard glass bulb for various intervals of time and found an increased rate of disappearance following parturition and surgical operations. Moolten and Vroman (1949) passed citrated blood through a glass-wool filter and measured the platelet loss, which they found to be increased in a variety of clinical disorders. In recent years, a number of investigators have studied the loss of platelets on passing whole blood or PRP through a column of glass beads: Hellem (1960) drove citrated blood or plasma through the column at constant speed and O'Brien (1961) used a similar system for native blood, while Salzman (1963a) drew blood directly from a vein through the column under negative pressure, with a progressively diminishing rate of flow.

It is probable that all these methods measure the same aspect of platelet behaviour; a recent comparison of Wright's method with a modification of that of Hellem, both carried out on citrated whole blood, showed close correlation of their results (Hirsh *et al.*, 1966). What is more difficult is to relate platelet "adhesiveness", as measured by these *in vitro* methods, to the rôles of platelets in hæmostasis and thrombosis. First, a word of caution must be given about the use of the terms "adhesiveness" and "stickiness" in this context. All these methods actually measure the proportion of platelets which *disappear* from the blood or plasma during some form of standard exposure to glass, and it does not follow either that they do so by direct adherence to the glass surface, or that the number of platelets lost depends solely on some intrinsic property of their own. There is good evidence, in fact, that a source of ADP, such, for example, as the red cells, is required for "normal platelet adhesiveness", and that the loss of platelets observed is attributable in large part to aggregation as well as to adhesion to the glass. The glass adhesiveness of platelets in the presence of red cells is greatly reduced by ADP antagonists such as adenosine (Caspary, 1965; Philp and Wright, 1965) and by the pyruvate kinase/phosphoenolpyruvate system, which removes ADP (Harrison and Mitchell, 1966); fibrinogen and divalent cations are necessary for glass adhesion, and thrombasthenic platelets are not removed from blood by contact with glass. For all these reasons, the property of platelet adhesiveness to glass must be regarded as quite distinct from the phenomenon of adhesion to connective tissue, which occurs normally in thrombasthenia and is independent of ADP, fibrinogen and divalent cations. Adhesion to glass has more in common with aggregation than with any other *in vivo* property of platelets.

If PRP is used for the determination of platelet adhesiveness, a standard amount of ADP must be added. Such a system suffers from the same disadvantages as methods for studying the aggregation of platelets in PRP, due to the effect of extraneous factors on the platelet yield, and the probability that the platelets in the sample of PRP tested are not truly representative of the whole-blood platelet population (see above). Such methods are not highly reproducible; the range of values found will vary widely with small differences of technique and must be established for each individual laboratory.

The use of whole blood ensures that a more representative sample of platelets is tested, but the "adhesiveness" will be proportional to the PCV, since red cells are the chief source of ADP in this system (Hellem, 1960). A correction for PCV must therefore be made if results obtained in different individuals are to be compared (Hirsh and McBride, 1965). The possibility should not be overlooked, however, as Harrison and Mitchell (1966) have pointed out, that the platelets in this system are acting merely as indicators of red-cell behaviour, and that the abnormal platelet adhesiveness observed in various conditions may relate to red-cell abnormalities affecting the release of ADP by contact with glass, rather than to changes in the platelets themselves.

Salzman's method of measuring platelet adhesiveness suffers from two major disadvantages: the rate of flow through the bead column is variable and cannot be accurately controlled, and the PCV cannot be corrected before testing. The first of these is particularly unfortunate, since in all these bead-column methods the rate of flow greatly influences the results. The attraction of Salzman's method lies in the fact that it has given subnormal results in von Willebrand's disease rather more consistently than other methods. The lack of reproducibility of glass-adhesion tests in this condition, however, and the failure to correlate the results of such tests with other evidence of a platelet abnormality, throws doubt on their significance.

Besides thrombasthenia, decreased platelet adhesiveness to glass has been observed in thrombocythæmia (Cronberg et al., 1965; McClure et al., 1966), afibrinogenæmia (Caen and Inceman, 1963; Gugler and Lüscher, 1963), severe uræmia (Hellem et al., 1964; Salzman and Neri, 1966), during cardiopulmonary by-pass (Salzman, 1963b), after infusion of dextrans (Weiss, 1967a) and in a variety of other bleeding states. No abnormality is seen in clotting factor deficiencies other than afibrinogenæmia. Increased adhesiveness has been reported in the post-operative period (Wright, 1942), after a fatty meal (McDonald and Edgill, 1958; Philp and Wright, 1965), in patients with venous thrombosis (Hirsh and McBride, 1965; Bygdeman et al., 1966), ischæmic heart disease (McDonald and Edgill, 1957) and diabetes (Bridges et al., 1965), in children with homocystinuria, a condition which predisposes to thrombosis (McDonald et al., 1964), and in multiple sclerosis (Caspary et al., 1965; Wright et al., 1965). The significance of these findings remains to be further explored, and much carefully controlled work on the phenomenon of platelet adhesiveness must be done before its usefulness as an indicator of the presence or absence of a thrombotic tendency is finally established. When studying possible increases in adhesiveness, it is appropriate to use relatively small glass-bead columns, with a correspondingly short contact time, in order to reduce the normal range of platelet loss and provide the opportunity for a more clear-cut increase in abnormal situations; conversely, a longer contact time is more appropriate for the study of conditions in which a decreased adhesiveness is expected.

Electrophoretic Mobility

Platelets carry a net negative charge and Bangham et al. (1958b) have suggested that platelet aggregation may be related to changes in this charge.

Hampton and Mitchell (1966a, b), using the capillary electrophoresis apparatus developed by Bangham *et al.* (1958a), have shown that the electrophoretic mobility of platelets in plasma falls on contact with glass and undergoes a biphasic change under the influence of aggregating agents: at concentrations which cause aggregation in a stirred system, ADP, ATP, noradrenaline, thrombin and collagen all cause a decrease in mobility, but at lower concentrations they produce an increase. Hampton and Mitchell suggest, as a possible explanation of these findings, that ADP, probably derived from the red cells or the platelets themselves during the preparation of PRP, becomes bound to the platelet surface, so increasing their negative charge; that the fall in mobility of platelets on contact with glass represents the removal of ADP from their surface; and that aggregating agents first increase the negative charge again as exogenous or endogenous ADP is readsorbed, and then, at higher concentrations, cause calcium to be adsorbed to the platelet surface, with a consequent reduction in charge, which diminishes the repulsive forces between the platelets and allows aggregation to take place.

In a variety of acute illnesses, including myocardial infarction and pneumonia, and after surgical operations, a striking increase in sensitivity of the platelets to both ADP and noradrenaline, as measured by the concentration of these reagents needed to induce the maximal increase in electrophoretic mobility, occurs within 12 hours of onset of the inflammatory state (Hampton and Mitchell, 1966c). In some patients with arterial disease, and with conditions thought to predispose to it (hypercholesterolæmia, diabetes mellitus and homocystinuria), increased sensitivity to ADP has been observed in association with normal sensitivity to noradrenaline (Hampton and Mitchell, 1966d); this increased sensitivity to ADP can be transferred to normal platelets by incubation with fresh platelet-poor plasma from abnormal subjects, suggesting that the platelets in this system are acting merely as indicators of the presence of a plasma factor. Bolton, Hampton and Mitchell (1967) have recently presented evidence that the active principle in the plasma is lysolecithin, derived from the action of a labile phospholipase on the lecithin fraction of low-density lipoproteins. In their patients with vascular disease, they have found at least five times the normal plasma concentration of this lecithin fraction. In multiple sclerosis, Bolton, Hampton and Phillipson (1968) have observed a similar abnormal sensitivity of the platelets to ADP, due in this case to an abnormality of the lysolecithin rather than the lecithin fraction of the patient's low-density lipoproteins.

While this method of studying platelet behaviour is clearly of great interest in relation to the physiological basis of platelet aggregation, and in the investigation of the pathogenesis of arterial disease, it is essentially a research procedure, which has no place in the routine diagnosis of thrombotic or hæmorrhagic disorders. The only bleeding disorder in which an abnormality has been reported in this system is *thrombasthenia*: in this condition, the electrophoretic mobility of platelets is completely unaffected by contact with glass or by any concentration of aggregating agents (Hampton and Hardisty, 1967). This finding, in common with other observations on thrombasthenic platelets, suggests that the essential defect in thrombasthenia may be an absence of ADP binding sites on the platelet membrane.

Platelet Factor 3

Phospholipid plays an essential part in the blood coagulation process, at the stage of conversion of prothrombin to thrombin by factor X, and possibly also in the activation of factor VIII by activated factor IX (see Fig. 1). The platelets provide the chief source of this phospholipid, and that part of the total lipid content of the platelets which contributes to the intrinsic blood coagulation process is termed platelet factor 3. Platelet lipid is not normally available for this purpose in the circulating blood, but becomes available when the platelets are activated by some appropriate stimulus, whether *in vivo* or *in vitro*. Complete disruption of the platelets, for example, by freezing and thawing or mechanical fragmentation, releases all their phospholipid, and lesser degrees of trauma *in vitro*, such as may be produced by rapid centrifugation and washing, make a variable proportion available. Such unphysiological procedures, however, provide no information about the means whereby platelet factor 3 is made available *in vivo*, nor the proportion of the total platelet phospholipid which normally contributes to the blood coagulation process.

Hardisty and Hutton (1966) have recently shown that platelet factor 3 becomes available whenever aggregation occurs: maximal aggregation of platelets makes about one-fifth as much of their lipid available, as judged by the effect on the Stypven time, as does total platelet lysis, and lesser degrees of aggregation result in the availability of correspondingly smaller proportions of the total lipid. Their findings suggest that platelet aggregation may well be the physiological stimulus which makes platelet factor 3 available and are consistent with the view of Marcus *et al.* (1966) that factor-3 activity is a property of the platelet membrane. It is probable that the membrane change associated with platelet aggregation also provides an active catalytic surface for the interaction of plasma coagulation factors, leading to local thrombin formation; this would lead in turn to consolidation of the platelet plug, with degranulation of the platelets and consequent release of further phospholipid into the surrounding plasma, to play a part in more widespread fibrin formation.

It follows from these observations that methods involving the use of washed platelet suspensions, such as modifications of the thromboplastin generation test, are unsuitable for the measurement of platelet factor-3 activity, as the preparation of such suspensions makes a variable and uncontrolled proportion of such activity available. Platelets should be studied for this purpose in platelet-rich plasma, subjected to the minimum amount of handling, and tested under standard conditions of activation. Two methods which fulfil these criteria are those of Hardisty and Hutton (1965) and Spaet and Cintron (1965), which are based respectively on the determination of the clotting time and Stypven time of PRP after incubation with a standard amount of kaolin. Comparison of the effect of kaolin and of ADP on the clotting activity of platelet-rich plasma suggests that both reagents activate the platelets through the same mechanism, involving their aggregation, and both make a similar proportion of their total phospholipid available (Hardisty, 1968). There is therefore reason to believe that these methods, involving activation of the platelets by kaolin, measure that proportion of their phospholipid which becomes available for coagulation *in vivo* during aggregation. Both can also be used as an index of total platelet lipid by freezing and thawing the platelet-rich plasma before testing, but there is no evidence that any bleeding disorder is attributable to an abnormality of total platelet lipid. The Stypven-time method (Spaet and Cintron, 1965) has the advantage that it eliminates the effect on the test results of variation in many of the plasma clotting factors, but this can also be done in either system by comparing a mixture of equal parts of patient's platelet-rich and control platelet-poor plasma with the opposite mixture. The results are conveniently expressed in the form of a "platelet factor-3 availability index" (Hardisty and Hutton, 1965), by comparing the platelet count of a plasma mixture containing the patient's platelets with that of a dilution of normal platelet-rich plasma which gives the same clotting time.

In practice, as might be expected, defects of the availability of platelet factor 3 have been demonstrated by these methods only in patients in whom platelet aggregation is also defective: in thrombasthenia (Hardisty *et al.*, 1964), afibrinogenæmia, in which the defects of aggregation and platelet factor 3 availability are corrected in parallel by the addition of fibrinogen (Hardisty and Hutton, 1966), and in some cases of uræmia (Castaldi *et al.*, 1966), in which a correlation between the degree of the aggregation and clotting abnormalities has recently been noticed (Hutton and O'Shea, 1968). Horowitz *et al.* (1967) have shown that the defect in uræmia is due to an inhibitory effect of uræmic plasma, and have produced evidence to suggest that the inhibitory substance may be guanidinosuccinic acid, a urea metabolite.

It seems likely, therefore, that platelet factor-3 availability is simply an indirect expression of the ability of platelets to aggregate, rather than a fundamentally separate index of platelet function. It thus becomes necessary to re-examine the concept that a bleeding disorder may be caused by an isolated defect of the clotting activity of the platelets. Braunsteiner (1955) proposed that the term "thrombopathia" should be used for a congenital bleeding disorder characterized by normal clot retraction but defective clotting function of the platelets, in contradistinction to thrombasthenia, in which clot retraction was defective but clotting function was thought to be normal. Since the fundamental defect of aggregation in thrombasthenia leads to a disorder of platelet clotting activity, this classification is no longer tenable. The term "thrombopathia" has subsequently continued to be applied to patients whose bleeding disorder, whether congenital or acquired, has been associated with some degree of abnormality of platelet clotting function, as determined by any of a wide variety of laboratory tests. In the light of present knowledge, however, it seems unwise to attribute a bleeding tendency solely to an abnormality of this aspect of platelet function unless it can be established that platelet aggregation is not also defective. Weiss (1967b) has recently used the term "thrombopathia" for a group of patients in whom diminished platelet factor-3 availability was associated with a failure of the platelets to release their ADP normally, and hence to aggregate, on incubation with connective tissue; aggregation occurred normally in response to extrinsic ADP, thus distinguishing this condition from thrombasthenia. A similar group of patients has been studied by Hardisty and Hutton (1967), who also found evidence of a defect of release of their platelet ADP when extrinsic ADP or noradrenaline was added. A defect of platelet factor-3 availability may thus apparently be secondary to a failure of the platelet either to react with ADP (thrombasthenia) or to release it (thrombopathia); there is as yet no evidence that it ever occurs as a primary abnormality.

In thrombocythæmia, defects of platelet thromboplastic function have been demonstrated by a variety of methods, most recently by McClure *et al.* (1966), who found that the defect was partially corrected by lysing the platelets, and suggested that it may have represented a failure of "the release of clotting components". Though they did not study platelet aggregation directly, they also observed a defect of *in vivo* and *in vitro* platelet adhesiveness in thrombocythæmia; this again suggests that platelet clotting function is related to adhesiveness, and hence to the reactivity of platelets with ADP. Platelet factor-3 availability has also been found to be reduced in macroglobulinæmia (Pachter *et al.*, 1959) and in patients receiving dextran (Ewald *et al.*, 1965), probably because of coating of the platelets by the large molecules.

Other Platelet Clotting Factors

Platelet Factor 1 is adsorbed plasma factor V. Various other plasma clotting factors, particularly factors VIII, XI and XII, have also been found to be adsorbed to the platelet surface, where they may help to accelerate thrombin formation, but there is no evidence that a bleeding tendency may result from a defect of such adsorption.

Platelet Fibrinogen. Washed platelets and platelet extracts have been shown to contain fibrinogen, by means of both coagulation and immunological methods, and there has been argument whether the fibrinogen is attached to the platelet surface—perhaps adsorbed from the plasma—or whether it forms an essential part of the internal structure of the platelet; both these views are probably correct (Castaldi and Caen, 1965). Although the presence of fibrinogen in the suspending medium appears to be necessary for normal platelet aggregation and adhesion to glass, the function of platelet fibrinogen is still not understood. Castaldi and Caen (1965) found a deficiency of platelet fibrinogen in six out of nine thrombasthenic patients and concluded, since the platelets of all nine patients failed to aggregate, that this latter abnormality could not be related to the fibrinogen content. They also found a deficiency of platelet fibrinogen in afibrinogenæmia and showed that transfused fibrinogen was adsorbed on to the platelets *in vivo*.

Platelet Factor 2 accelerates the conversion of fibrinogen to fibrin by thrombin, and **Platelet Factor 4** neutralizes the action of heparin. No bleeding or thrombotic tendency has been attributed directly to changes in the concentration of either of these active principles in the platelets.

Clot Retraction

Platelets, by virtue of their contractile protein, thrombosthenin (Bettex-Galland and Lüscher, 1961), are essential for clot retraction, in the course of which platelet ATP is broken down. Clot retraction is thus defective in thrombocytopenia and also in thrombasthenia, in which this was the earliest observed defect. Budtz-Olsen (1951) showed that the degree of retraction was also influenced by temperature, 40°C being the optimum, and was inversely related both to the PCV and to the mass of the fibrin clot, and hence to the plasma fibrinogen concentration. Quantitative determination of clot retraction should therefore take these variables into account, in addition to the platelet count. In practice, the measurement of clot retraction is of no value in the diagnosis of thrombocytopenia and has been superseded as a test for thrombasthenia by methods of studying platelet aggregation. The failure of clot retraction in thrombasthenia has not been fully explained, but may be related either to the failure of aggregation during clotting, or to an inability of thrombasthenic platelets to adhere to fibrin strands; there is no evidence of a failure of ATP breakdown in the platelets, as would be expected if thrombasthenin were deficient.

The ability to cause clot retraction is one of the properties of platelets which is lost fairly rapidly during storage, probably owing to the progressive fall in platelet ATP, which provides the energy for the process.

Pressor Amines

Platelets take up 5-hydroxytryptamine (5 HT) from the plasma against a concentration gradient, and provide the chief means of transporting it in the bloodstream. They release 5 HT during clotting, and in response to a variety of other stimuli, including contact with connective tissue particles, antigen-antibody complexes and glass surfaces. Although it is natural to suppose that 5 HT released from the platelets following vascular injury contributes to the hæmostatic mechanism by causing local vasoconstriction, this function of platelets is evidently not essential for normal hæmostasis. The best evidence for this is that profound depletion of platelet 5 HT by reserpine neither prolongs the bleeding time nor causes a bleeding tendency (Haverback et al., 1957). Determination of platelet 5 HT is thus of no practical value in the routine investigation of bleeding disorders.

Adrenaline and noradrenaline are also taken up by the platelets through an active transport mechanism, though less avidly than 5 HT. It is noteworthy that both these substances are powerful platelet-aggregating agents in vitro, and 5 HT rather less so; all these pressor amines may contribute to platelet plug formation in vivo, as well as to vasoconstriction.

Conclusion

The investigation of the various aspects of platelet function must still be regarded as predominantly a research procedure rather than an approach to the routine diagnosis of bleeding or thrombotic disorders. Much has already been learnt, by the use of the methods discussed here, about the complex rôles of the platelets in hæmostasis and thrombosis, and some of the inter-relationships between them. It is to be hoped that further work along these and similar lines may eventually help us to attach a specific pathophysiological meaning to the term "thrombotic tendency", and so lead to the control of vascular disease. Meanwhile, it is apparent that single platelet abnormalities may lead to disturbances of more than one aspect of platelet behaviour and that the results of many of the tests mentioned are affected by variables outside the platelets themselves, and should be interpreted in this knowledge.

References

BANGHAM, A. D., FLEMANS, R., HEARD, D. H. and SEAMAN, G. V. F. (1958a). An apparatus for microelectrophoresis of small particles. Nature, Lond., 182, 642.
BANGHAM, A. D., PETHICA, B. A. and SEAMAN, G. V. F. (1958b). The charged groups at the interface of some blood cells. Biochem. J., 69, 12.
BETTEX-GALLAND, M. and LÜSCHER, E. F. (1961). Thrombosthenin—a contractile protein from thrombocytes. Its extraction from human blood platelets and some of its properties. Biochim. Biophys. Acta, 49, 536.
BIZZOZERO, J. (1882). Über einen neuen Formbestandteil des Blutes und dessen Rolle bei der Thrombose und der Blutgerinnung. Virchows Arch., 90, 261.
BOLTON, C. H., HAMPTON, J. R. and MITCHELL, J. R. A. (1967). Nature of the transferable factor which causes abnormal platelet behaviour in vascular disease. Lancet, ii, 1101.

BOLTON, C. H., HAMPTON, J. R. and PHILLIPSON, O. T. (1968). Platelet behaviour and plasma phospholipids in multiple sclerosis. *Lancet*, **i**, 99.

BORCHGREVINK, C. F. (1960). A method for measuring platelet adhesiveness *in vivo*. *Acta med. scand.*, **168**, 157.

BORCHGREVINK, C. F. (1961). Platelet adhesion *in vivo* in patients with bleeding disorders. *Acta med. scand.*, **170**, 231.

BORN, G. V. R. (1956a). Adenosinetriphosphate (ATP) in blood platelets. *Biochem. J.*, **62**, 33P.

BORN, G. V. R. (1956b). The breakdown of adenosine triphosphate in blood platelets during clotting. *J. Physiol.*, **133**, 61P.

BORN, G. V. R. (1962). Aggregation of blood platelets by adenosine diphosphate and its reversal. *Nature, Lond.*, **194**, 927.

BORN, G. V. R. and CROSS, M. J. (1963). The aggregation of blood platelets. *J. Physiol.*, **168**, 178.

BORN, G. V. R., HONOUR, A. J. and MITCHELL, J. R. A. (1964). Inhibition by adenosine and by 2-chloroadenosine of the formation and embolization of platelet thrombi. *Nature, Lond.*, **202**, 761.

BRAUNSTEINER, H. (1955). Thrombopathie und Thrombasthenie. *Wien Z. inn. Med.*, **36**, 421.

BRIDGES, J. M., DALBY, A. M., MILLAR, J. H. D. and WEAVER, J. A. (1965). An effect of D-glucose on platelet stickiness. *Lancet*, **i**, 75.

BUDTZ-OLSEN, O. E. (1951). *Clot Retraction*. Oxford: Blackwell Scientific Publications.

BYGDEMAN, S., ELIASSON, R. and JOHNSON, S.-R. (1966). Relationship between postoperative changes in adenosine-diphosphate induced platelet adhesiveness and venous thrombosis. *Lancet*, **i**, 1301.

CAEN, J. P. and INCEMAN, S. (1963). Considérations sur l'allongement du temps de saignement dans l'afibrinogénémie congenitale. *Nouv. Rev. franç. Hémat.*, **3**, 614.

CAEN, J. P., SULTAN, Y. and LARRIEU, M.-J. (1968). A new familial platelet disease. *Lancet*, **i**, 203.

CASPARY, E. A. (1965). Effect of red blood-cells and adenosine on platelet adhesiveness. *Lancet*, **ii**, 1273.

CASPARY, E. A., PRINEAS, J., MILLER, H. and FIELD, E. J. (1965). Platelet stickiness in multiple sclerosis. *Lancet*, **ii**, 1108.

CASTALDI, P. A. and CAEN, J. (1965). Platelet fibrinogen. *J. clin. Path.*, **18**, 579.

CASTALDI, P. A., ROZENBERG, M. C. and STEWART, J. H. (1966). The bleeding disorder of uraemia. A qualitative platelet defect. *Lancet*, **ii**, 66.

CRONBERG, S., NILSSON, I. M. and GYDELL, K. (1965). Haemorrhagic thrombocythaemia due to defect platelet adhesiveness. *Scand. J. Haemat.*, **2**, 208.

EWALD, R. A., EICHELBERGER, J. W., YOUNG, A. A., WEISS, H. J. and CROSBY, W. H. (1965). The effect of dextran on platelet factor-3 activity: *in vitro* and *in vivo* studies. *Transfusion (Philad.)*, **5**, 109.

FRENCH, J. E., MACFARLANE, R. G. and SANDERS, A. G. (1964). The structure of haemostatic plugs and experimental thrombi in small arteries. *Brit. J. exp. Path.*, **45**, 467.

GAARDER, A., JONSEN, J., LALAND, S., HELLEM, A. and OWREN, P. A. (1961). Adenosine diphosphate in red cells as a factor in the adhesiveness of human blood platelets. *Nature, Lond.*, **192**, 531.

GRETTE, K. (1962). Studies on the mechanism of thrombin-catalysed haemostatic reactions in blood platelets. *Acta physiol. scand.*, **56**, Suppl. 195.

GUGLER, E. and LÜSCHER, E. (1963). Die Kongenitale Afibrinogenämie. *Ann. Paediat.*, **200**, 125.

HAMPTON, J. R. and HARDISTY, R. M. (1967). Platelet electrophoretic behaviour in thrombasthenia. *Nature, Lond.*, **213**, 400.

HAMPTON, J. R. and MITCHELL, J. R. A. (1966a). Effect of glass contact on the electrophoretic mobility of human blood platelets. *Nature, Lond.*, **209**, 470.

HAMPTON, J. R. and MITCHELL, J. R. A. (1966b). Effect of aggregating agents on the electrophoretic mobility of human platelets. *Brit. med. J.*, **i**, 1074.

HAMPTON, J. R. and MITCHELL, J. R. A. (1966c). Abnormalities in platelet behaviour in acute illnesses. *Brit. med. J.*, **i**, 1078.

HAMPTON, J. R. and MITCHELL, J. R. A. (1966d). A transferable factor causing abnormal platelet behaviour in vascular disease. *Lancet*, **ii**, 764.

HARDISTY, R. M. (1968). Platelet aggregation and platelet factor-3 availability in bleeding disorders. *Exp. Biol. Med.* (In press.)

HARDISTY, R. M., DORMANDY, K. M. and HUTTON, R. A. (1964). Thrombasthenia: studies on three cases. *Brit. J. Haemat.*, **10**, 371.

HARDISTY, R. M. and HUTTON, R. A. (1965). The kaolin clotting time of platelet-rich plasma: a test of platelet factor-3 availability. *Brit. J. Haemat.*, **11**, 258.

HARDISTY, R. M. and HUTTON, R. A. (1966). Platelet aggregation and the availability of platelet factor 3. *Brit. J. Haemat.*, **12**, 764.

HARDISTY, R. M. and HUTTON, R. A. (1967). Bleeding tendency associated with "new" abnormality of platelet behaviour. *Lancet*. **i**, 983.

HARRISON, M. J. G., EMMONS, P. R. and MITCHELL, J. R. A. (1966). The effect of white cells on platelet aggregation. *Thromb. Diath. haem.*, **16**, 105.

HARRISON, M. J. G., EMMONS, P. R. and MITCHELL, J. R. A. (1967). The variability of human platelet aggregation. *J. Atheroscler. Res.*, **7**, 197.

HARRISON, M. J. G. and MITCHELL, J. R. A. (1966). The influence of red blood-cells on platelet adhesiveness. *Lancet*, **ii**, 1163.

HAVERBACK, B. J., DUTCHER, T. F., SHORE, P. A., TOMICH, E. G., TERRY, L. L. and BRODIE, B. B. (1957). Serotonin changes in platelets and brain induced by small daily doses of reserpine; lack of effect of depletion of platelet serotonin in hemostatic mechanisms. *New Engl. J. Med.*, **256**. 343.

HELLEM, A. J. (1960). The adhesiveness of human blood platelets *in vitro. Scand. J. clin. Lab. Invest.*, **12**, Suppl. 51.

HELLEM, A. J., ÖDEGAARD, A. E. and SKÅLHEGG, B. A. (1964). Platelet adhesiveness in chronic renal failure. *Abstract K 1, Xth. Congr. Int. Soc. Haemat., Stockholm.*

HIRSH, J., CASTELAN, D. J. and LODER, P. B. (1967). Spontaneous bruising associated with a defect in the interaction of platelets with connective tissue. *Lancet*, **ii**, 18.

HIRSH, J. and MCBRIDE, J. A. (1965). Increased platelet adhesiveness in recurrent venous thrombosis and pulmonary embolism. *Brit. med. J.*, **ii**, 797.

HIRSH, J., MCBRIDE, J. A. and WRIGHT, H. P. (1966). Platelet adhesiveness: a comparison of the rotating bulb and glass-bead column methods. *Thromb. Diath. haem.*, **16**, 100.

HONOUR, A. J. and MITCHELL, J. R. A. (1964). Platelet clumping in injured vessels. *Brit. J. exp. Path.*, **45**, 75.

HONOUR, A. J. and ROSS RUSSELL, R. W. (1962). Experimental platelet embolism. *Brit. J. exp. Path.*, **43**, 350.

HOROWITZ, H. I., COHEN, B. D., MARTINEZ, P. and PAPAYOANOU, M. F. (1967). Defective ADP-induced platelet factor-3 activation in uremia. *Blood*, **30**, 331.

HOVIG, T. (1963). Release of a platelet-aggregating substance (adenosine diphosphate) from rabbit blood platelets induced by saline "extract" of tendons. *Thromb. Diath. haem.*, **9**, 264.

HUGUES, J. (1962). Accolement des plaquettes aux structures conjunctives périvasculaires *Thromb. Diath. haem.*, **8**, 241.

HUTTON, R. A. and O'SHEA, M. J. (1968). The haemostatic mechanisms in uraemia. *J. clin. Path.*, **21**, 406.

INCEMAN, S., CAEN, J. and BERNARD, J. (1966). Aggregation, adhesion and viscous metamorphosis of platelets in congenital fibrinogen deficiencies. *J. Lab. clin. Med.*, **68**, 21.

KÄSER-GLANZMANN, R. and LÜSCHER, E. F. (1962). The mechanism of platelet aggregation in relation to hemostasis. *Thromb. Diath. haem.*, **7**, 480.

MCCLURE, P. D., INGRAM, G. I. C., STACEY, R. S., GLASS, U. H. and MATCHETT, M. O. (1966). Platelet function tests in thrombocythaemia and thrombocytosis. *Brit. J. Haemat.*, **12**, 478.

MCDONALD, L., BRAY, C., FIELD, C., LOVE, F. and DAVIES, B. (1964). Homocystinuria, thrombosis, and the blood-platelets. *Lancet*, **i**, 745.

MCDONALD, L. and EDGILL, M. (1957). Coagulability of the blood in ischaemic heart-disease. *Lancet*, **ii**, 457.

MCDONALD, L. and EDGILL, M. (1958). Dietary restriction and coagulability of the blood in ischaemic heart-disease. *Lancet*, **i**, 996.

MACMILLAN, D. C. (1966). Secondary clumping effect in human citrated platelet-rich plasma produced by adenosine diphosphate and adrenaline. *Nature, Lond.*, **211**, 140.

MARCUS, A. J., ZUCKER-FRANKLIN, D., SAFIER, L. B. and ULLMAN, H. L. (1966). Studies on human platelet granules and membranes. *J. clin. Invest.*, **45**, 14.

MOOLTEN, S. E. and VROMAN, L. (1949). The adhesiveness of blood platelets in thromboembolism and hemorrhagic disorders. *Amer. J. clin. Path.*, **19**, 701.

MUCKLE, T. J. (1964). Low *in vivo* adhesive-platelet count in hereditary haemorrhagic telangiectasia. *Lancet*, **ii**, 880.

NIEWIAROWSKI, S., BAŃKOWSKI, E. and ROGOWICKA, I. (1965). Studies on the adsorption and activation of the Hageman factor (factor XII) by collagen and elastin. *Thromb. Diath. haem.*, **14**, 387.

O'BRIEN, J. R. (1961). The adhesiveness of native platelets and its prevention. *J. clin. Path.* **14**, 140.

O'BRIEN, J. R. (1962). Platelet aggregation. Part II. Some results from a new method of study. *J. clin. Path.*, **15**, 452.

O'BRIEN, J. R. (1967). Platelets: a Portsmouth syndrome. *Lancet*, **ii**, 258.

PACHTER, M. R., JOHNSON, S. A., NEBLETT, T. R. and TRUANT, J. P. (1959). Bleeding, platelets, and macroglobulinemia. *Amer. J. clin. Path.*, **31**, 467.

PHILP, R. B. and WRIGHT, H. P. (1965). Effect of adenosine on platelet adhesiveness in fasting and lipaemic bloods. *Lancet*, **ii**, 208.

SALZMAN, E. W. (1963a). Measurement of platelet adhesiveness. A simple *in vitro* technique demonstrating an abnormality in von Willebrand's disease. *J. Lab. clin. Med.*, **62**, 724.

SALZMAN, E. W. (1963b). Blood platelets and extracorporeal circulation. *Transfusion (Philad.)*, **3**, 274.

SALZMAN, E. W. and NERI, L. L. (1966). Adhesiveness of blood platelets in uremia. *Thromb. Diath. haem.*, **15**, 84.

SPAET, T. H. and CINTRON, J. (1965). Studies on platelet factor-3 availability. *Brit. J. Haemat.*, **11**, 269.

SPAET, T. H. and ZUCKER, M. B. (1964). Mechanism of platelet plug formation and rôle of adenosine diphosphate. *Amer. J. Physiol.* **206**, 1267.

WEISS, H. J. (1967a). The effect of clinical dextran on platelet aggregation, adhesion, and ADP release in man: *in vivo* and *in vitro* studies. *J. Lab. clin. Med.*, **69**, 37.

WEISS, H. J. (1967b). Platelet aggregation, adhesion and adenosine diphosphate release in thrombopathia (platelet factor-3 deficiency)—a comparison with Glanzmann's thrombasthenia and von Willebrand's disease. *Amer. J. Med.*, **43**, 570.

WEISS, H. J. and ALEDORT, L. M. (1967). Impaired platelet/connective-tissue reaction in man after aspirin ingestion. *Lancet*, **ii**, 495.

WRIGHT, H. P. (1941). The adhesiveness of blood platelets in normal subjects with varying concentrations of anti-coagulant. *J. Path. Bact.*, **53**, 255.

WRIGHT, H. P. (1942). Changes in the adhesiveness of blood platelets following parturition and surgical operations. *J. Path. Bact.*, **54**, 461.

WRIGHT, H. P., THOMPSON, R. H. S. and ZILKHA, K. J. (1965). Platelet adhesiveness in multiple sclerosis. *Lancet*, **ii**, 1109.

ZUCKER, M. B. (1964). Platelet adhesion, release and aggregation. *Thromb. Diath. haem.*, Suppl. **13**, 301.

F

Chapter 12

PREVENTION OF Rh IMMUNIZATION FOLLOWING PREGNANCY

P. L. Mollison and N. C. Hughes-Jones

It is now established that Rh immunization, which would otherwise occur in a proportion of Rh-negative women as a sequel to pregnancy, can be prevented by the passive administration of Rh antibody shortly after delivery. In this chapter, the development of this knowledge and the theoretical background of the subject will be discussed. As described later, it has been known for a long time that the simultaneous administration of antibody with antigen may inhibit immunization. However, it seems that the idea of trying to prevent Rh-immunization by injecting Rh-antibody was derived from another source, namely the observation of Levine (1943) that ABO incompatibility between husband and wife diminishes the likelihood of Rh hæmolytic disease in the offspring. Race and Sanger (1950) suggested that the mechanism of this protection was the rapid destruction of fœtal A or B Rh-positive red cells by anti-A or anti-B in the mother's circulation. A group of workers in Liverpool concluded that, if this were so, the deliberate destruction of Rh-positive ABO-*compatible* red cells by Rh antibody might also prevent Rh immunization (Finn, Clarke, Donohoe, McConnell, Sheppard, Lehane and Kulke, 1961). At about the same time, a group in New York began work on similar lines (Gorman, Freda and Pollack, 1962). Before describing these various experiments, present knowledge about Rh immunization in pregnancy will be briefly summarized.

Rh Immunization as a Consequence of Pregnancy

Among Caucasians, the combination: Rh(D*)-positive infant, Rh(D)-negative mother occurs in about 10 per cent of all pregnancies. The Rh antigen is found only on red cells so that the only way in which the fœtus can immunize its mother to Rh is by transplacental hæmorrhage. Most observers have found that fœtal red cells are only rarely demonstrable in the mother's blood during the first six months of pregnancy but are not uncommonly found in the last trimester, and that there is a tendency for the number of fœtal cells in the maternal circulation to increase during normal delivery (for a review see Mollison, 1967, page 314). The Liverpool group concluded that in two-thirds of cases in which fœtal cells were present in the mother's blood immediately after delivery, the "bleed" had occurred during delivery (Woodrow, Clarke, Donohoe, Finn, McConnell, Sheppard, Lehane, Russell, Kulke and Durkin, 1965). The same group concluded that about 16 per cent of women have 0·25 ml. or more of fœtal blood in their circulation immediately after delivery (Woodrow and Finn, 1966). Since transplacental hæmorrhage

---

* In this chapter "Rh" and "D" are used interchangeably.

seems to occur mainly at the time of delivery, it is not surprising that Rh antibodies are very seldom found during a first pregnancy with an Rh-positive fœtus but can often be detected for the first time three or six months after a first pregnancy (Weiner, Norris and Davidsohn, 1952; Woodrow *et al.*, 1966).

Results from Liverpool show clearly a relation between the number of fœtal red cells demonstrable in the mother's circulation immediately after delivery and the likelihood of immunization. Of Rh-negative primiparæ who had given birth to an Rh-positive, ABO-compatible infant and had no detectable fœtal red cells in their circulation immediately after delivery, only 3·1 per cent subsequently developed anti-Rh; of those who had detectable fœtal red cells equivalent to less than 0·25 ml. fœtal blood, 8·4 per cent developed anti-Rh; of those with 0·25 to 3 ml. fœtal blood, 20 per cent developed anti-Rh and of those with more than 3 ml., 50 per cent developed anti-Rh (McConnell, 1966).

Transplacental hæmorrhages of 0·25 ml. or more, which occur in about one-sixth of pregnancies, appear to account for about one third of all cases of Rh immunization in pregnancy. Thus: 8 per cent of primiparæ are Rh-negative women who give birth to an Rh-positive ABO-compatible infant, and about 16 per cent of these have 0·25 ml. or more of fœtal blood in their circulation at the time of delivery. Of these women, about one-fifth have detectable anti-Rh in their serum within six months and a further one-tenth have detectable anti-Rh in their serum during the succeeding pregnancy when (as in six out of eight cases), this is with an Rh-positive infant (J. C. Woodrow, personal communication). The number of affected infants resulting from second pregnancies in such women will thus be equivalent to approximately 0·3 per cent of all second pregnancies, which is about one third of the total incidence of Rh hæmolytic disease in second pregnancies.

It should not be overlooked that approximately two thirds of Rh-negative women become sensitized by a first pregnancy despite having less than 0·25 ml. of fœtal blood in their circulation at the time of delivery, and that some of these have no detectable fœtal red cells. The fact that many women become immunized to Rh by pregnancy without having demonstrable fœtal red cells in their circulation immediately after delivery suggests the possibility that less than 0·1 ml. of fœtal blood may constitute an adequate primary stimulus in some women—this being about the smallest amount that can be detected reliably. It is of course possible that in some of these cases larger amounts have been present in the mother's circulation earlier but have been eliminated.

ABO Incompatibility and Rh Immunization

Levine (1943) drew attention to the fact that ABO incompatibility between father and mother partially protected the mother against Rh immunization. Whereas in a random series of matings, 35 per cent were ABO-incompatible (father's red cells versus mother's serum) the percentage was only 24·7 per cent in matings between Rh-positive fathers and Rh-negative mothers resulting in the birth of infants affected with hæmolytic disease of the newborn; in a subsequent, more extensive series (Levine, 1958), the percentage was even lower (19·2 per cent). It should be pointed out that these figures for incompatibility apply to the father's red cells rather than to the infant's. Since a group-A father often has the genotype *AO* he will often be the father of a group-O infant, so that evidently Levine's findings imply that ABO incompatibility between infant and mother confers an even higher degree of protection against Rh immunization than the figures might suggest. Murray, Knox and Walker (1965) estimated that A incompatibility between infant and mother was 90 per cent protective and B incompatibility 55 per cent protective. Nevanlinna and Vainio (1956) investigated a series of families in which the mother was immunized to Rh but the father was ABO-incompatible and found that the healthy child immediately preceding the first affected child was almost four times more commonly ABO-compatible than incompatible. On the other hand, they found that once a mother had been immunized to Rh, ABO-incompatible infants were just as likely to be affected as ABO-compatible ones. The protection against primary Rh immunization afforded by ABO incompatibility was demonstrated directly in Rh-negative adult volunteers by Stern, Davidsohn and Masaitis (1956): of 17 subjects injected with ABO-compatible, Rh-positive cells, 10 developed anti-Rh (maximum titre 256 or more in 5 out of 10 subjects); by contrast, of 22 subjects injected with ABO-incompatible Rh-positive cells, only 2 developed antibody (titre 2–8).

The mechanism whereby ABO incompatibility protects against Rh immunization is discussed briefly in a later section.

The Effect of Passively Administered anti-Rh on the Survival of Rh-positive Red Cells

When anti-Rh, in the form of γ-globulin, is injected intramuscularly, substantial amounts reach the circulation within eight hours (Freda, Gorman and Pollack, 1964), but maximum values may not be reached even after 24 hours. If a small number of Rh-positive red cells is injected intravenously at the same time as the anti-Rh is injected intramuscularly, there is a delay of about six hours before the Rh-positive cells start to disappear (Mollison and Hughes-Jones, 1967; see Fig. 1). The subsequent rate of clearance is affected by the number of cells in the circulation as well as by the concentration of antibody.

There are two reasons why a small amount of red cells, say 0·3 ml. will be removed more rapidly than 10 ml. of cells. First, owing to the heterogeneity of the equilibrium constant of the antigen-antibody reaction, the average amount of antibody combined with each red cell increases as the total volume of cells in the circulation decreases. Secondly, because red cells coated with anti-Rh are removed predominantly in the spleen (Jandl, 1955; Mollison and Cutbush, 1955) the relatively small size of this organ must impose an upper limit on the amount of red cells which can be cleared from the circulation in unit time.

When amounts of Rh-positive red cells of the order of 0·3 ml. are injected it can be shown that the rate of clearance is proportional to approximately the square root of the amount of antibody on the red cells (Mollison and Hughes-Jones, 1967). In practice this means that very low concentrations of anti-Rh are capable of producing accelerated clearance of cells. With one particular example of anti-Rh ("Av") it was found that a total body content of 1 μg. was sufficient to produce a readily detectable increase in the rate of destruction of a small volume of Rh-positive red cells. Following the injection of 50 μg. of the same example of anti-Rh, red cells were cleared with a T½ of 3·5 hours. In experiments with another preparation of anti-Rh (pool N 46G prepared by Dr. W. d'A. Maycock at the Lister Institute) 50 μg. brought about the clearance at a distinctly slower rate (T½ 8·5 hours, see Fig. 2). The difference between "Av" and N 46 G was due at least partly to the higher equilibrium constant of the anti-D from the donor "Av", resulting in a greater average number of antibody molecules combined with each red cell.

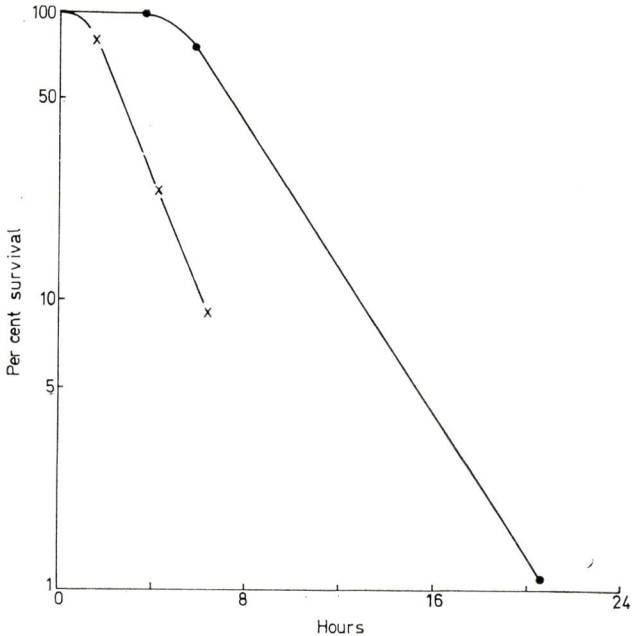

FIG. 1. "Clearance" of 0·3 ml. of ^{51}Cr-labelled Rh-positive red cells in two Rh-negative subjects injected with 250 μg anti-D.
×——× anti-D injected 24 hours before red cells
●——● anti D injected 10 minutes after red cells
(*From* Mollison and Hughes-Jones, 1967)

It seems probable that apart from the question of equilibrium constant there are other important qualitative differences between antibodies of the same serological specificity. Suggestive evidence relating to two different examples of anti-D was provided by Mollison and Hughes-Jones (1967), who also drew attention to examples of anti-C and anti-E which had been shown to be relatively ineffective in bringing about the clearance of red cells and to the example of anti-Xg^a described by Sausais, Krevans and Townes (1966) which appeared to be completely ineffective in bringing about the clearance of red cells.

As described below, there is much evidence that suppression of primary immunization depends on the amount of antibody combined with antigen and is thus only indirectly related to the rate of clearance of the cells.

Suppression of Rh Immunization by Passively Administered anti-Rh

Although most of our present knowledge on this subject has been obtained by injecting Rh-positive red cells and Rh antibody separately into Rh-negative volunteers, a highly relevant experiment was in fact performed somewhat earlier by Stern, Goodman and Berger (1961). Rh-positive red cells were coated *in vitro* with anti-Rh and injected into Rh-negative subjects. Of 16 subjects given a course of injections (usually five) of coated Rh-positive cells, not one produced anti-Rh; however, when ten of the subjects were, at a

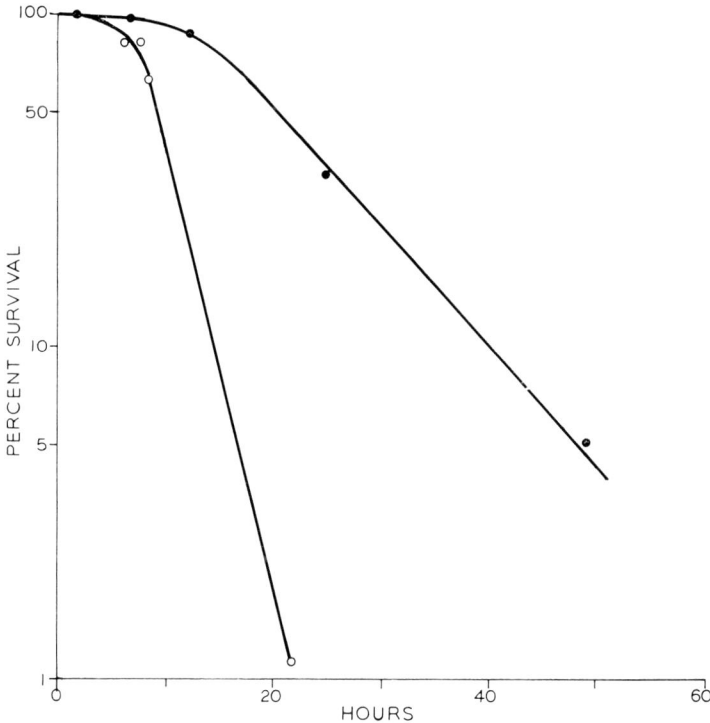

Fig. 2. "Clearance" of 0·3 ml. of ^{51}Cr-labelled Rh-positive red cells in two Rh-negative subjects injected 24 or 48 hours previously with 50 μg. of different anti-D preparations, "Av" and "N49G".

○———○ "Av"   ●———● N49G

later date, given injections of uncoated Rh-positive cells, five produced anti-Rh. In retrospect, this experiment does not seem to be different in any important way from later ones in which Rh antibody was given simultaneously with red cells.

An extensive series of experiments was reported by Clarke *et al.* (1963). In these experiments serum containing anti-Rh was injected intravenously into Rh-negative subjects immediately after injecting 5 ml. of Rh-positive blood. Many different batches of serum were used, some of which contained predominantly incomplete antibody (IgG) and some, predominantly Rh agglutinins (IgM). Of 21 subjects who received 35–50 ml. of potent incomplete anti-D on four occasions, following the intravenous injection of 5 ml. of Rh-positive blood, only 3 formed antibody, compared with 11 out of 21 controls who received Rh-positive blood alone. On the other hand, in a series in which 10–20 ml. of agglutinating Rh was given on each of two occasions with 5 ml. of Rh-positive blood, 8 out of 13 subjects formed antibody, compared with only 1 out of 11 control subjects given injections of Rh-positive blood alone; this experience suggested that agglutinating anti-Rh might actually enhance immunization, and the authors commented on the fact that, with the dose of agglutinating antibody which they used, only partial clearance of Rh-positive cells was achieved, about 50 per cent of the cells being cleared within 24 hours. Evidence that small amounts of IgM antibody, given simultaneously with red cells, may actually enhance immunization is considered later in this chapter.

In 1964, a New York group described experiments in which incomplete (IgG) anti-Rh was injected intramuscularly, in the form of a concentrate of γ-globulin, into subjects who also received 2 ml. of Rh-positive blood intramuscularly; after five successive injections of γ-globulin and blood, four out of four subjects remained unsensitized, whereas four out of five control subjects who received Rh-positive blood without γ-globulin formed potent anti-Rh (Freda *et al.* 1964).

Passive Administration of Rh Antibody to Recently Delivered Women

At the time of writing, trials of the efficacy of passively administered anti-Rh in preventing Rh immunization in recently delivered women are in progress in many parts of the world. In a combined study in which British and American workers have collaborated, only specially selected women have been treated, namely Rh-negative primiparæ who have given birth to an Rh-positive, ABO-compatible infant, and who, immediately after delivery, have had the equivalent of 0·25 ml. or more of fœtal blood in their circulation. Of 78 of such women treated with 5 ml. of anti-D γ-globulin, none was definitely immunized, whereas of 78 controls, 19 were immunized (A Combined Study, 1966). In a trial in New York and California, all Rh-negative women of whatever parity are included, provided only that they have given birth to an Rh-positive, ABO-compatible infant; the presence or absence of fœtal red cells in the mother's circulation is not taken into account. In this trial, of women treated with 5 ml. of anti-D γ-globulin, none out of 174 formed anti-Rh, compared with 20 out of 171 who formed antibody in the control series (Freda *et al.* 1967).

The evidence that anti-D, passively administered immediately after delivery, prevents the appearance of actively-formed anti-D during the subsequent six months now seems overwhelming. However, there has been some caution in accepting this evidence as indicating that immunization has been entirely prevented. Smith (1909) found that when a relatively small amount of antibody was given with antigen, primary immunization was delayed but eventually some antibody was produced and, following a second antigenic stimulus, there was a typical secondary response. Despite this finding of Smith (1909), there is reason to believe that when an adequate amount of anti-D is given with D-positive cells, primary immunization is entirely prevented. For example, in one series of experiments, when two successive injections of D-positive red cells were given without anti-D to D-negative subjects at an interval of six weeks, in approximately two-thirds of the subjects the second lot of red cells was rapidly cleared from the circulation indicating that primary immunization had occurred. By contrast, when D-positive red cells were given with anti-D and, at a later date, the recipient was "challenged" with D-positive red cells, survival was strictly normal, indicating that immunization had been completely prevented (Krevans, Woodrow, Nosenzo and Finn, 1964). Similarly Rh-negative mothers who have been protected by passively administered anti-Rh following a first pregnancy behave as if they are completely unsensitized to Rh, in the sense that in a subsequent pregnancy with an Rh-positive fœtus they do not form anti-Rh (A Combined Study, 1966).

The latest available figures (March, 1968) from centres in Britain, U.S.A., and Germany for 'subsequent' pregnancies are as follows: of 176 women untreated with anti-D γ-globulin at the time of their first delivery 33 formed anti-Rh in a subsequent pregnancy; by contrast, of 192 women treated with anti-D γglobulin at the time of their first delivery, only one formed anti-Rh in a subsequent pregnancy (C. A. Clarke, personal communication).

Administration of anti-Rh during Pregnancy. Although transplacental hæmorrhage seems to be commonest during delivery, it does also occur during pregnancy and particularly during the last trimester (Lewi, et al., 1961; Cohen and Zuelzer, 1964; Krevans et al., 1964; Woodrow and Finn, 1966). In view of this evidence it is surprising that the administration of anti-D only after delivery seems to be so universally successful in suppressing primary immunization. It seems possible that further experiments will show that primary immunization does sometimes occur before delivery and cannot be completely prevented by any treatment instituted after delivery.

In Canada the possibility of administering anti-D γ-globulin prophylactically during pregnancy is being explored. This treatment is potentially hazardous, since the anti-D (being IgG) will be transferred across the placenta and might set up a hæmolytic process in the infant. The intention in this trial is to give the mother an amount of anti-D which will suppress primary immunization without causing damage to the fœtus. 1 ml. of anti-D γ-globulin has been given at the beginning of the last trimester followed by 0·4 ml. every three weeks. Although an occasional infant has been born with a positive direct antiglobulin test, no signs of a hæmolytic process have been observed in any infant (Zipursky et al. 1966). It remains to be seen whether or not it is necessary to explore this method any further.

Mechanism of Suppression of Primary Immunization

The observation that passively administered antibody inhibits active antibody production may be found in a paper by Smith (1909), who showed that if antitoxin was administered at the same time as diphtheria toxoid, active antibody production was diminished and that the larger the dose of antitoxin, the greater the effect. It has subsequently been shown that passively administered antibody diminishes or prevents the antibody response to the following antigens: bovine serum albumin and globulin, ovalbumin, sheep red blood cells, poliomyelitis virus and bacteriophage (for reference see Uhr and Baumann, 1961). It is of course well recognized that the presence in newborn infants of a substantial titre of maternally derived diphtheria antitoxin interferes with active immunization (Barr, Glenny and Randall, 1950). It has only recently been realized that the suppression of active antibody production by passively administered antibody is probably a manifestation of the existence of a normal homeostatic mechanism ("feed-back") for control of antibody production (Uhr and Baumann, 1961).

Primary immunization can be prevented both by IgM and IgG antibody; both classes of antibody inhibit the primary response to sheep red cells injected into rats (Rowley and Fitch, 1964) and in mice (Möller and Wigzell, 1965), although the amount of IgM required is 100–200 times greater than the amount of IgG, based on hæmolytic titre (Möller and Wigzell, 1965). In rabbits, in whom the active production of IgG antibody has been inhibited by the administration of 6-mercaptopurine, the IgM response to bovine globulin can be inhibited by passively administered IgG antibody (Sahiar and Schwartz, 1964). The primary response can be inhibited when passive IgG antibody is given within 3–5 days following the injection of antigen (Uhr and Baumann, 1961; Finkelstein and Uhr, 1964; Möller and Wigzell, 1965; Freda *et al.*, 1966). Passively administered IgG antibody will produce some inhibition of the active production of IgG when given up to 40 days after the administration of antigen (Wigzell, 1966) Möller and Wigzell (1965) and Wigzell (1966) found that after administration of antibody there was a delay of 48–72 hours before the number of antibody-forming cells in the spleen began to fall. They interpreted this as indicating that passive antibody acted by removal of the stimulus and not by influencing cells already committed to divide and produce antibody.

It may be inferred that actively produced IgM and IgG inhibit the further production of antibody and it may be assumed that the ultimate level of plasma antibody is the resultant of the strength of the antigenic stimulus on the one hand and the degree of inhibition by "feed-back" on the other.

The mechanism of inhibition of the immune response by passive antibody remains a subject for speculation, but the most plausible theory is that suggested by Uhr and Baumann (1961) and supported by Möller and Wigzell (1965), namely that passive antibody acts by combining with antigen and diverting it away from the site where antibody production is initiated.

Diversion of antigen could occur at one or both of two stages: first, passive antibody could lead to the sequestration and breakdown of antigen at some anatomical site where antibody production is not stimulated. In rats it has been shown that the deposition of the protein flagellin in the spleen is different from that seen with carbon particles (Nossall *et al.*, 1966). It is thus possible that in the human spleen, antibody-coated red cells are treated differently from non-coated cells.

Secondly, diversion of antigen might occur after "processing" by phagocytes. There is evidence (Cohen, 1967) that small units of antigen combined with RNA are passed on by phagocytes to antibody-forming cells; passively administered antibody might combine with these small units and prevent them from stimulating antibody production. Very strong support for this theory is provided by the work of Brody, Walker and Siskind (1967). These authors showed that when animals were injected with two antigenic determinants carried on the same molecule, together with antibody against only the first determinant, the animal formed antibody against the second determinant. Evidently, if phagocytosis of the molecule was the important step in suppressing immunization there should have been no formation of antibody against either determinant.

There is evidence that suppression is also antigen-specific when two closely related antigens are carried on the same red cell. In Hg(A—F—)rabbits, injected with Hg (A + F +) red cells together with anti-Hg^A, the formation of anti-Hg^A but not of anti-Hg^F is suppressed (Pollack *et al.*, 1968).

Evidence that the amount of "passive" antibody required to inhibit the immune response is inversely proportional to its binding constant (Walker and Siskind, 1968) also strongly supports the idea that "passive" antibody competes with receptors on lymphocytes for available antigen and in this way may prevent antigen from triggering off an immune response.

The mechanism whereby ABO-incompatibility of Rh-positive red cells interferes with the initiation of the primary response is clearly different, since here the antibody (anti-A or anti-B) which suppresses has a specificity different from that of the antibody (anti-Rh) which is suppressed. Anti-A or anti-B usually produce predominantly intravascular lysis and the resulting red-cell stroma is probably cleared from the circulation chiefly in the reticulo-endothelial cells of the liver. It is known that the way in which antigen is presented to the antibody-forming cells is important in determing their response and it can only be surmised that the manner of presentation of Rh-antigen, following destruction of Rh-positive cells by anti-A and anti-B, is relatively unsuitable for stimulating anti-Rh production. There is, in fact, evidence that lysed red cells are less antigenic than intact red cells (Schneider and Preisler, 1966; Mollison, 1967, p. 203; Pollack et al., 1968).

Minimum Effective Dose of Passively Administered anti-Rh

The minimum dose of passively administered anti-D which will suppress immunization is not yet known, but seems certain to be related to the amount of Rh-positive cells injected. In the trials presented in a Combined Study (1966) in which anti-Rh was injected into Rh-negative women, most of whom had less than 1 ml. of Rh-positive foetal red cells in their circulation at the time of delivery, the dose of anti-Rh injected is now known to have been of the order of 750-1500 μg. (personal observations). It is known that doses lower than this are effective even when larger amounts of red cells are concerned. For example, of Rh-negative volunteers given 10 ml. of whole-group Rh-positive blood together with 300 μg. anti-Rh, on 3 successive occasions, none developed antibody whereas of 10 volunteers who received the same amount of blood without anti-Rh, 6 developed antibody (Pollack, Singher, Gorman and Freda, 1967). The same dose of anti-Rh was found to be effective when injected into Rh-negative women delivered of an ABO-incompatible Rh-positive child; only one out of 384 women developed antibody when tested six months later, compared to 17 out of 228 women who received no anti-Rh. Our own (unpublished) observations suggest that a dose of 75 μg. is probably effective in suppressing immunization when 1 ml. of group 0 R_1r red cells is injected.

If the action of anti-Rh is through diversion of D antigen away from antibody-forming cells, then the effectiveness of passively administered anti-D will depend on the extent to which it combines with the red cells or red-cell particles following phagocytosis. The extent of the reaction is dependent on the concentration of antibody in the plasma and extracellular fluid, and on the average value and degree of heterogeneity of the equilibrium constant of the antigen-antibody reaction. If these values are known, it is possible to calculate the number of antigen sites which are bound to antibody at equilibrium, using the binding equation given by Karush (1962). In our own observations, where 75 μg. anti-Rh was injected, it was estimated that less than 10 per cent of the antigen sites on 1 ml. of cells would have combined with antibody if the reaction had proceeded to equilibrium. If this estimate is correct it makes it very unlikely that passively admininstered anti-Rh acts simply by covering antigen sites; it is more probable either that red cells, or red-cell particles containing a few hundred antigen sites, are diverted away from or fail to penetrate antibody-forming cells when as few as 10 per cent of the Rh sites are covered with antibody following the injection of 1 ml. of red cells.

In defining the greatest amount of anti-D which has been shown to be *in*effective in suppressing primary immunization the observations of

Schneider and Preisler (1966) are helpful. These authors injected 0·5 ml. of Rh-positive blood together with 1 ml. of anti-D serum into Rh-negative subjects and, after two injections of both red cells and antibody, observed antibody formation in 5 out of 20 recipients, which was similar to the incidence of antibody formation in a control series. The titre of the anti-D serum which they used was approximately 128 so that the total amount of antibody given may have been of the order of 5 to 10 μg. (see Hughes-Jones, 1967). Of course, it is possible that the particular antibody used was relatively ineffective in clearing cells from the circulation and it seems premature to conclude that a dose of 5 to 10 μg. of anti-D will always be ineffective in suppressing primary immunization.

Augmentation of Antibody Production by Passively Administered Antibody

Augmentation of active immunization by relatively small amounts of passively administered antibody has been reported in mice, injected with human serum albumin combined with a relatively small amount of specific antibody (Terres and Wolins, 1959); and in rabbits injected with allogeneic red cells and relatively small amounts of passively administered specific iso-antibody (Cohen and Allton, 1962). In these experiments no evidence was presented about the class of Ig antibody responsible for the effect.

As already mentioned, there is some evidence that when Rh-positive red cells and agglutinating (IgM) anti-Rh are injected into Rh-negative subjects, active production of anti-Rh may be augmented (Clarke et al., 1963). Presumably this effect is due partly to the fact that the IgM antibody somehow renders the antigen more effective, possibly by concentrating, and partly to the fact that passively administered JgM antibody is relatively ineffective in suppressing active antibody production.

It is also possible that small amounts of IgG anti-Rh augment primary Rh immunization. Thus, in Rh-negative volunteers injected with 5ml. of Rh-positive (R_2R_2) blood together with varying amounts of anti-D immunoglobulin, the incidence of immunization was apparently increased in subjects receiving 10 μg. of anti-D (Pollack et al., 1968). On the other hand, in experiments not yet published we have obtained no evidence that a dose of 15 μg. anti-D augments immunization by 1ml. of Rh-positive (R_1r) red cells.

SUMMARY

In Rh-negative subjects, anti-Rh injected as an IgG concentrate prepared from human plasma containing potent Rh antibody will suppress primary immunization when it is given up to at least three days after a dose of Rh-positive red cells. When administered to a primiparous Rh-negative woman within 36 hours of delivery of an ABO-compatible Rh-positive infant it will suppress primary immunization which might otherwise have occurred as a result of the pregnancy. The minimum effective amount of anti-Rh is not known but is likely to be less than 200 μg. (equivalent very approximately to 2 ml. of an immunoglobulin concentrate with an incomplete anti-Rh titre of 5,000); with transplacental bleeds exceeding 10 ml. of Rh-positive blood it is possible that higher doses may be required.

References
A COMBINED STUDY FROM CENTRES IN ENGLAND AND BALTIMORE (1966). Prevention of Rh-Haemolytic Disease: Results of the Clinical Trial. *Brit. med. J.*, **2**, 1074.

BARR, M., GLENNY, A. T. and RANDAL, K. J. (1950) Diphtheria immunization in young babies. *Lancet*, **i**, 6.

BRODY, N. I., WALKER, J. G. and SISKIND, G. W. (1967). Studies on the control of antigenic competition and suppression of antibody formation by passive antibody on the immune response. *J. exp. Med.*, **126**, 81.

CLARKE, C. A., DONOHOE, W. T. A., McCONNELL, R. B., WOODROW, J. C., FINN, R., KREVANS, J. R., KULKE, W., LEHANE, D. and SHAPPERD, P. M. (1963). Further experimental studies on the prevention of Rh haemolytic disease. *Brit. med. J.*, **1**, 979.

COHEN, C. and ALLTON, W. H. Jr. (1962). Iso-immunization in the rabbit with antibody-coated erythrocytes. *Nature (Lond.)*, **193**, 990

COHEN, E. P. (1967). Conversion of non-immune cells into antibody-forming cells by RNA. *Nature (Lond.)*, **213**, 462.

COHEN, FLOSSIE and ZUELZER, W. W. (1964). Identification of blood group antigens by immunofluorescence and its application to the detection of the transplacental passage of erythrocytes in mother and child. *Vox Sang.*, **9**, 75.

FINKELSTEIN, M. S. and UHR, J. W. (1964). Specific inhibition of antibody formation by passively administered 19S and 7S antibody. *Science*, **146**, 67.

FINN, R. CLARKE, C. A., DONOHOE, W. T. A., McCONNELL, R. B., SHEPPARD, P. M., LEHANE, D. and KULKE, W. (1961). Experimental studies on the prevention of Rh haemolytic disease. *Brit. med. J.*, **1**, 1486.

FREDA, V. J., GORMAN, J. G. and POLLACK, W. (1964). Successful prevention of experimental Rh sensitization in man with an anti-Rh gamma₂ globulin antibody preparation: a preliminary report. *Transfusion (Philad.)*, **4**, 26.

FREDA, V. J., GORMAN, J. G. and POLLACK, W. (1966) Rh factor: prevention of immunization and clinical trial on mothers. *Science*, **151**, 828.

FREDA, V. J., GORMAN, J. G., POLLACK, W., ROBERTSON, J. G., JENNINGS, E. R. and SULLIVAN, J. F. (1967). Prevention of Rh-iso-immunization. Progress report of the clinical trial in mothers. *J. Amer. med. Ass.* **199**, 390.

GORMAN. J. G., FREDA, V. J. and POLLACK, W. (1962). Intramuscular injections of a new experimental gamma globulin preparation containing high levels of anti-Rh antibody as a means of preventing sensitization to Rh. *Proc. IX Congr. Int. Soc. Haemat.*, **2**, 545.

HUGHES-JONES, N. C. (1967). The estimation of the concentration and equilibrium constant of anti-D. *Immunology*, **12**, 565.

JANDL, J. H. (1955). Sequestration by the spleen of red cells sensitized with incomplete antibody and with metallo-protein complexes (abstract). *J. clin. Invest.*, **34**, 912.

KARUSH, F. (1962). Immunologic specificity and molecular structure in *Advances in Immunology*. Ed. W. H. Taliaferro and J. H. Humphrey. Acad. Press, New York.

KREVANS, J. R., WOODROW, J. C., NOSENZO, C. and FINN, R. (1964). Patterns of Rh-immunization. *Commun. 10th Congr. int. Soc. Haemat.*, Stockholm.

LEVINE, P. (1943). Serological factors as possible causes in spontaneous abortions. *J. Hered.*, **34**, 71

LEVINE, P. (1958). The influence of the ABO system on hemolytic disease. *Hum. Biol.*, **30**, 14.

LEWI, S., CLARKE, T. K., GUERITAT, P., WALTER, P. and MAYER, M. (1961). Les erythrocytes foetaux dans la circulation maternelle. *Bull. Gynec. Obstet.*, **13**, 355.

McCONNELL, R. B. (1966). The prevention of Rh haemolytic disease. *Ann. Rev. Med.*, **17**, 291.

MÖLLER, G. (1965). Survival of H-2 compatible mouse erythrocytes in untreated and iso-immune recipients. *Immunology*, **8**, 360.

MÖLLER, G. and WIGZELL, H. (1965) Antibody synthesis at the cellular level. Antibody-induced suppression at 19S and 7S antibody response. *J. exp. Med.*, **121**, 969.

MOLLISON, P. L. (1967). *Blood Transfusion in Clinical Medicine*, 4th edn. Blackwell Scientific Publications Ltd., Oxford.

MOLLISON, P. L. and CUTBUSH, MARIE (1955). The use of isotope-labelled red cells to demonstrate incompatibility *in vivo*, *Lancet*, **i**, 1290.

MOLLISON, P. L. and HUGHES-JONES, N. C. (1967). Clearance of Rh-positive red cells by low concentrations of Rh antibody. *Immunology*, **12**, 63.

MURRAY, SHEILAGH, KNOX, G. and WALKER, W. (1965). Haemolytic disease and the rhesus genotypes. *Vox Sang.*, **10**, 257.

NEVANLINNA, H. R. and VAINIO, T. (1956). The influence of mother-child ABO-incompatibility on Rh-immunization. *Vox. Sang. (Basel)*, **1**, 26.

NOSSAL, G. J. V., AUSTIN, CAROLINE, M., PYE, J and MITCHELL, JUDITH (1966). Antigens in Immunity XII. Antigen trapping in the spleen. *Int. Arch. Allergy*, **29**, 368.

POLLACK, W., GORMAN, J. G., HAGER, H. J., FREDA, V. J. and TRIPODI, D. (1968). Antibody-mediated immune suppression to the Rh factor: Animal models suggesting mechanism of action. *Transfusion (Philad.)* **8**, 134.

POLLACK, W., SINGHER, H. O., GORMAN, J. G. and FREDA, V. J. (1967). The prevention of isoimmunisation to the Rh factor by passive immunisation with Rho(D) immune globulin (human). American Association of Blood Banks, New York, Scientific exhibit.

RACE, R. R. and SANGER, RUTH. *Blood Groups in Man.* (1950) 1st edn. Blackwell, Oxford.

ROWLEY, D. A. and FITCH, F. W. (1964). Homeostasis at antibody formation in the adult rat. *J. exp. Med.,* **120**, 987.

SAHIAR, K. and SCHWATRZ, R. S. (1964). Inhibition of 19S antibody synthesis by 7S antibody, *Science,* **145**, 395.

SAUSAIS, LAIMA, KREVANS, J. R. and TOWNES, A. S. (1966) Characteristics of a third example of anti-Xg^{a}r. (In press).

SCHNEIDER, VON J. and PREISLER, O. (1966). Untersuchungen zur serologischen Prophylaxe der Rh sensibilisierung. *Blut,* **12**, 4.

SMITH, R. T. (1909). Active immunization produced by so-called balanced or neutral mixtures of diptheria toxin and antitoxin. *J. exp. Med.,* **11**, 241.

STERN, K., DAVIDSOHN, I., and MASIAITIS, LILIAN. (1956) Experimental studies on Rh immunization. *Amer. J. clin. Path.,* **26**, 833.

STERN, K., GOODMAN, H. S. and BERGER, MAYA. (1961) Experimental iso-immunization to hemoantigens in man. *J. Immunol.,* **87** 189.

TERRES, G. and WOLINS, L. (1959) Enhanced sensitization in mice by simultaneous injection of antigen specific rabbit antiserum. *Proc. Soc. Exp. Med.,* **102**, 632.

UHR, J. W. and BAUMANN, JOYCE, B. (1961) Antibody formation. 1. The Suppression of antibody formation by passively administered antibody. *J. exp. Med.,* **113**, 935.

WALKER, J. G. and SISKIND, G. W. (1968). Studies on the control of antibody synthesis. Effect of antibody affinity upon its ability to suppress antibody formation. *Immunology,* **14**, 21.

WEINER, W., NORRIS, VERA, and DAVIDSON, S. (1952). Transfusion treatment of women of child-bearing age: a statistical study of the incidence of anti-rhesus immunization. *Brit. med. J.,* **2**. 975.

WOODROW, J. C., CLARKE, C. A., DONOHOE, W. T. A., FINN, R., McCONNELL, R. B., SHEPPARD, P. M., LEHANE, D., RUSSELL, SHONA, H., KULKE, W. and DURKIN, CATHERINE, M. (1965). Prevention of Rh-haemolytic disease: A third report. *Brit. med. J.,* **1**, 279.

WOODROW, J. C. and FINN, R. (1966). Transplacental haemorrhage. *Brit. J. Haemat.,* **12**, 297.

WIGZELL, H. (1966). Antibody synthesis at the cellular level. Antibody-induced suppression of 7S antibody synthesis. *J. exp. Med.,* **124**, 953.

ZIPURSKY, A., POLLACK, J., YEOW, R., ISRAELS, L. G. and CHOWN, B. (1966). Studies of the pathogenesis and prevention of Rh isoimmunization in pregnant women. *Commun. 11th.Cong. int. Soc. Blood Transf.,* Sydney.

Chapter 13

THE DIAGNOSIS OF FOLATE DEFICIENCY

I. CHANARIN

THE liver in man contains about 10·5 mg. (7·0 μg. per g.) of folic acid; in patients with megaloblastic anæmia requiring therapy with folic acid the liver folate falls to about 1·5 mg. (1·0 μg. per g.). On the assumption that 100 μg. of folate is required each day, complete dietary deprivation will lead to folate deficiency of this order after 13 weeks. If folate in other tissues is also added to this figure, the time will be longer, and in the study described by Herbert (1962) on a folate-free diet, megaloblastic changes were noted after 20 weeks.

Usually the development of folate deficiency is accompanied by changes in laboratory tests used to assess folate deficiency and in some patients by morphological changes in the marrow, blood and epithelial surfaces. This pattern is not invariable. On occasion abnormal tests signifying folate deficiency may be found in patients in whom the folate content of the liver is within normal limits. The corollary of this is also found; that is, patients with megaloblastic anæmia who require folate therapy may, on occasion, fail to exhibit any of the usual biochemical abnormalities. Thus the diagnosis of folate deficiency depends on the assessment of all the features of a case; it must not be based on biochemical or microbiological data alone since the results of isolated abnormal tests of folate function generally have no clinical significance.

The diagnosis of folate deficiency may be considered under two main headings. First, when the marrow shows megaloblastic changes and, second, when the marrow is normal in appearance.

THE DIAGNOSIS OF FOLATE DEFICIENCY WITH MEGALOBLASTIC HÆMOPOIESIS

While it is essential to recognize the early changes in the blood and marrow indicating a megaloblastic process, on occasion such changes are diagnosed on slender grounds. The continued dependence on morphological criteria for the diagnosis of megaloblastic change remains a major weakness in this field for any marrow can be found to show some megaloblastic-like erythroblasts if sufficient bias is brought to bear upon the problem. Changes in the marrow must be clear-cut, and prolonged search for a few erythroblasts with a doubtfully open nuclear pattern hardly justifies this diagnosis. The presence of large metamyelocytes rests on even less certain ground as a diagnostic criterion for megaloblastic change, since not only does variation in normal metamyelocyte diameters overlap strikingly with the range seen in megaloblastic marrows but such abnormal metamyelocytes may be due to iron deficiency.

When megaloblastic hæmopoiesis is present, the diagnosis of folate deficiency can be made first, by the exclusion of vitamin B_{12} deficiency and, secondly, by the nature of the hæmatological response to treatment. Confirmatory evidence may be sought by assay of the folate content of serum and red cells and by measurement of the urinary excretion of formiminoglutamic acid. The order of these four criteria in the diagnosis of folate deficiency also indicates their relative importance in reaching a diagnosis.

The Exclusion of Vitamin B_{12} Deficiency

Since megaloblastic anæmia virtually implies deficiency of either folate or vitamin B_{12}, confident exclusion of one of these deficiencies must implicate the other substance as the missing factor. When the serum vitamin B_{12} level is within the normal range in a patient with megaloblastic anæmia, the cause is folate deficiency. Using *Lactobacillus leichmannii* as the test organism and preparing serum extracts in the presence of cyanide, the lower limit of the normal serum vitamin B_{12} concentration is 190 pg. per ml. Patients with untreated Addisonian pernicious anæmia have, before the development of any significant anæmia, been found to have serum vitamin B_{12} levels up to 180 pg. per ml. (Ardeman, Chanarin, Krafchick and Singer, 1966). There is no reason to suppose that different results are likely to be obtained with *Euglena gracilis* or other test organisms when these are used properly. Two independently collected serum samples should be assayed and reliance should not be placed solely on a single normal result.

It is essential to approach diagnosis in megaloblastic anæmia initially from the standpoint of vitamin B_{12} metabolism; prolonged treatment of vitamin B_{12} deficiency with folate may have unfortunate consequences in precipitating neurological disturbances. Demonstration of intrinsic factor antibody in serum and the absence of intrinsic factor and of acid from the gastric juice both point to a diagnosis of pernicious anæmia. These tests can be performed within an hour of receiving the gastric juice or serum sample and they provide rapid information as to the likely diagnosis.

A normal serum vitamin B_{12} level in megaloblastic anæmia enables one to make a confident diagnosis of folate deficiency, but an abnormally low serum vitamin B_{12} level requires more cautious interpretation. Folate deficiency *per se* has a significant effect on the serum concentration of vitamin B_{12}. The effect of folate deficiency is to reduce the serum vitamin B_{12} level and not uncommonly the level falls well into the range associated with true vitamin B_{12} deficiency. Folate therapy under these circumstances results in a rapid rise in the serum vitamin B_{12} level to within the normal range. Thus the finding of a reduced serum vitamin B_{12} level does not necessarily mean that the megaloblastic process is due to vitamin B_{12} deficiency. Nor does it mean that folate deficiency has been excluded. It has been suggested that vitamin B_{12} deficiency is likely if the serum level is below 80 pg. per ml., since this was the lowest serum vitamin B_{12} in a series of patients in whom megaloblastic anæmia was due entirely to folate deficiency (Mollins, Waters and Harriss, 1962). This is generally true although much lower serum vitamin B_{12} levels have been noted in megaloblastic anæmia in pregnancy and in association with the administration of anticonvulsant drugs, conditions which are almost invariably due to folate deficiency. Whatever the serum

developed in this short space of time. In the same way low serum folate levels may be found in comatose patients admitted with head injuries, and in patients who have lost their appetite because of a primary illness and reduced their folate intake. In general, low serum folate values are found in about one-third of unselected patients who have been admitted to hospital although relatively few of these patients have levels of less than 2 ng. per ml. In some disorders such as Crohn's disease, rheumatoid arthritis and carcinomatosis more than two-thirds of patients may have reduced serum folate values. The great majority of these patients have normoblastic hæmopoiesis. Many, but by no means all, will have reduced folate stores. Normal uncomplicated pregnancy too causes a fall in the serum folate level and at term about 60 per cent of women have serum folate levels between 1·5 and 4·5 ng. per ml. By contrast, the great majority of patients with well-developed megaloblastic anæmia due to folate-deficiency have serum folate levels of less than 2·0 ng. per ml.; patients with lesser degrees of anæmia, however, may have levels between 2 and 5 and occasionally the serum folate level is normal.

The value of the serum folate assay in the diagnosis of folate deficiency in patients with megaloblastic anæmia lies in the fact that the great majority of patients with pernicious anæmia (the major cause of vitamin B_{12} deficiency in patients of European origin) have either normal or even elevated levels. This, on the basis of current hypothesis, is a reflection of a failure to re-utilize methylfolate because of vitamin B_{12} deficiency and does not necessarily indicate normal folate tissue stores. Thus in patients with megaloblastic anæmia the serum folate level is likely to be within the normal range in those with vitamin B_{12} deficiency and low in those with folate deficiency.

Elevated serum folate values may also be found in patients with anatomical abnormalities of the small gut such as jejunal diverticulosis in whom there is a persistent bacterial flora in the normally sterile gut. In these patients it is supposed that folate originating from these bacteria is absorbed. The high folate intake in these patients probably explains why these patients almost invariably become vitamin B_{12} deficient, even to the extent of developing neurological lesions, but very rarely develop folate deficiency.

Red Cell Folate

The folate present in serum is fairly labile in so far as it may show fluctuations that do not strictly reflect body stores of folate. A better assessment of folate status may be obtained by the measurement of tissue folate and the most accessible tissue is the red blood cell. The red cell contains about 30 times as much folate as the serum. The greater part of this is 5-methyltetrahydrofolate in the polyglutamate form and exposure to normal serum at a pH of about 4.5 is required for the release of a monoglutamate. This takes place by simple dilution in aqueous ascorbate buffer. Considerable variation in the results of red cell folate assays have been reported; this is due partly to failure to release folate in the red cell in a form that is available to the microbiological assay organisms and partly to unexplained variation in assay media. The method giving the highest assay value is that described by Hoffbrand, Newcombe and Mollin (1966), wherein 1·0 ml. of whole blood (collected in heparin or sequestrene) is added to 9·0 ml. of 1 per cent ascorbate in distilled water. Thereafter the hæmolysate is stored at $-20°C$. until required for assay, when a further 1 in 10 dilution is made, this time in 0·1 M phosphate-ascorbate buffer at pH 5·7 containing 0·15 g. ascorbate per 100 ml. This is heated, as for serum, and the assay is carried out as described for serum.

Results should be expressed in terms of packed red cells. Thus it is necessary to know the hæmatocrit reading of the sample of blood used. It is usual to correct for folate content of the plasma although this is likely to be well within the range of error of the technique, the only exception being in cases where the serum folate value is high, as in some cases of pernicious anæmia. With this method healthy subjects have red cell folate values between 166 and 640 ng. per ml. with a mean of 316 (Hoffbrand, Newcombe and Mollin, 1966) and in the authors hands a range of 100 to 450 with a mean of 240 ng. per ml.

The results of the red cell folate values are influenced by two important factors. Firstly, the red cell folate is not in equilibrium with folate in other tissues and as the mean life-span of the red cells is 120 days, changes are relatively slow. Transfusion of normal red cells in an anæmic subject can produce marked elevation of the red cell folate values. Secondly, reticulocytes have a much higher folate content than older red cells and a persistently elevated reticulocyte count, as in patients with chronic hæmolysis, may result in a persistently normal red cell folate level although the patient has megaloblastic hæmopoiesis due to folate deficiency. With these limitations in mind, the red cell folate is a useful index of folate deficiency.

About 30 per cent of hospital patients with normal blood pictures and a low serum folate value also have reduced red cell folate values. Red cell folate shows a better correlation with the urinary formiminoglutamic acid excretion than the serum folate and, generally, where the red cell folate is low an elevated urinary excretion of formiminoglutamic acid can be expected. The red cell folate is generally low in megaloblastic anæmia requiring folate therapy and will be lowest in the most severely anæmic subjects. Unlike the serum folate levels, the red cell folate values decline in pernicious anæmia and about two-thirds of patients have reduced levels.

Pregnancy. The red cell folate declines in normal pregnancy from about 200 ng. per ml. before the 16th week to about 150 ng. per ml. at the 38th week. This decline can be prevented by an oral folate supplement of 100 μg. daily. Not all cases of megaloblastic anæmia in pregnancy have abnormally low red cell folate levels and this indicates a relatively rapid development of the deficiency. Nevertheless, there is a better correlation of megaloblastic anæmia in pregnancy with red cell folate than with any other parameter of folate deficiency (Hansen, 1964).

Urinary Excretion of Formiminoglutamic Acid

The major pathway for the breakdown of the amino-acid histidine is to urocanic acid, imidazole-5-propionic acid, formiminoglutamic acid and glutamic acid. The final step is accompanied by the release of a single-carbon fragment (C^2 of the imidazole ring of histidine) which is taken up by active folate to give 5-formiminotetrahydrofolate which is in turn changed to 10-formyltetrahydrofolate.

In folate deficiency there is a failure to accept this single carbon unit from histidine and thus formiminoglutamic acid accumulates and appears in the urine. Measurement of the urinary excretion of formiminoglutamic acid is thus a measure of a specific biochemical pathway for which folate is required and, in this respect, differs from most other methods which assess folate deficiency.

In practice relatively consistent elevation of the urinary excretion of formiminoglutamic acid in folate deficiency is only found if this metabolic pathway is put under stress by giving a large amount of histidine by mouth. 15 g. of 1-histidinemonohydrochloride (approximately 10 times the usual daily intake) as a single oral dose is satisfactory. Within two hours of this oral dose there is a rise and fall in the levels of blood and urinary histidine followed by an increased urinary excretion of formiminoglutamic acid which is complete in six hours. For this reason an eight-hour urine collection suffices. Formiminoglutamic acid, although stable at acid pH, undergoes rapid hydrolysis in alkali to yield glutamic acid and ammonia. Thus urine must be collected in the presence of between 2 and 5 ml. of N-HCl. Some patients find the oral dose of histidine unpleasant (it can be flavoured in solution with strong orange juice and sugar). Caution is necessary in hepatic failure where it may on occasion precipitate mental symptoms and even coma. In postgastrectomy patients who give a history of post-prandial (or dumping) symptoms, the oral histidine load can cause vaso-vagal collapse and it is therefore desirable to have these patients in bed when carrying out the test. Finally, it is as well to be aware that in some folate-deficient patients this dose of histidine can initiate a hæmatological response.

Formiminoglutamic acid can be separated by chromatography and electrophoresis (low voltage and high voltage) either as formiminoglutamic acid itself or after conversion to glutamic acid by alkali treatment. Its property of staining with ninhydrin only after alkali treatment, which exposes a free-NH_2 group in the glutamic acid moiety is used for its positive identification in most of these procedures. Unfortunately these methods give only qualitative or at the best semiquantitative results and their uncritical application has brought the test into some disrepute. This is partly because the method reflects urinary concentration of formiminoglutamic acid rather than total output and, although a high output is usually associated with a reasonable concentration, a normal output in a small urine volume may also give a positive result. For this reason a quantitative method of assay is recommended and the method employing chick-liver enzyme described by Chanarin and Bennett (1962) is the simplest. Details of the method are set out at the end of this section. Following 15 g. of 1-histidine-mono-hydrochloride by mouth, healthy subjects excrete 1 to 17 mg. in the urine with a mean output of 9 mg. In folate deficiency the output may be increased to as much as 1,500 mg. in eight hours.

Elevated formiminoglutamic acid excretion, like low serum folate levels, is common in patients admitted to hospital with a variety of complaints such as thyrotoxicosis, neoplastic disorders, hæmolytic anæmia, congestive cardiac failure, Crohn's disease and rheumatoid arthritis. The overall correlation between the serum folate level and the urinary excretion of formiminoglutamic acid in selected groups of patients is good (Chanarin, 1964; Mollin and Hoffbrand, 1965). The results in patients with pernicious anæmia, however, need special consideration. In this disorder there is a tendency for the serum folate level to be unusually high and in a small proportion of cases to be elevated above the normal range (Waters and Mollin, 1961). This is convenient from the viewpoint of distinguishing vitamin B_{12} deficiency from folate deficiency, since pernicious anæmia is due primarily to vitamin B_{12} deficiency. There is good reason to suspect, however, that in pernicious anæmia the serum folate level is not a reliable index of folate stores and abnormal results are obtained more often when other tests of folate status are considered. Thus in pernicious anæmia the urinary excretion of formiminoglutamic acid is often elevated and the folate content of the red cells may be low.

The urinary excretion of formiminoglutamic acid is also of little value as a test of folate function in pregnancy. This is due to the physiological changes in renal and intestinal function in pregnancy and to the increased utilization of amino acids for protein synthesis. After histidine the mean excretion of formiminoglutamic acid before the 16th week of pregnancy is 21 mg. and about one-third of patients have abnormally high values at this time. The mean output then declines to reach 7 mg. at 35 weeks and 8 mg. at 39 weeks, and only about 5 per cent of women have increased excretion at this time. There is a rise in formiminoglutamic acid excretion after delivery with an elevated output in about one-third of post-natal women. This declining formiminoglutamic acid excretion during pregnancy is probably due to increased incorporation of histidine into protein with less being catabolized to give formiminoglutamic acid and glutamic acid. But altered histidine metabolism in pregnancy also results in increased loss of histidine in the urine due to a lowered renal threshold which on the average accounts for a loss of 20 per cent of the oral dose as compared to a urine loss of about 3–4 per cent in non-pregnant controls. There is also a very slow and prolonged pattern of absorption of histidine from the gut in pregnancy, possibly a consequence of the loss of tone of smooth muscle, including that of the small gut, in pregnancy. Finally, passage of histidine and its breakdown products across the placenta to the fœtus has been demonstrated.

Formiminoglutamic acid excretion in folate deficiency occurring in patients on *antiepileptic drugs* is also frequently normal although the serum folate level is low. The explanation for this is not obvious.

The conversion of histidine to formiminoglutamic acid involves a number of biochemical steps and it is therefore not surprising that this pathway may be interrupted at levels other than a failure of 5-formiminotransferase to transfer the formimino-group to tetrahydrofolate. The vulnerable link in this pathway is the enzyme urocanase which converts urocanic acid to imidazolone-5-propionic acid. There is a defect at this stage in a number of conditions not primarily associated with folate malfunction. The most important conditions are liver disease and protein malnutrition as, for example, in kwashiorkor in infancy and, less commonly, in adults in the malnutrition which may follow partial gastrectomy. Here there is a failure to carry histidine breakdown beyond urocanic acid and this is then excreted into the urine. Nevertheless, in a minority of cases with high urocanic excretion the depression of urocanase is the result of a feed-back inhibition due to high tissue levels of formiminoglutamic acid. Thus formiminoglutamic acid excretion may alternate with, or be replaced by, urocanate excretion. The method of assay recommended measures both urocanate and formiminoglutamic acid. Heating the urine at alkaline pH destroys the latter, leaving behind the stable urocanate which can then be assayed alone. Most urine samples contain both urocanate and formiminoglutamic acid.

When specific therapy is given in megaloblastic anæmia due to folate deficiency the formiminoglutamic acid excretion declines in 3 to 5 days although entirely normal values may not be found for about 10 days. In vitamin B_{12} deficiency, such as untreated pernicious anæmia, the elevated formiminoglutamic acid excretion declines in the same way in response to therapy with either vitamin B_{12} or folic acid.

Other Methods

The Folate Clearance Test. This experimental manœuvre involves measurement of the rate of removal of folate from the blood after a standard dose of folic acid of 15 μg. per kg. of body weight. In practice it is adequate to take a single blood sample 15 minutes after the intravenous injection of folate. The folate content of the 15-minute sample is assayed microbiologically. *Str. fæcalis* is used as the test organism since it is desired to measure only the injected pteroylglutamic acid persisting in the bloodstream. Healthy subjects have a folate level of 21 to 80 ng. per ml. (mean 40) at 15 minutes. In folate deficiency the 15-minute level is less than 21 ng. per ml. and frequently is zero. The results of the folate clearance test show an excellent correlation with the results of other tests of folate deficiency and they are not bedevilled by the many difficulties of technique and interpretation that have been mentioned in relation to these tests.

Hepatic Folate. Since the liver is the main folate store and indeed the site of the important biochemical reactions in which folate co-enzymes participate, measurement of folate content of the liver is the final court of appeal in the diagnosis of folate deficiency. In general, liver tissue is not likely to be available for assay, but on occasion material from a liver biopsy (15 mg. is adequate) may be available. The "wet weight" of the liver specimen is determined, the specimen transferred to a small hand tissue-grinder and 1 ml. of 0·1 M potassium phosphate buffer pH 6·0 containing 1·0 per cent ascorbate, is added for every 2 mg. of liver present. The liver suspension is frozen in dry-ice and rapidly thawed on four occasions and homogenized to a uniform consistency in the tissue-grinder. The suspension is transferred to a screw-capped container, autoclaved at 116°C for 10 minutes and finally filtered through No. 1 Whatman paper. The filtrate is assayed microbiologically using *L. casei* as the test organism.

Patients with normal serum folate values and normal formiminoglutamic acid excretion have from 5·2 to 10·0 μg. of folate per g. of wet liver (mean 6·9). Very few observations are available in patients with megaloblastic anæmia due to folate deficiency, but in these the level has been of the order of 1·0 μg. of folate per g. of wet liver. Reduced hepatic folate levels have been noted in hospital patients. These have been as low as the values found in patients with megaloblastic anæmia although blood and marrow findings in these were entirely normal. Thus even severe folate deficiency is not necessarily accompanied by any abnormality in blood and marrow.

Excretion of C^{14}-labelled Histidine in Man. Fish, Pollycove and Fleichtmeir (1963) showed that a rapid distinction between vitamin B_{12} deficiency and folate deficiency in man could be made by injecting 0·5 mg. of histidine abelled with ^{14}C in position 2 of the imidazole ring. Normally maximum $^{14}CO_2$ output in the expired air occurred in 20 to 25 minutes. In folate deficiency it took place in 140 to 240 minutes. Patients with vitamin B_{12} deficiency showed a normal excretion pattern.

THE DIAGNOSIS OF FOLATE DEFICIENCY IN THE PRESENCE OF NORMAL BLOOD AND MARROW

It is clear from what has been said that the laboratory tests that may prove of value in establishing a diagnosis of folate deficiency in a megaloblastic patient are far less likely to be of value in hæmatologically normal subjects.

Abnormal results are encountered in over one-third of unselected hospital patients when the serum folate level or the urinary excretion of formimino-glutamic acid is measured. In some groups of patients, such as those with neoplastic disease, the proportion of abnormal results is even higher. Chanarin, Hutchinson, McLean and Moule (1966) have shown that in some of these patients with low serum folate levels and elevated formiminoglutamic acid excretion the liver folate stores may be normal. Thus neither of these tests should be used to diagnose folate deficiency in normoblastic subjects. Assay of the red cell folate may prove to be more reliable, but correlation with hepatic folate levels has yet to be carried out. A reduced liver folate level is unequivocal evidence of folate deficiency.

In the present state of our knowledge abnormal results pointing to folate deficiency in the absence of megaloblastic hæmopoiesis are of no clinical significance and are not an indication for folate therapy.

APPENDIX

MICROBIOLOGICAL ASSAY OF SERUM AND RED CELL FOLATE

Organism. *Lactobacillus casei* N.C.I.B. 8010. From Torrey Research Station, Aberdeen, Scotland.

Stock Culture. As a stab in Bacto micro assay culture agar.

Propagate Organism. On Bacto micro Inoculum Broth.

Racks. Metal racks holding 48 tubes are an advantage. Use metal caps or a metal tray to cover the tubes in preference to cottonwool plugs.

Tubes. 19×150 mm. Pyrex rimless tubes.

Assay Medium. This can be purchased in dehydrated form and 1·0 g. of ascorbate should be added to each 500 ml. of reconstituted medium before use. The *p*H should be between 6·6 and 6·8. The medium can also be assembled from stock solutions of the ingredients; details are given by Toepfer *et al.* (1951).

Folic Acid Solution. Dry folic acid in a Petri dish in an oven at $\pm 100°C$ for 2 hours, and store in a desiccator under P_2O_5 in the dark. Weigh out 100 mg. accurately. Bring into solution by adding 10 ml. distilled water and N-NaOH dropwise. Make up to 100 ml.

STANDARD CURVE

Tubes (triplicate) ng. folic acid	Solution No.	ml.	Water ml.
0·0	...	0·0	2·0
0·05	E	0·25	1·75
0·1	E	0·5	1·5
0·2	E	1·0	1·0
0·3	E	1·5	0·5
0·4	E	2·0	0·0
0·5	D	0·5	1·5
0·75	D	0·75	1·25
1·0	D	1·0	1·0
wash tube 1	...	...	5·0
wash tube 2	...	...	5·0
wash tube 3	...	...	5·0
Inoculum 4	...	...	2·0
Zero setting 5	...	...	2·0

Solution A. Take 10·0 ml. folic acid solution and make it up to 1,000 ml. in 25 per cent ethanol. This can be stored in the cold.

Solution B. 25 ml. A to 1,000 ml. water.

Solution C. 20 ml. B to 500 ml. water.

Solution D. 10 ml. C to 100 ml. (1·0 ng./ml.).

Solution E. 20 ml. D to 100 ml. (0·2 ng./ml.).

Add 5·0 ml. medium to wash tubes 1, 2 and 3; 2·0 ml. medium to all other tubes. The Zero tube is NOT inoculated.

Preparation of Serum

Phosphate Ascorbate Buffer pH 5·7

$$NaH_2PO_4 . H_2O \qquad 27·6 \text{ g. to } 1,000 \text{ ml. (A)}$$
$$Na_2HPO_4 . 12H_2O \quad 71·6 \text{ g. to } 1,000 \text{ ml. (B)}$$

Add 212·5 ml. of A to 37·5 ml. of B.

Add 150 mg. of ascorbic acid per 100 ml. buffer and readjust pH to 5·7.

Add 9·8 ml. of ascorbate buffer to a 25 ml. screw-capped container and add 0·2 ml. of serum being tested (1 in 50 dilution). Autoclave 10 pounds 10 minutes. Retain the clear filtrate.

Preservation of Serum. Unhæmolysed serum is required. Add a "pinch" (5–10 mg.) of dry ascorbic acid to the serum before storage. This serum *cannot* be used for vitamin B_{12} assay.

Preparation for Red Cell Folate Assay

Blood collected in either heparin or sequestrene is suitable. The PCV of the sample or of a blood count taken at the same time is required and, preferably, serum for serum folate assay as well.

A. Whole blood   1·0 ml.⎫
   1 per cent ascorbic acid in water 9·0 ml.⎭ store frozen

B. To extract folates add 1·0 ml. of solution A to 9·0 ml. of 0·1 M phosphate buffer containing 150 mg. ascorbate (as for serum) and heat as for serum. Retain filtrate.

C. Dilute filtrate 1 in 5 for assay, i.e. add 0·4 ml. of B to each tube in the assay and make up to 2·0 ml. with ascorbate-phosphate buffer.

The Inoculum

The organism is passaged through three to four broths over the course of a few days and a further broth is inoculated on the morning of the assay. This is removed from the incubator six to seven hours later, centrifuged and the organisms resuspended with the contents of wash tube 1. This is repeated on two further occasions and the deposited organisms finally resuspended in 4·0 ml. single-strength medium (tube 4).

The Assay

Set up the standard curve.

For each serum set up three tubes and add 2·0 ml. filtrate to each tube. Add 2·0 ml. medium to all tubes other than the "wash tubes" which receive 5·0 ml. Autoclave at 10 pounds pressure for 10 minutes and allow to cool. The inoculum is prepared and each tube inoculated with one drop from a sterile 50 dropper pipette. *Do not inoculate zero tube.* Incubate for 18–20 hours at 35°–37°C.

Next day add 5·0 ml. water to all tubes. Shake well and allow to stand for 20 minutes to get rid of small air-bubbles, Most colorimeters are adequate for reading. The zero setting is made with the "zero setting tube" in position. Read the optical density of all the other tubes and average the values of the triplicates, any single result that is markedly different from the other two being discarded. Plot folate content of the standard curve against optical density on arithmetic squared paper. Read the folate value of the filtrates from the standard curve.

Calculation. *Serum*, e.g. optical density is 0·1; this corresponds to 0·2 ng. on standard curve.

Thus serum folate $= \dfrac{\text{reading} \times \text{dilution}}{\text{volume of filtrate}}$

$= \dfrac{0 \cdot 2 \times 50}{2}$

$= 5$ ng./ml.

Normal range $= 5$ to 16.

Red Cell Folate. e.g. optical density $= 0 \cdot 2$ and this corresponds to $0 \cdot 4$ ng. on standard curve.

Thus whole blood folate $= \dfrac{0 \cdot 4 \times 500}{2} = 100$ ng.

Subtract 60 per cent of serum folate value, say $4 = 96$ ng. per ml.

Red cell folate $= \dfrac{96 \times 100}{\text{PCV}}$ ng.

Folate per ml. red cells $= \dfrac{96 \times 100}{40} = 240$ ng. per ml.

Normal range $= 166$ to 650.

A SPECTROPHOTOMETRIC METHOD FOR ESTIMATING FORMIMINOGLUTAMIC ACID

Materials

Principle. A crude liver-enzyme preparation is employed firstly to reduce folic acid to the active form, and secondly to transfer the formimino group of formiminoglutamic acid to this active form of folic acid. The end-product of the reaction is converted to 5-10-methenyl-tetrahydrofolic acid with HCl and read spectrophotometrically.

Water. All water used is passed through an ion-exchange resin. (Indicator bio-deminrolit-permutit.)

Substrate Solution. KH_2PO_4, 20 m-mole (2·72 g.); citric acid 2 m-mole (0·42 g.); $MgSO_4 \cdot 7H_2O$, 2 m-mole (0·49 g.); TPN, 12 μmole (0·02 g.); folic acid, 55 μmole (0·024 g.). The KH_2PO_4 and citric acid is brought into solution and the pH adjusted to 6 with KOH. The folic acid is brought into solution with the minimum amount of KOH, the TPN and $MgSO_4$ added, the volume made up to 100 ml., and the solution is stored at $-20°$C. Check that the final pH is 6·0.

0·1 M Potassium Phosphate Buffer pH 6

          a. KH_2PO_4 6·8   g. to 500 ml.

          b. K_2HPO_4 1·742 g. to 100 ml.

Use 425 ml. of *a* to 75 ml. of *b*.

Enzyme Preparation. All operations are carried out at 2–4°C. Frozen chicken liver is sliced into 2-mm. slices with a scalpel, added to 1·3 volumes of 0·1 M potassium phosphate buffer pH 6, and homogenized for 15 seconds in an M.S.E. homogenizer. The homogenate is centrifuged for 10 minutes at 33,000 g and the supernatant dialysed against distilled water overnight. The pH is adjusted to 6 and the insoluble residue removed by centrifugation. The extract is stored at $-20°$C.

Standard Solutions. Formiminoglutamic acid solution containing 0·5 μmole/ml. at pH 6 is prepared. Urocanic acid, which is fully active and more readily available than formiminoglutamic acid, can be used as a standard instead of formiminoglutamic acid. Dissolve 87·0 mg. of urocanic acid in 100 ml. water with addition of N/HCl and heat ($= 5 \cdot 0$ μM./ml.). Dilute this 1 in 10 in pH 6·0 phosphate buffer for use ($= 0 \cdot 5$ μM./ml.).

Urine Samples. Urine is collected direct into "polythene" containers, containing 5 ml. of N/HCl. Collection is restricted to eight hours after an oral dose 15 g. histidine hydrochloride.

Method

One part of liver extract is mixed with two parts of substrate solution: 3·0 ml. of the solution is distributed into 12 × 125 mm. glass tubes and incubated at 37°C for two hours. The urine being tested is then added to each tube. The amount of formiminoglutamic acid in the sample should not exceed 0·2 μmole, the urine volume varying from 0·01 to 0·4 ml. Distilled water is added to make the volume 3·4 ml., the tube being gently inverted three times and incubated for a further two hours. At the end of this time 1·5 ml. of 3 N/HCl is added to each tube, mixed, and allowed to stand for 15 minutes. The mixture is filtered and the clear filtrate read on a spectrophotometer at 350 mμ, using a 1-cm. light path.

The test and controls are set out in Table I. Controls are treated in the same manner as the test. The tube containing the test urine (A) is read against the enzyme blank (B). The corresponding urine blank (C) is read against water, and this value is subtracted from the test.

TABLE I

Tests and Controls in estimating Formiminoglutamic Acid

	A Test	B Enzyme blank	C Urine blank	D Standard
Substrate solution	Yes	Yes	No	Yes
Liver enzyme	Yes	Yes	No	Yes
Urine	Yes	No	Yes	No
Formiminoglutamic acid	No	No	No	0·05 and 0·1 μmole
Water	Volume to 3·4 ml. with water			

The amount of formiminoglutamic acid (A-C) is calculated from the reading of the standard formiminoglutamic acid or urocanic acid solution (D).

Preparation of Urine for Urocanate Assay. To 4·0 ml. urine add measured amounts of 1·5 N KOH until pH is about 9·5 (use indicator paper). Heat the urine at 116°C for 10 minutes. Add the equivalent amount of 1·5 N HCl to adjust the pH to approximately its original value. Assay as for formiminoglutamic acid multiplying the final answer by the appropriate factor to allow for the dilution brought about during the adjustment of pH, e.g. if 0·5 ml. alkali and subsequently 0·5 ml. acid was added, multiply final result, e.g. 24 mg. by $\frac{5}{4}$ i.e. $\frac{24 \times 5}{4}$=30 mg. of urocanate.

Note. Molecular weight for formiminoglutamic acid is 174 and that of urocanic acid is 138. The combined excretion of urocanic acid and formiminoglutamic acid in urine is expressed in terms of mg. of formiminoglutamic acid by multiplying the value (in μM.) by 174. When urocanic acid alone is estimated the mg. value is obtained by multiplying by the value (in μM.) by 138.

General References

CHANARIN, I. (1967). Folic acid and derivatives. In *The International Encyclopedia of Pharmacology and Therapeutics, Haematopoietic Agents.* Eds. J. C. Dreyfus and B. Dreyfus. Pergamon Press, Oxford.

FRIEDKIN, M. (1963) Enzymatic Aspects of Folic Acid. In *Annu. Rev. Biochem*, Vol. **32**, Eds. E. E. Snell and J. M. Luck. Annu. Rev. Inc. Palo Alto, California.

JOHNS, D. G. and BERTINO, J. R. (1965). Folates and Megaloblastic Anaemia: A review. *Clin. pharm. Therap.*, **6**, 372.

METZ, J. (1963). Folates in megaloblastic anaemia. *Bull. Wld Hlth Org.*, **28**, 517.

O'BRIEN, J. S. (1962). The Role of the Folate Coenzymes in Cellular Division. A review. *Cancer Res.*, **22**, 267.

RABINOWITZ, J. C. (1960) Folic Acid. In *The Enzymes*, Vol 2. Ed. P. D. Boyer, M. Lardy and K. Myrback. Academic Press, New York.

Other References

ARDEMAN, S., CHANARIN, I., KRAFCHICK, B. and SINGER, W. (1966). Addisonian pernicious anaemia and intrinsic factor antibodies in thyroid disorders. *Quart. J. Med.*, **35**, 421.

CHANARIN, I. (1964). Studies on urinary formiminoglutamic acid excretion. *Proc. roy. Soc. Med.* **57**, 384.

CHANARIN, I. and Bennett, M. C. (1962). A spectrophotometric method for estimating formiminoglutamic acid and urocanic acid. *Brit. med. J.*, **i**, 27.

CHANARIN, I., DACIE, J. V. and MOLLIN, D. L. (1959), Folic-acid deficiency in haemolytic anaemia. *Brit. J. Haemat.*, **5**, 245.

CHANARIN, I., HUTCHINSON, M., MCLEAN, A. and MOULE, M. (1966), Hepatic folate in man. *Brit. med. J.*, **i**, 396.

DELLER, D. J., IBBOTSON, R. N. and CROMPTON, B. (1964). Metabolic effects of partial gastrectomy with special reference to calcium and folic acid. **5**, 225.

HANSEN, H. A. (1964). *On the Diagnosis of Folic Acid Deficiency*. Almqvist and Wiskell, Stockholm.

HERBERT, V. (1961). The assay and nature of folic acid activity in human serum. *J. clin. Invest.*, **40**, 81.

HERBERT, V. (1962). Experimental nutritional folate deficiency in man. *Trans. Ass. Amer. Physiol.*, **65**, 307.

HOFFBRAND, A. V., NEWCOMBE, B. F. A. and MOLLIN, D. L. (1966). Method of assay of red cell folate activity and the value of the assay as a test for folate deficiency. *J. clin. Path.*, **19**, 17.

MOLLIN, D. L. and HOFFBRAND, A. V. (1965). The diagnosis of folate deficiency. In *Vitamin B_{12} and Folic Acid*. Ed. S. E. Bjorkman. Munksgaard, Copenhagen

MOLLIN, D. L., WATER, A. H. and HARRISS, E. (1962). Clinical aspects of the metabolic interrelationship between folic acid and vitamin B_{12}. In *Vitamin B_{12} und Intrinsic Faktor*. 2, *Europäisches Symposion*, Hamburg, 1961. Ed. H. C. Heinrich. F. Enke, Stuttgart.

Sturgis, C. C. and Isaacs, R. (1938). Pernicious anemia. In *Handbook of Hematology*, Vol. III, p. 2261. Ed. H. Downey. Hamilton, London.

TOEPFER, E. W., ZOOK, E. G., ARR, M. L. and RICHARDSON, L. R. (1951). Folic acid content of foods. Microbiological assay by standardized method and compilation of data from the literature. *Agriculture Handbook*, No. 29. U.S. Dept. of Agriculture, Washington.

WATERS, A. H. and MOLLIN, D. L. (1961). Studies on the folic acid activity of human serum. *J. clin. Path.*, **14**, 335.

Chapter 14

THALASSÆMIA AND SICKLE-CELL DISEASE

D. J. WEATHERALL

SINCE the review of the abnormal hæmoglobin field which appeared in this series four years ago (Lehmann, 1964), a considerable number of hæmoglobin variants have been isolated and their structure determined. Furthermore, a start has been made in trying to relate these structural alterations to changes in function in those abnormal hæmoglobins which are associated with disease states. The other area of particular current interest in this field is that of control mechanisms in hæmoglobin synthesis. For this reason the thalassæmia syndromes, a series of inherited disorders characterized by a defective rate of hæmoglobin synthesis, have received much attention in the last few years.

By far the commonest hæmoglobinopathies encountered in clinical practice are the sickling disorders and the thalassæmias. In this chapter both these groups of disorders will be considered with particular reference to the light which they throw on structure-function relationships and abnormal genetic regulatory mechanisms.

As an introduction to these topics, the genetic control of hæmoglobin synthesis and the current clinical classification of the abnormal hæmoglobin syndromes will be summarized.

THE STRUCTURE AND GENETIC CONTROL OF NORMAL HÆMOGLOBIN

Hæmoglobin is a spherical protein consisting of a globin fraction and four hæm units. Globin is made up of four peptide chains, each chain having a single hæm group suspended between two histidine residues (for references see Huehns and Shooter, 1965). The hæm units lie in deep clefts in the surface of the molecule and the globin chains, and hence the hæm groups, alter their spatial orientation during oxygenation (Muirhead and Perutz, 1963). These spatial re-arrangements are essential to the normal functioning of hæmoglobin as an oxygen carrier, i.e. the production of a physiological oxygen dissociation curve and Bohr effect.

In normal adults hæmoglobin is a heterogenous mixture of proteins consisting of a major component, hæmoglobin A, and a minor component, hæmoglobin A_2, which comprises about 2·5 per cent of the total hæmoglobin. In fœtal life the major hæmoglobin component is hæmoglobin F, although small amounts of hæmoglobin A are present from the age of about 15 weeks. At birth, hæmoglobin F synthesis ceases in normal individuals, only traces of it being detectable after 6 months. There is probably a primitive embryonic hæmoglobin which precedes hæmoglobin F and which disappears at about the 12th week of development.

The globin fraction of hæmoglobin A consists of a pair of α-chains and a pair of β-chains and is written $α_2β_2$. Each α-chain consists of 141 amino acid residues and each β-chain 146 amino acid residues, the full sequence of the amino acids in each chain having been worked out (for references see Baglioni, 1963). Hæmoglobin A_2 also has two α-chains, in this case paired with two structurally distinct δ-chains $(α_2δ_2)$. The δ-chains differ from the β-chains by only 10 amino acid residues. Fœtal hæmoglobin has 2 α-chains paired with 2 γ-chains $(α_2γ_2)$, the γ-chains showing many chemical differences from the β-chains. The globin chains may be separated and purified by a variety of electrophoretic and chromatographic techniques or by counter-current distribution.

Genetic Control

The genetic control of the structure of human hæmoglobin is now worked out although the factors which control its rate of synthesis may remain to be elucidated.

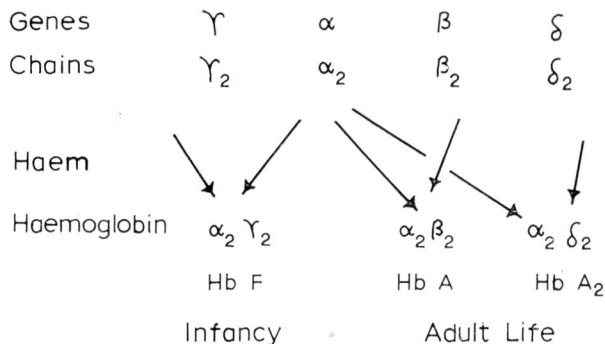

FIG. 1. The genetic control of haemoglobin synthesis.

There is good evidence, obtained from the study of families carrying more than one gene for structural hæmoglobin variants, that separate pairs of genes control the synthesis of α-, β-,and δ-chains and probably γ-chains (Fig. 1). Thus, in intrauterine life, α-chains combine with γ-chains to form hæmoglobin F $(α_2γ_2)$ and, in normal children, γ-chain synthesis is "turned off" at birth. At that time the β- and δ-chain loci become fully activated, α-chains now combining with β- and δ-chains to form hæmoglobins A $(α_2β_2)$ and A_2 $(α_2δ_2)$ respectively. In this scheme, a single α-chain gene controls α-chain synthesis in fœtal and adult life and hence mutations at this locus will result in abnormalities of both fœtal and adult hæmoglobin synthesis. On the other hand, mutations at the β-chain locus will only affect adult hæmoglobin synthesis and so not become apparent until after the first few months of life.

The chromosomal location of the hæmoglobin genes has not yet been determined. The β- and δ-chain loci are closely linked on the same chromosome while the α-chain locus does not appear to be closely linked to the β-locus. The relationship of the γ-locus to the other hæmoglobin loci is not known. Although most of the fundamental experimental work on the early stages of protein synthesis has been carried out in micro-organisms and in rabbit reticulocytes, the principles which result from these studies can probably be applied to the human red cell precursors (Fig. 2).

The sequence of amino acids in the globin chains is determined by the sequence of base pairs which constitute the DNA of the gene which controls that particular chain. Each amino acid is determined by a single triplet of bases, this information being transferred from the cell nucleus to the cytoplasm by means of a species of RNA (messenger RNA) with bases exactly complimentary to those of the DNA of the gene.

Globin chains are synthesized on groups of ribosomal particles, or

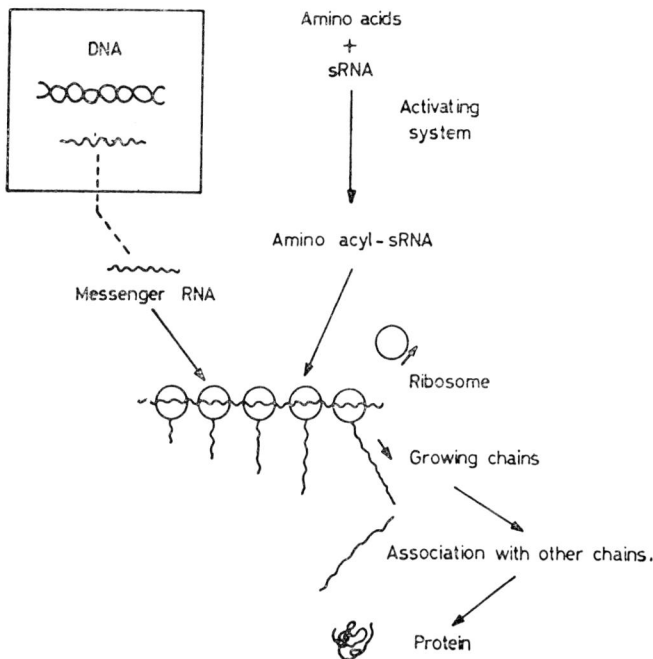

FIG. 2. An outline of the organisation of protein synthesis; from Weatherall (1965) with permission of the publishers.

polysomes, the polysome containing five ribosomes being the commonest type in rabbit reticulocytes (Fig. 2). The amino acids which are to constitute the globin chain are activated and carried to the ribosomes attached to a specific form of RNA, called transfer RNA. Each amino acid has one or more specific transfer RNAs. The ribosomal particles, carrying the growing peptide chains, move across the messenger RNA strand, the appropriate amino acid being put in place in the growing chain by virtue of the bases of the transfer RNA being complementary to those of the messenger RNA, The globin chains are synthesized by stepwise addition of amino acids starting from the amino-terminal end. The mechanism of protein synthesis has been the subject of several recent reviews (see Wiseman, 1965).

The way in which this series of synthetic steps are controlled is not yet understood (Itano, 1965). Clearly the rate of production of a peptide chain could be modified at any one of several stages. The rate of messenger RNA production, the rate of laying down of amino acids and their binding in peptide linkage and the availability of different types of transfer RNA could all modify the rate of chain synthesis. Furthermore, since hæm can stimulate globin chain production and since there is evidence of variable affinity between the different types of globin chains, control can also be mediated at the level of hæm-globin or globin-subunit association.

Hæm is synthesized through a series of enzymic steps following the condensation of glycine and active succinate. Finished hæm can, by feed-back inhibition, depress the early steps in this pathway, thus regulating its own rate of synthesis (London *et al.*, 1964). It seems likely that a similar "feed-back" mechanism exists for the regulation of globin chain synthesis although no experimental evidence for the existence of such a mechanism has yet been reported. The answers to some of these problems of protein synthetic control may well be obtained from a study of abnormal hæmoglobin synthesis, particularly as seen in thalassæmia.

THE INHERITED HÆMOGLOBINOPATHIES

Inherited defects of globin synthesis fall into two main groups (Table I). In the first group there is an inherited alteration in the structure of globin

TABLE I

The Inherited Hæmoglobinopathies

Structural variants	Defects in synthetic rate of globin chains
α-chain, e.g. Hb I	α-thalassæmia
β-chain, e.g. Hb S	β-thalassæmia
δ-chain, e.g. Hb A$_2^1$	δ-thalassæmia
γ-chain, e.g. Hb Texas	γ-thalassæmia

usually following a single amino acid substitution or deletion in either the α- or the β-chain. In the second group the structure of the globin chains is normal, but their rate of synthesis is grossly retarded. The latter group of anæmias are associated with the clinical picture of thalassæmia and are known as the thalassæmia syndromes.

Many of the structural hæmoglobin variants have been observed as chance findings in population surveys and are of no clinical significance. They have nearly all been observed in the heterozygous state and, since the letters of the alphabet have been long used up to describe new hæmoglobins, are now usually known by their place names (see Huehns and Shooter, 1965). A few of the structural hæmoglobin variants are, however, associated with disease states (Table II). The mechanisms whereby a single amino acid substitution in a globin chain can result in a hæmatological disorder are just beginning to be worked out (Table II). In some cases the abnormal hæmoglobin results in a shortened red cell survival and hæmolytic anæmia. A second group of hæmoglobinopathies is associated with defects in oxygen transport and a third group is associated with anæmia resulting from a defective rate of synthesis of globin due to the associated structural alteration. These clinical disorders are summarized in Table II.

In the hæmolytic anæmia group there are several different mechanisms responsible for shortened red cell survival. In hæmoglobin S or C disease there is deformation of the red cell due to the physical properties of the abnormal hæmoglobin, and it seems likely that there is a secondary increase in membrane permeability with shortening of red cell survival. In the presence of an unstable hæmoglobin such as hæmoglobin Zurich or Köln, red cell inclusion bodies are formed due to precipitation of the unstable molecules.

TABLE II

Structural Hæmoglobin Variants associated with Disease

Hæmoglobin	Chain affected	Change	Clinical findings
S	β	6 Glu → Val	Hæmolytic anæmia
C	β	6 Glu → Lys	Mild hæmolytic anæmia
D Punjab	β	121 Glu → Glm	Mild hæmolytic anæmia
Zurich	β	63 His → Arg	Drug induced hæmolysis
Seattle	β	70 or 76 Ala → Glu	Mild hæmolytic anæmia
E	β	26 Glu → Lys	Hæmolytic anæmia
M Hyde Park	β	92 His → Tyr	Congenital cyanosis
M Saskatoon	β	63 His → Tyr	Congenital cyanosis
M Milwaukee	β	67 Val → Glu	Congenital cyanosis
Kansas	β	102 Asp → Thr	Congenital cyanosis
Freiburg	β	23 Val → O	Cyanosis and anæmia
C-Harlem	β	6 Glu → Val 73 Asp → Asp NH_2	Sickling. Defective renal concentrating power in heterozygotes
Köln	β	98 Val → Met	Heinz body anaemia
Hammersmith	β	98 Phe → Ser	Heinz body anaemia
Gun Hill	β	92 et seq → 0	Mild hæmolytic anaemia
M Boston	α	58 His → Tyr	Congenital cyanosis
M Iwate	α	87 His → Tyr	Congenital cyanosis
Chesapeake	α	92 Arg → Leu	Congenital polycythæmia

It is probable that such denatured hæmoglobin is removed from the red cells in the spleen with resultant membrane damage, or that cells containing denatured hæmoglobin are actually sequestered in the spleen. Certainly both *in vivo* and *in vitro* kinetic studies of patients heterozygous for hæmoglobin Zurich have shown that the rate of synthesis of hæmoglobin Zurich is similar to that of hæmoglobin A. The fact that it occurs as only about 30 per cent of the total hæmoglobin in red cell lysates suggests that it is being preferentially removed from the red cells (Rieder *et al.*, 1965). Similar kinetic data have been obtained from a patient with another unstable hæmoglobin by Grimes and his co-workers (1964).

Defects in oxygen transport due to single amino acid substitutions also result from a variety of mechanisms. Hereditary methæmoglobinæmia may result from any one of several different amino acid substitutions at or near either of the two hæm-related histidine residues. Recently a form of familial

G

polycythæmia has been described in which there was an associated hæmoglobin variant named hæmoglobin Chesapeake (Charache *et al.*, 1966) Hæmoglobin Chesapeake has an arginine → leucine substitution at position 92 in the α-chain, an area of the molecule of critical importance in the movement of the β-subunits in relationship to the α-subunits during oxygenation.

Studies of these rare structural hæmoglobin variants are thus providing much information about structure-function relationships in abnormal proteins. From a clinical view, however, by far the most important structural hæmoglobin variants are those associated with the sickle-cell disorders.

The Sickling Disorders

The sickling disorders include sickle-cell anæmia and the clinical disorders resulting from the combination of hæmoglobin S and another structural hæmoglobin variant, or thalassæmia, in the same individual. This group of conditions are summarized in Table III. The most frequently occurring

TABLE III

The Sickling Disorders

Disorder	Genotype	Clinical findings
Sickle-cell disease	$\alpha\alpha\ \beta^S\beta^S$	Severe hæmolytic anæmia
S-C disease	$\alpha\alpha\ \beta^S\beta^c$	Moderate hæmolytic anæmia
Sickle-cell thalassæmia	$\alpha\alpha\ \beta^S\beta^{thal}$	Variable—depending on type of associated thalassæmia gene
S-D (Punjab) disease	$\alpha\alpha\ \beta^S\beta^D$	Moderate hæmolytic anæmia
S-J (Baltimore) disease	$\alpha\alpha\ \beta^S\beta^J$	No clinical abnormality
S-K disease	$\alpha\alpha\ \beta^S\beta^k$	No clinical abnormality
S-hereditary persistence of Hb F heterozygosity	$\alpha\alpha\ \beta^S\beta^-$	No clinical abnormality*
S-E disease	$\alpha\alpha\ \beta^S\beta^E$	Moderate hæmolytic anæmia
Hæmoglobin Memphis-S	$\alpha^{Mem}\alpha\ \beta^S\beta^S$	Mild hæmolytic anæmia†
Haemoglobin G (Philadelphia) S	$\alpha\alpha^G\ \beta^S\beta^S$	Mild haemolytic anaemia
S-O disease	$\alpha\alpha\ \beta^S\beta^O$	Moderate haemolytic anaemia
S-D (Ibadan) disease	$\alpha\alpha\ \beta^S\beta^D$	No clinical abnormalities

* It is assumed that one β-locus remains inactive with persistent γ-chain synthesis.

† This disorder was described by Kraus *et al.* (1966). The presence of this α-chain variant in an individual homozygous for hæmoglobin S seems to reduce the tendency to sickling. This is not so in the case of hæmoglobin G (Philadelphia).

sickling disorders are sickle-cell disease, hæmoglobin S-C disease and sickle-cell thalassæmia.

Clinical and Hæmatological Characteristics. The clinical manifestations of the sickling syndromes result from two main mechanisms:

1. The blockage of small vessels with aggregations of sickled erythrocytes with subsequent tissue infarction.

2. Shortened red cell survival resulting from deformation due to intravascular sickling.

Both these mechanisms depend on the level of hæmoglobin S in each red cell and the interaction or lack of interaction between sickle hæmoglobin and the other hæmoglobin components. Thus in sickle-cell trait there are normally no symptoms or hæmatological abnormalities, since the level of hæmoglobin S is only in the 30–40 per cent range. Splenic infarction may occur, however, in response to a marked hypoxia such as may occur in unpressurized aircraft or during anæsthesia.

The clinical picture of sickle-cell anæmia usually becomes manifest after the first few months of life when β-chain synthesis is fully activated. The earliest manifestation is often a painful symmetrical swelling of the hands and feet, the so-called "hand-foot" syndrome. As the child grows older the typical sickle-cell habitus is developed which is characterized by a disproportionately long lower segment and asthenic build. The course in childhood is one of chronic anæmia interspersed with severe exacerbations or "crises". Most of the clinical features can be related to tissue infarction. Many patients have chronic indolent leg ulcers and the spleen is usually enlarged in early childhood, but, following repeated small infarctions, regresses during development and is rarely palpable in adult life. This phenomenon may be partly responsible for the increased susceptibility to pneumococcal infection, particularly meningitis, which is found in this disorder. Hepatomegaly is very common in childhood, particularly during crises, and occasionally a picture of hepatomegaly with rapidly progressive liver failure is encountered in adult sicklers. Recurrent pulmonary infarction is not uncommon while focal neurological symptoms also result from local tissue anoxia. Bone pain occurs in practically all cases and is particularly related to crises. Radiological evidence of bone infarction is not uncommon and aseptic necrosis of the humeral and femoral heads occurs very commonly in hæmoglobin S-C disease. Extensive bone marrow necrosis has been recently encountered during crises associated with extreme bone pain in an individual with hæmoglobin S-D disease (Charache, 1966). There is a marked susceptibility to infection, particularly with the salmonella group, and typhoid osteomyelitis quite frequently follows local bony destruction. Some degree of cardiomegaly is almost invariably found and less commonly right heart failure occurs secondary to severe pulmonary fibrosis. Remarkable tortuosity of the retinal vessels is found in sickle-cell anæmia while hæmoglobin S-C disease is often associated with proliferation of the retinal vessels with a tendency to intra-ocular hæmorrhage and permanent visual disturbance.

The hæmatological findings in sickle-cell anæmia are those of a chronic hæmolytic anæmia. The packed cell volume is usually in the 20–30 per cent range while there is invariably an elevated reticulocyte count in the 15–30 per cent range. A stained blood smear reveals marked anisopoikilocytosis and usually sickle forms can be seen in the tail of the smear. The sickled cells associated with many target cells and intracellular crystals which are found in hæmoglobin S-C disease often enable the diagnosis to be made from the blood film. The level of serum bilirubin is raised, serum haptoglobins are usually absent and the Schumm's test positive. The presence of a sickling disorder can be confirmed by the demonstration of sickling in a sealed cover-slip preparation with freshly prepared 2 per cent sodium metabisulphite.

The acute exacerbations or crises which occur in sickle-cell anæmia may be associated with either thrombosis, hæmolysis or marrow failure or any combination of these mechanisms. Severe bone pain or abdominal pain is extremely common and is often associated with intercurrent infection. Hæmolysis is usually increased and may be associated with a marked leuco-cytosis. A rapid fall in packed cell volume associated with progressive splenomegaly and splenic sequestration of red cells is frequently observed in children during a sickle-cell crisis. An even more serious form of crisis is that associated with temporary red cell aplasia in which the patient may become profoundly anæmic over a period of a few hours. Occasionally a severe and rapidly progressive anæmia may result from intercurrent folic acid deficiency.

The prognosis in the sickling disorders depends on the socio-economic background of the patient and the particular form of sickling condition. It is clear that homozygous sickle-cell anæmia is compatible with survival into adult life provided that such complications as anæmia, infection, folate deficiency and cardiac decompensation can be controlled. A recent follow-up of patients with sickle-cell disease in the U.S.A. has stressed the importance of infection as the cause of death in this condition at all age-groups (Charache and Richardson, 1964). However, practically all patients with sickle-cell anæmia require careful follow-up and intermittent periods of hospital admission. Hæmoglobin S-C disease is not usually so severe and is compatible with a normal life, while hæmoglobin S-D (Punjab) disease behaves in a similar way to sickle-cell disease.

The survival of patients with sickle-cell anæmia into adult life means that the problem of pregnancy and sickling disorders is not uncommon. Pregnancy in sickle-cell anæmia is not particularly hazardous, provided that folic acid deficiency is prevented. Similarly, early reports of a very high maternal mortality in hæmoglobin S-C disease seem to have been exaggerated, although a recent survey in Ibadan has suggested a 2 per cent mortality rate mainly due to thrombo-embolic disease or hæmolytic crisis occurring late in pregnancy (Fullerton *et al.*, 1965).

The Mechanism of Sickling. It is clear from the preceding section that the clinical manifestations of sickle-cell anæmia can all be accounted for by the change in red cell configuration which occurs during deoxygenation. It is still not certain how the substitution of a valine residue for a glutamic acid residue in the 6th position of the β-chain can so profoundly alter the physical properties of hæmoglobin, but some recent progress has been made in this field.

It has been observed that a concentrated solution of hæmoglobin S forms a gel at 38° but remains liquid at 0°C, whereas a similar solution of hæmoglobin A remains in solution at both temperatures (Murayama, 1964). Furthermore, optical rotatory studies in the gelled state suggest that an intramolecular ring structure is formed and Murayama has suggested that this represents a hydrophobic bond between the valine in position 6 and that in position 1. Such a bond could produce a cyclical configuration at the end of the β-chain which would act as a "key" and would "fit" into a space, formed during the spatial alterations which occur during deoxygenation, in the α-chain of a neighbouring molecule. Finally, such a "lock" arrangement occurring in a series of molecules would result in the production of linear stacks of hæmoglobin molecules, the occurrence of such stacks in the long axis of sickled cells having already been deduced by studies of their behaviour in polarized light (Harris, 1950). The presence of such intramolecular bond formation awaits confirmation, however, and it is possible that the normal changes in spatial orientation of the β-chains during deoxygenation may be so profoundly altered by the substitution of a hydrophobic valine for a hydrophilic glutamic acid residue, that such "molecular stacking" will occur without any bond formation.

Studies of blood viscosity have shown that the clinical severity of the sickling disorders can be clearly related to the rate of increase of blood viscosity which occurs during deoxygenation (Charache and Conley, 1964). Such viscosity changes depend on the packed cell volume, the level of hæmoglobin S in the red cell and on the degree of interaction with other hæmoglobins which may be present in those heterozygous for the sickle-cell gene and another hæmoglobin variant. The most marked increase in viscosity for any given reduction in oxygen tension occurs in the presence of hæmoglobins S and D (Punjab) while no such interaction occurs between hæmoglobins S and F. Hæmoglobins C, J and A all interact with hæmoglobin S to a varying degree. These observations are in agreement with the clinical finding that hæmoglobin S-D disease is characterized by a severe course with many crises while those individuals heterozygous for the sickle-cell and persistent fœtal hæmoglobin genes (S-F), though having similar levels of hæmoglobins S and F to many patients with sickle-cell anæmia, have no clinical disability (Conley et al., 1963). In sickle-cell disease the fœtal hæmoglobin is heterogenously distributed throughout the red cells whereas in the S-F combination *each red cell* carries about 25 per cent hæmoglobin F. Because of the lack of interaction between hæmoglobins S and F, such a uniformly high level of the latter in each red cell protects against sickling with remarkable efficiency. It is possible that the variable degree of intracellular interaction between hæmoglobin S and other hæmoglobin types depends on differences in the configurational changes which occur between their constituent α- and β-chains during deoxygenation. Thus, the lack of interaction between hæmoglobins S and F and the interaction between hæmoglobins S and A may reflect the fact that the β-chains of hæmoglobin S find complementary "locks" in the α-chains of hæmoglobin A, but not in those of hæmoglobin F. This mechanism may, in turn, reflect the different spatial configuration between α- and β-chains of hæmoglobin A and α- and γ-chains of hæmoglobin F (Heller, 1965).

It has been shown that viscosity of sickle-cell blood is approximately proportioned to the square of the packed cell volume, a finding which may explain the occurrence of crises in sicklers after blood transfusion or in those heterozygous for the sickle-cell gene and another β-chain hæmoglobin variant, who have relatively high packed cell volumes (Charache and Conley, 1964).

The Treatment of the Sickling Disorders. The management of the sickling disorders must be based upon a knowledge of the patho-physiology of sickling as outlined in the previous sections. In between crises most patients with sickle-cell anæmia manage fairly well with a packed cell volume in the 25 per cent range. They should be maintained on regular folic acid supplements. Since crises are most frequently related to intercurrent infection it has recently been suggested that young children should receive long-term prophylactic antibiotic therapy combined, in malarious areas, with malarial prophylactic drugs (Warley *et al.*, 1965). It is too soon to assess whether such measures are of real value, but, since so many affected children who live in Europe or North America appear to have increased numbers of crises in the winter months following upper respiratory infection, it seems reasonable to cover this period of time with a broad-range antibiotic. Since the course of sickle-cell anæmia is so variable, properly conducted double-blind trials using this type of régime are badly needed.

The place of transfusion in sickle-cell anæmia is fairly clear. Unless there has been a rapid fall in packed cell volume following a hæmolytic or thrombotic crisis there is no indication for blood transfusion. In fact, such a procedure may often precipitate a thrombotic crisis, since it raises the packed cell volume to about 30 per cent, at which level there is a marked increase in blood viscosity for any given reduction in oxygen tension. Small blood transfusions produce this effect by raising the hæmatocrit to a dangerous level without significantly reducing the number of sickle cells. Thus for major surgical procedures, including grafting of leg ulcers resistant to local therapy, or in periods of repeated crises, it is much better to perform a partial exchange transfusion. If the level of cells capable of sickling can be reduced to below 60 per cent, and maintained at this level by frequent small transfusions, so depressing endogenous red cell production, symptoms can be prevented for very long periods of time.

Crises should be managed with adequate analgesia, warmth, oxygen, antibiotics in the presence of infection, and frequent estimations of the packed cell volume. Transfusion should be withheld unless the packed cell volume falls to a dangerously low level, but sometimes the use of a plasma volume expander may be helpful. Régimes using alkalis and magnesium, low molecular weight dextrans, phenothiazines, hyperbaric oxygen and many other forms of therapy have been advocated for the treatment or prevention of crises. Because of the natural tendency for all crises to settle it has been extremely hard to assess such régimes. However, double blind trials have shown that phenothiazines and low molecular weight dextrans probably have no place in the treatment of sickle-cell anaemia. There have been more promising reports, however, of the use of alkalis and magnesium, and this type of régime (Lehmann, 1963) will be well worth studying by a carefully designed double blind trial in the future.

Patients with a sickle-cell or hæmoglobin S-C disease who are pregnant should be followed most carefully, both before and after delivery, since there is an increased incidence of thrombotic episodes near term and in the immediate post-natal period (Fullerton *et al.*, 1965). The same precautions should be taken regarding transfusion as in the non-pregnant sickler, i.e. they should be avoided unless the hæmatocrit is dangerously low. Severe crises at term in patients with S-C disease have been treated with exchange transfusion and heparinization with some success. If a pregnant patient with hæmoglobin S-C disease commences with severe bone pain or a picture of toxæmia of pregnancy near term or after delivery, it is advisable to perform an exchange transfusion, since these phenomena frequently precede the development of severe thrombo-embolic complications (Fullerton *et al.*, 1965).

HÆMOGLOBINOPATHIES ASSOCIATED WITH A DEFECTIVE RATE OF GLOBIN CHAIN
 SYNTHESIS

The Thalassæmia Syndromes

The thalassæmias are a group of inherited anæmias characterized by a defective rate of synthesis of normal hæmoglobin (Weatherall, 1965). The division of the disorder into major, intermediate and minor forms has been useful at a clinical level, but such a classification has little genetic meaning since a similar clinical picture of thalassæmia can result from several distinct inherited abnormalities of hæmoglobin synthesis.

The thalassæmias are now classified according to the associated hæmoglobin patterns (Ingram and Stretton, 1959). In the thalassæmias with elevations of hæmoglobin F or A_2 levels it is assumed that there is an inherited defect in β-chain synthesis: β-thalassæmia. The hæmoglobin level is maintained in part by the production of the γ-chains of hæmoglobin F and the δ-chains of hæmoglobin A_2. In some patients with thalassæmia there is no increase in hæmoglobin F or A_2 levels, but small quantities of hæmoglobin composed entirely of normal β-chains (β_4 or hæmoglobin H), or of normal γ-chains (γ_4 or hæmoglobin Bart's) are found. It is thought that these thalassæmias result from defective α-chain synthesis, α-thalassæmia, the level of hæmoglobins A, F and A_2 being equally depressed since they all have α-chains, the structure of which is directed by a single genetic locus. In the absence of sufficient α-chains an excess of β-chains or γ-chains are formed which aggregate to form hæmoglobins H (β_4) or Bart's (γ_4) respectively.

The β-thalassæmias

This is the group of thalassæmias associated with the severe anæmias of infancy and early childhood which were first described by Cooley and Lee in 1925. The hæmoglobin patterns of these children are characterized by levels of hæmoglobin F in the 20–60 per cent range while in some cases no hæmoglobin A is detectable, the hæmoglobin pattern consisting of F and A_2 only.

Studies of the parents of children with these severe types of β-thalassæmia have shown that the affected children may be either homozygous for one type of β-thalassæmia gene or heterozygous for two different β-thalassæmia genes. These studies and the studies of the hæmoglobin electrophoretic patterns of individuals heterozygous for both the β-thalassæmia gene and a β-chain hæmoglobin variant have resulted in the definition of several distinct variants of β-thalassæmia (Table IV).

β-thalassæmia with increased levels of hæmoglobin A_2: true β-thalassæmia. In the homozygous state this condition is associated with the clinical picture of Cooley's anæmia and hæmoglobin F levels in the 20–60 per cent range. The hæmoglobin A_2 value is usually normal or low, although it is elevated if expressed as a percentage of hæmoglobin A. The presence of small quantities of free α-chain can be demonstrated on starch gel electrophoresis of fresh hæmolysates from some of these patients and inclusion bodies consisting of denatured α-chain can be found in the red cell precursors (Fessas, 1963; Fessas and Loukopolous, 1964).

The clinical findings in the heterozygous state are very variable, ranging from a completely normal hæmatological picture to one characterized by moderate anæmia, jaundice and hepato-splenomegaly. The hæmoglobin pattern is characterized by an elevated level of hæmoglobin A₂ and, in about 50 per cent of cases, a slight elevation in hæmoglobin F in the 2–6 per cent range. Quite exceptionally, heterozygotes for this type of thalassæmia have higher levels of hæmoglobin F and this type represents a separate genetic entity (see Weatherall, 1965). The fœtal hæmoglobin is quite heterogenously distributed throughout the red cells in the β-thalassæmias.

β-δ-thalassæmia. This is a much rarer β-thalassæmia variant and the

TABLE IV

The β-thalassæmias

Type of thalassæmia	Homozygous state	Heterozygous state
β-thalassæmia (with some hæmoglobin A production)	Severe anæmia. High proportion of Hb F in most cases	Increased level Hb A₂. Slight increase in Hb F in 50 per cent cases
β-thalassæmia (with no hæmoblogin A production)	Severe anæmia. Hæmoglobin consists of F and A₂ only	Identical to above
β-δ-thalassæmia*	Moderate anæmia. Hæmoglobin consists of F only	Normal or reduced Hb A₂. Hb F in 5–20 per cent range, heterogeneously distributed
Hæmoglobin Lepore thalassæmia	Severe anæmia. Hæmoglobin consists of F and Lepore only	Normal or reduced level of Hb A₂. Hb Lepore and F present
β-thalassæmia with normal levels of Hb F and A₂	Not described	Thalassæmia-like blood picture with normal levels of Hb A₂ and F

* Probably also occurs in a form with some β- and δ-chain synthesis on affected chromosome.

homozygous state has only recently been encountered (Brancati and Baglioni, 1966). The clinical picture in homozygotes is that of a moderately severe thalassæmia; the associated hæmoglobin pattern consists of hæmoglobin F only, no hæmoglobin A or A₂ being detectable. The fundamental genetic defect would, therefore, seem to be an inherited inability to synthethize β- or δ-chains, with persistent synthesis of fœtal hæmoglobin at a rate insufficient to maintain a normal hæmoglobin level. The heterozygous state is characterized by little or no anæmia, the diagnosis depending on morphological changes of the red cells associated with hæmoglobin F levels in the 5–20 per cent range and normal or slightly reduced levels of hæmoglobin A₂. Again the fœtal hæmoglobin is quite heterogenously distributed among the red cells.

Individuals who receive the true (high A₂) β-thalassæmia gene from one parent and the β-δ-thalassæmia gene from the other have the clinical picture of severe Cooley's anæmia with levels of hæmoglobin F in the 80–90 per cent range, normal or reduced levels of hæmoglobin A_2 and little detectable hæmoglobin A.

Hæmoglobin Lepore Disorders. A disorder clinically indistinguishable from the β-thalassæmia trait associated with the presence of about 10 per cent of a slow-moving hæmoglobin was found in one parent of a child with typical thalassæmia major (Gerald and Diamond, 1958). Hæmoglobin variants of this type, named Lepore after the first family, have been found in many different racial groups, and thus named Lepore (Washington), Lepore (Hollandia), Lepore (Pylos), etc., after their places of origin (for references see Weatherall, 1965). Chemical studies of hæmoglobin Lepore have revealed that it has normal α-chains combined with two chains consisting of the amino terminal residues of the δ-chain and the carboxyl terminal residues of the β-chain (Baglioni, 1962). It is believed that such a composite δ-β-chain has arisen as an accident following unequal genic crossing over during meiosis, part of the δ-chain gene becoming attached to part of the β-chain gene. The composite δ-β-gene gives rise to a peptide chain which is synthesized ineffectively with the resulting clinical picture of thalassæmia (Baglioni, 1962).

The hæmoglobin Lepore gene has been found in the homozygous state and in the heterozygous state, either alone or in association with β-thalassæmia or hæmoglobin S. The clinical picture in the homozygous state is that of severe thalassæmia with complete absence of hæmoglobin A or A_2 synthesis, the predominant hæmoglobin being hæmoglobin F with small quantities of hæmoglobin Lepore.

β-thalassæmia associated with β-chain hæmoglobin variants. β-thalassæmia has been found in association with many β-chain hæmoglobin variants (see Weatherall, 1965), and the clinical results of such a combination depend on the degree of suppression of normal β-chain synthesis and the physical properties of the associated hæmoglobin variant. These principles are well illustrated by the most common disorder in this group, sickle-cell thalassæmia.

In some patients with sickle-cell thalassæmia the hæmoglobin pattern is characterized by the presence of about 30 per cent hæmoglobin A, the remainder being hæmoglobin S with about 5 per cent hæmoglobin A_2. In other patients no hæmoglobin A can be detected, the hæmoglobin consisting of about 90 per cent hæmoglobin S, 5 per cent hæmoglobin A_2 and some hæmoglobin F. The presence or absence of hæmoglobin A runs true within families and varies markedly between racial groups. This suggests that there are two distinct varieties of β-thalassæmia gene, one with complete failure of β-chain synthesis, the other with partial failure. Although there are exceptions, the type of sickle-cell thalassæmia associated with hæmoglobin A production is generally milder than that with no hæmoglobin A production. This probably reflects the more marked reduction in hæmoglobin synthesis and higher mean level of hæmoglobin S per red cell in the "non-hæmoglobin A producing" variety of the disorder.

The correlation between the chemical type of β-thalassæmia and the associated clinical severity is seen in the other β-thalassæmia–β-chain hæmoglobin variant combinations. Thus, hæmoglobin C-thalassæmia in the

Negro population is usually associated with some hæmoglobin A production and is a very mild disorder, whereas in the Mediterranean region, where it has been found with the non-hæmoglobin A producing type of β-thalassæmia it is much more severe.

Hæmoglobin E-thalassæmia is very common in S.E. Asia, and is characterized by a clinical picture of thalassæmia major. The hæmoglobin pattern consists of hæmoglobin E and F, hæmoglobin A not being found. Thus the severity of this condition may well result from the high frequency of the non-hæmoglobin A producing type of β-thalassæmia in S.E. Asia.

The α-thalassæmias

Like the β-thalassæmias there is evidence of a genetic heterogenity within the group of disorders associated with defective α-chain synthesis.

Homozygous α-thalassæmia. There are now many reports from S.E. Asia of stillborn infants with the clinical picture of hydrops fœtalis, the associated hæmoglobin pattern consisting of about 80 per cent hæmoglobin Bart's (Lie-Injo et al., 1962). It is now assumed that this condition represents the homozygous state for a severe form of α-thalassæmia, the gross defect in α-chain synthesis resulting in a great excess of γ-chains which aggregate to form γ_4 molecules. The parents of these infants have not been anæmic and their blood smears have shown very mild morphological changes of the red cells. The hæmoglobin patterns have been normal and no cases have been reported in which hæmoglobin H inclusion bodies have been found. It is, therefore, impossible to prove that these infants are homozygous for the α-thalassæmia gene until a method exists for recognizing the heterozygous carrier state in adults. It does seem likely, however, that these infants have inherited a severe defect in α-chain synthesis which is incompatible with fœtal survival and that α-thalassæmia is a frequent source of fœtal wastage in S.E. Asia.

Hæmoglobin H thalassæmia. Hæmoglobin H disease is characterized by a moderate degree of anæmia, the red cell morphological appearances of thalassæmia and the presence of a variable amount of hæmoglobin H, usually in the 10–20 per cent range. In addition, after incubation with brilliant cresyl blue, the red cells show numerous inclusion bodies representing denatured hæmoglobin H. In addition to hæmoglobin H, red cell lysates from many patients with hæmoglobin H disease contain variable amounts of hæmoglobin Bart's and a component consisting entirely of the δ-chains of hæmoglobin A_2. In this disorder there is a defect in α-chain synthesis, the rate of β-chain production being about two to three times that of α-chain production (Weatherall et al., 1965). The excess of β-chains form a large intracellular pool and presumably aggregate to form β_4 molecules. If γ-chain synthesis persists, hæmoglobin Bart's is formed rather than hæmoglobin F because of the overall deficit of α-chains. In addition to the underlying defect in hæmoglobin synthesis there is a marked hæmolytic element in hæmoglobin H disease. Hæmoglobin H is unstable and tends to precipitate in old red cells. The resulting large, single intracellular inclusions, which can be demonstrated only in the peripheral blood after splenectomy, are probably removed by the spleen, with subsequent shortening of red cell survival. Whether such hypothetical "pitting" of inclusion bodies results in damage to the cell membrane is uncertain, but recent evidence suggests that the erythrocytes are "leaky" in this disorder (Nathan and Gunn, 1966).

The inheritance of hæmoglobin H disease is still uncertain. One parent usually shows the mild morphological abnormalities of the red cells which characterize the α-thalassæmic carrier state while the other parent is normal. It is probable that the condition results from the interaction of two α-thalassæmia genes, one of which is completely "silent" with the limited techniques currently available for studying hæmoglobin synthesis.

The α-thalassæmia carrier state. It is probably impossible to recognize this condition with certainty in adult life. At the most there are mild morphological changes of the red cells, slightly diminished red cell osmotic fragility, occasional cells containing inclusion bodies on incubation with brilliant cresyl blue, or the presence of traces of hæmoglobin H or Bart's on starch gel electrophoresis in a phosphate buffer at pH 7·0. All these findings may easily be overlooked and are inconstant and it is probable that the condition can only be recognized with certainty in the neonatal period when it is associated with levels of hæmoglobin Bart's in the 5–20 per cent range.

When the α-thalassæmia trait is found in association with α-chain hæmoglobin variants there is clear evidence of interaction and the α-chain variant has been found either in association with about 30 per cent hæmoglobin A or there has been complete suppression of hæmoglobin A production. This suggests that, as in β-thalassæmia, two kinds of α-thalassæmia exist, one in which there is complete suppression of α-chain synthesis and a second with a partial defect of α-chain production.

The Nature of the Defect in Thalassæmia. Recent *in vitro* studies of hæmoglobin synthesis in thalassæmic reticulocytes have confirmed that there is a defective rate of β-chain synthesis in β-thalassæmia and of α-chain production in α-thalassæmia. The synthetic level at which there is defective peptide chain synthesis has not yet been determined although it seems likely that at least one type of β-thalassæmia results from a quantitative abnormality of the messenger RNA for the β-peptide chain (Weatherall *et al.*, 1965; Bank and Marks, 1966).

It is now clear that, based upon this primary defect in globin chain synthesis, there are many complex secondary abnormalities of hæmoglobin synthesis and red cell survival. In β-thalassæmia α-chain synthesis proceeds unimpaired and excess α-chains, with their attached hæm units, are deposited as inclusion bodies in the red cell precursors. It is likely that the removal of these bodies results in a shortening of red cell survival either by membrane damage or sequestration of inclusion-containing cells within the spleen. "Leaky" cell membranes have recently been demonstrated in this disorder and the number of inclusions which can be demonstrated in the peripheral blood is markedly increased after splenectomy (Nathan and Gunn, 1966). Consequent to the defect in globin synthesis there is a secondary defect in hæm synthesis in which the excess of hæm inhibits the early steps of its biosynthetic pathway. Similarly there is evidence that excessive iron will also inhibit the early steps of hæm synthesis.

The hæmatological findings in thalassæmia are thus the end-result of a series of secondary phenomena based on a primary defect in globin chain production. The nature of this defect remains unknown and it is likely that there are several different mechanisms which operate in the different clinical forms of thalassæmia.

The Diagnosis and Management of Thalassæmia

The diagnosis of thalassæmia depends on a clinical and hæmatological assessment, backed by studies of the associated hæmoglobin pattern. The hæmoglobin studies should include a careful search for hæmoglobin H inclusions after incubation of the cells with brilliant cresyl blue, an estimation of fœtal hæmoglobin, electrophoretic studies of the hæmoglobin pattern and a quantitation of the level of hæmoglobin A_2 by either starch block or cellulose acetate electrophoresis followed by elution of the major and minor components (for methods see Weatherall, 1965).

It is still not clear whether children with severe thalassæmia should have their hæmoglobin maintained at a level of about 8 Gm. with relatively infrequent transfusions or have very frequent transfusions in an attempt to maintain a completely normal hæmoglobin level. It is claimed that better growth and all round development follows the second course (Wolman, 1964). The major problem encountered in thalassæmic children is that of generalized iron deposition, particularly in the myocardium and, until it is decided if this occurs more frequently in those children who receive very frequent transfusion, it seems safer to transfuse only as often as is needed to maintain a safe hæmoglobin level.

The main forms of treatment are still, therefore, folic acid supplements, intermittent transfusions, early treatment of infection and the occasional use of splenectomy where the spleen is shown to be active in sequestration or destruction of red cells or causing symptoms due to size alone. The use of the newer chelating agents, desferrioxamine and DTPA, is still under study in several countries (Sephton-Smith, 1964). Although considerable amounts of iron can be removed using a régime of intravenous DTPA with each transfusion and intramuscular desferrioxamine between transfusions, it is still not certain whether severe iron deposition can be prevented. In addition, the long-term toxic effects of these agents have yet to be fully assessed.

References

BAGLIONI, C. (1962). The fusion of two peptide chains in hemoglobin Lepore and its interpretation as a genetic deletion. *Proc. Nat. Acad. Sci. U.S.A.*, **48**, 1880.

BAGLIONI, C. (1963). Correlations between genetics and chemistry of human hemoglobins. In: *Molecular Genetics*, Part I, p. 405, ed. New York, Academic Press.

BANK, A. and MARKS, P. A. (1966). Protein synthesis in a cell-free human reticulocyte system: ribosome function in thalassemia. *J. Clin. Invest.*, **45**, 330.

BRANCATI, C. and BAGLIONI, C. (1966). Homozygous β-δ Thalassaemia (βδ Microcythaemia). Nature, **212**, 262.

CHARACHE, S. (1966). Personal communication.

CHARACHE, S. and CONLEY, C. L. (1964). Rate of sickling of red cells during de-oxygenation of blood from persons with various sickling disorders. Blood, **24**, 25.

CHARACHE, S. and RICHARDSON, S. N. (1964). Prolonged survival of a patient with sickle cell anemia. *Arch. Int. Med.*, **113**, 844.

CHARACHE, S., WEATHERALL, D. J. and CLEGG, J. B. (1966). Polycythemia associated with a hemoglobinopathy. *J. Clin. Invest.*, **45**, 813.

CONLEY, C. L., WEATHERALL, D. J., RICHARDSON, S. N., SHEPARD, M. K. and CHARACHE, S. (1963). Hereditary persistence of fetal hemoglobin: a study of 79 affected persons in 15 Negro families in Baltimore. *Blood*, **21**, 261.

COOLEY, T. B. and LEE, P. (1925). A series of cases of splenomegaly in children with anemia and peculiar bone changes. *Trans. Amer. Pediat. Soc.*, **37**, 29.

FESSAS, P. (1963). Inclusions of hemoglobin in erythroblasts and erythrocytes of thalassemia. *Blood*, **21**, 21.

FESSAS, P. and LOUKOPOULOS, D. (1964). Alpha-chain of human hemoglobin: occurence *in vivo*. *Science*, **143**, 590.

FULLERTON, W. T., HENDRICKSE, J. P. De v. and Watson-Williams, E. J. (1965). In Abnormal Haemoglobins in Africa, p. 411, ed. Jonxis, J. H. P. Blackwell, Oxford.

GERALD, P. S. and DIAMOND, L. K. (1958). The diagnosis of thalassemia trait by starch block electrophoresis. *Blood*, **13**, 61.

GRIMES, A. J., MEISLER, A. and DACIE, J. V. (1964). Congenital Heinz body anaemia: further evidence on the cause of Heinz-body production in red cells. *Brit. J. Haemat.*, **10**, 281.

HARRIS, J. W. (1950). Studies of the destruction of red blood cells. VIII Molecular orientation in sickle-hemoglobin solutions. *Proc. Soc. Exper. Biol. N.Y.*, **75**, 197.

HELLER, P. W. (1965). The molecular basis of the pathogenicity of the abnormal hemoglobins—some recent developments. *Blood*, **25**, 110.

HUEHNS, E. R. and SHOOTER, E. M. (1965). Human haemoglobins. *J. med. Genet.*, **2**, 48.

INGRAM, V. M. and STRETTON, A. O. W. (1959). The genetic basis of the thalassaemia diseases. *Nature*, **184**, 1903.

ITANO, H. A. (1965). The synthesis and structure of normal and abnormal hemoglobins. In: Abnormal Haemoglobins in Africa, p. 3, ed. Jonxis, J. H. P., Blackwell, Oxford.

KRAUS, L. M., MIYAJI, T., IUCHI, I. and KRAUS, A. P. (1966). Characterization of $\alpha^{23GluNH_2}$ in hemoglobin Memphis. Hemoglobin Memphis/S, a new variant of molecular disease. *Biochem.*, **5**, 3701.

LEHMANN, H. (1963). Treatment of sickle-cell anaemia. *Brit. Med. J.*, **1**, p. 1158.

LEHMANN, H. (1964). Recent Advances in Clin. Path. p. 152. ed. Dyke, S. C. Churchill, London.

LIE INJO LUAN ENG, LIE HONG GHIE, AGER, J. A. M. and LEHMANN, H. α-Thalassaemia as a cause of hydrops foetalis. *Brit. J. Haemat.* **8**, 1.

LONDON, I. M., BRUNS, G. P. and KARIBIAN, O. (1964). The regulation of hemoglobin synthesis and the pathogenesis of some hypochromic anemias. *Medicine (Baltimore)*, **43**, 789.

MUIRHEAD, H. and PERUTZ, M. F. (1963). Structure of haemoglobin. A three-dimensional Fourier synthesis of reduced human haemoglobin at 5·5Å resolution. *Nature*, **149**, 633.

MURAYAMA, M. (1964). A molecular mechanism of sickled erythrocyte formation. *Nature*, **202**, 258.

NATHAN, D. G. and GUNN, R. B. (1966). Thalassemia: the consequences of unbalanced hemoglobin synthesis. *Amer. J. Med.*, **41**, 815.

RIEDER, R. F., ZINKHAM, W. H. and HOLTZMAN, N. A. (1965). Hemoglobin Zurich. *Amer. J. Med.*, **39**, 4.

SEPHTON-SMITH, R. (1964). Chelating agents in the diagnosis and treatment of iron overload in thalassemia. *Ann. New York Acad. Sci.*, **119**, 776.

WARLEY, M. A., HAMILTON, P. J. S., MARSDEN, P. D., BROWN, R. E., MERSELIS, J. G. and WILKS, N. (1965). Chemoprophylaxis of homozygous sicklers with antimalarials and long-acting penicillin. *Brit. med. J.*, **2**, 86.

WEATHERALL, D. J. (1965). *The Thalassemia Syndromes*. Blackwell, Oxford.

WEATHERALL, D. J., CLEGG, J. B., NAUGHTON, M. A. (1965). Globin synthesis in thalassaemia. An *in vitro* study. *Nature*, **208**, 1061.

WISEMAN, A. (1965). *Organisation for Protein Synthesis*. Blackwell, Oxford.

WOLMAN, I. J. (1964). Transfusion therapy in thalassaemia. Growth and health as related to long-range hemoglobin levels. A progress report. *Ann. New York Acad. Sci.*, **119**, 736.

Chapter 15

RED CELL METABOLISM AND CONGENITAL HÆMOLYTIC ANÆMIAS

G. C. DE GRUCHY and A. J. GRIMES

Introduction — Normal Red Cell Metabolism — Pentose Phosphate Pathway Abnormalities — Embden-Meyerhof Pathway Abnormalities

INTRODUCTION

IT is now recognized that a number of hæmolytic disorders of previously uncertain ætiology are due to hereditary enzyme deficiencies affecting the red cell; these disorders are collectively known as the enzyme deficiency hæmolytic anæmias or hereditary enzymopathies. Biochemically, the hereditary enzymopathies fall into two broad groups, namely those associated with abnormalities of the pentose phosphate pathway (PPP) and glutathione metabolism, and the Embden-Meyerhof pathway (EMP).

Clinically, they cause two main types of hæmolytic disease.

Drug-induced Hæmolytic Anæmia. In this disorder, clinical hæmolysis is intermittent and occurs only following the ingestion of certain drugs. Glucose-6-phosphate dehydrogenase (G6PD) deficiency is the main cause of this type of hæmolysis, but it may be caused also by glutathione reductase deficiency.

Non-spherocytic Congenital Hæmolytic Anæmia with Continuing Hæmolysis. This is due most often to pyruvate kinase (PK) deficiency, occasionally to G6PD deficiency, and rarely to triosephosphate isomerase deficiency, diphosphoglycerate mutase deficiency, glyceraldehyde-3-phosphate dehydrogenase deficiency, hexokinase deficiency and deficiency of glutathione or glutathione reductase. It should be realized, however, that not all drug-induced hæmolytic anæmias are due to red cell enzyme deficiencies, and that in some non-spherocytic congenital hæmolytic anæmias no specific enzyme deficiency has been demonstrated (Dacie, 1964; Loder and de Gruchy, 1965).

In addition to the hæmolytic disorders in which a specific enzyme deficiency has been identified, it has been shown that metabolic abnormalities may occur in other hæmolytic anæmias in which it is not considered that the primary defect is an enzyme deficiency of the glycolytic pathways or glutathione metabolism. The abnormalities have been mainly changes in the red cell phosphates, particularly ATP, and it is thought that they are secondary to other more basic defects, which have not yet been precisely identified. These disorders include hereditary spherocytosis (Jacob, 1966; Loder, Barbarczy and de Gruchy, 1967) and hereditary elliptocytosis (de Gruchy, Loder and Hennessy, 1962). The group of unstable hæmoglobinopathies, which includes hereditary Heinz-body anæmia, is a further

example of hæmolytic anæmia with associated red cell metabolic ab-
normalities but no specific enzyme defect (Dacie, Grimes, Meisler, Steingold,
Hemsted, Beaven and White, 1964; Grimes, Meisler and Dacie, 1964b;
Vaughan Jones, Grimes, Carrell and Lehmann, 1967).

Red cell enzyme deficiencies may occur also without an associated
hæmolytic anæmia, e.g. catalase deficiency (Takahara, 1951, 1952; Takahara
et al., 1960; Jacob, Ingbar and Jandl, 1965), diaphorase deficiency (Gibson,
1948; Scott and Hoskins, 1958), or hexokinase deficiency. Finally there
exist defects in the cell which apparently do not account for the hæmolytic
anæmia which is present, e.g. acetylcholinesterase deficiency in paroxysmal
nocturnal hæmoglobinuria (De Sandre, Ghiotto and Mastella, 1956;
De Sandre and Ghiotto, 1960).

This chapter gives a brief description of normal red cell metabolism,
followed by clinical and chemical considerations of those red cell defects
directly concerned with the glycolytic pathways.

THE METABOLISM OF NORMAL HUMAN RED CELLS

The normal human mature red cell is non-nucleated and is sustained
throughout its 120-day life-span by a simplified metabolic organization
comprising anærobic glycolysis (Embden-Meyerhof pathway, EMP) and
aerobic glycolysis (pentose phosphate pathway, PPP). The rate of glucose

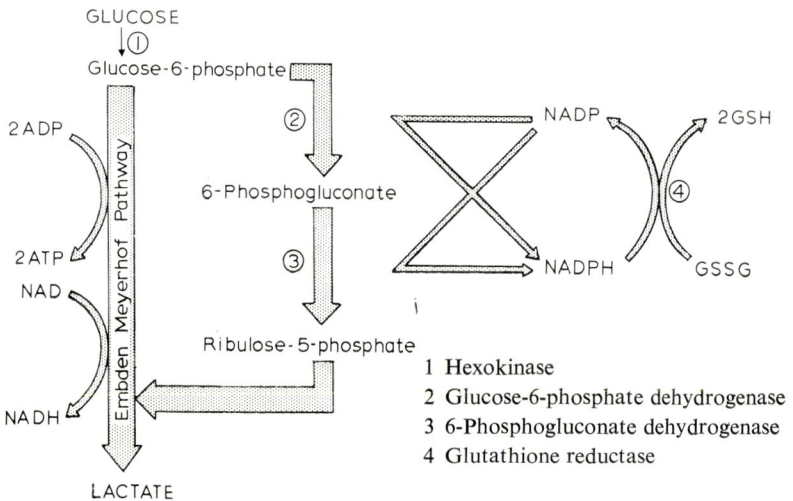

FIG. 1. Production of key intermediates in red cell glycolysis.

consumption *in vitro* varies with the incubation medium used, but is of the
order of 2 m.moles/litre RBC/hour at 37°C. The EMP pathway utilizes over
90 per cent of consumed glucose while the PPP metabolizes the remainder.
These two pathways yield, or are associated with, four key intermediates,
namely, adenosine triphosphate (ATP), reduced glutathione (GSH), reduced
nicotinamide-adenine dinucleotide (NADH) and reduced nicotinamide-

adenine dinucleotide phosphate (NADPH) (Fig. 1). ATP acts as the cells energy source whilst the other three compounds confer reducing potential which functions in protection of hæmoglobin, enzymes and membrane against oxidation, e.g. by drugs; this reducing potential may lessen with increasing cell age.

Much of the reported data on red cell enzymes or intermediates are obtained using venous blood freed, as far as is practicable, from white cells, platelets and sometimes plasma. Such blood contains red cells whose ages range from 1 to 120 days. A continuous decay of many red cell enzymes takes place during ageing and thus most of the data on red cells are average values (See Table 1).

Energy Requirements. Hydrolysis of the terminal energy-rich phosphate bond of ATP yields ADP with the simultaneous liberation of sufficient energy for normal requirements of the red cell. ADP is reconverted into ATP during anærobic glycolysis which yields two moles of ATP and two moles of lactate per mole of glucose consumed. Glucose and lactate can diffuse through the cell wall without energy exchange, but ATP, in common with other phosphorylated intermediates, is non-diffusible. Gas exchange, the prime function of red cells, is not energy-dependent.

An alternative route for ATP breakdown is catalysed by adenylate kinase which is known to be present in the mammalian red cell (Tatibani, Nakao and Yoshikawa, 1958; Kashket and Denstedt, 1958; Cerletti and Bucci, 1960), although its quantitative contribution remains unknown.

$$ATP + AMP \rightarrow 2ADP$$

ADP and AMP are present in small amounts only in fresh red cells compared with ATP.

The energy yield from ATP hydrolysis is utilized primarily to maintain the sodium pump which is located in the membrane. The constituents are ATPase, ATP, Mg^{2+}, K^+ and Na^+, and the pump operates to sustain the high intracellular K^+ and low Na^+ content. The high extracellular Na^+ results in passive diffusion of this ion into the cell, an influx which is reversed by pumping Na^+ out with the concomitant entry of K^+. A continuous Na^+ and K^+ flux thus occurs yielding a steady state of intracellular Na^+ and K^+. Clearly, maintenance of this steady state depends upon ATP availability and thus upon glycolysis.

Reducing Potential. *NADH.* A steady state of oxidized and reduced NAD(H) is maintained by anaerobic glycolysis (Fig. 2). No synthesis *de novo* of this nucleotide occurs in the mature cell, and the two states are available in the amounts shown in Table I. Apart from the co-enzyme function of NADH in the pyruvate-lactate reaction catalysed by lactate dehydrogenase, it serves also as co-enzyme to diaphorase. Diaphorase catalyses the reduction of methæmoglobin to hæmoglobin using NADH as electron donor (Gibson, 1948). Hæm iron in methæmoglobin is in the ferric state and lacks oxygen-carrying capacity. Reconversion to divalent ferrous iron yields functional hæmoglobin. In the absence of a reducing system hæmoglobin forms methæmoglobin *in vivo* at a rate of 0·5–3·0 per cent per day (Eder, Finch and McKee, 1949) and even with the normal reducing system large amounts may be formed by oxidant drug action (see later). A normal red cell population can, however, reduce large amounts of methæmoglobin *in vitro* (Grimes, 1965).

NADPH. Both oxidized (NADP) and reduced (NADPH) forms of this nucleotide are present in steady-state concentrations (Table I) and NADP is the co-enzyme for the first two reactions in metabolic sequence in the PPP (Fig. 1). The co-enzyme product (NADPH) is re-oxidized by two systems:

(i) *Methæmoglobin Reductase.* A system complementary to diaphorase and differing from it by its NADPH co-enzyme specificity. The quantitative contribution of this enzyme *in vivo* is probably small compared with diaphorase (Scott, Duncan and Ekstrand, 1965).

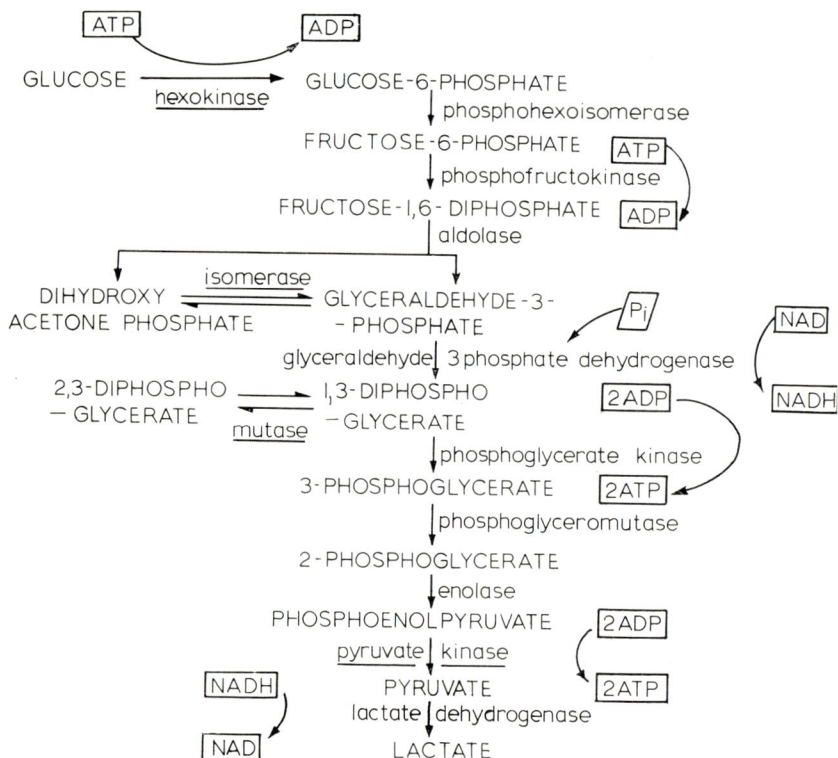

FIG. 2. Embden-Meyerhof pathway. Enzymes underlined have been reported as deficient.

(ii) *Glutathione Reductase.* The reduced form of glutathione (GSH) is present in high concentration whilst the oxidized form (GSSG) is the minor fraction of the two (Table I). GSH is readily oxidized spontaneously, by oxidant drugs, or in protecting protein -SH groups against oxidation. GSH reductase maintains the GSH level and utilizes NADPH as co-enzyme (Fig. 1).

GSH. The GSH measured in whole blood is almost exclusively from red cells and, together with the activity of most red cell enzymes, falls with age of the cell (Sass, Caruso and O'Connell, 1965). GSH is a tripeptide of glutamic acid, glycine and cysteine and the -SH group of cysteine provides the primary protection for the sulphydryl groups of globin, enzymes and membrane protein. In effecting this protection GSH is oxidized to the dimer (GSSG) which lacks reducing power. GSH reductase converts GSSG

TABLE I

Levels of Key Intermediates in Normal, Human Red Cells

Substance	Concentration (μmoles/litre packed red cells)	Reference
NAD + NADH	6·4 (13 males) 7·4 (8 females) 6·2 (2 subjects)	Bishop, Rankine and Talbot (1959) Mills and Summers (1959)
NADP + NADPH	1·3 –1·6 2·5 (13 males) 2·7 (8 females) 3·6 (2 subjects)	Bartlett (1959) Bishop et al. (1959) Mills and Summers (1959)
ATP	3·94–4·15 (Firefly method)* 90–123 (Column chromatography) 84–110 (Column chromatography) 75–88 (Column chromatography) 75–125 (Hexokinase)	Beutler and Mathia (1967) Bartlett (1959) Robinson, Loder and de Gruchy (1961) Nathan, Oski, Sidel and Diamond (1965)
2,3-DPG	348–440 360–501 310–453 356–406	Keitt (1966) Bartlett (1959) Robinson et al. (1961) Grimes, Meisler and Dacie (1964a)
GSH	173–274 (Nitroprusside) 160–300 (Nitroprusside) 195–319 (Iodimetric) 192–343 (Amperometric)	Zinkham (1959) Jocelyn (1960) Farmer and Maizels (1939) Grimes and Meisler (1962)
GSSG (% GSH + GSSG)	0–6 10–25 7–22	Jocelyn (1960) Bhattacharya, Robson and Stewart (1955) Koj (1962)

* Units are μmoles ATP per gm. Hb.

to GSH as mentioned earlier. Synthesis de novo of GSH in red cells does occur (Miller and Horiuchi, 1962; Sass, 1963), but its quantitative contribution is not clear.

The Oxidation of Red Cells. A variety of compounds, mainly oxidant (see Table II), will, in adequate amount, damage red cells. Older cells, in which glycolysis has been diminished by age, are more susceptible to oxidative change than younger cells. The three foci of oxidation are:

$$2GSH \rightarrow GSSG$$
$$Fe^{2+} \rightarrow Fe^{3+} + 1e^-$$
$$Protein—SH \rightarrow Protein—S—S—$$

These reactions are shown by the broken arrows in Figure 3. The reverse reactions, all linked to glycolysis, are able to reinstate the reducing potential of the cell, shown also in Figure 3.

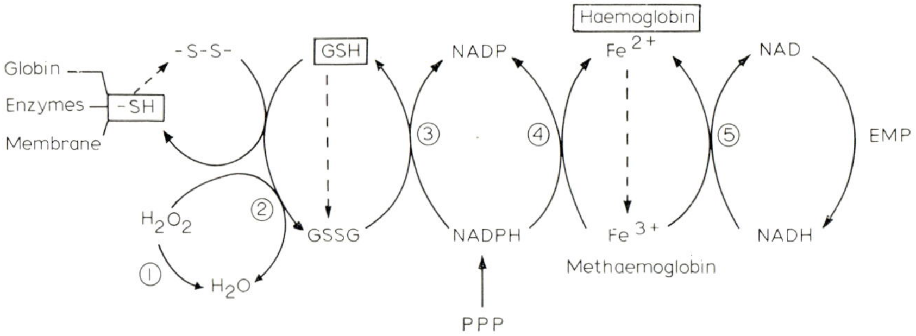

FIG. 3. The Oxidation-Reduction System. Boxed moieties are foci for oxidation while broken arrows indicate oxidation products. For details see text. (1) Catalase, (2) GSH peroxidase, (3) GSH reductase, (4) NADPH-linked methaemoglobin reductase, (5) diaphorase.

In G6PD deficiency (see later) the reducing power of the cell is diminished and the cell is accordingly abnormally sensitive towards oxidant drugs. This arises because maintenance of GSH levels depends, via NADPH, upon PPP activity which is restricted in this deficiency. The presence of an oxidant drug or its metabolites leads to oxidation of GSH of which there is inadequate regeneration. Without the protection of GSH other -SH groups are liable to oxidize and changes culminating in hæmolysis can occur. NADH is the sole reducing system unimpaired in the cell and methæmoglobin reduction can occur.

Hæmoglobin. The globin moiety comprises approximately 98 per cent of the protein complement of the red cell and this preponderance has permitted intensive study of the degradative changes which occur during oxidation. The sequence of events culminating in Heinz body formation has been described (Allen and Jandl, 1961). Methæmoglobin formation occurs readily and is, probably, the initial step. This is followed by a reversible oxidation of the two accessible β-chain -SH groups. Subsequent steps are irreversible and involve the remaining four -SH groupings. Continued oxidation yields progressively denatured and insoluble protein which eventually precipitates within the cell as an inclusion or Heinz body, visualized with methyl violet stain.

Hydrogen Peroxide. This powerful oxidant may be decomposed in red cells by catalase or by glutathione peroxidase

$$\text{Catalase: } 2H_2O_2 \longrightarrow 2H_2O + O_2$$

GSH peroxidase:

The source of H_2O_2 under normal conditions is not clear, but it may be formed (Cohen and Hochstein, 1962; Jacob et al., 1965) during the action of certain drugs (primaquine, pamaquin) or of ascorbic acid upon red cells. That catalase is important in breaking down H_2O_2 is shown by the ready formation of methæmoglobin in H_2O_2-treated cells either congenitally deficient in catalase (Takahara, 1960) or with a catalase inhibitor present (Cohen and Hochstein, 1962). The alternative route for destruction of H_2O_2 uses GSH peroxidase, an enzyme first described (Mills, 1957) in bovine and rat cells and later by some (Cohen and Hochstein, 1963; Hill, Haut, Cartwright and Wintrobe, 1964; Jacob et al., 1965), but not all, workers (Szeinberg and Marks, 1961) in human red cells. Peroxidation of H_2O_2 by this reaction is linked to the PPP since GSH becomes oxidized and requires reduction by GSH reductase using NADPH as co-enzyme. Study of the relative importance of the two reactions suggests that under normal conditions catalase disposes of H_2O_2, but peroxidation offers an alternative route (Jacob et al., 1965).

The Ageing Process

Reticulocytes possess enzyme systems essential to the nucleated cell developing in the marrow. Some are residual in the reticulocyte and disappear with its maturation. For example, vestigial activity is demonstrable of enzymes concerned with protein synthesis, respiration and oxidative phosphorylation. In addition, reticulocytes contain many enzymes having no apparent relevance for the mature cell yet which persist, at a declining level, throughout its life-span, e.g. glyoxalase, transaminases.

The two glycolytic pathways essential to the mature cell are present at elevated activity in reticulocytes. Membrane lipid is present also in greater amount than in mature cells. With ageing of the cell there is a decline of enzymic activity, possibly exponential, each enzyme decaying at a characteristic rate. In parallel with this fall there is a loss of surface lipid (van Gastel, van den Berg, de Gier and van Deenen, 1965). Eventually glycolysis cannot be sustained, the pump fails and the effect of elution of surface constituents yields an effete cell which is removed by the reticulo-endothelial system.

HÆMOLYTIC ANÆMIAS ASSOCIATED WITH ABNORMALITIES OF THE PENTOSE PHOSPHATE PATHWAY AND GLUTATHIONE METABOLISM

GLUCOSE-6-PHOSPHATE DEHYDROGENASE (G6PD) DEFICIENCY

Four types of hæmolytic disorder have been described in association with G6PD deficiency:

> Drug (primaquine) sensitive hæmolytic anæmia
> Favism
> Icterus neonatorum
> Congenital non-spherocytic hæmolytic anæmia

Drug (Primaquine) Sensitive Hæmolytic Anæmia. Favism.
Icterus Neonatorum

In 1952 Hockwald and his collaborators noted that between 5 and 10 per cent of otherwise healthy American Negro troops developed an acute hæmolytic anæmia after the administration of the 8-aminoquinoline anti-malarial drug primaquine.

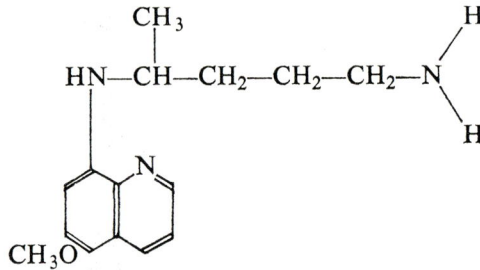

$$HN-\underset{\underset{|}{CH_3}}{CH}-CH_2-CH_2-CH_2-N\underset{H}{\overset{H}{<}}$$

PRIMAQUINE
8-(4-Amino-1-methylbutylamino)-6-methoxyquinoline

Before exposure to the drug there was no evidence of hæmolysis in these sensitive Negroes and their red cells were morphologically normal. Subsequent study of sensitive Negro subjects has shown (Carson, Flanagan, Ickes and Alving, 1956) that they have a genetically determined red cell abnormality,

TABLE II

Drugs which may cause Hæmolysis in G6PD-Deficient Subjects

Antimalarials
Primaquine
Pamaquin ("Plasmoquine")
Mepacrine ("Quinacrine", "Atebrin")

Sulphones
Dapsone ("Avlosulphon")
Sulphoxone ("Diasone")
Thiazosulphone ("Promizole")

Sulphonamides
Sulphanilamide
Sulphacetamide ("Albucid", "Sulamyd")
Sulphafurazole ("Gantrisin")
Sulphamethoxypyridazine ("Lederkyn",
    "Midicel", "Kynex")

Nitrofurans
Nitrofurantoin ("Furadantin")
Furazolidone ("Furoxone")
Nitrofurazone ("Furacin")

Analgesics
Acetylsalicyclic acid
Acetophenetidin (Phenacetin)
Acetanilide

Miscellaneous
Vitamin K (water-soluble
    analogues)
Naphthalene (moth balls)
Probenecid ("Benemid")
Dimercaprol (BAL)
Methylene blue
Quinine*
Quinidine*
Chloramphenicol*
Acetylphenylhydrazine
Phenylhydrazine
p-Aminosalicyclic acid

* Not shown to be hæmolytic in Negroes.

namely, a deficiency of the enzyme glucose-6-phosphate dehydrogenase (G6PD). Most of the experimental work elucidating the nature of this red cell defect has involved studying the effect of primaquine on sensitive individuals, and so the disorder is sometimes called primaquine sensitive hæmolytic anæmia (Tarlov, Brewer, Carson and Alving, 1962). However, it has been demonstrated that a number of other drugs, mainly oxidants, may cause hæmolysis in G6PD-deficient subjects, leading to an explanation of the cause of many previously unexplained drug-induced hæmolytic anæmias and also of the disorder favism (see Table II).

The known red cell abnormalities associated with G6PD deficiency are shown in Table III. The possible mechanism whereby this deficiency renders the red cell more susceptible to hæmolysis are discussed in the preceding section on red cell metabolism.

TABLE III

Associated Red Cell Abnormalities in G6PD Deficiency

Enzyme or intermediate	Level	Reference
GSH	Low or low-normal	Beutler, Dern, Flanagan and Alving (1955)
GSH stability	Low	Beutler, Dern and Alving (1955)
GSH reductase	High	Schrier, Kellermeyer, Carson, Ickes and Alving (1958)
GSH synthesis *de novo*	Slow incorporation of ^{14}C-glycine	Szeinberg, Adam, Ramot, Sheba and Myers (1959)
Catalase	Low	Tarlov and Kellermeyer (1961)
Aldolase	High	Schrier, Kellermeyer, Carson, Ickes and Alving (1959)
NAD	Slightly raised	}Schrier, Kellermeyer and Alving
NADP	High	} (1958)
Oxygen consumption	Low	Johnson and Marks (1958) Kellermeyer, Carson, Schrier Tarlov and Alving (1961)
MetHb reductase	Low	Bonsignore, Fornaini, Segni and Fantoni (1960)

Racial and Genetic Features. The defect has a high incidence in Negroes; it also occurs in a number of non-Negro races and is seen most commonly in Mediterranean peoples, namely Italians, particularly Sardinians and some Greeks. Values recorded in various population studies include American Negroes (13 per cent), Nigerians (10 per cent), Sardinian males (4–30 per cent) and Greeks (0·7–3 per cent). It is common in Sephardic (dark-complexioned Oriental) Jews but rare in Ashkenazic Jews (light-complexioned Jews from eastern, central and western Europe). Other races shown to be affected include Indians, Chinese, Malays, Thais, Filipinos, Melanesians (see Beutler, 1966a, for references). In general, the deficiency of the enzyme is more marked in non-Negroes. It is estimated that the trait is present in more than one hundred million people in the world. There is evidence to suggest that the defect confers some protection against falciparum malaria; thus it may represent a biological advantage where this disorder is endemic, in that it may lessen the severity of malarial infections in young children and infants (Motulsky, 1965).

The disorder is genetically transmitted by a sex-linked gene of intermediate dominance. Full expression of the trait occurs in hemizygous males, in whom the single X chromosome carries the mutant gene, and in homozygous females in whom both sex chromosomes (XX) carry a mutant gene. Intermediate expression is found in heterozygous females, in whom expression is variable. Female heterozygotes have been shown to have two populations of red cells, one with normal enzyme activity and one with markedly deficient activity (Beutler and Baluda, 1964). The relative proportion of the two populations present in different heterozygotes results in G6PD activities which may vary from almost normal to those found for hemizygotes. Full expression occurs in from 10 to 15 per cent of American Negro males and in 1 to 2 per cent of American Negro females. Intermediate expression has been described in about 16 per cent of American Negro females, but because of the difficulty in identifying heterozygote females, especially with screening tests, this value may be too low. It has been demonstrated that the disorder shows a close linkage with colour blindness (Adam, 1961; Porter, Schulze and McKusick, 1962). The genetics of the disorder are reviewed in detail by Beutler (1966a).

Starch gel electrophoresis of hæmolysates from American Negroes yields two bands with G6PD activity, a fast A and a slower B band (Boyer, Porter and Weilbacher, 1962). Normal males have A+ or B+, normal females have A+, B+ or AB+, whilst G6PD-deficient males show, with rare exceptions, only the A band which is designated A−. Normal Caucasians yield only B+. Some reports are available of mildly affected heterozygous males in Greece (Stamatoyannopoulos, Panayotopoulos and Papayannopoulou, 1964), in an American male Negro (Tarlov and Kellermeyer, 1961) and in two males of Italian ancestry (Marks, Gross and Banks, 1961; Marks, Banks and Gross, 1962). In addition, some females with activities near the low values for male hemizygotes are described (Carson and Frischer, 1966).

Clinical Features. The nature and severity of the hæmolytic disorder shows some variation with the racial group involved. There are three clinical manifestations, namely, drug-sensitive hæmolytic anæmia, favism, and icterus neonatorum. In Negro subjects the chief manifestation is drug-sensitive hæmolysis, while in Mediterranean subjects and in certain other races favism and icterus neonatorum also occur. There is some evidence to suggest that the hæmolytic episodes tend to be more severe in Mediterranean subjects and possibly also in other non-Negro races.

Drug-induced Hæmolysis. *The Hæmolytic Episode.* The severity of the hæmolytic episode induced by a particular drug is, in general, related to its dose. The most detailed study of the clinical course has been in primaquine-sensitive Negro volunteers, receiving 30 mg. of primaquine per day. This results in a self-limiting hæmolysis, beginning in two to three days and lasting for about seven days, and followed by a return of the hæmoglobin value to normal between the twentieth and thirtieth day despite continued drug administration (Dern, Beutler and Alving, 1954). Clinically some patients have only darkening of the urine, but the more severely affected complain of weakness, abdominal and back pain, and are found to be jaundiced and to pass black urine. The self-limiting nature of the hæmolysis is because cell drug sensitivity is a function of cell age; older cells are destroyed, while younger cells are resistant (Beutler, Dern and Alving, 1954). Hæmolysis ceases when the older population of cells has been destroyed and only the younger cells remain. However, the resistance of younger cells is relative, as a second hæmolysis can be induced if the dose is suddenly greatly increased. In some non-Negro subjects the hæmolysis does not appear self-limiting; in such subjects withdrawal of the drug is of paramount importance.

Drugs which may cause Hæmolysis. A large number of compounds may cause a hæmolytic reaction in sensitive subjects. They include antimalarials, sulphonamides, nitrofurans, sulphones, analgesics and water-soluble vitamin K analogues (Table II). Some drugs, e.g. chloramphenicol, quinine and quinidine, do not cause hæmolysis in Negroes but may in certain other affected races (Beutler, 1966a).

The degree of hæmolysis varies from mild to severe. There is a consistent relationship between the dose of a particular drug and the degree of hæmolysis it produces. Dose response is discussed in detail by Kellermeyer, Tarlov, Brewer, Carson and Alving (1962).

Predisposing Factors—Infection, Diabetic Acidosis, Renal Impairment. Infections, both bacterial and viral, may cause hæmolysis in sensitive subjects without the administration of drugs, or may accentuate the hæmolysis due to drugs. Infections recorded as causing hæmolysis include upper respiratory tract infection, influenza, pneumonia, typhoid, viral hepatitis and infectious mononucleosis. Diabetic acidosis has also been recorded as both causing hæmolysis and accentuating drug-induced hæmolysis.

In persons with impaired renal function there may be reduced drug elimination, leading to a higher blood concentration of a drug at a particular dosage and therefore to more severe hæmolysis. This point is of particular importance in relation to drugs used in treating urinary tract infections, e.g. "furadantin", "lederkyn" and "gantrisin", as renal function is sometimes impaired by the infection.

Favism

Favism is a disorder characterized by an acute hæmolytic anæmia of sudden onset, often with hæmoglobinuria, which occurs in persons sensitive to the fava bean (*Vicia faba*), either on ingestion of the uncooked or lightly cooked bean or on inhalation of the pollen from the blossom of the plant (McCrae and Uller, 1933); attacks occur most commonly in the spring when the beans are fresh and the pollen is in the air. When due to pollen inhalation hæmolysis may be fulminating and begin within a few minutes, but when due to bean ingestion there is commonly a latent period of 6 to 24 or more hours before onset of hæmolysis. The hæmolysis varies in severity, but the anæmia is often severe; attacks usually last from two to six days, followed by spontaneous recovery, but death occurs occasionally. Certain other plants may also cause hæmolysis (Larizza, Brunetti and Grignani, 1960; Motulsky, 1965).

Favism occurs mainly in Sardinia, Sicily, southern Italy and Greece. However, cases are now being reported in the U.S.A., Great Britain, Australia and other countries in persons of Mediterranean descent; thus it should be realized that the fava bean is the common European broad bean, which is widely grown and eaten in temperate climates. Although favism occurs typically in Mediterranean subjects it may also occur in certain non-Mediterranean subjects with G6PD deficiency, including Chinese and Jews. It has recently been described in several English subjects in whom there was no apparent history of descent from races known to carry the disorder (Brodribb and Worssam, 1961; Davies, 1961).

Persons susceptible to favism have a deficiency of G6PD, but it appears that some other factor(s) (possibly hypersensitivity) are involved in the hæmolytic attack which follows exposure to fava beans (Panizon and Vullo, 1962). Some G6PD-deficient Mediterraneans can eat fava beans without hæmolysis occurring (Roth and Frumin, 1960).

In an extensive study of 500 G6PD-deficient Greek subjects, Kattamis (1967) has several noteworthy findings: (a) some 10 per cent of G6PD-deficient subjects studied experienced hæmolytic crises following ingestion of fava beans, (b) susceptibility to fava beans decreased with age and was uncommon in adults, (c) a seasonal variation existed in the distribution of favism which was most frequent in May. This may be related to variation in the potency of the bean with age, for in May the fresh bean becomes available. (d) G6PD activity in the red cells of affected subjects was nil. During hæmolytic crises the activity rose only slightly and was always considerably lower than the values found with primaquine-sensitive American male Negroes.

Icterus Neonatorum

It has been demonstrated that in Mediterranean and Chinese full-term infants G6PD deficiency may cause icterus neonatorum (Doxiadis and Valaes, 1964; Yue and Strickland, 1965); it is probable also that the deficiency causes this disorder in other non-Negro races. The icterus is sometimes accentuated by the administration of water-soluble vitamin K analogues, or by exposure to naphthalene. It is considered that G6DP deficiency does not cause the disorder in full-term Negro infants—nevertheless, recent evidence suggests that it may in premature Negro infants (Oski, Eshaghpour and Williams, 1966).

The clinical aspects of icterus neonatorum associated with G6PD deficiency are well discussed by Doxiadis and Valaes (1964). In their large series of cases they found that in affected infants jaundice usually appeared on the second or third day of life and thus could not be distinguished from "physiological" jaundice; occasionally jaundice appeared later or in the first 24 hours. The jaundice was frequently severe and kernicterus was common.

Hæmatological Features. In the absence of exposure to drugs the blood peripheral picture is normal; in particular there is no evidence of hæmolysis. A slightly shortened red cell life span has been demonstrated and electron microscopy has shown an abnormality of the stroma resembling that seen in normal red cell ageing (Danon, Sheba and Ramot, 1961). During hæmolytic episodes there is the usual evidence of hæmolysis, namely a fall of hæmoglobin, reticulocytosis, polychromasia and hyperbilirubinæmia. Heinz bodies are seen in the early phases of hæmolysis but not alter; the red cells contain no excess methæmoglobin. The osmotic fragility is either normal or slightly decreased; the mechanical fragility is normal as is the Ham acid hæmolysis test. The antiglobulin (Coombs') test is negative. There is no abnormal hæmoglobin, no excess fœtal hæmoglobin and the sickle-cell test is normal.

Laboratory Detection of Sensitive Individuals. The first tests used to detect sensitive subjects were the Heinz body test and GSH stability test. These tests have been superseded by more specific screening tests.

The Heinz Body Test. The principle of this test is that when G6PD-deficient red cells are incubated with acetylphenylhydrazine they develop more Heinz bodies and in a greater proportion of cells than do normal cells. Details are given by Dacie and Lewis (1963). While this test is simple to perform and is consistently positive in subjects with marked G6PD deficiency, it has certain disadvantages, including difficulty of standardization. Furthermore, it occasionally gives false positive results in patients with thalassæmia and in normal non-anæmic subjects (Beutler, 1966a).

Glutathione (GSH) Stability Test. The principle of this test, introduced by Beutler (1957), is that incubation of G6PD-deficient cells with acetylphenyl-hydrazine for a period of two hours results in a marked decrease in red cell GSH, but little or no fall in normal cells. Recently Beutler, Duron and Kelly (1963) have published an improved method of GSH assay. Although in general there is a good correlation between the GSH stability test and enzyme assays, occasional discrepancies occur. Thus false positive results have been described in Hb E-thalassæmia disease, congenital nonspherocytic hæmolytic anæmia due to glutathione reductase deficiency and renal insufficiency (Beutler, 1966a).

Screening Tests. (a) *Dye Screening Tests.* The principle of these tests is that the decolourization of a dye (usually brilliant cresyl blue) is used to measure NADP reduction in a test system. A red cell hæmolysate is incubated in the presence of excess glucose-6-phosphate as substrate and NADP as co-enzyme, together with brilliant cresyl blue dye. Dehydrogenation of glucose-6-phosphate, catalysed by G6PD in the reaction mixture, results in the reduction of NADP to NADPH. The added dye is reduced to a colourless compound in proportion to the amount of NADPH formed. Absence or deficiency of the enzyme results in a significantly prolonged dye-decolouriza-tion time. Details of the test, which is essentially that of Motulsky, Kraut, Thieme and Musto (1959), are given by Dacie and Lewis (1963).

(b) *Methæmoglobin Reduction Test.* In this test nitrite is used to oxidize hæmoglobin to methæmoglobin and the reduction of methæmoglobin in the presence of methylene blue, which stimulates the shunt pathway, is used as an indication of G6PD activity. Details are given by Brewer, Tarlov and Alving (1962).

The screening tests will satisfactorily detect hemizygous males and homozygous females. The proportion of female heterozygotes detected by these tests varies, but is up to 80 per cent with the methæmoglobin reduction test. The problem of detection of female heterozygotes is discussed in detail by Motulsky (1965).

Enzyme Assay. The method is based on that of Kornberg and Horecker (1955) and measures spectrophotometrically the rate of reduction of NADP to NADPH. Values in fully expressed hemizygous males range from 0 to approximately 15 per cent of normal, activity in Negroes being generally from 3 to 15 per cent and in Mediterranean and Oriental subjects from 0 to 8 per cent (Carson and Frischer, 1966). As mentioned, there is a wide variation of activity in heterozygote females.

Spot Tests. A spot test was introduced by Fairbanks and Beutler in 1962; recently a new fluorescent spot test which is apparently technically superior has been described (Beutler, 1966b).

Diagnosis. The possibility of drug-induced hæmolysis due to G6PD deficiency or favism should be considered in any patient with an unexplained acute hæmolytic anæmia in which the antiglobulin (Coombs') test is negative, especially in persons of Negro, Mediterranean or Oriental ancestry. When the diagnosis is suspected on clinical grounds a screening test should be performed and, if possible, an enzyme assay. In fully expressed subjects the timing of the assay is not important, but it may be in heterozygotes. It has been pointed out that young cells have a higher G6PD activity than mature cells. The increase in younger cells occurring during a hæmolytic episode may therefore mask a G6PD deficiency in a heterozygote female. In fully expressed subjects with severe deficiency the rise, if it occurs at all, is not sufficient to obscure diagnosis (Carson and Frischer, 1966). The assay should be repeated two to four months after the hæmolytic episode in patients in whom the diagnosis of G6PD deficiency is definitely suspected, despite a normal G6PD activity on assay during or shortly after hæmolysis.

Differential Diagnosis. Not all cases of drug-induced hæmolysis are due to G6PD deficiency. Some can be shown to have an immunological basis, e.g. quinidine, while in other cases the mechanism is uncertain (de Leeuw, Shapiro and Lowenstein, 1963; Beutler, 1964). A few cases have been shown to be associated with other metabolic abnormalities, e.g. glutathione reductase deficiency and the hæmoglobinopathy associated with hæmoglobin Zürich (Frick, Hitzig and Betke, 1962).

Treatment. Treatment consists of withdrawal of the drug or of fava beans, blood transfusion as necessary and, with severe hæmolytic reactions, measures designed to prevent oliguria. No drug has been shown to be therapeutically effective in limiting the hæmolysis.

Congenital Non-spherocytic Hæmolytic Anæmia

In recent years a small number of cases of congenital non-spherocytic hæmolytic anæmia have been described in children with deficiency of G6PD; references to original case reports are given by Loder and de Gruchy (1965) and Beutler (1966a). In general, affected subjects have a chronic mild to moderate anæmia present from birth; the anæmia may be exacerbated by the administration of drugs or by infection. Some cases have presented with neonatal jaundice. Most reported cases have been in Caucasians, mainly of Northern European origin, in whom the disorder has been transmitted as a sex-linked character. The enzyme has been shown to be more labile in subjects with chronic hæmolytic anæmia than in other types of G6PD deficiency (Kirkman, McCurdy and Naiman, 1964) and this may possibly explain the fact that hæmolysis is continuous rather than intermittent.

Most cases appear to belong to the Type I group of non-spherocytic hæmolytic anæmias, but it should be realized that this group includes congenital hæmolytic anæmias due to at least several other defects (Dacie, 1964; Loder and de Gruchy, 1965).

Other Features of G6PD

Occurrence of Variants. The practicability of electrophoretic separation of G6PD into iso-enzyme fractions has permitted identification, partial purification and kinetic studies to be carried out on hæmolysate material. Using such criteria as electrophoretic mobility, Michaelis constants with natural and abnormal substrates, temperature lability, storage stability and activation energy a variety of mutants of G6PD have now been documented. Current data are tabulated by Carson and Frischer (1966).

G6PD Deficiency in Tissues other than Red Cells. Red cell G6PD deficiency in Negroes is accompanied by low values for this enzyme in lens tissue (Zinkham, 1961) and platelets (Wurzel, McCreary, Baker and Gumerman, 1961), both tissues being non-nucleated. An association between this enzyme deficiency and cataract has been reported (Kinoshita, 1964). Nucleated cells appear to be normal in this respect. Affected Caucasians, however, demonstrate sub-normal G6PD activities in many tissues, viz. leucocytes (Marks and Gross, 1959; Ramot, Fisher, Szeinberg, Adam, Sheba and Gafni, 1959a), platelets (Ramot et al., 1959b), liver (Brunetti, Rosetti and Broccia, 1960), skin (Gartler, Gandini and Cepellini, 1962), saliva (Ramot, Sheba, Adam and Ashkenazi, 1960), and kidney and adrenals (Chan, Todd and Wong, 1965).

Elevated Activities of GP6D. Recently there was reported (Dern, 1966) a family in which four males had red cell G6PD activities approximately four times the normal mean value and six females had elevated intermediate activities. Inheritance followed the expected pattern, there were no clinical or other hæmatological abnormalities and the chromosome pattern of an affected male subject was normal. Leucocyte G6PD activity of another affected male was increased also to approximately four times the normal mean value. Apart from reticulocytosis, the only other known situation yielding elevated red cell G6PD activity is hyperthyroidism (Pearson and Druyan, 1961) in which levels approximately twice the normal value may occur.

OTHER HÆMOLYTIC DISORDERS ASSOCIATED WITH ABNORMALITIES OF THE PENTOSE PHOSPHATE PATHWAY

Hæmolytic Anæmia associated with Glutathione Reductase Deficiency

A new syndrome of hereditary glutathione reductase deficiency associated with hæmatological and neurological abnormalities has been described by Waller, Löhr, Zysno, Gerok, Voss and Strauss (1965). Hæmatologically there is thrombocytopenia, non-spherocytic hæmolytic anæmia or pancytopenia. The pancytopenia may become dangerously severe after prolonged therapy with phenopyrine derivatives, primaquine or chloroquine, and may cause death. The liver and spleen are always enlarged. Neurologically all patients from four families with the enzyme defect showed spastic signs and abnormal EEG findings, and in one family there was oligophrenia. The disorder appears to be transmitted as an autosomal dominant. There is no successful therapy for these patients; drugs which cause accentuation of the hæmatological abnormalities should be avoided. Glutathione reductase deficiency is found in red cells, white cells and platelets. The GSH content of the red cells is normal and the GSH stability test normal or slightly impaired. The Heinz body test is markedly positive. Fornaini, Bianchini, Leoncini and Fantoni (1964) briefly report a case of non-spherocytic congenital hæmolytic anæmia associated with glutathione reductase deficiency but no neurological abnormalities are described.

Desforges, Thayer and Dawson (1959) report a case of sulfoxone-induced hæmolytic anæmia in which there was a moderate reduction of glutathione reductase activity; however, the significance of this reduction in relation to the hæmolysis is uncertain. Carson, Brewer and Ickes (1961) also report a patient with an approximately 50 per cent reduction of glutathione reductase activity and increased susceptibility to hæmolysis with 8-aminoquinolines.

Non-spherocytic Congenital Hæmolytic Anæmia associated with GSH Deficiency

Reports of red cell GSH deficiency (Waller and Gerok, 1964; Oort, Loos and Prins, 1961) without G6PD deficiency have been followed by a more extensive study of five affected members of a Dutch family, all with a fairly well compensated hæmolytic anæmia (Prins, Oort, Loos, Zürcher and Beckers, 1966). The disorder appears to be inherited as an autosomal recessive. Osmotic fragility, glycolytic activity and ATP of the deficient red cells were normal and the cells showed little morphological abnormality apart from slight anisocytosis and slight hypochromia. In the Heinz body formation test a number of comparatively small Heinz bodies was produced. The rate of hæmolysis *in vivo* was increased by administration of primaquine. Apart from a diminished GSH, the red cells exhibited a low activity of glyoxalase, an enzyme which requires GSH as co-factor.

The ability of the cells to sustain GSH produced artificially by hæmolysates supplemented with GSSG was demonstrated. However, the cells were unable to synthesize ^{14}C-GSH in incubates supplemented with ^{14}C-glycine and containing adequate glutamate and cysteine, whereas normal red cells were competent in this respect. In addition the GSH-deficient cells were incapable of synthesizing ^{14}C-labelled GSH when ^{14}C-glutamine replaced the poorly permeable glutamate, whereas normal cells yielded radioactive GSH. It was suggested that the primary defect in GSH deficiency is an inability of the red cells to synthesize GSH. Synthesis of GSH occurs in two stages, viz. glutamyl-cysteine formation followed by glycine fixation to yield the tripeptide. A separate study of two cases of congenital GSH deficiency (Boivin and Galand, 1965) suggests that the second stage, the attachment of glycine, is defective.

6-Phosphogluconic Dehydrogenase Deficiency

The screening of 1,148 unrelated subjects revealed a partial deficiency of red cell 6-phosphogluconate dehydrogenase in two Caucasians and three American Negroes (Brewer and Dern, 1964a, b; Dern, Brewer, Tashian and Shows, 1966). In deficient subjects the activities were 42–65 per cent of normal values and an autosomal inheritance was demonstrated. In one family the data suggested that affected subjects were heterozygous for the mutant gene. None of the five deficient subjects had any physical or hæmatological abnormalities and one subject gave no response to 60 mg. primaquine daily, a dose level provoking severe hæmolysis in primaquine-sensitive subjects. In two affected subjects studied the leucocytes contained 6PGD activities significantly less than normal values. Starch-gel electrophoresis revealed that the affected subjects had diminished levels of the normal enzymes rather than a mutant enzyme.

Starch gel electrophoresis studies have revealed the existence of several variants of the enzyme, not, apparently, associated with hæmatological abnormalities (Parr, 1966; Bowman, Carson, Frischer and DeGaray, 1966). A recent exception is a report (Scialom, Najean and Bernard, 1966) of a male with partial 6PGD deficiency accompanied by a congenital non-spherocytic hæmolytic anæmia. Autohæmolysis yielded a Type I value, GSH and GSH stability were normal, and pentose phosphate pathway activity was probably somewhat depressed when corrected for the young red cell population. Stimulation of this pathway by methylene blue was also less than normal.

HÆMOLYTIC ANÆMIAS ASSOCIATED WITH ABNORMALITIES OF THE EMBDEN-MEYERHOF PATHWAY

Pyruvate Kinase (PK) Deficiency Hæmolytic Anæmia

The association of PK deficiency with non-spherocytic congenital hæmolytic anæmia was first described by Valentine and his collaborators (Valentine, Tanaka and Miwa, 1961; Tanaka, Valentine and Miwa, 1962). Since then reports of at least 80 cases have been published, the literature being reviewed by Keitt (1966). Most cases have the hæmatological characteristics of Type II non-spherocytic congenital hæmolytic anæmia described by Selwyn and Dacie (1954), but it is now realized that there is a much wider range of clinical severity than in the cases originally described.

Clinical Features. There is considerable variation in the severity of the disorder, the clinical picture ranging from that of a severe hæmolytic anæmia presenting in early infancy to a fairly well compensated hæmolytic disorder of adults. However, in general, the defect appears to be fairly severe and, in many reported cases, the clinical onset has been in infancy or early childhood; in some cases jaundice has been present at birth. Less commonly the disorder presents in late childhood or early adult life. The common manifestations of a congenital hæmolytic anæmia, namely jaundice and slight to moderate splenomegaly, are usual, but in less severely affected subjects presenting in the second or third decades clinical icterus may be absent. Hepatomegaly is common, especially in patients who have had numerous transfusions; cholelithiasis is also common. In general, the clinical and hæmatological features tend to remain fairly constant in the individual patient, but there may be variation in severity in the same family; intercurrent infection or surgery may cause a temporary increase in anæmia. There is evidence to suggest that there may be a relatively high mortality rate in the first few years of life. Nevertheless, survival to adult life is common even in patients presenting in infancy, and those surviving to adult life may lead fairly normal active lives.

Inheritance. The disorder is transmitted as an autosomal recessive trait and it has been shown that both parents of an affected subject show a moderate reduction in PK activity. Most, but not all, reported cases have been in persons of Northern European origin; both sexes are equally affected. Heterozygous subjects have no clinical manifestations of the disorder and their peripheral blood picture is normal.

Hæmatological Features. Reported hæmoglobin values show considerable variation, ranging from 5 to 12 g. per 100 ml. The increase in reticulocyte count also varies from patient to patient; before splenectomy it is usually slight to moderate, but after splenectomy high values, e.g. 50 per cent or more, are common. In most reported cases the red cells have shown a fairly uniform round macrocytosis, of moderate to marked degree; the macrocytes show only a mild variation in size and little or no poikilocytosis. The cells are either normally hæmoglobinized or very slightly hypochromic; polychromasia is usual and a variable number of nucleated red cells may be

present. A few cells with irregularly crenated or contracted margins, some
of which are smaller than normal and stain slightly more deeply than normal
are usually present. Post-splenectomy, siderocytes and Pappenheimer bodies
are commonly present and are often numerous.

Oski, Nathan, Sidel and Diamond (1964) reported the case of a child
with severe congenital non-spherocytic hæmolytic anæmia associated with
PK deficiency and marked abnormalities of red cell morphology which were
in some respects similar to those seen in acanthocytosis; however, in
contrast to the situation in acanthocytosis the serum β-lipoprotein was
normal. The patient was atypical in that the increased hæmolysis in the
autohæmolysis test was not reduced by ATP. Both parents were shown to be
carriers of the PK-deficiency trait, but the mother was also a carrier of the
G6PD-deficiency trait.

The osmotic fragility of fresh blood is normal or slightly decreased; the
fragility of incubated blood is usually but not invariably increased. The
autohæmolysis test classically shows a marked increase of hæmolysis
uncorrected by glucose but corrected by ATP (de Gruchy, Santamaria,
Parsons and Crawford, 1960). However, in mildly affected subjects the
degree of hæmolysis in blood alone may be within the normal range, although
added glucose does not reduce the amount of hæmolysis as in normal subjects
(Grimes et al., 1964a). The antiglobulin (Coombs') test is negative, as is the
Ham acid hæmolysis test and the test for Heinz bodies. No abnormal type
of hæmoglobin has been demonstrated nor has any increase of fœtal or
A$_2$ hæmoglobin.

Diagnosis. The diagnosis should be considered in any case of non-
spherocytic congenital hæmolytic anæmia, especially when the clinical
features suggest recessive inheritance. Estimation of the red cell PK activity
will establish the diagnosis; further confirmatory evidence may be obtained
by the demonstration of typical heterozygote values in parents and other
relatives. Recently a screening test for PK deficiency has been described
(Beutler, 1966b).

Pyruvate Kinase Values. Values in affected homozygous subjects usually
range from less than 10 to 40 per cent of the normal mean value (Grimes
et al., 1964a) but occasionally are higher. In rare cases values are in the
lower normal range, but are nevertheless abnormally low if the increase of
reticulocytes is allowed for; in such cases estimation of the 2,3-DPG values
of fresh and incubated cells may give strong supportive diagnostic evidence
(Loder and de Gruchy, 1965). There is no correlation between the enzyme
level and the apparent severity of the hæmolytic anæmia. Heterozygotes
commonly show about one-half normal mean values (Tanaka et al., 1962).

Rarely the PK value is moderately decreased in other disorders. Loder and
de Gruchy (1965) measured PK activity in over 70 patients with anæmia of
varying degree, including a number of other types of hæmolytic anæmia;
values were normal or increased in all but two cases, namely one case of
hereditary spherocytosis and one case of paroxysmal nocturnal hæmoglobinuria in an aplastic phase, which showed a moderate decrease; diagnosis
must therefore be based on a consideration of the clinical and hæmatological
features as well as on the PK values.

Treatment. The main form of treatment is blood transfusion as required for symptomatic comfort. Requirements vary significantly and may be heavy; nevertheless, some patients reach adult life without requiring transfusion. Originally splenectomy was not considered to be of benefit, but more recent evidence suggests that it may cause improvement even though the hæmolysis persists. Nathan and Gardner (1965) in transfusion experiments showed that the intrinsic cell defect is worsened by passage through the spleen which "tempers" the cells for hepatic destruction, and that removal of the spleen improves the survival of PK-deficient cells. Furthermore, there are a number of reports of improvement following splenectomy with lessening of transfusion requirements and rise of hæmoglobin, together with subjective improvement and increased exercise tolerance (Keitt, 1966). Thus splenectomy should be considered in any patient with significant transfusion requirements. Infection, when present, should be treated promptly and adequately.

Associated Abnormalities in PK-deficient Red Cells. In addition to enzymopenia, these red cells have markedly elevated levels of 2,3-DPG (Loder and de Gruchy, 1965) and usually, though not invariably, a low ATP content (Robinson et al., 1961; Grimes et al., 1964a; Nathan et al., 1965; Keitt, 1966). Abnormal leakage of potassium occurs from cells incubated in vitro (Selwyn and Dacie, 1954; Nathan et al., 1965) and there is a normal or depressed glucose consumption (Grimes et al., 1964a; Keitt, 1966). Incubation in vitro over a period of several hours results in an abnormally rapid fall of ATP (Robinson et al., 1961; Nathan et al., 1965).

A second interesting feature of PK-deficient red cells is their ability to consume glucose with the production of ATP and lactate despite a gross block in the Embden-Meyerhof pathway. It is possible that the diminished PK activity is nevertheless adequate to permit glycolysis for the short period that these red cells survive. This restricted survival time results in large numbers of reticulocytes which are the preponderant cells in more severely affected patients. Reticulocytes are known to contain residual oxidative phosphorylation activity and this pathway is an alternative source of ATP. Keitt (1966) has proposed that in PK deficiency this pathway is in fact used and his relevant studies on a severely affected patient with a reticulocyte count of 68–85 per cent may be summarized thus: (a) PK-deficient red cells maintained ATP levels during short-term incubation in the absence of glucose. (b) ATP disappeared when the cells were treated with cyanide, an inhibitor of oxidative phosphorylation, whereas normal red cells were apparently unaffected by this treatment. (c) Blood rich in reticulocytes but metabolically not defective was treated with fluoride, an inhibitor of enolase, thus simulating PK-deficient blood in containing a high proportion of reticulocytes together with a block in anærobic glycolysis. Such treated blood further resembled PK deficiency in that ATP was not lost upon short-term incubation unless cyanide was present. The author concluded that in PK deficiency the reticulocytes survive by utilizing oxidative phosphorylation as a means of producing ATP, but on maturation, when this route disappears, the cell is doomed by its dependence solely upon the impaired EMP.

It has been suggested by several authors that in addition to the enzyme deficiency there exists a membrane defect. Some support for this is offered by the gross in vitro hæmolysis that may occur after prolonged incubation.

H

OTHER ANÆMIAS ASSOCIATED WITH ABNORMALITIES OF THE EMBDEN-MEYERHOF PATHWAY

Triosephosphate Isomerase (TPI) Deficiency Hæmolytic Anæmia

Valentine and his colleagues (1966) have described severe hæmolytic anæmia in two infants with a deficiency of the enzyme triosephosphate isomerase (TPI) in the red cells. Triosephosphate isomerase activity was reduced in the patients' red cells to less than 10 per cent of normal and in the parents and other siblings to approximately 50 per cent of normal, suggesting an autosomal recessive mode of inheritance; the heterozygote subjects were clinically normal. The osmotic fragility of fresh blood was normal. The white cells also showed TPI deficiency, values being approximately 10 to 20 per cent of normal; however, they were normal in morphology. In addition to the hæmolytic anæmia the patients suffered from recurrent infections and progressive neurological disease. The nature of the neurological abnormality and the mechanism of the increased susceptibility to infection are unexplained; possibly they indicate a widespread enzyme deficiency.

Diphosphoglycerate Mutase Deficiency Hæmolytic Anæmia

Prankerd (1961) reported evidence of deficiency of the enzyme diphosphoglycerate mutase in two cases of hæmolytic anæmia (a father and son), and Löhr and Waller (1963) have reported evidence indicating a deficiency of the enzyme in three unrelated patients; an associated feature described by the latter authors was mesobilifuscinuria. Schröter (1965) reports studies on the family of a case of a severe fatal congenital non-spherocytic anæmia, observed between the fourth and twelfth weeks of life. In the erythrocytes of the asymptomatic parents, the sister, and the father's mother the 2,3-DPG content was diminished by 50 per cent, and the 2,3-diphosphoglycerate mutase activity by 55 to 60 per cent. Because of numerous transfusions, enzyme assays were not performed on the blood of the propositus. It is considered that the defect was transmitted as an autosomal recessive trait. Schröter points out that his case varies in mode of inheritance and clinical picture from cases previously described.

Hæmolytic Anæmia associated with Glyceraldehyde-3-phosphate Dehydrogenase Deficiency

The occurrence of compensated hæmolytic disease in a father and son with red cells deficient in the enzyme glyceraldehyde-3-phosphate dehydrogenase (GAPD) has been reported by Harkness and Yunis (1966). The peripheral blood films revealed macrocytes, target cells, burr cells and polychromasia. Osmotic fragility was normal. Red cell autohæmolysis was increased but was corrected by glucose and ATP. Glutathione levels and stability were normal. The erythrocytes of both father and son contained 20 to 30 per cent of the normal levels of GAPD; values for all other glycolytic enzymes, including the hexose monophosphate pathway and glutathione reductase were either normal or moderately elevated.

Hexokinase Deficiency

Recently Valentine and his colleagues (1967) have described a patient with congenital hæmolytic anæmia associated with a specific deficiency of hexokinase in the red cells; this was shown to result in decreased metabolism of glucose via the Embden-Meyerhof pathway. The leucocytes showed normal enzyme activity and indirect studies suggested that the activity was probably normal also in the platelets. Family studies, although not conclusive, suggested an autosomal recessive mode of inheritance.

Hexokinase deficiency has also been described in the red cells of patients with Fanconi-type pancytopenia (Löhr and Waller, 1965); the deficiency was associated with a decrease of red cell ATP levels and lactate production. Chromosome aberrations were also demonstrated (Schroder, Anschütz and Kropp, 1964). Although this disorder is not characterized by hæmolytic anæmia, it may represent an example of an hereditary enzymopathy.

References

ADAM, A. (1961). Linkage between deficiency of glucose-6-phosphate dehydrogenase and colour-blindness. *Nature, Lond.*, **189**, 686.

ALLEN, W. and JANDL, J. H. (1961). Oxidative hemolysis and precipitation of hemoglobin. II. Role of thiols in oxidant drug action. *J. clin. Inv.*, **40**, 454.

BARTLETT, G. R. (1959). Human red cell glycolytic intermediates. *J. biol. Chem.*, **234**, 449.

BEUTLER, E. (1957). The glutathione instability of drug-sensitive red cells: A new method for the *in vitro* detection of drug sensitivity. *J. Lab. clin. Med.*, **49**, 84.

BEUTLER, E. (1964). Drug-induced blood dyscrasias. III. Hemolytic anaemia. *J. Amer. med. Ass.*, **189**, 143.

BEUTLER, E. (1966a). Glucose-6-phosphate dehydrogenase deficiency. In *The Metabolic Basis of Inherited Disease* (Eds. Stanbury, J. B., Wyngaarden, J. B. and Fredrickson, D. S.), 1060. New York: McGraw-Hill.

BEUTLER, E. (1966b). A series of new screening procedures for pyruvate kinase deficiency, glucose-6-phosphate dehydrogenase deficiency, and glutathione reductase deficiency. *Blood*, **28**, 558.

BEUTLER, E. and BALUDA, M. C. (1964). The separation of glucose-6-phosphate dehydrogenase deficient erythrocytes from the blood of heterozygotes for glucose-6-phosphate dehydrogenase deficiency. *Lancet*, **i**, 189.

BEUTLER, E., DERN, R. J. and ALVING, A. S. (1954). The hemolytic effect of primaquine. II. A study of primaquine-sensitive erythrocytes. *J. Lab. clin. Med.*, **44**, 177.

BEUTLER, E., DERN, R. J. and ALVING, A. S. (1955). The hemolytic effect of primaquine. VI. An *in vitro* test for sensitivity of erythrocytes to primaquine. *J. Lab. clin. Med.*, **45**, 40.

BEUTLER, E., DERN, R. J., FLANAGAN, C. L. and ALVING, A. S. (1955). The haemolytic effect of primaquine. VII. Biochemical studies of drug-sensitive erythrocytes. *J. Lab. clin. Med.*, **45**, 286.

BEUTLER, E., DURON, O. and KELLY, B. M. (1963). Improved method for the determination of blood glutathione. *J. Lab. clin. Med.*, **61**, 882.

BHATTACHARYA, S. K., ROBSON, J. S. and STEWART, C. P. (1955). The determination of glutathione in blood and tissues. *Biochem. J.*, **60**, 696.

BISHOP, C., Rankine, D. M. and TALBOT, J. H. (1959). The nucleotides in normal human blood. *J. biol. Chem.*, **234**, 1233.

BOIVIN, P. and GALAND, C. (1965). La synthèse du gluthathion au cours de l'anémie hémolytique congénitale avec deficit en glutathion réduit. *Nouv. rev. fr. d'Hémat.*, **5**, 707.

BONSIGNORE, A., FORNAINI, G., SEGNI, G. and FANTONI, A. (1960). Glutathione-reductase and methaemoglobin reductase in erythrocytes of human subjects with a case history of favism. *Ital. J. Biochem.*, **9**, 345.

BOWMAN, J. E., CARSON, P. E., FRISCHER, H. and DE GARAY, A. L. (1966). Genetics of starch-gel electrophoretic variants of human 6-phosphogluconic dehydrogenase. population and family studies in the United States and in Mexico. *Nature, Lond,*: **210**, 811.

BOYER, S. H., PORTER, I. H. and WEILBACHER, R. G. (1962). Electrophoretic heterogeneity of glucose-6-phosphate dehydrogenase and its relationship to enzyme deficiency in man. *Proc. nat. Acad. Sci.*, **48**, 1868.

BREWER, G. J. and DERN, R. J. (1964a). Study of a kindred with a new inherited enzymatic deficiency of erythrocyte 6-phosphogluconic dehydrogenase (6-PGD) deficiency. *Clin. Res.*, **12**, 215.

BREWER, G. J. and DERN, R. J. (1964b). A new inherited enzymatic deficiency of human erythrocytes: 6-phosphogluconate dehydrogenase deficiency. *Amer. J. hum. Genet.*, **16**, 471.

BREWER, G. J., TARLOV, A. R. and ALVING, A. S. (1962). The methaemoglobin reduction test for primaquine-type sensitivity of erythrocytes. *J. amer. med. Ass.*, **180**, 386.

BRODRIBB, H. S. and WORSSAM, A. R. H. (1961). Favism in an Englishman. *Brit. med. J.*, **i**, 1367.

BRUNETTI, P., ROSSETTI, R. and BROCCIA, G. (1960). Nuovo acquisizimi in tema di bio-enzimologia del favismo ittero-emoglobinurico. Nota III. l'attivita glucose-6-fosato deidaogenasica del parenchima epalico. *Rass. fisiopat. Clin. Terap.*, **32**, 338.

CARSON, P. E., BREWER, G. J. and Ickes, C. (1961). Decreased glutathione reductase with susceptibility to hemolysis. *J. Lab. clin. Med.*, **58**, 840.

CARSON, P. E., FLANAGAN, C. L., ICKES, C. E. and ALVING, A. S. (1966). Enzymatic deficiency in primaquine-sensitive erythrocytes. *Science*, **124**, 484.

CARSON, P. E. and FRISCHER, H. (1966). Glucose-6-phosphate dehydrogenase deficiency and related disorders of the pentose phosphate pathway. *Amer. J. Med.*, **41**, 744.

CERLETTI, P. and BUCCI, E. (1960). Adenylate kinase of mammalian erythrocytes. *Biochem. biophys. Acta*, **38**, 45.

CHAN, T. K., TODD, D. and WONG, C. C. (1965). Tissue enzyme levels in erythrocyte glucose-6-phosphate dehydrogenase deficiency. *J. Lab. clin. Med.*, **66**, 937.

COHEN, G. and HOCHSTEIN, P. (1962). Primaquine-induced generation of hydrogen peroxide in erythrocytes. (Abstr.) *Blood*, **20**, 785.

COHEN, G. and HOCHSTEIN, P. (1963). Glutathione peroxidase: the primary agent for the elimination of hydrogen peroxide in erythrocytes. *Biochemistry*, **2**, 1420.

DACIE, J. V. (1964). The hereditary non-spherocytic haemolytic anaemias. *Acta haemat.*, **31**, 177.

DACIE, J. V. and LEWIS, S. M. (1963). *Practical Haematology*. London: Churchill.

DANON, D., SHEBA, CH. and RAMOT, B. (1961). The morphology of glucose-6-phosphate dehydrogenase deficient erythrocytes: electron-microscopic studies. *Blood*, **17**, 229.

DAVIES, P. (1962). Favism: a family study. *Quart. J. Med.*, **31**, 157.

DE GRUCHY, G. C., LODER, P. B. and HENNESSY, I. V. (1962). Haemolysis and glycolytic metabolism in hereditary elliptocytosis. *Brit. J. Haemat.*, **8**, 168.

DE GRUCHY, G. C., SANTAMARIA, J. N., PARSONS, I. C. and CRAWFORD, H. (1960). Non-spherocytic congenital haemolytic anemia. *Blood*, **16**, 1371.

DE LEEUW, N. K. M., SHAPIRO, L. and LOWENSTEIN, L. (1963). Drug-induced haemolytic anaemia. *Ann. intern. Med.*, **58**, 592.

DERN, R. J. (1966). A new hereditary quantitative variant of glucose-6-phosphate dehydrogenase characterised by a marked increase in enzyme activity. *J. Lab. clin. Med.*, **68**, 560.

DERN, R. J., BEUTLER, E. and ALVING, A. S. (1954). The hemolytic effect of primaquine. II. The natural course of the hemolytic anemia and the mechanism of its self-limited character. *J. Lab. clin. Med.*, **44**, 171.

DERN, R. J., BREWER, G. J., TASHIAN, R. E. and SHOWS, T. B. (1966). Hereditary variation of erythrocytic 6-phosphogluconate dehydrogenase. *J. Lab. clin. Med.*, **67**, 255.

DE SANDRE, G. and GHIOTTO, G. (1960). An enzymic disorder in the erythrocytes of paroxysmal nocturnal haemoglobinuria: a deficiency in acetylcholinesterase activity. *Brit. J. Haemat.*, **6**, 39.

DE SANDRE, G. GHIOTTO, G. and MASTELLA, G. (1956). L'acetil-colinesterasi eritrocitaria. II. Rapporti con le malatti emolitiche. *Acta med. patav.*, **16**, 310.

DESFORGES, J. F., THAYER, W. W. and DAWSON, J. P. (1959). Hemolytic anemia induced by sulfoxone therapy, with investigations into the mechanisms of its production. *Amer. J. Med.*, **27**, 132.

DOXIADIS, S. A. and VALAES, T. (1964). The clinical picture of glucose-6-phosphate dehydrogenase deficiency in early infancy. *Arch. Dis. Childh.*, **39**, 545.

EDEN, H. A., FINCH, C. A. and McKEE, R. W. (1949). Congenital methemoglobinemia. A clinical and biochemical study of a case. *J. clin. Inv.*, **28**, 265.

FAIRBANKS, V. F. and BEUTLER, E. (1962). A simple method for detection of erythrocyte glucose-6-phosphate dehydrogenase (G-6-PD spot test). *Blood*, **20**, 591.

FARMER, S. N. and MAIZELS, M. (1939). Organic anions of human erythrocytes. *Biochem. J.*, **33**, 280.

FORNAINI, G., BIANCHINI, E., LEONCINI, G. and FANTONI, A. (1964). Metabolic aspects of red cells in congenital non-spherocytic haemolytic anaemia. *Brit. J. Haemat.*, **10**, 23.

FRICK, P. G., HITZIG, W. H. and BETKE, K. (1962). Hemoglobin Zürich. I. A new hemoglobin anomaly associated with acute hemolytic episodes with inclusion bodies after sulfonamide therapy. *Blood*, **20**, 261.

GARTLER, S. M., GANDINI, E. and CEPELLINI, R. (1962). Glucose-6-phosphate dehydrogenase deficient mutant in human cell culture. *Nature, Lond.*, **193**, 602.

VAN GASTEL, C., VAN DEN BERG, D., DE GIER, J. and VAN DEENEN, L. L. (1965). Some lipid characteristic of normal red blood cells of different age. *Brit. J. Haemat.*, **11**, 193.

GIBSON, O. H. (1948). The reduction of methaemoglobin in red blood cells and studies in the cause of idiopathic methaemoglobinaemia. *Biochem. J.*, **42**, 13.

GRIMES, A. J. (1965). Chemical aspects of haemolysis. *Proc. Roy. Soc. Med.*, **58**, 19.

GRIMES, A. J. and MEISLER, A. (1962). Possible cause of Heinz bodies in congenital Heinz-body anaemia. *Nature, Lond.*, **194**, 190.

GRIMES, A. J., MEISLER, A. and DACIE, J. V. (1964a). Hereditary non-spherocytic haemolytic anaemia. A study of red-cell carbohydrate metabolism in twelve cases of pyruvate kinase deficiency. *Brit. J. Haemat.*, **10**, 403.

GRIMES, A. J., MEISLER, A. and DACIE, J. V. (1964b). Congenital Heinz body anaemia. Further evidence on the cause of Heinz-body production in red cells. *Brit. J. Haemat.*, **10**, 281.

HARKNESS, D. R. and YUNIS, A. A. (1966). A new erythrocytic enzyme defect with hemolytic anemia: glyceraldehyde-3-phosphate dehydrogenase deficiency. *J. Lab. clin. Med.*, **68**, 879.

HILL, A. S., HAUT, A., CARTWRIGHT, G. E. and WINTROBE, M. M. (1964). The role of nonhemoglobin proteins and reduced glutathione in the protection of hemoglobin from oxidation *in vitro*. *J. clin. Inv.*, **43**, 17.

HOCKWALD, R. S., ARNOLD, J., CLAYMAN, C. B. and ALVING, A. S. (1952). Status of primaquine. IV. Toxicity of primaquine in negroes. *J. Amer. med. Ass.*, **149**, 1568.

JACOB, H. S. (1966). Abnormalities in the physiology of the erythrocyte membrane in hereditary spherocytosis. *Amer. J. Med.*, **41**, 734.

JACOB, H. S., INGBAR, S. H. and JANDL, J. H. (1965). Oxidative hemolysis and erythrocyte metabolism in hereditary acatalasia. *J. clin. Inv.*, **44**, 1187.

JOCELYN, P. C. (1960). The reduction of oxidized glutathione in erythrocyte haemolysates in pernicious anaemia. *Biochem. J.*, **77**, 363.

JOHNSON, A. B. and MARKS, P. A. (1958). Glucose metabolism and oxygen consumption in normal and glucose-6-phosphate dehydrogenase deficient human erythrocytes. *Clin. Res.*, **6**, 187.

KASHKET, S. and DENSTEDT, O. F. (1958). The metabolism of the erythrocyte. XV. Adenylate kinase of the erythrocyte. *Canad. J. Biochem. Physiol.*, **36**, 1057.

KATTAMIS, C. A. (1967). Personal communication.

KEITT, A. S. (1966). Pyruvate kinase deficiency and related disorders of red cell glycolysis. *Amer. J. Med.*, **41**, 762.

KELLERMEYER, R. W., CARSON, P. E., SCHRIER, S. L., TARLOV, A. R. and ALVING, A. S. (1961). The hemolytic effect of primaquine. XIV. Pentose metabolism in primaquine-sensitive erythrocytes. *J. Lab. clin. Med.*, **58**, 715.

KELLERMEYER, R. W., TARLOV, A. R., BREWER, G. J., CARSON, P. E. and ALVING, A. S. (1962). Haemolytic effect of therapeutic drugs: clinical considerations of the primaquine-type hemolysis. *J. Amer. med. Ass.*, **180**, 388.

KINOSHITA, J. H. (1964). Selected topics in opthalmic biochemistry. *A.M.A. Ardi. Opthal.*, **72**, 554.

KOJ, A. (1962). Biosynthesis of glutathione in human blood cells. *Acta Biochim. Polonika*, **9**, 11.

KORNBERG, A. and HORECKER, B. L. (1955). Glucose-6-phosphate dehydrogenase. In *Methods in Enzymology* (Eds. Colowick, S. P. and Kaplan, N.O.), Vol. 1, p. 323, New York: Academic Press.

LARIZZA, P., BRUNETTI, P. and GRIGNANI, F. (1960). Anemie emolitiche enzimopeniche. *Haematologica (Pavia)*, **45**, 1, 129.

LODER, P. B., BARBARCZY, G. and DC GRUCHY, G. C. (1967). Red-cell metabolism in hereditary spherocytosis. *Brit. J. Haemat.*, **13**, 95.

LODER, P. B., and DE GRUCHY. (1965). Red-cell enzymes and co-enzymes in non-spherocytic congenital haemolytic anaemias. *Brit. J. Haemat.*, **11**, 21.

LÖHR, G. W. and WALLER, H. D. (1963). Zur biochemie einiger angelborener hämolytischen anämien. *Folia haemat.*, N.F. **80**, 377.

LÖHR, G. W., WALLER, H. D., ANSCHÜTZ, F. and KNOPP, A. (1965). Biochemische defekte in den blutzellen bein fämiliaren panmyelopathie (Type Fanconi). *Human genetik*, **1**, 383.

MCCRAE, T. and OLLERY, J. C. (1933). Favism Report of a case. *J. Amer. med. Ass.*, **101**, 1389.

MARKS, P. A. and GROSS, R. T. (1959). Erythrocyte glucose-6-phosphate dehydrogenase deficiency: evidence of difference between Negroes and Caucasians with respect to this genetically determined trait. *J. clin. Inv.*, **38**, 2253.

MARKS, P. A., GROSS, R. T. and BANKS, J. (1961). Evidence for heterogeneity among subjects with glucose-6-phosphate dehydrogenase deficiency. *J. clin. Inv.*, **40**, 1060.

MILLER, A. and HORIUCHI, M. (1962). Erythrocyte glutathione. I. *In vitro* incorporation of radioactive amino acid precursors into the glutathione of human erythrocytes. *J. Lab. clin. Med.*, **60**, 756.

MILLS, G. C. (1957). Haemoglobin catabolism. I. Glutathione peroxidase, an erythrocyte enzyme which protects hemoglobin from oxidative breakdown. *J. biol. Chem.*, **229**, 189.

MILLS, G. C. and SUMMERS, L. B. (1959). The metabolism of nucleotides and other phosphate esters in erythrocytes during *in vitro* incubation at 37°. *Arch Biochem. Biophys.*, **84**, 7.

MOTULSKY, A. G. (1965). Theoretical and clinical problems of glucose-6-phosphate dehydrogenase deficiency. In *Abnormal Haemoglobins in Africa* (Ed. Jonxis, J. H. P.), p. 143. Oxford: Blackwell Scientific Publications.

MOTULSKY, A. G., KRAUT, J. M., THIEME, W. T. and MUSTO, P. E. (1959). Biochemical genetics of glucose-6-phosphate dehydrogenase deficiency. *Clin. Res.*, **7**, 89.

NATHAN, D. G. and GARDNER, F. H. (1965). The removal of pyruvate kinase deficient (PK) erythrocytes from the circulation of normal and splenectomized individuals. *Blood*, **26**, 896.

NATHAN, D. G., OSKI, F. A., SIDEL, V. W. and DIAMOND, L. K. (1965). Extreme hemolysis and red-cell distortion in erthrocyte pyruvate kinase deficiency. II. Measurements of erythrocyte glucose consumption, potassium flux and adenosine triphosphate stability. *New Engl. J. Med.*, **282**, 118.

OORT, M., LOOS, J. A. and PRINS, H. K. (1961). Hereditary absence of reduced glutathione in the erythrocytes—a new clincial and biochemical entity. *Vox Sang.*, **6**, 370.

OSKI, F. A., ESHAGHPOUR, E. and WILLIAMS, M. L. (1966). Red-cell glucose-6-phosphate dehydrogenase deficiency as a cause of hyperbilirubinemia in the premature infant. *J. Paed.*, **69**, 903.

OSKI, F. A., NATHAN, D. G., SIDEL, V. W. and DIAMOND, L. K. (1964). Extreme hemolysis and red-cell distortion in erythrocyte pyruvate kinase deficiency. I. Morphology, erythrokinetics and family enzyme studies. *New Engl. J. Med.*, **270**, 1023.

PANIZON, F. and VULLO, C. (1962). Effects of the administration of fava beans and primaquine on G6PD-deficient erythrocytes labelled with Cr51. *Haematologica*, **47**, 205.

PARR, C. W. (1966). Erythrocyte phosphogluconate dehydrogenase polymorphism. *Nature, Lond.*, **210**, 487.

PEARSON, H. A. and DRUYAN, R. (1961). Erythrocyte glucose-6-phosphate dehydrogenase activity related to thyroid activity. *J. Lab. clin. Med.*, **57**, 343.

PORTER, I. H., SCHULZE, J. and McKUSICK, V. A. (1962). Genetical linkage between the loci for glucose-6-phosphate dehydrogenase deficiency and colour-blindness in American Negroes. *Ann. hum. Genet.*, **26**, 107.

PRANKERD, T. A. J. (1961). The nature of the erythrocyte defect and the haemolytic mechanism in hereditary spherocytosis and hereditary nonspherocytic haemoytic anaemia. In *Hämolyse und hämolytische Erkrankungen*, 7th Freiburger Symposium, 1959. Schubothe, H. (hisg.), p. 136. Berlin-Gottingen-Heidelberg: Springer-Verlag.

PRINS, H. K., OORT, M., LOOS, J. A., ZÜRCHER, C. and BECKERS, T. (1966). Congenital nonspherocytic hemolytic anemia, associated with glutathione deficiency of the erythrocytes. Haematologic, biochemical and genetic studies. *Blood*, **27**, 145.

RAMOT, B., FISHER, S., SZEINBUERG, A., ADAM, A., SHEBA, CH. and GAFNI, D. (1959a). A study of subjects with erythrocyte glucose-6-phosphate dehydrogenase deficiency. II. Investigation of leukocyte enzymes. *J. clin. Inv.*, **38**, 2234.

RAMOT, B., SHEBA, CH., ADAM, A. and ASHKENAZI, I. (1960). Erythrocyte glucose-6-phosphate dehydrogenase deficient subjects: Enzyme level in saliva. *Nature, Lond.*, **185**, 931.

RAMOT, B., SZEINBERG, A., ADAM, A., SHEBA, CH. and GAFNI, D. (1959b). A study of subjects with erythrocyte glucose-6-phosphate dehydrogenase deficiency: investigation of platelet enzymes. *J. clin. Inv.*, **38**, 1659.

ROBINSON, M. A., LODER, P. B. and DE GRUCHY, G. C. (1961). Red-cell metabolism in non-spherocytic congenital haemolytic anaemia. *Brit. J. Haemat.*, **7**, 327.

ROTH, K. L. and FRUMIN, A. M. (1960). Studies on the haemolytic principle of the fava bean. *J. Lab. clin. Med.*, **56**, 695.

SASS, M. D. (1963) Utilization of alpha ketoglutarate by red blood cells for glutathione synthesis. *Nature, Lond.*, **200**, 1209.

SASS, M. D., CARUSO, C. J. and O'CONNELL, D. J. (1965). Decreased glutathione in ageing red cells. *Clin. Chim. Acta*, **11**, 334.

SCHRIER, S. L., KELLERMEYER, R. W. and ALVING, A. S. (1958). Coenzyme studies in primaquine-sensitive erythrocytes. *Proc. Soc. exp. biol. Med.*, **99**, 354.

SCHRIER, S. L., KELLERMEYER, R. W., CARSON, P. E., ICKES, C. E. and ALVING, A. S. (1958). The haemolytic effect of primaquine. IX. Enzymatic abnormalities in primaquine-sensitive erythrocytes. *J. Lab. clin. Med.*, **52**, 109.

SCHRIER, S. L., KELLERMEYER, R. W., CARSON, P. E., ICKES, C. E. and ALVING, A. S. (1959). The hemolytic effect of primaquine. X. Aldolase and glyceraldehyde-3-phosphate dehydrogenase activity in primaquine-sensitive erythrocytes. *J. Lab. clin. Med.*, **54**, 232.

SCHRÖDER, T. M., ANSCHUTZ, F. and KNOPP, A. (1964). Spontaneous chromosomen aberrationen bei familiärer panmyelopathie. *Human gentik*, **1**, 194.

SCHRÖTER, W. (1965). Kongenitale nichtsphärocytäre hamolytische anemia bei 2, 3,-diphosphoglyceratmutase-mangel der erythrocyten im frühen sänglingsalten. *Klin. Wschr.*, **43**, 1147.

SCIALOM, C., NAJEAN, Y. and BERNARD, J. (1966). Anémie hémolytique congénitale non spherocytaire avec déficit incomplet en 6-phosphogluconate déshydrogenase. *Nouv. rev. fr. d'Hemat.*, **6**, 452.

SCOTT, E. M., and HOSKINS, D. D. (1958). Hereditary methemoglobinemia in Alaskan eskimos and Indians. *Blood*, **13**, 795.

SELWYN, J. G. and DACIE, J. V. (1954). Autohaemolysis and other changes resulting from the incubation in vitro of red cells from patients with congenital haemolytic anaemia. *Blood*, **9**, 414.

STAMATOYANNOPOULOS, G. PANAYOTOPOULOS, A. and PAPAYANNOPOLOU, TH. (1964). Mild glucose-6-phosphate dehydrogenase deficiency in Greek males. *Lancet*, **ii**, 932.

SZEINBERG, A., ADAM, A., RAMOT, B., SHEBA, CH. and MEYERS, F. (1959). Incorporation of isotopically labelled glycine into glutathione of erythrocytes with glucose-6-phosphate dehydrogenase deficiency. *Biochim. biophys. Acta*, **36**, 65.

SZEINBERG, A. and MARKS, P. A. (1961). Substances stimulating glucose catabolism by the oxidative reactions of the pentose phosphate pathway in human erythrocytes. *J. clin. Inv.*, **40**, 914.

TAKAHARA, S. (1951). Acatalasemia (lack of catalase in blood) and oral progressive gangrene. *Proc. Jap. Acad.*, **27**, 295.

TAKAHARA, S. (1952). Progressive oral gangrene probably due to lack of catalase in the blood (acatalasaemia). *Lancet*, **ii**, 1101.

TAKAHARA, S., HAMILTON, H. B., NEEL, J. V., KOBARA, T. Y., OGURA, Y. and NISHIMURA, E. T. (1960). Hypocatalasemia: a new genetic carrier state. *J. clin. Inv.*, **39**, 610.

TANAKA, K. R., VALENTINE, W. N. and MIWA, S. (1962). Pyruvate kinase (PK) deficiency hereditary non-spherocytic hemolytic anemia. *Blood*, **19**, 267.

TARLOV, A. R., BREWER, G. J., CARSON, P. E. and ALVING, A. S. (1962). Primaquine sensitivity: Glucose-6-phosphate dehydrogenase deficiency: an inborn error of metabolism of medical and biological significance. *Arch. int. Med.*, **109**, 209.

TARLOV, A. R. and KELLERMEYER, R. W. (1961). The hemolytic effect of primaquine: XI. Decreased catalase activity in primaquine-sensitive erythrocytes. *J. Lab. clin. Med.*, **58**, 204.

TATIBANI, M., NAKAO, M. and YOSHIKAWA, H. (1958). Adenylate kinase in human erythrocytes. *J. Biochem. (Tokyo)*. **45**, 1037.

VALENTINE, W. N., SCHNEIDER, A. S., BAUGHAN, M. A., PAGLIA, D. E. and HEINS, H. L. (1966). Hereditary hemolytic anemia with triosephosphate isomerase deficiency. *Amer. J. Med.*, **41**, 27.

VALENTINE, W. N., TANAKA, K. R. and MIWA, S. (1961). A specific erythrocyte glycolytic enzyme defect (pyruvate kinase) in three subjects with congenital non-spherocytic hemolytic anemia. *Trans. Ass. Amer. Phys.*, **74**, 100.

VAUGHAN JONES, R. V., GRIMES, A. J., CARRELL, R. W. and LEHMANN, H. (1967). Köln Haemoglobinopathy. Further data and a comparison with other hereditary Heinz body anaemias. *Brit. J. Haemat.*, **13**, 394.

WALLER, H. D. and GEROK, W. (1964). Schwere strahleninduzierte hämolyse bei hereditören mangel an reduziertem glutathion in blutzellen. *Klin. Wschr.*, **42**, 948.

WALLER, H. D., LÖHR, G. W., ZYSNO, E., GEROK, W., VOSS, D. and STRAUSS, G. (1965). Glutathionereduktasemangel mit hämatologischen und neurologischen stonungen (Autosomal dominant vererbliche Bildung eines pathologischen Enzyms). *Klin Wschr.*, **43**, 413.

WURZEL, H., MCCREARY, T., BAKER, L. and GUMERMAN, L. (1961). Glucose-6-phosphate dehydrogenase activity in platelets. *Blood*, **17**, 314.

YVE, P. C. K. and STRICKLAND, M. (1965). Glucose-6-phosphate dehydrogenase deficiency and neonatal jaundice in Chinese male infants in Hong Kong. *Lancet*, **i**, 350.

ZINKHAM, W. H. (1959). An *in vitro* abnormality of glutathione metabolism in erythrocytes from normal newborns. *Paed.*, **23**, 18.

ZINKHAM, W. H. (1961). A deficiency of glucose-6-phosphate dehydrogenase activity in lens from individuals with primaquine-sensitive erythrocytes. *Bull. Johns Hopkins Hosp.*, **109**, 206.

Chapter 16

TREATMENT OF HÆMOLYTIC DISEASE OF THE NEWBORN BY INTRA-UTERINE TRANSFUSION

C. A. HOLMAN and JADWIGA KARNICKI

INTRODUCTION

HÆMOLYTIC disease of the newborn is the result of immune antibodies to a blood group antigen passing from a pregnant woman to her fœtus and reacting with that same antigen on the fœtal red cells. The attachment of the antibody to the fœtal red cells leads to a hæmolytic process with red cell destruction, increased bilirubin production, increased red cell production, increase in extra-medullary hæmopoietic tissue with consequent hepato-splenomegaly and, when destruction exceeds production, to anæmia. The anæmia produces little disturbance in the fœtus until the hæmoglobin level drops to about 7–8 gm./100 ml. when cardiac failure, presumably from in-adequate oxygen supply, appears and is followed by fœtal œdema. This condition, known as hydrops fœtalis, has long been recognized in its fully developed form in which there is generalized gross œdema of the fœtus, ascites, pleural and pericardial effusions and a considerable enlargement of the placenta with gross hydropic changes. More recently, because of attempts to alter the course of the disease, we have seen the condition in the course of its development and found very varied pictures in which either fœtus or placenta may be more severely affected than the other. As hydrops appears, the fœtal movements diminish in strength, sometimes after a period of excessive activity, and disappear altogether although the fœtal heart may continue to beat for days or weeks. With intra-uterine death the fluid may be gradually absorbed leaving a macerated fœtus and a disproportion-ately heavy placenta.

The degree of affection of the fœtus depends partly on the quantity of immune, 7–S, antibody gamma-globulin reaching it and partly on the duration of the process. There remains much that is not known about the antibodies and the fœtal reaction to them, so that apparently similar con-ditions may yield widely different results.

In the last twenty years considerable advances have been made in the treatment of this disease by the use of exchange transfusions and induction of labour. Kernicterus has been largely eliminated by careful exchange transfusions guided by bilirubin levels. Cardiac failure and respiratory embarrassment have responded to venesection and the consequent lowering of the raised venous pressure together with a raising of the hæmoglobin level during exchange transfusion. The number of stillborn and hydropic fœtuses was significantly reduced by premature induction of labour at about 36 weeks. Although earlier induction was attempted, even at 32 weeks, the hazards of prematurity added to severe hæmolytic disease led to a low survival rate in this group so that the perinatal mortality was not appreciably further diminished. This left a stillbirth rate of 7·5 per cent (Holman, 1966) and a perinatal mortality rate of 14·9 per cent.

The fact that the liquor amnii was sometimes markedly jaundiced had been recognized for years, but visual assessment had proved of little value in the early days. Bevis (1956), however, persisted in his study of the amniotic fluid and showed that much more valuable results could be obtained by spectrophotometric examination. Liley (1961) in New Zealand followed Bevis's work, performed many amniocenteses and correlated the bilirubin levels in the liquor with the cord hæmoglobin of the fœtus. Many workers had concluded that the fœtus was lost from severe anæmia and the possibility of transfusing before birth had been considered and generally rejected because operative interference was likely to precipitate labour and defeat the purpose of the transfusion. Liley (1963b), however, realized that he could needle the fœtal abdomen *in utero* and that intraperitoneal transfusion often worked well in young babies; he therefore attempted intraperitoneal transfusion of the fœtus *in utero*. He reported the first successful intra-ut rine transfusion in 1963 and since then other workers have attempted the procedure with varying degrees of success.

Two new techniques were therefore available. Firstly, amniocentesis and estimation of the bilirubin in the liquor amnii giving hope of a reliable assessment of the degree of fœtal disease and, secondly, intra-uterine transfusion to correct fœtal anæmia, prevent stillbirth and allow continued development until the fœtus was mature enough to be born safely. Our team has now had over three years experience with these techniques and what follows represents our views and practice early in 1967.

AMNIOCENTESIS

The literature on this subject gives the impression that it is a simple, harmless procedure and this is possibly true if it be performed by an expert on a pregnancy of about 34 weeks. At this stage in pregnancy it is usually possible to tell by palpation where the fœtal small parts are and whether the placenta is likely to be in an anterior position: before 30 weeks this is difficult if not impossible. We have reported our earlier experiences (Holman and Karnicki, 1964; Karnicki and Holman, 1966), in which we had seen fœtuses lost by exsanguination following puncture of a vessel on the fœtal aspect of the placenta. Since then we have performed about 1600 more amniocenteses without loss of a fœtus.

We recommend that the puncture be attempted with a $1\frac{1}{2}$ in. intravenous needle mounted on a sterile disposable 10 ml. syringe and aimed between the fœtal small parts. This is expected either to enter a pool of liquor or to enter but not pass through the placenta. The risk of puncturing a large placental vessel is much diminished but still exists if the placenta is thin or one has the misfortune to needle the edge of it. If a longer needle is used it is quite possible to pass it through the placenta unwittingly and to obtain a clear sample of liquor; on the next attempt, however, one may find that the liquor is full of old blood. There is also a risk that placental puncture may cause a leak of blood from fœtus to mother and thus boost the antibody

titre so that the fœtus may be far more seriously affected than if amniocentesis had not been performed at all. An example of this is shown in
Figure 1. We do not regard this as a very serious risk, since we believe that
an anterior implantation of the placenta always carries a greater risk of
damage and of fœto-maternal transfusion than any other site and that this
trouble is as likely to follow normal ante-natal examination as it is to follow
amniocentesis.

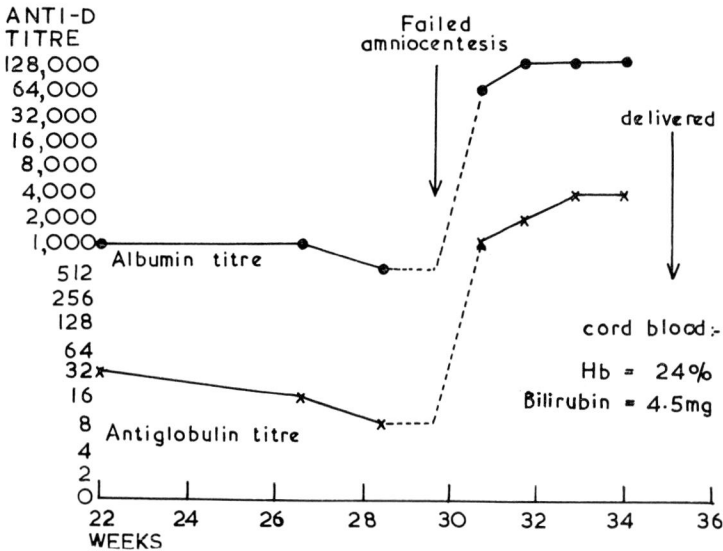

FIG. 1. Puncture of anterior placenta at amniocentesis. Blood drawn at attempted
amniocentesis was group O, Rh positive, direct Coombs' positive and 75 per cent
fœtal.

We do not think it wise to perform routine amniocentesis on all patients
with Rhesus isoimmunization. Our patients have been selected for this
investigation either because they have a history of stillbirth or severe hæmolytic disease in a previous pregnancy or because they have an antiglobulin
titre of 1/32 or more. An analysis of our results for 1966 (Fig. 2) shows that
we delivered 183 mothers of fœtuses affected by anti-D antibodies. Of the
72 who had antiglobulin titres of 1/16 or less eight had amniocentesis on
account of their previous history and four of them were sufficiently seriously
affected to require intra-uterine transfusion. Of the remaining 64 patients
only one would have been excluded from amniocentesis by these criteria
and would have suffered thereby. This patient had a first affected pregnancy,
an antiglobulin titre of 1/16 and an albumin titre of 1/512 and was not
referred to us until she was 37 weeks maturity. By this time the fœtal movements had so diminished in strength that we suspected hydrops fœtalis.
Amniocentesis was performed and an exceptionally high bilirubin peak was
found indicating imminent fœtal death by any standards. From our analysis
it is c ear that the addition of a further indication for amniocentesis, viz.
an albumin titre of 1/256, would have allowed us to select all seriously
affected fœtuses.

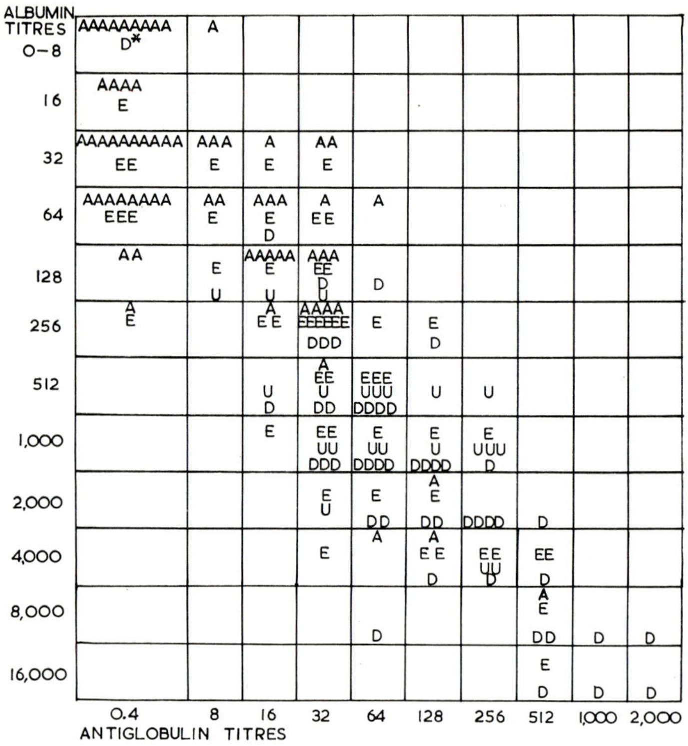

ALBUMIN TITRES	0.4	8	16	32	64	128	256	512	1000	2000
0–8	AAAAAAAAA D*	A								
16	AAAA E									
32	AAAAAAAAA EE	AAA E	A E	AA E						
64	AAAAAAA EEE	AA E	AAA E D	A EE	A					
128	AA	E U	AAAAA E U A	AAA EE D U	D					
256	A E		EE	AAAA EEEEE DDD	E	E D				
512			U D	A EE U DD	EEE UUU DDDD	U	U			
1,000			E	EE UU DDD	E UU DDDD	E U DDDD A	E UUU D			
2,000				E U	E E DD A	E DD A	DDDD	D		
4,000				E	E	A EE D	A EE UU D	EE UU D A E		
8,000						D		A E DD	D	D
16,000								E D	D	D

ANTIGLOBULIN TITRES

FIG. 2. Results in 183 infants affected by anti-D antibodies. Each symbol represents an infant and indicates titres at delivery.

A = Survivor without transfusion.
E = Survivor after exchange transfusion.
U = Survivor after intra-uterine transfusion.
D = Death intra-uterine or neonatal.
* = Unrelated to haemolytic disease.

Our indications for amniocentesis now are:

(a) previous stillbirth or severe hæmolytic disease.
(b) antiglobulin titre of 1/32 or more.
(c) albumin titre of 1/256 or more.

Since methods and titres vary from laboratory to laboratory each group of workers must determine their own significant antibody levels and see that methods and reagents are standardized.

If, because of the history or the antibody level, there is a clear indication for amniocentesis the question is when to do it. Certainly it must be done before the maturity at which a previous infant died *in utero* and, if treatment is to be effective, it must be before hydrops fœtalis supervenes. When the indication is clear early in pregnancy we like to see the patient at about four months and check the maturity. Nowadays many patients become pregnant as soon as they stop taking contraceptive pills and can offer no guidance as to the maturity of the pregnancy. We usually perform the first amniocentesis between 22 and 26 weeks and not less than one month before the maturity at which the last infant died.

Once the decision has been made that amniocentesis is advisable the obstetrician must examine the mother and ascertain the position of the fœtus and whether there are clinical indications to suggest the presence of an anterior placenta. Generally the fœtus will face the placenta and the presence of an anterior placenta will interfere with the palpation of the fœtal parts. When it is fairly certain that the placenta is posterior a favourable place for amniocentesis is selected by separating the fœtal small parts with the fingers of one hand and introducing the needle between the fingers. It then enters directly into the amniotic cavity and a clear sample of liquor is easily obtained. If by chance blood is drawn or the placenta is thought to be anterior it must be localized as accurately as possible by the best means available. We have preferred placental arteriography and have been guided reasonably accurately by it; thereafter amniocentesis has usually been performed with safety. Some workers (Gottesfeld, Thompson, Holmes and Taylor, 1966) are now using an ultrasonic device to localize the placenta and the early reports suggest that this may be satisfactory; it can also be used to monitor the fœtal heart rate. A number of different radio-isotope methods have been used with varying degrees of success. Urografin placento-graphy is very helpful but may alter the bilirubin values of the liquor (Fig. 9), so that its routine use is inadvisable.

When the sample has been aspirated it should be placed in a dark bottle and sent to the laboratory where it should be promptly centrifuged and filtered to remove debris, red cells, etc. If blood contamination occurs a further sample should be drawn into a fresh syringe. It is wise to retain all blood and liquor that is aspirated and to keep all samples separate. Any blood collected should be examined by the acid-elution technique for fœtal cells, and should have the direct Coombs' test, ABO and Rhesus group checked. From such samples it is sometimes possible to know that the infant is Rhesus negative and unaffected or is certainly affected. Any sample that appears to be whole blood should have a hæmoglobin estimation, as it is occasionally possible to know that the fœtal hæmoglobin is not below a certain level. Maternal blood is often drawn from the uterine sinuses, the fœtus is occasionally pricked and its blood contaminates the liquor; placental blood may be maternal or have any proportion of fœtal cells in it.

Occasionally, attempted amniocentesis yields a fluid other than liquor amnii. Although we insist that the mother's bladder be emptied beforehand we have once drawn maternal urine in avoiding a large anterior placenta. Liley (1963a) reports the aspiration of fœtal ascitic fluid and also fluid from amniotic cysts.

Examination of Liquor Amnii. At least 5 ml. of liquor should have been collected and immediately protected from light; it should then be centrifuged to free it from squamous debris, vernix and any red cells that may be present. At this stage the specimen may be stored or sent by post so long as it is protected from light, undue heat and freezing. Before examination it should be cleared and this can be done by centrifugation in a Hemming filter. The sample is then placed in a spectrophotometer and readings of the optical density are taken over the range of 300 to 700 mμ and plotted on semi-logarithmic graph paper. Normal liquor yields a nearly straight curve and the introduction of bilirubin adds a peak with its maximum at about 450 mμ; the height of this peak is proportional to the concentration of bilirubin and is measured in terms of optical density from the theoretical straight line of bilirubin-free liquor (Fig. 3).

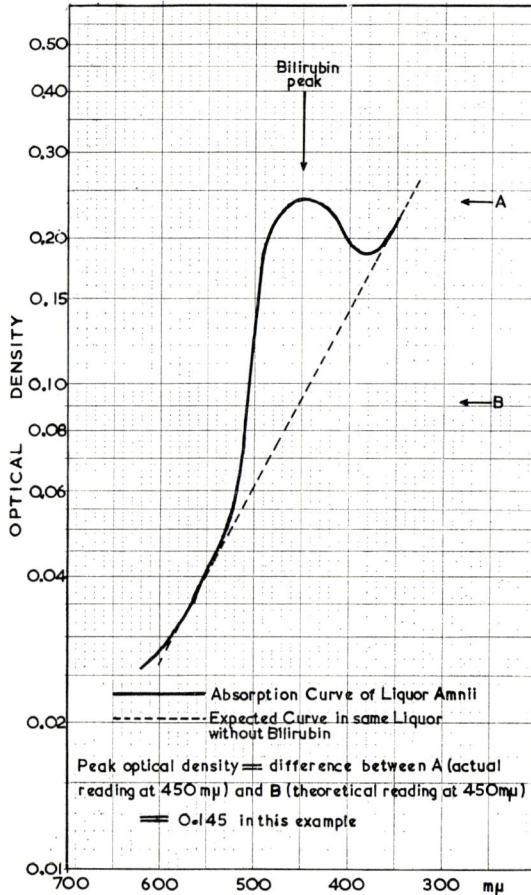

FIG. 3. Optical density curve of amniotic fluid illustrating bilirubin peak.

No real difficulties arise unless hæmoglobin or its degradation products are also present. Hæmoglobin produces a peak at 410 to 415 mμ which alters the baseline and may overlap the bilirubin peak giving an unreliable result (Fig. 4). The segment of the curve between 490 and 520 mμ is, however, usually unaffected by hæmoglobin (Knox et al., 1965) and bears a regular relation to the 450 mμ peak. Our colleague, Dr. D. N. Whitmore, has examined a large number of these curves and has shown that, on average, the difference between the optical density readings at 490 and 520 mμ multiplied by a factor of 1·49 is equal to the 450 mμ peak. It is our practice to take both these measurements and, if they are nearly equal, accept them: if they differ the curve must be examined carefully and it will usually be found that a hæmoglobin peak is present and that the 490-520 calculation is the more reliable. Less commonly the hæmoglobin concentration is so great that the 450 mμ peak is swamped by the 410 mμ hæmoglobin peak and that the lesser hæmoglobin peak at 540 mμ has spread and interfered with the 520 mμ section of the bilirubin curve so that no estimation of the bilirubin concentration is possible except by extraction techniques. The term "bilirubin" is used throughout to represent the complex of bilirubin-like pigments found in the amniotic fluid.

Apart from those due to the presence of hæmoglobin, errors may occur from plasma contaminating the liquor after the red cells have been removed (Liley, 1963a). We were misled on one occasion by a 450 mμ peak with an optical density of 0·330 and did not know that an appreciable quantity of red cells had been present. Two days later an optical density peak of 0·080 was found.

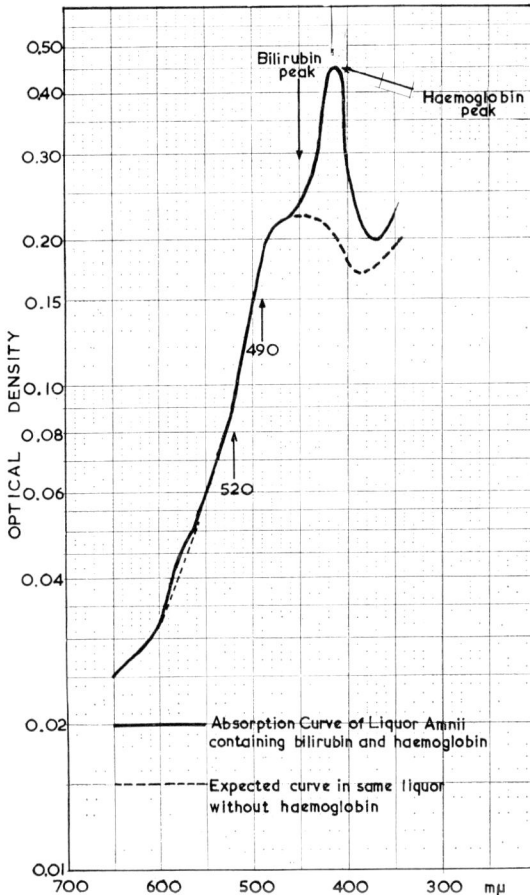

FIG. 4. Note that the hæmoglobin peak at 410 mμ overlaps the bilirubin peak at 450 mμ interfering with the method of reading described in Fig. 1. The segment of the curve between 520 and 490 mμ is unaltered by the presence of hæmoglobin.

The presence of meconium in the liquor is not a common finding in hæmolytic disease and has its usual implication of fœtal distress. In large quantity it is obvious but in small quantity it may suggest severe hæmolytic disease on naked eye examination; the absorption curve is, however, characteristically different (Liley, 1963a).

Assessment of Amniocentesis Results

This method of measuring the bilirubin peak in terms of its optical density was introduced by Liley (1961) and has been adopted by most workers in this field; he found that the peak optical densities in normals, plotted against the maturity of the fœtus, showed a steady diminution as the fœtus became more mature and from these the lower sloping line in Figure 5 was constructed. The upper sloping line was drawn parallel to the lower one in such a position as to separate as far as possible the group of results from live-born infants and the group of results from hydropic and stillborn infants. Liley's chart was based on amniocentesis readings from 27 weeks maturity onwards and the extrapolation of his lines to 20 weeks does not yet rest on a sufficient accumulation of reliable data although many workers use it.

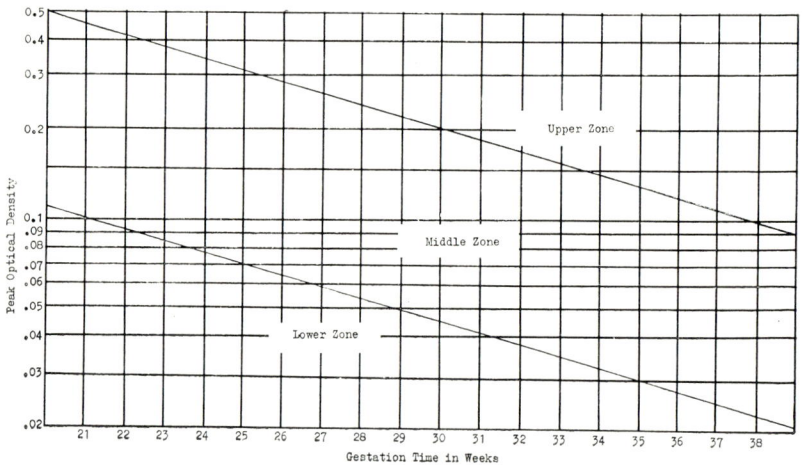

FIG. 5. Relationship of peak optical density, fœtal maturity and probable outcome. This chart is derived from that produced by Liley, but is extended backwards from 27 to 20 weeks. Peak optical densities falling in the Upper Zone indicate the likelihood of hydrops fœtalis or stillbirth. Those in the Middle Zone a likelihood of live infants with hæmolytic disease, of severity proportional to peak height. Results in the Lower Zone indicate probable normality of infants.

In practice results that fall in the lower and the upper zone usually give reliable advice on the state of the fœtus at that time Results falling in the middle zone were acknowledged by Liley to be of less value but even so we have been surprised by the degree of overlap found in our groups of patients. We have plotted results from groups of infants having approximately the same degree of severity, as measured by their need for exchange transfusion. Although the means of these results do show a steady rise through the middle zone the results of individual infants range so widely as to be of little prognostic value. As an example Figures 6 and 7 show respectively results from (a) Rhesus negative, unaffected infants of immunized mothers and (b) Rhesus positive infants requiring three or four exchange transfusions. It is clearly not possible to know whether infants with results in the lower middle zone are affected or not unless one has other evidence such as the blood group, a rising antibody titre or a rising bilirubin peak as a guide. This test is, of course, empirical and it is surprising that it

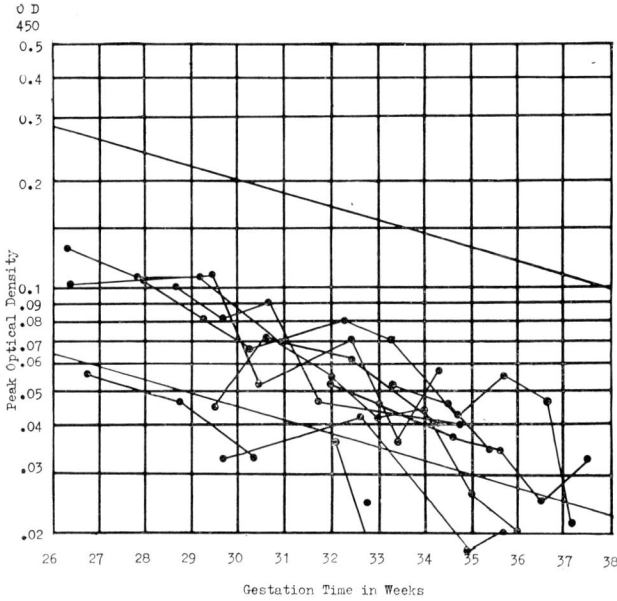

FIG. 6. (a) Serial amniocentesis results in Rhesus-negative infants of Rh-immunized mothers.

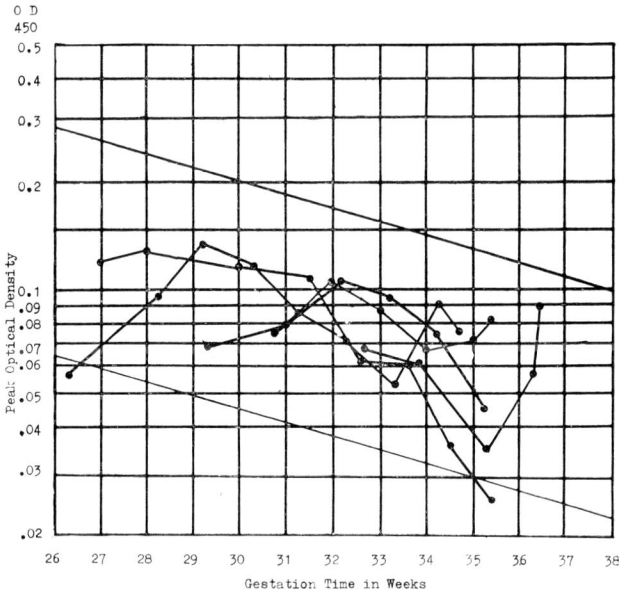

FIG. 7. (b) Serial amniocentesis results in infants needing 3-4 exchange transfusions.

provides guidance. The total amount of bilirubin in the liquor of a severely affected fœtus can be estimated to be about 3 mg. This quantity is about one-sixth of the amount a normal fœtus produces every day and a much smaller fraction of that produced when a hæmolytic state exists. How the bilirubin gets into the liquor and where it goes is not known. We have collected several samples of fœtal urine from severely jaundiced fœtuses and have found it to be a clear, water-white fluid in which no bilirubin could be detected. It is most likely that bilirubin diffuses from fœtal blood through the mucosa of the respiratory or alimentary tract (Walker, Fairweather and Jones, 1964), becomes protein bound and is finally deposited in the gut in meconium.

We followed Liley's chart in deciding when to perform intra-uterine transfusion because it appeared to be based on a sufficiently large number of observations. Other workers have since offered other criteria, e.g. Freda (1965), Knox, Fairweather and Walker (1965), Robertson (1966). Initially we regarded any result above Liley's upper line as an indication for intra-uterine transfusion or induction of labour. We have been misled on three occasions: twice when the parents were both of West-Indian extraction and once when the mother was an Italian married to an American Negro. This indication, however, failed to warn us that hydrops fœtalis could occur when the peak optical density was below the upper line. Since loss of the fœtus is due to anæmia and the bilirubin peak is at best related to the rate of destruction of red cells it is surprising that the correlation was good. It is to be expected that an appreciable variation from the average will occur and will lead to deaths with low bilirubin peaks and survivals with high peaks.

Most workers will agree that decisions should not rest on single estimations. When a series of results are plotted for patients they usually run parallel to Liley's lines or rise relative to them. The rate of change is important and failure to repeat amniocentesis sufficiently soon can lead to the loss of the infant. The most rapid rates of change seen are shown in Figure 8. It is clear that after a normal result not more than two weeks should elapse before repeating the test and in many cases the intervals should be a week or less. It should be noted that the introduction of urografin into the amniotic cavity is sometimes followed by a significant drop in the bilirubin level (Fig. 9). The cause of this has not yet been established.

INTRA-UTERINE TRANSFUSION

Technique. Our present technique starts with the injection of 15–20 ml. of contrast medium (76 per cent urografin) into the amniotic cavity on the day before that planned for the transfusion. This is preferably done with an arteriography trocar and cannula so that there is no risk of injecting into the fœtal tissues. As the fœtus drinks the liquor the contrast medium becomes concentrated firstly in the small intestine and later in the large bowel. This can be visualized with the aid of an image-intensifier and television screen linked to the X-ray apparatus. If the contrast medium cannot be seen it is probable that the fœtus has not swallowed because it is hydropic; alternative causes such as anencephaly or duodenal atresia are possible, but it can also happen that a normal fœtus does not swallow on one occasion but does so on another. On the day of the transfusion the mother is asked to lie quietly on her back in the hope that the fœtus will settle into the hollow beside

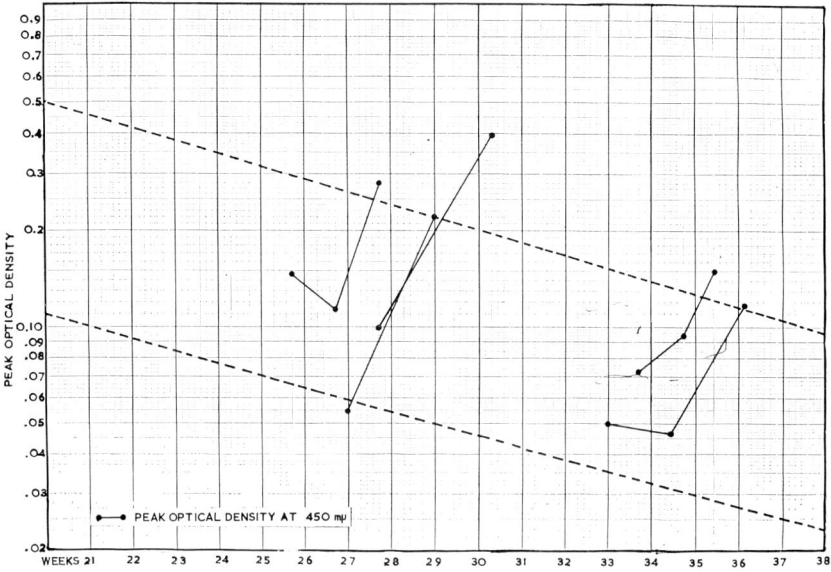

FIG. 8. Examples of rapid increase in peak optical density.

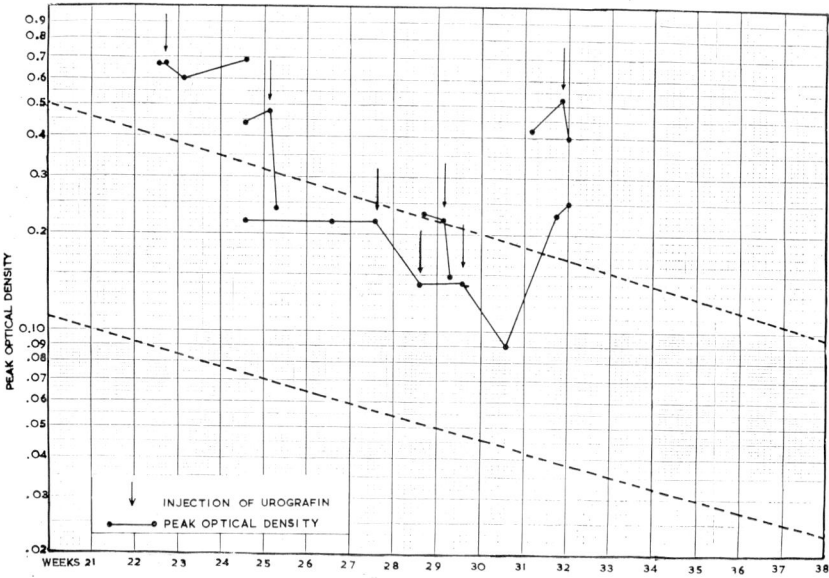

FIG. 9. Examples of fall in peak optical density after injection of urografin into the liquor amnii.

the maternal spine. It will then be in the lateral position, which offers the easiest approach to the fœtal abdomen. Premedication consists of pethidine 100 mg, and Promazine 50 mg. intramuscularly one hour before transfusion. Antibiotic cover is provided by four mega-units of penicillin and one gram of streptomycin divided into four doses over 24 hours.

The operation takes place in the X-ray department with strict aseptic precautions. A local anæsthetic is given through a 1½ in. needle at the site chosen for the puncture. This is determined by the position of the placenta, which must be avoided, and the position of the fœtus, in which the target area is the right or left lower quadrant of the abdomen. This area may be impossible of access because of the lie of the fœtus relative to the placenta or because the fœtal back is anterior: under such circumstances the operation should be postponed until the fœtus has turned into a more favourable position. A breech presentation is not favourable, as the thighs overlap the abdomen and the position may be fixed. The mother's skin is nicked with a knife and a 6 in. Tuohy needle is introduced into the uterine cavity. This needle must have been prepared previously by blunting the sharp edges on all aspects of the orifice and testing for size and bluntness with a nylon catheter. Under television screening the needle is directed towards the fœtal abdomen, by-passes the limbs and can often be felt and seen to enter the fœtal abdomen which offers little resistance. In some cases ascitic fluid can be aspirated and is easily recognized since it is more deeply pigmented and froths more than the liquor. When the needle is in the fœtal peritoneal cavity the catheter will pass through it easily. We use a 24 in. "Pink Portex" nylon catheter, O.D. 1·02 mm. If the needle is in fœtal tissue the catheter cannot be pushed in at all and the needle must be withdrawn and the puncture repeated. Before passing the catheter 2 ml. of contrast medium (60 per cent Conray) is injected through the needle and a characteristic picture of it between the coils of gut (Fig. 10), under the diaphragm and outlining the fœtal abdomen, is seen on the television screen. The catheter is then passed, more contrast medium is injected to check that the catheter is in and the Tuohy needle is then gently withdrawn leaving the bulk of the catheter in the fœtal abdomen. Blood can now be injected together with such other substances as may be indicated. Until recently, if a further transfusion was likely to be required we injected 2–3 ml. of an inert oily contrast medium (Myodil) which remained in the peritoneal cavity indefinitely and provided a target for a Tuohy needle weeks later. We have now abandoned the use of Myodil because of a suspicion that it may cause an inflammatory reaction.

The puncture is not always straightforward or easy. For example a small fœtus can be very mobile and attempt to elude the needle, in which case it may need to be transfixed through the buttock with a separate needle. The liver and spleen are large in this disease and occupy the whole upper abdomen whilst the bladder occupies a large central part of the lower abdomen. Sometimes this latter organ will be punctured and a clear fluid will be expelled from the needle, the catheter will only pass with difficulty and contrast medium will reveal the bladder (Fig. 11). This has happened to a sufficient number of infants without sequelæ for us to feel untroubled about it. Puncture of many other organs and tissues has now been recorded

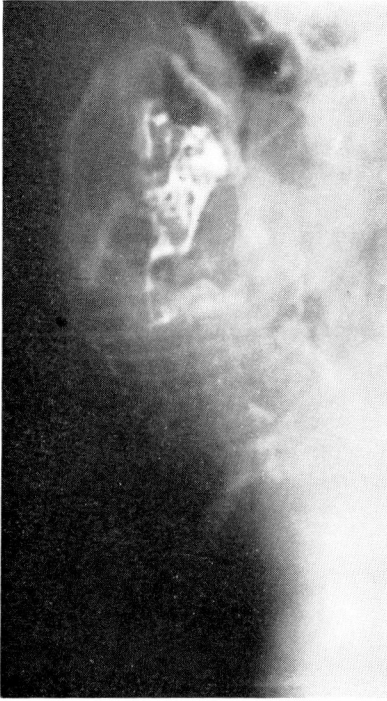

FIG. 10. Contrast medium in fœtal peritoneal cavity.

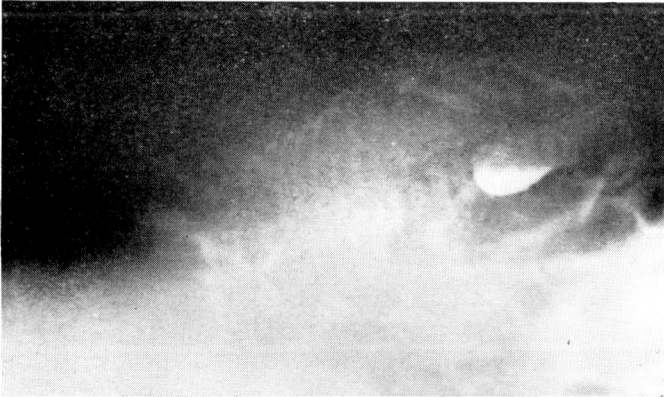

FIG. 11. Contrast medium in fœtal bladder.

by one centre or another and in general little harm has come to the fœtus. It is probably most at peril from puncture of the spleen leading to severe intraperitoneal hæmorrhage; a puncture of the liver usually clots and heals well.

The amount of blood introduced varies with the size of the fœtus. We try to estimate the weight by palpation or, failing that, from maturity tables and give the appropriate amount of concentrated rhesus negative red cells of the same ABO group as the mother: this concentrate usually has a hæmoglobin level of 20–22 g.,/100 ml. The fœtal abdomen will safely accept about 30–35 ml. for every pound of body weight (66–77 ml./kg.) and this amount will be absorbed via the subdiaphragmatic lymphatics in the course of a few days. The hæmoglobin level achieved is lower the less mature the fœtus, since the placenta is proportionately larger earlier in pregnancy than later. All the early transfusions were given by a disposable syringe connected by a two-way tap to the catheter and a drip set. After finding that the presence of ascitic fluid could lead to complete clotting of the transfused blood we used 3·8 per cent sodium citrate in quantities of 4 to 12 ml. to reduce the risks of clotting. This was not, however, adequate to prevent clotting when the fœtus bled into its peritoneal cavity. Since this not only caused adhesions but also led to a layer of fibrin over the diaphragm which prevented blood absorption we have more recently given 5,000 units of Urokinase at each transfusion and have seen less cases with clotted blood or adhesions since.

Because each transfusion carries a risk to the fœtus we sought to diminish the number of transfusions by using a self-retaining catheter made by our colleague Dr. J. D. Irving (1966), which allowed us to put in less blood on a single occasion but to repeat it several times. We have now abandoned the use of the self-retaining catheter having found that leakage of donor blood from the fœtal abdomen was much more common than with the single transfusion and simple catheter and that the survival rate was much lower.

Results of Intra-uterine Transfusion

Between November 1963 and December 1966 we transfused 103 fœtuses. In the first year and a half we were chiefly treating our own patients and had a survival rate of about 60 per cent. Since then, although we believe our skill and knowledge has increased, our survival rate dropped to 40 per cent and is now fairly stable at a little above that level (Table I). This change is due

TABLE I

Cumulative Results of Intra-uterine Transfusion
from November 1963

	No. of I.U.T.	No. of Patients	Survivors	Losses
September 1965	46	34	20 (59·9%)	14 (40·1%)
March 1966	84	54	27 (50%)	27 (50%)
September 1966	135	76	32 (40·8%)	44 (59·2%)
December 1966	170	103	43 (41·8%)	60 (58·2%)

in part to the large number of patients referred on account of a history of early stillbirth and in part to patients being referred when the disease has already passed the optimal time for intra-uterine transfusion. Since December 1966 an additional 69 patients have been treated, another 105 intra-uterine transfusions have been given and the survival rate is still approximately 40 per cent.

When the results are considered in relation to a history of previous hæmolytic disease or none (Table II) it is clear that there is no significant

TABLE II

Comparison of Results in First and subsequent
affected Pregnancies

Group	No. of Cases	Survivors	Losses
First affected pregnancy	27	11 (40·7%)	16 (59·3%)
Previous infant(s) affected	76	32 (42·1%)	44 (57·9%)

difference in the proportion of survivors. Within the group with previous hæmolytic disease the degree of affection of the previous pregnancy is of significance since those who have never lost a child from hæmolytic disease have twice as good a chance as those who have lost one (Table III). This guidance is not available in the first affected pregnancies, a group which yields about one-third of all fœtal losses from hæmolytic disease (Liley, 1961).

We have at times chosen to perform intra-uterine transfusion when the peak optical density was below Liley's upper line. Usually we were guided in this by the previous history, diminished fœtal movements, a rapidly rising bilirubin peak or a rapidly rising antibody titre and we were often disconcerted to find that the fœtus was already hydropic. We have plotted these peak optical densities for survivors (Fig. 12) and losses (Fig. 13)

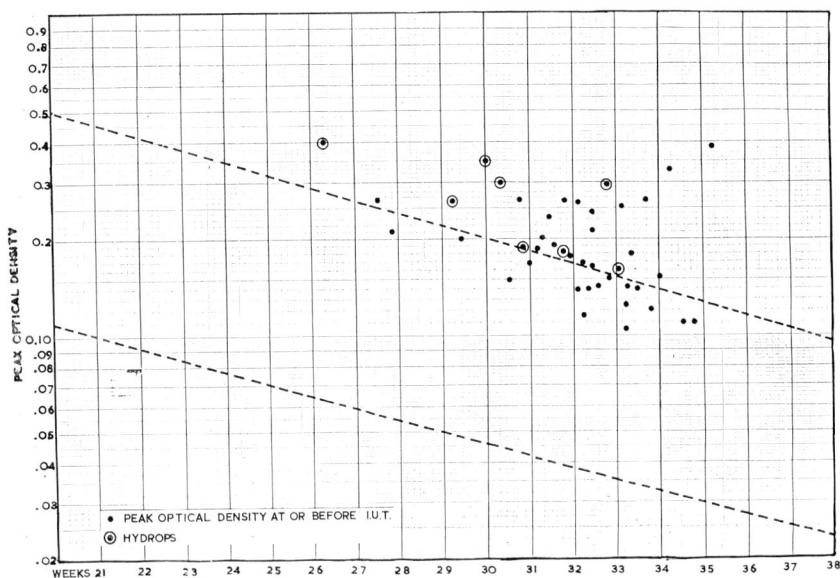

FIG. 12. Intra-uterine transfusion: all survivors.

and derived from the latter and Figure 6 a new chart for our guidance (Fig. 14).

The development of hydrops fœtalis carries a serious prognosis. Out of 59 infants that certainly had it only eight (13·5 per cent) survived whereas of the other 44 infants 35 (79 per cent) survived. Our observations make it

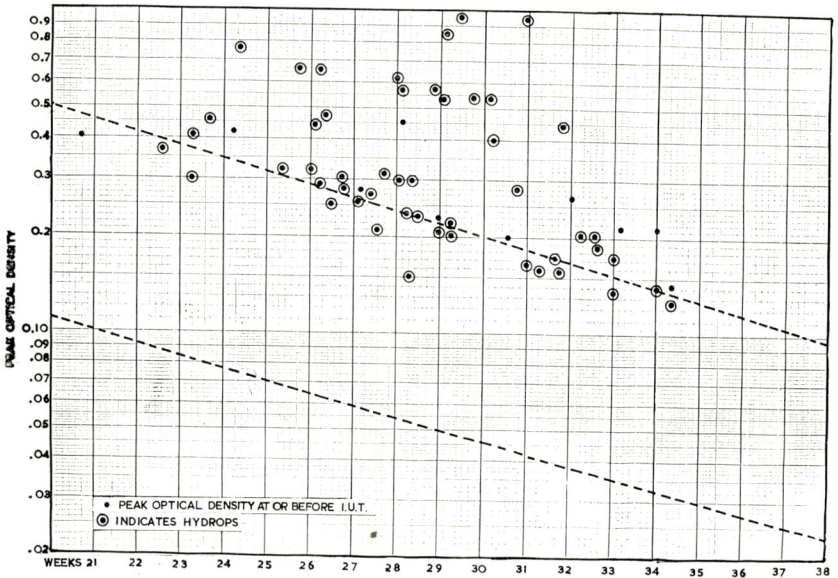

FIG. 13. Intra-uterine transfusion: all losses.

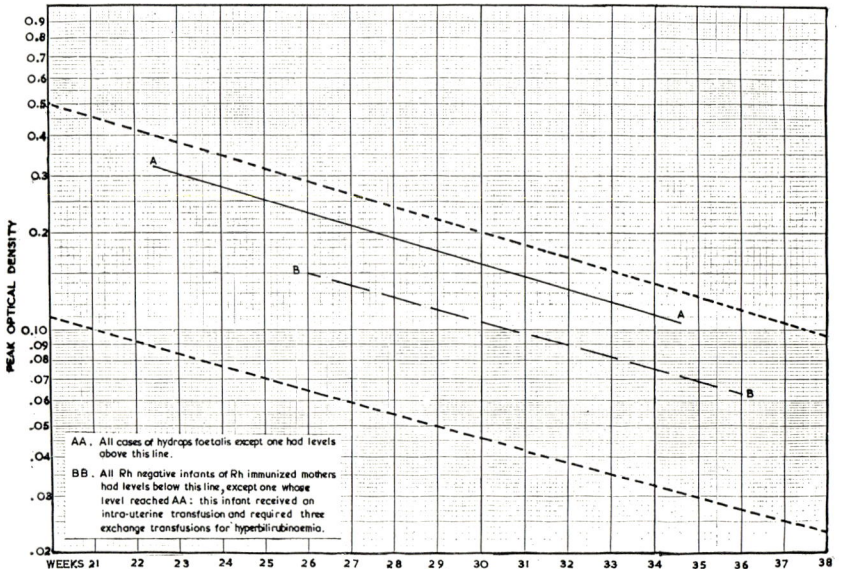

FIG. 14. New chart for interpretation of peak optical density.

clear that an hydropic fœtus with gross ascites can absorb blood from its peritoneal cavity, may have its hæmoglobin level raised to normal yet may die in an hydropic state. We had hoped that correction of anæmia would lead to a disappearance of œdema, but this was not the case: even those who survived were œdematous at birth. This has been observed by other workers and a variety of treatments have been attempted without success:

TABLE III

Results in Cases with previous affected Pregnancy

Group	No. of Cases	Survivors	Losses
Previous stillbirth or neonatal death	44	13 (29·5%)	31 (70·5%)
Previous hæmolytic disease with survival	32	18 (59·3%)	13 (40·7%)

we, for example, knowing that some seriously affected fœtuses had hypo-albuminæmia introduced human albumin into the fœtal peritoneal cavity but without effect. We now think that the likely explanation is that, although the anæmia has been corrected and blood oxygen carriage is normal, the placenta has become so diseased that trans-placental oxygen transfer is inadequate and that the œdema is thereby maintained.

When the figures are analysed to separate the hydropic fœtuses from the others (Table IV) the differences are clear.

TABLE IV

Proportion of Cases with Hydrops Fœtalis

	Miscarriage	Stillbirth	Neonatal death	Survivors
Definite hydrops	8	31	12	8
Other	2	2	5	35
Total	10	33	17	43

Two-thirds with hydrops were lost *in utero* and one-third born alive: allowing that two, with neonatal death due to accidental pyocyaneus infection, would otherwise have survived, the best expectation of survival is one-sixth. On the other hand only 9 per cent of the other group died *in utero*, and accepting that two neonatal deaths were due to accidents and one to an error of judgement the best expectation would have been 86 per cent survival. These last figures imply that if hydrops has not developed only about 14 per cent of pregnancies will be lost from the present technique or, since 66 intra-uterine transfusions were performed on these 44 fœtuses, a risk of about 9 per cent per transfusion.

In the group of hydropic fœtuses a few were lost from trauma: two had their spleens punctured and bled into the peritoneal cavity and one had a puncture hole in its colon which became epithelialized and through which a meconium peritonitis arose. Several were found to have clotted blood and fibrin deposits in the peritoneal cavity without other evidence of puncture of a vessel or a viscus: in these cases fœtal hæmorrhage from the puncture may have interfered with the absorption of donor blood. Nearly one half of the intra-uterine deaths occurred within a day or two of intra-uterine transfusion: post-mortem examination usually revealed incomplete absorption of the blood and a hydropic fœtus without serious damage from the transfusion. Although some of these babies could have died from their disease the proportion lost in this way is so great as to suggest that the transfusion was the final insult.

Spontaneous premature labour occurred in 39 of the 103 infants and was more than twice as frequent in the hydropic as in the non-hydropic group. In Table V, which shows the causes of neonatal death, the cases in

TABLE V

Causes of Neonatal Death

Hydrops fœtalis		and Prematurity
with cardiac failure	4	...
with hæmorrhagic condition	2	1
with injury to spleen	1	...
with injury to colon	1	1
with prematurity	2	2
with pseudomonas septicæmia	2	2
Injury to heart		
by cardiac massage	1	...
Ruptured umbilical artery		
during exchange transfusion	1	1
Prematurity		
alone	1	1
with respiratory distress	1	1
with bronchopneumonia	1	1

which prematurity was a contributory factor are indicated. How far hydrops or intra-uterine transfusion were factors in precipitating labour is not clear. About two-fifths of the cases of premature labour in hydropic fœtuses occurred in the first five days after transfusion whereas none of the non-hydropic fœtuses were affected before the sixth day, and this suggests that hydrops was a significant factor. The presence of blood in the liquor was more often noted in cases of spontaneous premature labour whether due to leakage of donor blood from the fœtal abdomen or to damage to the placenta.

We have analysed our results in a number of different ways: there is a suggestion that the optimal maturity for delivery might be 35 weeks (Table VI) and the optimal weight $5\frac{1}{2}$ to $6\frac{1}{2}$ pounds (Table VII). It is clear that the earlier intra-uterine transfusion is required the greater the risk of losing the infant and Figure 15 shows that the prognosis is far better if it

TABLE VI

Results in Live-born Infants related to Maturity

Weeks Maturity	29	30	31	32	33	34	35	36	37
Survived	0	1	1	2	3	6	15	13	2
Died	1	1	2	0	3	2	2	5	1

TABLE VII

Results in Live-born related to Birth Weight

Birthweight in lbs.	$2\frac{1}{2}-3\frac{1}{2}$	$3\frac{1}{2}-4\frac{1}{2}$	$4\frac{1}{2}-5\frac{1}{2}$	$5\frac{1}{2}-6\frac{1}{2}$	$6\frac{1}{2}-7\frac{1}{2}$
Survived	3	6	9	18	7
Died	2	5	3	2	4

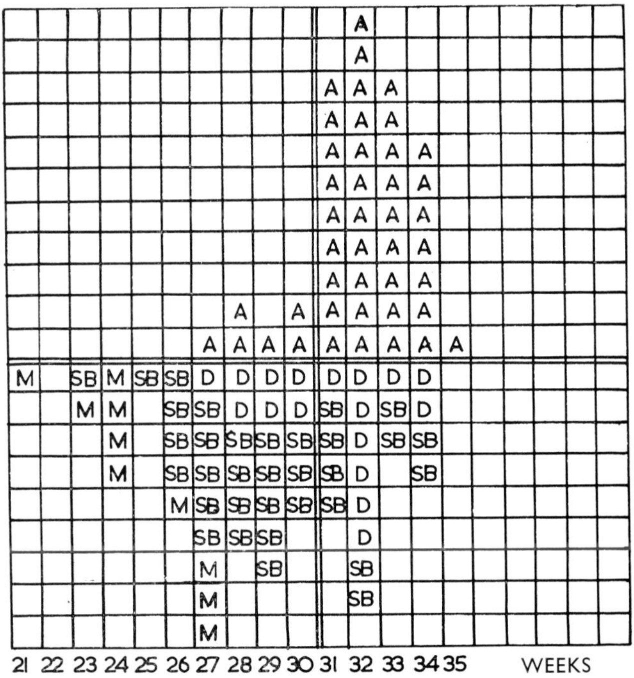

FIG. 15. Results of I.U.T. according to maturity when first transfusion was given.

A = Survivor.
D = Neonatal death.
SB = Stillbirth.
M = Miscarriage.

is not needed until after the thirtieth week. Although these numbers are rather small for analysis the percentage born alive and the percentage surviving suggest an increasing chance of success from the twenty-seventh week onwards.

The survivors did not all escape without complications, the most severe were prolonged jaundice in two, infection in one, non-infective plastic peritonitis and meconium obstruction in one and bilateral scrotal herniæ full of organized blood clot in one.

Neonatal Care

The neonatal care of these babies requires much skill and attention from the pædiatric service. In assessing them the blood group findings must be ignored since most have little Rh positive blood left and some appear to have only Rh negative blood and a negative Direct Coombs' Test. Many are more jaundiced than usual but do not always have as rapid a rate of increase in bilirubin levels as usual. We have been guided in our exchange transfusions by bilirubin levels and one is often obliged to check them several times a day. The 43 survivors required in all 76 one-pint units of blood for exchange transfusion. Since antibody levels were in general high and the exchange transfusions fewer than in comparable infants without pre-natal transfusion, we were not surprised to find that antibodies persisted in sufficient quantity to cause severe anæmia at about six weeks after birth: in all, 10 of the survivors required a further simple transfusion. Feeding was often slow and œdema and jaundice persisted in some. When, however, the first weeks were past the infants appeared to thrive and become normal children. We have so far no evidence of late complications.

Maternal complications have been surprisingly few and have been largely due to anterior position of the placenta. One patient had an intraperitoneal hæmorrhage as a result of puncture of the uterine wall directly over the placental site with a Tuohy needle. The uterine musculature at the site of placental attachment is more vascular and can contract less well than elsewhere. Two patients became shocked when the Tuohy needle pierced the placenta but responded to blood transfusion. We believe that it is necessary to know the position of the placenta and to avoid puncturing it.

We have sought for evidence of infection but have found none. Some workers in this field are very concerned about the risks of infection and regard it as a contra-indication to intra-uterine transfusion: many others with considerable experience have never seen infection. We have heard of two cases infected with *Cl. welchii*, but have no details. Some workers are opposed to the prophylactic use of antibiotics, others introduce them into the amniotic cavity or the fœtus: we prefer to give them to the mother.

Amniotic fluid embolism is a theoretical risk which we have not seen. We have, however, refrained from performing intra-uterine transfusion on patients who have "maternal syndrome", viz. œdema, albuminuria and hypertension associated with hydrops fœtalis, because we think the risk is greatest in them and that the chance of fœtal survival is minute.

One risk that is not generally appreciated is that the donor cells may pass into the maternal circulation. In one case a new antibody (anti-Jk^a) appeared in the mother after an intra-uterine transfusion with Rhesus negative, Jk^a positive blood and made the selection of a further donor difficult (Kelly and Kenwright, 1966).

COMMENTS

This new approach has revealed our ignorance of many aspects of fœtal life. We knew little about the ratio of placental blood volume to that of the fœtus and nothing at all about the way in which bilirubin enters the liquor or how the concentration of it is related to the hæmolytic process in the fœtus. Much interest has been stimulated and a variety of investigations made. Walker *et al.* (1964), knowing that the protein concentration of liquor fell as pregnancy progressed and that the bilirubin was probably protein-bound considered various refinements but did not think that their assessment of severity was improved. Cherry, Kochwa and Rosenfield (1965), however, measured the ratio of bilirubin to protein in the hope that this would give a consistent guide irrespective of the maturity of the pregnancy or the dilution of the liquor and concluded that it was useful. Their contention has been supported by Morris, Murray and Ruthven (1967), who reported that their assessment had been improved by the use of this method. There is still disagreement and uncertainty about the value of all tests and we feel that one should gather all available information about the mother and fœtus and judge each cases on its merits, expecting that some data will be misleading. On at least two occasions we have performed serial amniocenteses on an Rh negative fœtus when the husband was undoubtedly homozygous.

It is clear that the major problem is hydrops fœtalis and that, although we have had success in about 13 per cent of such cases, we are often too late. Sometimes this is because we see the patient too late but in other cases the condition has become established whilst we were waiting for an indication to perform intra-uterine transfusion. In a few cases this has been associated with a rapid rise in the bilirubin peak, suggesting rapid hæmolysis and we have found ascites present when the peak optical density has only just reached the level associated with hydrops fœtalis. We do not know at what stage in fœtal life the fœtus is able to destroy sensitized red cells, but it would seem likely that it cannot do so in the early months of pregnancy since the fœtus is rarely lost before 20 weeks, however much antibody is present. Our observations suggest that the ability is probably developed in the period between 16 and 24 weeks.

All the spectroscopy referred to was performed manually on a Hilger Uvispek. In the present year we have changed to a Unicam SP800A recording spectrophotometer and found that our calculated value from 590–520 mμ no longer agreed with the 450 mμ peak. Dr. Whitmore has examined these curves and found that 485 mμ–515 mμ multiplied by 1·5 gives the best correlation. It is obviously necessary to consider the particular machine used before depending on the answers derived.

In any large unit antibodies other than anti-D will be found and their effect on the fœtus must be considered. We have seen a number of other Rh antibodies and found that they behaved similarly to anti-D of the same titre. An immune anti-Vw with an antiglobulin titre of 1/128 produced a severely affected fœtus requiring intra-uterine and exchange transfusion.

Finally the question has to be asked as to whether intra-uterine transfusion is justified. In most of the patients we treat, the prospect of survival of the fœtus without intervention is minute and our hope of success small.

Nevertheless the patients prefer active treatment to no treatment and we feel that the risks to the mother are not likely to be greater than those of permitting the disease to progress and possibly producing "maternal syndrome" or acute defibrination. The alternative treatment of hysterotomy and direct transfusion of the fœtus carries so great a risk of prompt delivery that we have not been prepared to subject our patients to it. We do, however, seriously consider the alternative of induction of labour once the fœtus has reached 34 weeks, since we consider its prospects of survival greater if its size is reasonable, than if it received an intra-uterine transfusion and has a prompt premature labour with an abdomen distended with donor blood.

The work on these mothers and babies has involved most of the staff of the obstetric, pædiatric, pathological and radiological departments of Lewisham Hospital and we are indebted to them for their help, patience and tolerance. Miss A. Austin, Dr. M. Ata, Dr. B. Gans, Dr. J. D. Irving, Dr. N. D. Morrison and Dr. D. N. Whitmore have been closely associated with the work throughout and our thanks are due to them and to numerous other colleagues who have helped us with particular problems. We are indebted to the Editor of the *Postgraduate Medical Journal* for permission to reproduce Figures 3, 4 and 5.

References

BEVIS, D. C. A. (1956). Blood pigments in haemolytic disease of newborn. *J. Obstet. Gynae. Brit. Emp.*, **63**, 68.

CHERRY, S. H., KOCHWA, S. and ROSENFIELD, R. E. (1965). Bilirubin-protein ratio in amniotic fluid as an index of the severity of erythroblastosis foetalis. *Obstet. and Gynae.*, **26**, 826.

FREDA, V. J. (1965). The Rh problem in obstetrics and a new concept of its management using amniocentesis and spectrophotometric scanning of amniotic fluid. *Amer. J. Obstet.*, **92**, 341.

GOTTESFELD, K. R., THOMPSON, H. E., HOLMES, J. H. and TAYLOR, E. S. (1966). Ultrasonic placentography—a new method for placental localization. *Amer. J. Obstet.*, **96**, 538.

HOLMAN, C. A. and KARNICKI, J. (1964). Intrauterine transfusion for haemolytic disease of the newborn. *Brit. med. J.*, **ii**, 594.

IRVING, J. D. (1966). A self-retaining catheter for intra-uterine foetal transfusion. *Brit. med. J.*, **1**, 1228.

KARNICKI, J. and HOLMAN, C. A. (1966). Intrauterine transfusion. *Postgrad. med. J.*, **42**, 755.

KELLY, J. and KENWRIGHT, M. G. (1966). Personal communication.

KNOX, E. G., FAIRWEATHER, D. V. I. and WALKER, W. (1965). Spectrophotometric measurements on liquor amnii in relation to the severity of haemolytic disease of the newborn. *Clin. Sci.*, **28**, 147.

LILEY, A. W. (1961). Liquor amnii analysis in the management of the pregnancy complicated by rhesus sensitization. *Amer. J. Obstet.*, **82**, 1359.

LILEY, A. W. (1963a). Errors in the assessment of haemolytic disease from anmiotic fluid. *Amer. J. Obstet.*, **86**, 485.

LILEY, A. W. (1963b). Intrauterine transfusion of foetus in haemolytic disease. *Brit. med. J.*, **ii**, 1107.

MORRIS, E. D., MURRAY, J. and RUTHVEN, C. R. J. (1967). Liquor bilirubin levels in normal pregnancy: a basis for accurate prediction of haemolytic disease. *Brit. med. J.*, **ii**, 352.

Report of 53rd Ross Conference on Paediatric Research. Ross Laboratories, September 1966.

ROBERTSON, J. G. (1966). Evaluation of the reported methods of interpreting spectrophotometric tracings of amniotic fluid in rhesus iso-immunization. *Amer. J. Obstet.*, **95**, 120.

WALKER, W., FAIRWEATHER, D. V. I. and JONES, P. (1964). Examination of liquor amnii as a method of predicting severity of haemolytic disease of newborn. *Brit. med. J.*, **ii**, 141.

Chapter 17

SIDEROBLASTIC ANÆMIA

D. L. MOLLIN and A. V. HOFFBRAND

SIDEROBLASTIC anæmia may be defined as a dyshæmopoietic anæmia in which there is defective synthesis of hæmoglobin associated with an abnormal accumulation of ionizable iron granules in the erythroblasts, some of which show a "ring" or "collar" of iron granules around the nucleus. The stained peripheral blood shows a variable number of hypochromic cells. The anæmia may be inherited or acquired, and the acquired form may be primary or secondary to other conditions. In spite of the wide variety of conditions in which sideroblastic anæmia is found, it is possible that the underlying cause is always the same, i.e. defective synthesis of hæm.

The purpose of this review is to describe the hæmatological features and classification of the anæmia and to discuss its pathogenesis. Other recent reviews are those by Heilmeyer (1963), Harris and Horrigan (1964), Morrow and Goldberg (1965), Dacie and Mollin (1966), Kierkegaard-Hansen (1966) and Verloop (1967). Before describing sideroblastic anæmia it might be wise to say something about siderocytes and normal and abnormal sideroblasts and their relation to sideroblastic anæmia.

Siderocytes and Sideroblasts

Morrow and Goldberg (1965) refer to Bizzozero (1883) as first describing Prussian-blue staining granules in erythrocytes. However, the first detailed study of these bodies was made by Grüneberg (1941a and b), who demonstrated granules of iron, stainable by Perl's reaction, in erythrocytes of mouse, rat and human embryos, and in the erythrocytes and erythroblasts of mice with a congenital anæmia. Soon afterwards they were observed in some of the erythrocytes of patients who had undergone splenectomy (Doniach *et al.*, 1943). Subsequently these granules were reported in the erythrocytes and erythroblasts of the bone marrow (and the peripheral blood after splenectomy) of patients with certain severe anæmias (Dacie and Doniach, 1947; McFadzean and Davis, 1947, 1949). In most instances the granules staining positively for iron were also demonstrable as small discrete basophilic bodies in the Romanowsky stain, so-called Pappenheimer bodies (Pappenheimer *et al.*, 1945).

These iron-staining granules were originally considered to be a fœtal or pathological phenomenon. However, small numbers were noted by McFadzean and Davis (1947) in some of the erythroblasts of a small proportion of normal adult subjects. In the early 'fifties Douglas and Dacie (1953) and Kaplan *et al.* (1954) made a detailed study of the occurrence of siderotic granules and reported their presence both in marrow reticulocytes and in a significant proportion of the erythroblasts of normal subjects as well as in the erythrocytes and erythroblasts in a wide variety of hæmatological disorders. Both groups of workers noted that the number and size of the siderotic granules varied. They were small and difficult to see in normal subjects, absent in iron deficiency, but numerous and increased in size in conditions where there was evidence of defective hæmoglobin synthesis or where the serum iron concentration was increased. Siderotic granules are also absent from the erythroblasts of patients with the anæmia of infection, but in this condition, in contrast to iron deficiency, the marrow iron stores are normal or only slightly reduced.

In normal erythroblasts and in the erythroblasts of most of the patients referred to in the papers by Douglas and Dacie (1953) and Kaplan *et al.* (1954) mentioned above, the siderotic granules were distributed throughout the cytoplasm of the cells. However, the distribution of the iron granules was altered in one of the patients referred to by the first authors. Instead of being scattered throughout the cytoplasm of the erythroblast, the siderotic granules were concentrated as a ring in the perinuclear zone. This patient was considered (at the time of writing) to have "an acquired defect of hæmoglobin synthesis", but undoubtedly suffered from sideroblastic anæmia (Dacie and Mollin, 1966). A similar distribution of iron granules was illustrated by McFadzean and Davis (1949) in erythroblasts of guinea-pigs poisoned by lead.

Nomenclature. The term "siderocyte" and "siderotic granule" are appropriate descriptive terms and universally used. The term "sideroblast" was introduced by Kaplan and his co-workers in 1954 to describe a nucleolated red cell containing iron granules visible under the light microscope. It has since been used widely to describe cells in which *pathological* amounts of iron are present. Perhaps the term "sideroblast" should be restricted to a normal cell. We use the term "abnormal or pathological sideroblast" to indicate a cell containing more iron than normal and "ring sideroblast" (Bowman, 1961) to refer to the cell which is characteristic of so-called "sideroblastic anæmia" (Fig. 1).

Types of Sideroblast

It is therefore possible to recognize three varieties of siderotic granulation in erythroblasts, i.e. three types of sideroblast (Table I).

The *first type* is the sideroblast seen in normal marrow; the iron-containing granules are few in number, difficult to see and very difficult to photograph. They are visible in only a proportion of erythroblasts. The granules are not localized in the perinuclear zone, but are scattered through the cytoplasm.

The *second type* of sideroblast is found in conditions in which the percentage of saturation of transferrin is increased; that is, in conditions in which there is dyshæmopoiesis, usually without selective defect in hæm or globin synthesis, or in which there is excessive hæmolysis, or in which the body stores of iron are increased. The siderotic granules in such conditions are larger and more numerous than normal, but as in normal erythroblasts, the granules are diffusely scattered throughout the cytoplasm. In this group of conditions (Table I, 2) the percentage of erythroblasts showing siderotic granules and the number and size of the siderotic granules are directly proportional to the percentage saturation of transferrin (Bainton and Finch, 1964).

The *third type* of sideroblast (Table I, 3) is found in conditions in which there is defective synthesis of globin, as in thalassæmia, and probably of hæm, as in the primary and secondary sideroblastic anæmias. The granules are usually larger and much more numerous than in the conditions mentioned above. All the erythroblasts usually show siderotic granulation, and there is no correlation between the percentage saturation of transferrin and the number of granules and proportion of affected erythroblasts in thalassæmia (Bainton and Finch, 1964) or in sideroblastic anæmia (Dacie and Mollin, 1966).

TABLE I

Types of Sideroblast

1. **Normal Sideroblasts**
> granules few in number,
> difficult to see,
> randomly distributed throughout the cytoplasm.

2. **Abnormal Sideroblasts**
> (*a*) Increased granulation directly proportional to percentage saturation of transferrin.
>> granules larger and more numerous, easily visible with "normal" distribution in the cytoplasm as in:
>>> hæmolytic anæmia
>>> megaloblastic anæmia
>>> hæmochromatosis
>>> hæmosiderosis
> (*b*) Increased granulation *not* directly proportional to percentage saturation of transferrin.
>> granules more numerous and usually large.
>>> (i) With "normal" distribution of granules
>>>> thalassæmia
>>>> other conditions with defective globin synthesis.
>>> (ii) "Ring" sideroblasts
>>>> primary and secondary sideroblastic anæmia.

Modified from Dacie and Mollin (1966), *Acta med. scand.*, supp. 445, **179**, 235.

The pathological sideroblasts found in thalassæmia differ strikingly from those found in sideroblastic anæmia. In the great majority of erythroblasts in thalassæmia the distribution of siderotic granules is similar to that found in the conditions described previously, i.e. they are scattered throughout the cytoplasm. Characteristically in sideroblastic anæmia they are concentrated in a complete or partial ring around the nucleus. Why the iron granules are concentrated in this perinuclear zone is uncertain. Bessis and Breton-Gorius (1959), Sorenson (1962) and Bessis and Jensen (1965) have shown that in some instances at least the iron granules in this position are attached to perinuclear mitochondria (see later). The proportion of erythroblasts that show this characteristic ring form varies. In primary ("idiopathic") sideroblastic anæmia it is usual to find that the majority of the erythroblasts are "ring" sideroblasts. On the other hand in secondary sideroblastic anæmia

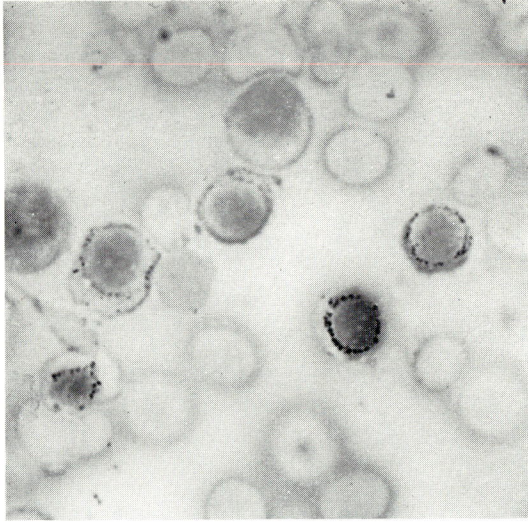

FIG. 1

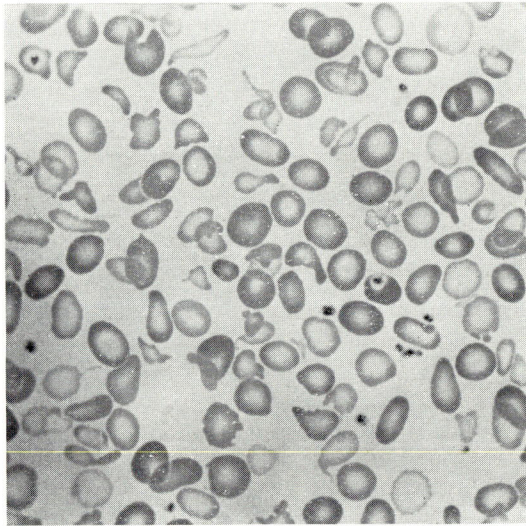

FIG. 2

Fig. 1. Ring sideroblast showing typical appearance of a cell containing excess iron.

Fig. 2 Blood picture from a male with severe inherited sideroblastic anaemia.

only a small proportion of the erythroblasts may be affected. In such patients the remaining erythroblasts may contain numerous large siderotic granules even when the percentage saturation of transferrin is normal or only slightly increased.

Rôle of the Spleen

It is well known that after splenectomy large numbers of siderocytes may appear in the peripheral blood of patients with certain hæmatological

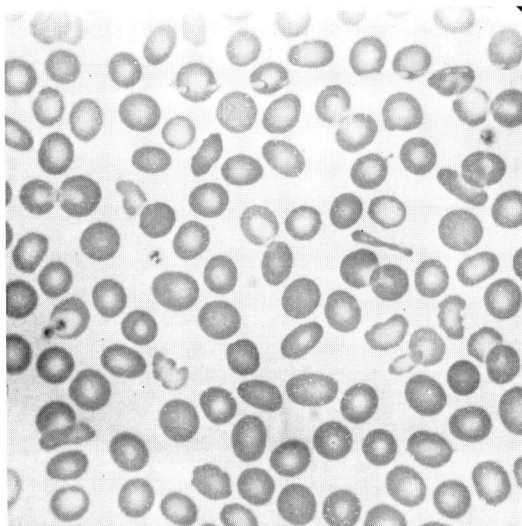

Fig. 3

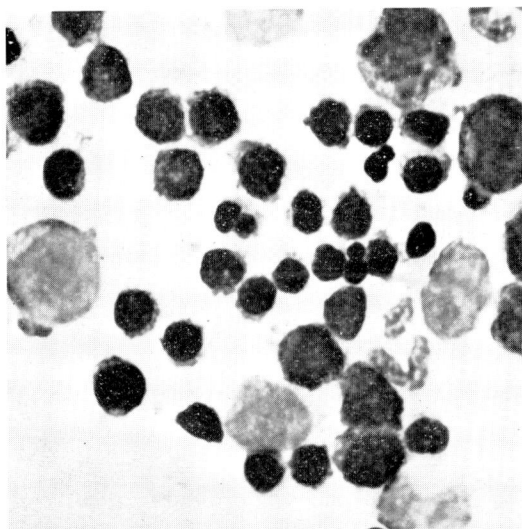

Fig. 4

Fig. 3. Blood picture from a female showing mild sideroblastic anaemia (compare with Fig. 2).

Fig. 4. Primary sideroblastic anaemia (Romanowsky stains) showing usual appearance of erythroblasts (contrast with Fig. 5).

disorders whose pre-splenectomy blood contains few if any siderocytes. Small numbers of siderocytes may also be found in the blood of normal subjects whose spleen has been removed for traumatic rupture. Two splenic mechanisms appear to play a part in removal of iron from red cells. Normal reticulocytes, after leaving the bone marrow, spend some time—a matter of hours perhaps—in the spleen and, while sequestered there, hæmoglobin formation is completed and iron visible by the light microscope is utilized. Thus, when these cells again circulate in the peripheral blood they are free from easily demonstrable iron granules, with the result that the siderocyte count of normal peripheral blood is zero. In conditions in which erythropoiesis is greatly increased and reticulocytes are released prematurely from the marrow, small amounts of iron may be utilized in the peripheral blood even in the absence of the spleen (Deiss *et al.*, 1966).

In pathological states in which the developing normoblasts contain iron in excess of that needed for hæm synthesis, excess iron must persist in reticulocytes and in non-reticulated erythrocytes unless a mechanism other than metabolic usage removes it. As demonstrated by Crosby (1957) the spleen has the power of removing large foreign bodies which may be present in erythrocytes; in particular, it can remove large siderotic granules without destroying the cells themselves. Hence the virtual absence of siderocytes in the peripheral blood of patients with, for example, refractory sideroblastic anæmia, who have intact spleens. After splenectomy, however, siderocytes circulate in large numbers in this condition, partly because the cells which contain siderotic granules are unable to metabolize the iron further and partly because no mechanism other than the spleen appears to exist in the body for their removal.

SIDEROBLASTIC ANÆMIA

Nomenclature. As we have already mentioned, we use the term "sideroblastic anæmia" to describe a dyshæmopoietic anæmia characterized by the presence of ring sideroblasts in the bone marrow. This term is not entirely satisfactory because it does not indicate either that the distribution of iron is abnormal or that abnormal amounts of iron are present. It does, however, emphasize the possible analogy of this condition to megaloblastic anæmia, another condition in which a particular morphological change in the erythroblasts may be brought about by a number of different mechanisms. Other terms have been suggested, notably "sideroachrestic anæmia" (Heilmeyer *et al.*, 1958). The disadvantage of this term is that it also fails to emphasize the morphological features of the condition and it draws attention to a feature present in other dyshæmopoietic anæmias. The term "refractory normoblastic anæmia" was used by Dacie *et al.* (1959), but the anæmia is not invariably refractory or normoblastic. Other names which have been used are chronic refractory hypochromic anæmia with disturbed hæm synthesis (Garby *et al.*, 1957), hypochromic anæmia with secondary iron loading (Crosby and Sheehy, 1950), dyshæmopoietic anæmia (Goldberg, 1965), and dyssideroblastic anæmia (Bowman, 1967).

Classification. The sideroblastic anæmias are classified according to MacGibbon and Mollin (1965) in Table II. They are not a single disorder; there are both inherited and apparently acquired types. The acquired type may be divided into primary (or idiopathic) and secondary acquired sideroblastic anæmia. The latter may be the result of drugs or toxins or may be associated with malabsorption, nutritional deficiency or with conditions causing increased cellular proliferation.

<h3 style="text-align:center">TABLE II</h3>

Classification of Sideroblastic Anæmia

Hereditary:		Sex-linked hypochromic anæmia
Acquired:		
	Primary:	"Refractory sideroblastic anæmia"
	Secondary:	Anti-tuberculous drugs
		Malnutrition, Malabsorption, etc.
		Drugs and Toxins
		Myeloproliferative conditions
		Malignant diseases
		Hæmolytic anæmia, etc.

<h3 style="text-align:center">Primary Sideroblastic Anæmia</h3>

Hereditary Sideroblastic Anæmia. This is a rare disorder which was first described, though not at the time recognized as sideroblastic anæmia, by Cooley (1945) and Rundles and Falls (1946). Many examples have subsequently been described and recent reviews include those of Bourne *et al.* (1965), Losowsky and Hall (1965), MacGibbon and Mollin (1965) and Elves *et al.* (1966). The hæmatological features are summarized in Table III.

<h3 style="text-align:center">TABLE III</h3>

Inherited Sideroblastic Anæmia

Age of onset: 6–30 years	**Sex**: usually male
Family history: characteristic	
Anæmia: hypochromic, often dimorphic	
M.C.H.C.: 22–28 per cent	**M.C.V.**: 74–84 cu.μ
Reticulocytes: 1–4 per cent	**Siderocytes**: many after splenectomy
Hb-F: absent or a trace	**Hb-A$_2$**: reduced
^{51}CrT$_{\frac{1}{2}}$: slightly decreased	**G-6-PD**: increased
Serum Fe: raised	**T.I.B.C.**: usually normal
	Per cent saturation: usually but not invariably almost completely saturated

The disorder presents as a chronic hypochromic anæmia, particularly affecting males. Erythroblasts may occasionally be seen in the peripheral blood film but never in large numbers. The serum iron concentration is usually increased and the plasma transferrin is usually saturated. The anæmia may be severe enough to require transfusion or the abnormality may be unrecognized unless the patient either develops folate deficiency or a pyridoxine-responsive anæmia, or is given one of the drugs which precipitates sideroblastic change. A typical example of the blood picture in a male with severe inherited sideroblastic anæmia is shown in Figure 2. The inheritance typically follows a sex-linked, apparently partially recessive, pattern (Cooley, 1945; Rundles and

Falls, 1946; Bourne *et al.*, 1965; Losowsky and Hall, 1965; Elves *et al.*, 1966). Females are less severely affected and the changes are usually very mild (Fig. 3). Occasionally females may be severely anæmic, however, with a dimorphic blood picture (Cooley, 1945; Rundles and Falls, 1946), which may be more striking than in the male (Pinkerton, 1967). This is shown in Figure 8, which is a microphotograph of the blood film of the patient shown in Figure 6 of MacGibbon and Mollin (1965) who was a woman with the inherited condition. Diagnosis is usually made in adolescence but may be made as early as the first year of life. Because of the striking hypochromasia (the MCHC is usually less than 28 per cent, and is sometimes very low), the anæmia is often misdiagnosed as iron-deficiency anæmia or, where a dimorphic picture is striking, as deficiency of iron and B_{12} and/or folate. However, it is readily differentiated by the level of the serum iron, by the excess of iron in the marrow, and of course by the failure to respond to iron therapy. Furthermore, small numbers of siderocytes are usually present in the peripheral blood and, if splenectomy has been performed, poorly hæmoglobinated siderocytes are present in large numbers.

Patients with sideroblastic anæmia also usually have increased amounts of the "i" antigen on the surface of their erythrocytes, whereas in iron-deficiency anæmia, the "i" antigen content of the erythrocytes is usually normal (Cooper, 1968). This antigen is only rarely present on the surface of normal human adult erythrocytes. In certain pathological conditions, however, principally those in which there is "marrow stress" or ineffective erythropoiesis, the "i" antigen is found in high titre on adult erythrocytes. For instance, increased amounts of the "i" antigen are also found on the erythrocytes in thalassæmia and megaloblastic anæmia (Hillman and Giblett, 1965; Cooper *et al.*, 1967).

Sideroblastic anæmia is distinguished from β-thalassæmia and hæmoglobin H disease by the presence of the ring sideroblasts in the marrow of the patients with sideroblastic anæmia. Furthermore, the mode of inheritance of the disease is different, hæmolysis is mild, the level of fœtal hæmoglobin low, and the level of hæmoglobin A_2 is normal or subnormal (Reed and Mollin, 1967).

Acquired Sideroblastic Anæmia. The main features of this condition are summarized in Table IV. This table summarizes the findings in 35 patients studied by MacGibbon and Mollin (1965) at Hammersmith Hospital during the last 16 years. Details of the first seven patients have been published elsewhere (Dacie *et al.*, 1959). Unlike the inherited condition, this is not a rare disease. However, cases will only be recognized if bone marrow films are routinely stained for iron. The disease most commonly affects middle-aged and elderly subjects and both sexes are affected. Patients usually present with symptoms attributable to anæmia, which extend back over a period of months or years. Often they will have been previously diagnosed as megaloblastic anæmia and treated unsuccessfully with B_{12} and/or folic acid. The condition may also be an incidental finding in a patient who presents with some unrelated complaint. Physical examination is usually unrewarding, but occasionally the spleen may be just palpable. At a late stage the clinical features of hæmochromatosis may develop.

The peripheral blood is characteristic and, if one is aware of the significance of the changes, permits a tentative diagnosis to be made. The abnormality which suggests sideroblastic anæmia is the presence of hypochromic erythrocytes amid many more or less normal looking cells. The proportion of hypochromic cells varies from patient to patient: they are never absent unless the condition is complicated by severe megaloblastic anæmia. However, they do not dominate the picture as in the inherited cases, so the MCHC is rarely very low (Table IV). Macrocytosis is present and is usually sufficiently severe to raise the mean cell volume above the upper limit of normal. Erythroblasts are seldom seen in the peripheral blood and the leucocyte and platelet counts are usually normal. Siderocytes are typically absent from the peripheral blood unless there is a fairly marked degree of

TABLE IV

Primary Acquired Sideroblastic Anæmia

Age of onset: 30–80 years	**Sex**: either sex
Family history: none	
Anæmia: Characteristically dimorphic: hypochromic cells ± to + +	
M.C.H.C.: 30–34 per cent	**M.C.V.**: 100–120 cu.μ
Reticulocytes: 0·8–8·0 per cent	**Siderocytes**: many after splenectomy
Hb-F: absent or a trace	**Hb-A$_2$**: reduced
^{51}CrT$_{\frac{1}{2}}$: slightly decreased	**G-6-PD**: normal or slightly increased
Serum Fe: normal or raised	**T.I.B.C.**: usually normal or reduced
	Per cent saturation: normal or slightly increased

hypochromasia. Even so they are present only in very small numbers unless the spleen has been removed, when extremely hypochromic cells, containing large siderotic granules, will be present in large numbers. In contrast to the findings in the inherited form of the disease, the serum iron concentration is frequently not increased and the percentage saturation of transferrin may be normal or only slightly raised.

Bone Marrow Appearance in Primary Sideroblastic Anæmia. In both inherited and acquired primary sideroblastic anæmia the bone marrow is characteristically hypercellular with erythropoiesis predominating. Nearly every erythroblast shows an excess of siderotic granules, almost all of them being ring forms, and the marrow particles also contain an excess of iron. In the inherited form the erythroblasts, when stained with Romanowsky stains, usually appear small with ragged, deficient cytoplasm and resemble the erythroblasts of thalassæmia or iron deficiency (Fig. 4). This micronormoblastic change may be so severe that it may mask the changes of an associated folate deficiency. In contrast, erythroblasts in the acquired form are macronormoblastic, that is, larger than normal, and may even be megaloblastic (Fig. 5). This megaloblastic change is sometimes due to an associated folate deficiency (see below), and in such patients the marrow may be indistinguishable from pernicious anæmia. But in other patients

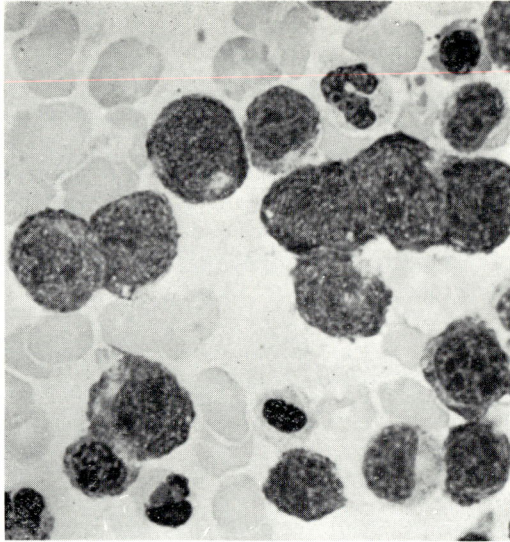

FIG. 5

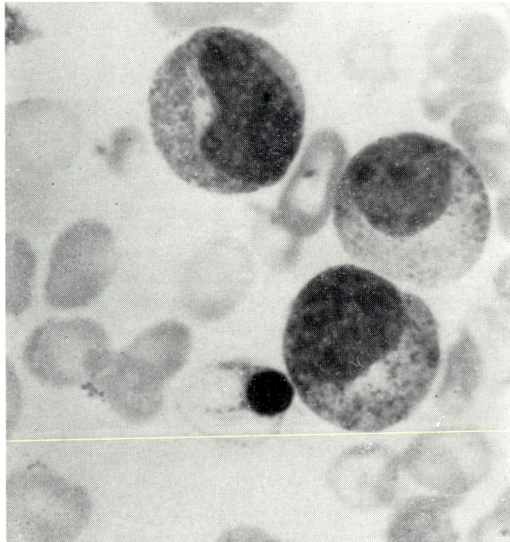

FIG. 6

FIG. 5. Acquired sideroblastic anaemia showing abnormally large erythroblasts.

FIG. 6. Marrow from a female patient with inherited sideroblastic anaemia
(MacGibbon and Mollin, 1965).

deficiency of folate or B_{12} is not the cause of the megaloblastic change for it persists in spite of treatment with B_{12} or folic acid. In both the acquired and the inherited types the percentage of hæmocytoblasts and pronormoblasts is strikingly increased when the anæmia is severe, a feature which may also suggest a diagnosis of megaloblastic anæmia or even erythroleukæmia. A

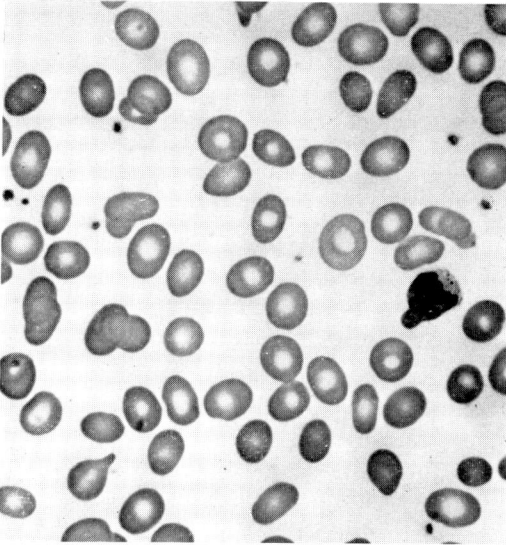

FIG. 7

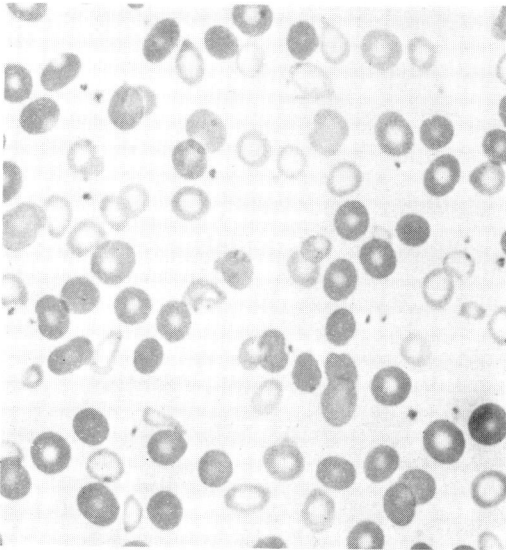

FIG. 8

FIG. 7. Peripheral blood film in inherited sideroblastic anaemia with folate deficiency, before treatment.

FIG. 8. Dimorphic appearance in a severe case of inherited sideroblastic anaemia, after folic acid therapy. Same case as Figs. 6 and 7.

valuable diagnostic finding in the bone marrow in sideroblastic anæmia is the presence of late normoblasts with characteristic vacuolated cytoplasm. These cells were first described by Dacie et al. (1959) and are shown in Figure 6.

The intensely erythroid bone marrow in the presence of a low hæmoglobin concentration and low peripheral reticulocyte count and the finding of abnormal, pyknotic dying erythroblasts in the marrow suggest that there is a considerable degree of ineffective erythropoiesis in sideroblastic anæmia. This is supported by the finding in some patients of raised fæcal urobilinogen excretion despite the relatively minor degree of peripheral hæmolysis (Dacie et al., 1959; Verloop et al., 1962), and of increased iron turnover but reduced incorporation of iron into circulating hæmoglobin (Dacie et al., 1959; Barry and Day, 1964). Wickramasinghe et al. (1968) who made cytochemical and autoradiographical studies on three patients with sideroblastic anæmia suggest that there is interference with the progress of early polychromatic cells through interphase probable leading to marrow death. In view of the considerable evidence of ineffective erythropoiesis in sideroblastic anæmia a surprising finding is that the serum lactic dehydrogenase activity, which is raised in other conditions asociated with significant degrees of ineffective erythropoiesis is normal in sideroblastic anæmia (Hoffbrand et al., 1966). The explanation for this discrepancy is unknown.

The Effect of Folate Deficiency on the Hæmatological Findings. As mentioned above, some degree of megaloblastic overlay due to folate deficiency is not uncommon in primary sideroblastic anæmia, and changes due to this deficiency may produce a striking alteration in the peripheral blood film. Figures 7 and 8 show the peripheral blood films of a patient with inherited sideroblastic anæmia before and after folic acid therapy. Hypochromic cells are absent from the peripheral blood before therapy and appear for the first time when folic acid is given. The initial absence of hypochromic cells suggests that the abnormal erythroblasts which produce them are particularly susceptible to folate deficiency, perhaps because they have an increased rate of mitosis and DNA synthesis.

Deficiency of Folate, Pyridoxine and of other Factors in Primary Sidero-blastic Anæmia. *Folate Deficiency.* There is biochemical, morphological and therapeutic evidence of folate deficiency in this condition. Subnormal serum folate levels were found in 80 per cent of the patients with primary sideroblastic anæmia by MacGibbon and Mollin (1965). The serum folate level is, however, a very sensitive test of folate deficiency and it is difficult to assess the severity of the deficiency from the result of this test alone. In a smaller group of patients the FIGLU excretion test was also carried out; 75 per cent of those who were tested gave positive results. However, although increased excretion of FIGLU in uncomplicated folate deficiency indicates that the deficiency is severe, the test is less specific than the serum assay. In particular, it is very frequently positive in patients with liver disease, and this is not infrequent in sideroblastic anæmia (Brain and Herdan, 1965). In liver diseases, excess excretion of FIGLU is often accompanied by an excessive excretion of the other histidine metabolite, urocanic acid, and both metabolites have indeed been found in the urine of about 15 per cent of patients with sideroblastic anæmia, including some with normal serum folate levels (Hoffbrand, Newcombe and Mollin, unpublished observations).

Morphological and therapeutic studies also give confusing results in patients with sideroblastic anæmia. Thus the appearance of the bone marrow is a poor criterion of the severity of folate deficiency. It may be normoblastic in patients with sideroblastic anæmia who have low serum folate levels and who respond excellently to treatment with small doses of the vitamin (MacGibbon and Mollin, 1965). In other patients, particularly in those with primary acquired sideroblastic anæmia, the marrow may show gross megaloblastic change, yet the hæmatological response may be insignificant despite the fact that the marrow reverts to normoblastic. Presumably in such patients the defect which causes sideroblastic anæmia inhibits the response to folic acid. It is probable that the most precise information about the severity of folate deficiency in sideroblastic anæmia will be obtained by studies of the folate content of red cells. Preliminary results show that between 20 and 30 per cent of the patients have subnormal red cell folate levels (Hoffbrand and Mollin, unpublished observations) but detailed results are not yet available.

In spite of these reservations about the significance of the different tests of folate deficiency, it is clear that this deficiency is rarely the main cause of anæmia in patients with primary sideroblastic anæmia. Only about one-third of the patients respond to treatment with folic acid and usually the response is small—frequently no more than a significant reticulocytosis associated with a small increase in the hæmoglobin concentration (Mollin and Dacie, 1960; MacGibbon and Mollin, 1965). However, a few respond more dramatically (Mollin and Dacie, 1960; Hines and Harris, 1964; MacGibbon and Mollin, 1965), and one should always be aware of the possibility that folate deficiency may aggravate the anæmia in these patients. As folate deficiency may develop at any stage of the disease, it is probably advisable to give daily supplements of folic acid to all patients with sideroblastic anæmia whether or not they show any initial response to this hæmatinic. If this is to be done, the serum B_{12} level should be checked, particularly in elderly patients, as sideroblastic anæmia may occasionally be found in association with syndromes which cause B_{12} deficiency.

Deficiency of Pyridoxine: "Pyridoxine-responsiveness". An anæmia closely resembling sideroblastic anæmia may develop in patients or experimental animals given anti-tuberculous drugs which interfere with B_6 metabolism (see later) and abnormalities of B_6 metabolism frequently occur in primary sideroblastic anæmia. Approximately 50 per cent. of the patients with primary sideroblastic anæmia excrete abnormal amounts of xanthurenic acid after a loading dose of 4 g. of L-tryptophan by mouth (MacGibbon and Mollin, 1965). A similar proportion of patients have low serum pryidoxine concentrations (Anderson and Mollin, unpublished observations). Other biochemical abnormalities found in B_6 deficiency have also been reported in sideroblastic anæmia, e.g. the serum cholesterol and serum lipid concentrations may be markedly reduced in pyridoxine-responsive patients with sideroblastic anæmia (Spitzer et al., 1966). In addition, approximately 37 per cent of patients with primary sideroblastic anæmia respond to treatment with large doses of pyridoxine. The responses are often minimal, but in some patients, usually with the inherited disease, the response was considerable and normal hæmoglobin concentrations are sometimes reached (Harris et al., 1965; Bishop and Bethell, 1959; Bourne et al., 1965; Losowsky and Hall, 1965; MacGibbon and Mollin, 1965). However, even in the latter patients abnormalities persist in the peripheral blood and ring sideroblasts persist, albeit in reduced numbers, in the bone marrow. In some patients in whom the initial hæmatological response to pyridoxine is minimal, treatment with large doses over a period of months may be associated with small, but clinically valuable, increases in hæmoglobin concentration. Patients who respond to treatment note a marked increase in energy and well-being. Similar subjective improvement is often reported by patients who show little or no hæmatological response.

The relationship between the biochemical evidence of pyridoxine deficiency and the clinical finding of pyridoxine responsiveness is uncertain. The fact that large and unphysiological doses of B_6 may be required to produce a hæmatological response (Harris and Horrigan, 1964; Gehrmann, 1965) suggests that the abnormality is not deficiency of B_6. Furthermore, there is no predictable correlation between the excretion of xanthurenic acid after a tryptophan load and the response to treatment with pyridoxine; patients with negative tests may respond to pyridoxine in large doses or vice versa. A more detailed study of the metabolism of B_6 on lines suggested by Linkswiler's (1967) review of the biochemical effects of B_6 deficiency is needed before the significance of these observations is understood.

There is a large literature on *pyridoxine-responsive anæmia*—the hypochromic anæmia which responds to treatment with large doses of pyridoxine. The subject has recently been reviewed by Horrigan and Harris (1964) and Gehrmann (1965). It is doubtful if these anæmias need to be placed in a separate category from the sideroblastic anæmias; hæmatologically they appear to be identical with patients discussed above (Mollin and Dacie, 1960). The most striking responses are found in patients suffering from the inherited condition.

"Deficiency" of other Factors. Occasionally patients with sideroblastic anæmia show a hæmatological response to ascorbic acid (Verloop and Rademaker, 1960; Vuylsteke *et al.*, 1961) or to a crude liver extract (Horrigan *et al.*, 1957; Mollin and Dacie, 1960; MacGibbon and Mollin, 1965) after failing to respond to either pyridoxine or folic acid. More recently, Hadnagy and Huszar (1966) have reported a patient with "sideroachrestic anæmia" who apparently showed reticulocyte responses to riboflavine and niacin as well as to pyridoxine. In other patients one factor alone fails to elicit a response, but a combined treatment with two factors, e.g. pyridoxine and liver extract (Horrigan and Harris, 1964), produces a significant rise in hæmoglobin. The nature of the factor present in crude liver extract which produces the response is unknown, but studies to date indicate that it is non-protein, of small molecular weight, and contains an intact indole ring (Horrigan and Harris, 1964). The existence of another active humoral factor which is a stable protein is suggested by the observations of Erslev *et al.* (1960). Their patient showed reticulocyte responses to transfusions of packed erythrocytes, fresh plasma and a plasma protein substance, and transfusion of whole blood produced a sustained rise in hæmoglobin, more than could be accounted for by the amount of cells given. Ultimately, however, their patient became refractory to these forms of therapy and his anæmia responded to pyridoxine.

Tissue Iron Stores in Primary Sideroblastic Anæmia. An increase in tissue iron stores, chiefly in the liver and bone marrow, is an almost invariable finding in primary sideroblastic anæmia. In some patients this increase in tissue iron may be attributed in part at least to long continued iron therapy or to repeated blood transfusions. In others the degree of iron loading far exceeds that which can be explained by therapy and in these the main source of the excess iron is probably increased absorption of dietary iron, since this occurs in many chronic anæmias associated with increased bone marrow activity (Bothwell *et al.*, 1958). Increased iron absorption was found by Brain and Herdan (1965) in one patient with sideroblastic anæmia, while a further ten patients absorbed normal amounts of iron despite having increased tissue iron stores. Increased iron absorption in the face of excess iron stores such as occurs in idiopathic hæmochromatosis has also been found in sideroblastic anæmia by Verloop *et al.* (1964) and Losowsky and Hall (1965).

In many of the patients with primary sideroblastic anæmia, hæmosiderosis is extremely severe (Brain and Herdan, 1965), and fully developed hæmochromatosis may occur in these patients. It is particularly frequent in the patients who show a hæmatological response to pyridoxine. For instance, Hathaway *et al.* (1967), who studied liver samples from 31 patients with pyridoxine-responsive anæmia, found that as many as one-third showed features of hæmochromatosis, i.e. excessive iron deposits, portal fibrosis and disordered architecture of the liver lobules with nodular regeneration. The high incidence of hæmochromatosis in patients who develop pyridoxine-responsive anæmia may be related to the length of history of these patients, for B_6 deficiency may be a late manifestation of the disease. It may also be that the derangement of pyridoxine metabolism damages the liver cells directly, apart from any effect of iron overload, since pyridoxine deficiency is known to cause liver damage with cirrhosis in the experimental animal (Wizgird *et al.*, 1965). In some of the patients the histological findings in the liver are extremely bizarre, resembling those caused by B_6 deficiency in the experimental animal or associated with extreme malnutrition (Mollin and Harrison, unpublished observations).

Treatment of Iron Overload. Because of the danger of hæmochromatosis and also because it has been suggested that iron overload may aggravate the anæmia (Bishop and Bethell, 1959; Harriss *et al.*, 1965), a number of workers have attempted to reduce iron overload in patients with sideroblastic anæmia, either by repeated venesection (Crosby and Sheehy, 1960; Verloop *et al.*, 1964) or by the use of the iron-chelating agent, desferrioxamine (Verloop *et al.*, 1964; Brain and Herdan, 1965; Lee *et al.*, 1966; Malpas, 1966). There is as yet no definite evidence that either of these methods of treatment benefits the anæmia, though they may well help to prevent or delay the onset of hæmachromatosis in some patients.

Secondary Sideroblastic Anæmia

Sideroblastic anæmia, or more frequently sideroblastic change, may be found in patients suffering from conditions listed in Table V. In many instances the sideroblastic change contributes only minimally to the anæmia from which the patient suffers, but in some instances it is the major cause of anæmia. The hæmatological features most commonly resemble those seen in inherited sideroblastic anæmia, but the blood picture may resemble that in the primary acquired condition. In either case, the hæmatological features will be modified to a variable extent by the associated condition.

Severe hypochromic sideroblastic anæmia may occur in patients receiving pyridoxine antagonists for the treatment of tuberculosis. Isoniazid alone or with para-aminosalicyclic acid (PAS) is a rare cause of the anæmia (Kohn *et al.*, 1962; Redleaf, 1962; McCurdy, 1963; McCurdy and Donohue, 1966). However, these drugs, if given for more than a few months, frequently produce abnormal sideroblasts in the bone marrow, sometimes with characteristic ring forms (Roberts *et al.*, 1966). Cycloserine and pyrazinamide, on the other hand, readily produce the anæmia (Harriss *et al.*, 1965; Verwilghen *et al.*, 1965). The sideroblastic anæmia is usually cured if the drugs are stopped or if pyridoxine is given.

TABLE V

Secondary Acquired Sideroblastic Anæmia

	No. of cases
Anti-tuberculosis therapy (Isoniazid, PAS, Cycloserine, etc.)	4
Malabsorption syndrome	5
Partial gastrectomy	3
Nutritional megaloblastic anæmia	1
Chronic alcoholism	5
Phenacetin, Paracetamol	6
Lead	3
Polycythæmia, thrombocythæmia or myelofibrosis	8
Leukæmia (usually myeloid)	5
Carcinoma	6
Myeloma	2
Hæmolytic anæmia (Hereditary spherocytosis, elliptocytosis)	3
Pernicious anæmia	1
Myxœdema	2
Rheumatoid arthritis	8
Total	62

Modified from Dacie and Mollin (1966), *Acta Med. Scand.*, Supp. 445, **179**, 235.

Sideroblastic change, and more rarely sideroblastic anæmia, is occasionally seen in patients with nutritional megaloblastic anæmia, malabsorption syndrome or chronic alcoholism. The cause of sideroblastic anæmia in these patients is uncertain, but it is possible that it is due to deficiency of pyridoxine, due to a defective diet with or without defective absorption. In these patients sideroblastic anæmia is always associated with megaloblastic anæmia due to folate deficiency. When they are treated with folic acid and given a normal hospital diet, both the megaloblastic anæmia and the sideroblastic anæmia disappear rapidly (Mollin, Hines, Booth and Waters, unpublished observations). It is possible that during treatment with folic acid the increased dietary intake of pyridoxine or some other factor consequent on their improved appetite may allow absorption of enough of the active compound to cure the associated sideroblastic anæmia. However, in one patient with idiopathic steatorrhœa who developed megaloblastic anæmia due to folate deficiency and sideroblastic anæmia, who was also receiving isoniazid and PAS for pulmonary tuberculosis, folic acid therapy did not reverse the sideroblastic change (Fig. 9). It is clear that more precise therapeutic studies are needed in this group to elucidate the cause of anæmia. If sideroblastic anæmia in these patients is due to nutritional deficiency of some factor like pyridoxine, it may appear surprising that sideroblastic change is so rare in these con-

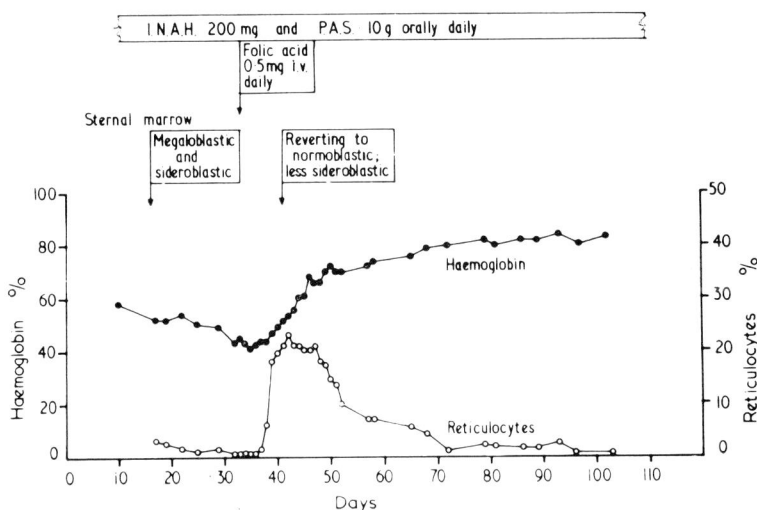

FIG. 9

ditions. This may be because, as Dawson et al. (1964) pointed out, the defect is masked by the presence of iron-deficiency anæmia which is almost invariably present in malabsorption syndrome and in nutritional megaloblastic anæmia. Certainly we have only found sideroblastic anæmia in patients with the malabsorption syndrome who have been given an intramuscular course of iron some time before we investigated them.

Drugs which may produce sideroblastic anæmia are listed in Table V. Lead, which inhibits the synthesis of hæm at several points in its synthetic pathway (Goldberg et al., 1956), is a well-recognized cause. Sideroblastic change may also occur in patients with partial gastrectomy or blind loop syndrome who have taken large doses of phenacetin or paracetamol (Table V). Sideroblastic anæmia in these latter patients is usually associated with folate deficiency and hæmolytic anæmia, and sideroblastic change has also been reported in association with intravascular hæmolysis in mechanical hæmolytic anæmia (Petz and Goodman, 1966).

Finally, sideroblastic anæmia may develop in conditions in which there is increased proliferation of cells (Table V). It is noteworthy that these are the disorders in which secondary folate deficiency has also been reported (Chanarin et al., 1958; Mollin and Hoffbrand, 1965). In some of these patients it seems possible that sideroblastic anæmia is also due to a conditioned deficiency of some factor, possibly pyridoxine, for, as in other diseases listed in Table V, the condition is frequently reversed by treatment with folic acid alone and/or pyridoxine. However, in some patients, particularly in some of those with myeloproliferative disorders and leukæmia, sideroblastic change may persist after treatment, suggesting that the change is due to irreversible disordered cell function.

THE PATHOGENESIS OF SIDEROBLASTIC ANÆMIA

As we pointed out earlier, the sideroblastic anæmias are a diverse group of conditions characterized by an abnormal accumulation of iron on peri-nuclear mitochondria and by a defect in the synthesis of hæmoglobin. Both the reason for the abnormal distribution of iron and the nature of the defect in hæmoglobin synthesis is uncertain, but possible explanations have been discussed earlier in this paper and in a number of previous papers, for example, by Mollin and Dacie (1960), Harris and Horrigan (1964), Horrigan and Harris (1964), and Dacie and Mollin (1966).

Hæm and Globin Synthesis and Pyridoxine Metabolism in Sideroblastic Anæmia. It has been suggested that the primary defect may be a failure in the synthesis of globin (Heller et al., 1965) However, defective synthesis of globin in thalassæmia does not produce the characteristic changes of sideroblastic anæmia, and the evidence for a *primary* defect in globin synthesis in sidero-blastic anæmia is unconvincing. Others have suggested that the anæmia is due to defective synthesis of hæm—the result of defects in the mitochondrial enzymes concerned with this synthesis. A pyridoxal co-enzyme is known to be required for the synthesis of delta-aminolævulinic acid (ALA) from glycine and succinyl co-enzyme A and it is suggested that in pyridoxine-responsive anæmia there is an acquired or inherited enzyme defect interfering with the synthesis of ALA (Vogler and Mingioli, 1965) which may be partially over-come if relatively enormous doses of pyridoxine are given. Frimpter (1965) has shown that in children with cystathionuria, the apo-enzyme cystathionase is present in liver tissue but not active until the cellular concentration of the co-enzyme pyridoxine is greatly elevated. It may be that an analogous situation occurs in some patients with pyridoxine-responsive anæmia (Scrivener, 1967). Lee and his colleagues (1966) have suggested that there may also be a block in the incorporation of iron into protoporphyrin in those patients with sidero-blastic anæmia who do not respond to treatment with pyridoxine, but, as they point out, direct evidence for this and for the other hypotheses explaining the defect in sideroblastic anæmia is lacking. In some cases of secondary sideroblastic anæmia, pyridoxine may overcome the defect in ALA synthesis by correcting a deficiency of the vitamin or by overcoming the effect of known pyridoxine antagonists. In the experimental animal at least, nutritional deficiency of pyridoxine or the administration of pyridoxine antagonists can produce an anæmia resembling sideroblastic anæmia (Harriss et al., 1965; Deiss et al., 1966). But direct evidence for this and for other hypotheses is lacking, thus Vavra and Poff (1967) were unable to detect any deficiency in activity of any step between aminolævulinic acid and hæm. Nor were they able to demonstrate any defect in synthesis of hæm beyond the stage of coproporphyrin. They pointed out that the synthesis of ALA was not ade-quately studied but concluded that no serious inhibition was present.

Iron Accumulation on Mitochondria. It is claimed that, in normal erythro-blasts, free iron granules are not associated with the mitochondria. In cells in which ring or partial perinuclear rings are found, the iron seems to be associated with mitochondria. This intense accumulation of iron on the mitochondria in sideroblastic anæmia and the persistence of these bodies in the perinuclear situation may be a direct consequence of the block in hæm synthesis. These changes are unlikely to be due to a failure to synthesize hæmoglobin, since this massive accumulation of iron is rarely if ever seen in the poorly hæmoglobinated erythroblasts found in uncomplicated thalassæmia. Iron may accumulate on some of the mitochondria in some patients with thalassæmia (Bessis et al., 1958) and has also been reported to occur on mitochondria in patients with chloramphenicol poisoning and porphyria cutanea tarda (Goodman and Hall, 1967), in mechanical hæmolytic anæmia (Petz and Goodman, 1966) and in lead poisoning in the experimental animal (Jensen and Moreno, 1964). Ring sideroblasts also may occur in these conditions, but the incidence of ring sideroblasts is much lower than in primary sideroblastic anæmia.

It has been suggested that pyridoxal phosphate also affects the mobiliza-tion of iron from the mitochondria (Cooper et al., 1963) and it is possible that this vitamin also directly or indirectly affects the rate of entry of iron into the erythroblasts. It is uncertain whether the presence of excess amounts of iron in the cells and on the mitochondria interferes with pyridoxine metabolism and with the synthesis of hæmoglobin. One curious fact that is unexplained is that pyridoxine dependency may develop during the course of the disease. Brown (1958) showed that excess iron could inhibit the synthesis of delta-aminolaevulinic acid by chicken erythrocyte preparations, and Bishop and Bethell (1959) therefore suggested that pyridoxine dependency was due to a direct toxic effect of excess iron in the erythroblast. Drug-induced sideroblastic anæmia in mice and guinea-pigs tends to be more severe if the animals are given an iron supplement, but there is no evidence that this iron supplement caused a further increase in accumulation of iron in the abnormal erythroblasts (Harriss et al., 1965). Moreover, the removal of the excess iron from patients with primary sideroblastic anæmia associated with iron overload by phlebotomy (Crosby and Sheehy, 1960; Verloop et al., 1962), or by the use of desferrioxamine (Lee et al., 1966), does not usually lead to a significant improvement in the anæmia. This is perhaps not surprising as ring sideroblasts remain until the body stores of iron are exhausted and iron deficiency develops.

Aetiology of Folate Deficiency in Sideroblastic Anæmia. Folate deficiency is very common in sideroblastic anæmia, and is often the main cause of the anæmia in the secondary form. In fact, it is so common in the latter that it is possible that it is a factor contributing to the production of sideroblastic change. However, there is no experimental evidence in support of this view (Harris *et al.*, 1965). In the primary condition the deficiency is probably due to an increased requirement for folate caused by the greatly increased, though largely ineffective, erythropoiesis. In some patients inadequate intake of the vitamin also plays a part. It is possible that abnormal pyridoxine function also contributes to the megaloblastic anæmia and "folate deficiency" found in these patients, for some of the enzymatic reactions in which folate is concerned are pyridoxine-dependent.

The Inherited Condition. In a proportion of patients with sideroblastic anæmia, the condition is obviously genetically determined. In other patients with the apparently acquired forms of the condition it may well be that susceptibility to the disease is also genetically determined but the overt disease only becomes apparent when secondary factors, e.g. pyridoxine or folate deficiency, drugs or hæmolysis, put an additional stress on the marrow. The gene responsible for the inherited condition may be linked to the X chromosome, and the striking dimorphic blood picture which may be found in the heterozygous female carrier has led Pinkerton (1967) to suggest that there may be X chromosome inactivation in such patients, "the abnormal erythrocytes stemming from cells in which the maternal X chromosome has been inactivated and the normal cells from those in which the paternal X chromosome has been 'turned off' ". On the other hand, Losowsky and Hall (1965) did not consider that the presence of two populations of red cells in the carrier state can be taken as evidence in favour of X chromosome inactivation since, as they and others have noted, an obviously dimorphic film may be found in males with the overt disease.

Sideroblastic Anæmia and Myeloproliferative Diseases. The relationship of leukæmia and in particular erythroleukæmia with sideroblastic anæmia is of special interest and has received a good deal of attention (Dameshek, 1965). However, ring sideroblasts are not commonly found in leukæmia (Dacie and Mollin, 1966). Occasionally ring sideroblasts may be found in some patients and exceptionally many ring sideroblasts occur. In these rare instances the distinction between the chronic Di Guglielmo's disease and primary sideroblastic anæmia may be difficult. One distinctive feature is that severe folate deficiency and rapid clearance of folic acid are unusual in the former disease but are frequent in the latter (Mollin, unpublished observations). Furthermore, we have not seen a patient with primary sideroblastic anæmia develop the typical hæmatological features of acute Di Guglielmo's disease. Nevertheless, three of our patients who apparently suffered from typical primary acquired sideroblastic anæmia developed myeloblastic leukæmia after a period of years, and similar cases have been previously reported by Björkman (1956) and Reimann *et al.* (1965). The leucocytes of a patient of Petz *et al.* (1966) showed an acquired Pelger-Huët-like anomaly which is usually associated with leukæmia. Sideroblastic change is not uncommon in patients with myelofibrosis, and may occur occasionally in patients with polycythæmia (Table V). In this connection it is interesting that De Grouchy *et al.* (1966) observed a chromosome abnormality in patients they considered to be suffering from "idiopathic acquired sideroblastic anæmia" similar to that which Kay *et al.* (1966) found in patients with polycythæmia rubra vera.

In some instances, therefore, it appears that sideroblastic anæmia and sideroblastic change are a part of a leukæmic or leukæmia-like process. It may be that the presence of sideroblastic anæmia and the consequent long-continued increased and disordered marrow cell turnover increases the patient's susceptibility to develop myeloproliferative disorders of the marrow. Moreover, iron overload itself may at least in the experimental animal produce malignant change. It is unlikely, however, that the majority of patients with either inherited or primary acquired sideroblastic anæmia have leukæmia, Di Guglielmo's disease, or myelofibrosis. However, until the pathogenesis of sideroblastic anæmia is understood, such a statement must remain a matter of opinion.

Treatment of Sideroblastic Anæmia

In general, treatment of sideroblastic anæmia is unsatisfactory. As we have pointed out, a small proportion of the patients respond almost completely to folic acid or pyridoxine, but this is exceptional. A small hæmatological improvement occurs more commonly in response to these vitamins and more rarely to ascorbic acid or crude liver extract. These drugs should therefore be tried and may sometimes be successful in combination when one alone fails to elicit a response. Blood transfusion may be necessary in patients whose anæmia is severe, but this should be used sparingly in order to reduce the danger of iron overload. Desferrioxamine and, in patients with relatively mild anæmia, repeated venesections may also be used in an effort to reduce iron stores (Crosby and Sheehy, 1960; Verloop *et al.*, 1962; Karabus and Fielding, 1967); iron therapy should be avoided. Finally, in patients with secondary sideroblastic anæmia, treatment of the associated disease and/or discontinuation of the drug or toxin that is causing or aggravating the condition may improve the anæmia.

References

BAINTON, D. F. and FINCH, C. A. (1964). The diagnosis of iron deficiency anemia. *Amer. J. Med.*, **37**, 62.

BARRY, W. E. and DAY, H. J. (1964). Refractory sideroblastic anemia. *Ann. int. Med.*, **61**, 1029.

BESSIS, M. C., ALAGILLE, D. and BRETON-GORIUS, J. (1958). Particularités des erythroblastes et des erythrocytes dans la maladie de Cooley. Etude au microscope électronique. *Rev. hémat.*, **13**, 37

BESSIS, M. C. and BRETON-GORIUS, J. (1959). Ferritin and ferruginous micelles in normal erythroblasts and hypochromic hypersideremic anemias. *Blood*, **14**, 423.

BESSIS, M. C. and JENSEN, W. N. (1965). Sideroblastic anaemia, mitochondria and erythroblastic iron. *Brit. J. Haemat.*, **11**, 49.

BISHOP, R. C. and BETHELL, F. H. (1959). Hereditary hypochromic anemia with transfusion hemosiderosis treated with pyridoxine. *New Engl. J. Med.*, **261**, 486.

BIZZOZERO, G. (1883). Cited by P. EHRLICH. Zur Physiologie und Pathologie der Blut scheiben. *Charite-Ann.*, **10**, 136.

BJÖRKMAN, S. E. (1965). Chronic refractory anemia with sideroblastic bone marrow: a study of four cases. *Blood*, **11**, 250.

BOTHWELL, T. H., PIRZIO-BIROLI, G. and FINCH, C. A. (1958). Iron absorption: 1. Factors influencing absorption. *J. Lab. clin. Med.*, **51**, 24.

BOURNE, M. S., ELVES, M. W. and ISRAËLS, M. C. G. (1965). Familial pyridoxine-responsive anaemia. *Brit. J. Haemat.*, **11**, 1.

BOWMAN, W. D. (1961). Abnormal ("ringed") sideroblasts in various hematologic and non-hematologic disorders. *Blood*, **18**, 662.

BOWMAN, W. D. (1967). Reversible sideroblastic anemia during infectious mononucleosis. *Rocky Mountain med. J.*, **64**, 46.

BRAIN, M. C. and HERDAN, A. (1965). Tissue iron stores in sideroblastic anaemia. *Brit. J. Haemat.*, **11**, 107.

BROWN, E. G. (1958). Evidence for the involvement of ferrous iron in the biosynthesis of amino levulinic acid by chicken erythrocyte preparations. *Nature*, **182**, 313.

CHANARIN, I., MOLLIN, D. L. and ANDERSON, B. B. (1958). Folic acid deficiency and the megaloblastic anaemias. *Proc. roy. Soc. Med.*, **51**, 757.

COOLEY, T. B. (1945). A severe type of hereditary anemia with elliptocytosis. Interesting sequence of splenectomy. *Amer. J. med. Sci.*, **209**, 561.

COOPER, A. G., HOFFBRAND, A. V. and WORLLEDGE, S. M. (1968). Increased agglutinability by anti "i" of red cells in sideroblastic and megaloblastic anaemia. *Brit. J. Haemat.* (in press).

COOPER, R. G., WEBSTER, L. T. and HARRIS, J. W. (1963). A role of mitochondria in iron metabolism of developing erythrocytes. (Abstract.) *J. clin. Invest.*, **42**, 926.

CROSBY, W. H. (1957). Siderocytes and the spleen. *Blood*, **12**, 165.

CROSBY, W. H. and SHEEHY, T. W. (1960). Hypochromic iron-loading anaemia: Studies on iron and haemoglobin metabolism by means of vigorous phlebotomy. *Brit. J. Haemat.*, **6**, 56.

DACIE, J. V. (1963). *The Haemolytic Anaemias*. Part I, The Congenital Anaemias. London: Churchill.

DACIE, J. V. and DONIACH, I. (1947). The basophilic property of the iron-containing granules in siderocytes. *J. Path. Bact.*, **59**, 884.

DACIE, J. V. and MOLLIN, D. L. (1966). Siderocytes, sideroblasts and sideroblastic anaemia. *Acta med. scand.*, Suppl., **445**, 237.

DACIE, J. V., SMITH, M. D., WHITE, J. C. and MOLLIN, D. L. (1959). Refractory normo-blastic anaemia: a clinical and haematological study of seven cases. *Brit. J. Haemat.*, **5**, 56.

DAMESHEK, W. (1965). Sideroblastic anaemia: Is this a malignancy? *Brit. J. Haemat.*, **11**, 52.

DAWSON, A. M., HOLDSWORTH, D. D. and PITCHER, C. S. (1964). Sideroblastic anaemia in adult coeliac disease. *Gut*, **5**, 304.

DE GROUCHY, J., DE NAVA, C., ZITTOUN, R. and BOUSSER, J. (1966). Analyses chromo-somiques dans l'anémie sidéroblastique idiopathique acquise. *Nouv. Rev. franc. d'Hemat.*, **6**, 367.

DEISS, A., KURTH, D., CARTWRIGHT, G. E. and WINTROBE, M. M. (1966). Experimental production of siderocytes. *J. clin. Invest.*, **45**, 353.

DONIACH, I., GRÜNEBERG, H. and PEARSON, J. E. G. (1943). The occurrence of siderocytes in adult human blood. *J. Path. Bact.*, **55**, 23.

DOUGLAS, A. S. and DACIE, J. V. (1953). The incidence and significance of iron-containing granules in human erythrocytes and their precursors. *J. clin. Path.*, **6**, 307.

ELVES, M. W., BOURNE, M. S. and ISRAËLS, M. C. G. (1966). Pyridoxine-responsive anaemia determined by an X-linked gene. *J. med. Genet.*, **3**, 1, 1966.

ERSLEV, A. J., LEAR, A. A. and CASTLE, W. B. (1960). Pyridoxine-responsive anemia. *New Engl. J. Med.*, **262**, 1209.

FRIMPTER, G. (1965). Cystathionuria: nature of the defect. *Science*, **149**, 1095.

GARBY, L., SJÖLIN, S. and VAHLQUIST, B. (1957). Chronic refractory hypochromic anaemia with disturbed haem-metabolism. *Brit. J. Haemat.*, **3**, 55.

GEHRMANN, G. (1965). Pyridoxine-responsive anaemias. *Brit. J. Haemat.*, **11**, 86.

GOLDBERG, A. (1965). Sideroblastic anaemia: a commentary. *Brit. J. Haemat.*, **11**, 114.

GOLDBERG, A., ASHENBRUCKER, H., CARTWRIGHT, G. E. and WINTROBE, M. M. (1956). Studies on the biosynthesis of heme *in vitro* by avian erythrocytes. *Blood*, **11**, 821.

GOODMAN, J. R. and HALL, S. G. (1967). Accumulation of iron in mitochondria of erythro-blasts. *Brit. J. Haemat.*, **13**, 335.

GRÜNEBERG, H. (1941a). Siderocytes: a new kind of erythrocytes. *Nature, Lond.*, **148**, 114.

GRÜNEBERG, H. (1941b). Siderocytes in man. *Nature, Lond.*, **148**, 469.

HADNAGY, C. S. and HUSZAR, I. (1966). Effect of pyridoxine, riboflavine and niacin on sideroachrestic anaemia. *Proc. 11th Congr. Int. Soc. Haemat.*, *Sydney*. Abstracts, p. 349.

HARRIS, J. W. and HORRIGAN, D. L. (1964). Pyridoxine-responsive anemia—prototype and variations on a theme. In *Vitamins and Hormones*, **22**, 721. New York and London: Academic Press.

HARRIS, J. W., WHITTINGTON, R. N., WEISMAN, R. (Jr.) and HORRIGAN, D. L. (1956). Pyridoxine responsive anemia in the human adult. *Proc. Soc. exp. Biol.* (*N.Y.*), **91**, 427.

HARRISS, E. B., MacGIBBON, B. H. and MOLLIN, D. L. (1965). Experimental sideroblastic anaemia. *Brit. J. Haemat.*, **11**, 99.

HATHAWAY, D., HARRIS, J. W. and STENGER, R. J. (1967). Histopathology of the liver in pyridoxine responsive anemia. *Arch. Path.*, **83**, 175.

HEILMEYER, L. (1963). Symposium on sideroachrestic anaemias, introd. by L. Heilmeyer. In: *Proc. 9th Congr. europ. Soc. Haemat., Lisbon*, 1963, p. 240. Basel/New York: S. Karger.

HEILMEYER, L., KEIDERLING, W., BILGER, R. and BERNAUER, H. (1958). Uber chronische refraktäre Anämien mit sideroblastichem Knochenmark (Anaemia refractoria sideroblastica). *Folia Haemat. (Frankfurt)*, N. F. **2**, 49.

HELLER, P., STONE, J. V., APPLE, D. and COLEMAN, R. D. (1965). Defective globin synthesis in hypochromic hypersideremic anemia (⌐-thalassemia?). *Blood*, **25**, 635.

HILLMAN, R. S. and GIBLETT, E. R. (1965). Red cell membrane alteration associated with "marrow stress". *J. clin. Invest.*, **44**, 1730.

HINES, J. D. and HARRIS, J. W. (1964). Pyridoxine-responsive anemia. Description of three patients with megaloblastic erythropoiesis. *Amer. J. clin. Nutr.*, **14**, 137.

HOFFBRAND, A. V., KREMENCHUZKY, S., BUTTERWORTH, P. J. and MOLLIN, D. L. (1966). Serum lactic dehydrogenase activity and folate deficiency in myelosclerosis and other haematological diseases. *Brit. med. J.*, **i**, 577.

HORRIGAN, D. L. and HARRIS, J. W. (1964). Pyridoxine-responsive anemia: an analysis of 61 cases. *Advanc. intern. Med.*, **12**, 103.

HORRIGAN, D. L., WHITTINGTON, R. M., WEISMAN, R. and HARRIS, J. W. (1957). Hypochromic anemia with hyperferricemia responding to oral crude liver extract. *Amer. J. Med.*, **22**, 99.

JENSEN, W. N. and MORENO, G. (1964). Les ribosomes et le ponctuations basophules des erythrocytes dans l'intoxication par le plomb. *C.R. Acad. Sci. (Paris)*, **258**, 3596.

KAPLAN, E., ZUELZER, W. W. and MOURIQUAND, C. (1954). Sideroblasts. A study of stainable nonhemoglobin iron in marrow normoblasts. *Blood*, **9**, 203.

KARABUS, C. D. and FIELDING, J. (1967). Desferrioxamine chelatable iron in haemolytic, megaloblastic and sideroblastic anaemias. *Brit. J. Haemat.*, **13**, 924.

KAY, H. E. M., LAWLER, S. D. and MILLARD, R. E. (1966). The chromosomes in polycythaemia vera. *Brit. J. Haemat.*, **12**, 507.

KIERKEGAARD-HANSEN, A. (1966). Sideroblastanaemier: En oversigt og to tilfaelde af primaer akvisit sideroblastanaemi. *Saertryk af Ugeskrift for Laeger*, **128**, 1532.

KOHN, R., HEILMEYER, L. and CLOTTEN, R. (1962). Reversible pyridoxin-sensible symtomatische sideroachrestische Anämie unter Isoniazidbehandlung bei einer käsigen Lymphknotentuberkulose mit Pleuritis exsudativa. *Dtsch. med. Wschr.*, **87**, 1765.

LEE, G. R., CARTWRIGHT, G. E., and WINTROBE, M. M. (1966). The response of free erythrocyte protoporphyrin to pyrodoxine therapy in a patient with sideroachrestic (sideroblastic) anemia. *Blood* **27**, 557.

LINKSWILER, H. (1967). Biochemical and physiological changes in vitamin B6 deficiency *Amer. J. clin. Nutr.*, **20**, 547.

LOSOWSKY, M. S. and HALL, R. (1965). Hereditary sideroblastic anaemia. *Brit. J. Haemat.*, **11**, 70.

MCCURDY, P. R. (1963), Isoniazid conditioned pyridoxine responsive anemia. *Clin. Res.*, **11**, 59.

MCCURDY, P. R. and DONOHOE, R. F. (1966). Pyridoxine-responsive anemia conditioned by isonicotinic acid hydrazide. *Blood*, **27**, 352.

MCFADZEAN, A. J. S. and DAVIS, L. J. (1947). Iron-staining erythrocytic inclusions with especial reference to pernicious haemolytic anaemia. *Glas. med. J.*, **28**, 237.

MCFADZEAN, A. J. S. and DAVIS, L. J. (1949). On the nature and significance of stippling in lead poisoning, with reference to the effect of splenectomy. *Quart. J. Med.*, **18**, 57

MACGIBBON, B. H. and MOLLIN, D. L. (1965). Sideroblastic anaemia in man: observations on seventy cases. *Brit. J. Haemat.*, **11**, 59.

MALPAS, J. S. and CALLENDER, S. (1967). Studies on sideroblastic anaemia. (To be published.)

MOLLIN, D. L. and DACIE, J. V. (1960). Further observations on refractory normoblastic anaemia. *Proc. 7th Congr. europ. soc. Haemat., London*, 1959, Part 2, p. 74. Basel: S. Karger.

MOLLIN, D. L. and HOFFBRAND, A. V. (1965). The diagnosis of folate deficiency. *Series Haemat.*, **1**, 3. Copenhagen: Munksgaard.

MORROW, J. J. and GOLDBERG, A. (1965). The sideroblastic anaemias. *Postgrad. med. J.* **41**, 740.

PAPPENHEIMER, A. M., THOMPSON, W. P., PARKER, D. D. and SMITH, K. E. (1945). Anemia associated with unidentified erythrocytic inclusions, after splenectomy. *Quart. J. Med.*, **14**, 75.

PETZ, L. D. and GOODMAN, J. R. (1966). Ringed sideroblasts and intramitochondrial iron, in cases of mechanical hemolytic anemia. *Ann. intern. Med.*, **64**, 635.

PETZ, L. D., GOODMAN, J. R., HANN, S. G. and FINK, D. J. (1966). Refractory normoblastic ("sideroblastic") anemia. *Amer. J. clin. Path.*, **45**, 581.

PINKERTON, P. H. (1967). X-linked hypochromic anaemia. *Lancet*, **i**, 1106.

REDLEAF, P. D. (1962). Pyridoxine-responsive anemia in a patient receiving isoniazid. *Dis. Chest*, **42**, 222.

REED, L. J. and MOLLIN, D. L. (1967). A₂ haemoglobin levels in sideroblastic anaemia. (In preparation.)

REIMANN, F., ERDOGAN, G. and TANGÜN, Y. (1965). Ein fall von sideroblastischer Anaemie mit besonderem chromosomenbefund. *Proc. 10th Congr. europ. Soc. Haemat., Strasbourg*, 1964. Basel: S. Karger.

ROBERTS, P. D., HOFFBRAND, A. V. and MOLLIN, D. L. (1966). Iron and folate metabolism in tuberculosis. *Brit. med. J.*, **ii**, 198.

RUNDLES, R. W. and FALLS, H. F. (1946). Hereditary (? sex-linked) anemia. *Amer. J. med. Sci.*, **211**, 641.

SCRIVENER, C. R. (1967). Pyridoxine deficiency and dependency. *Amer. J. Dis. Child.* **113**, 109.

SORENSON, G. D. (1962). Electron microscopic observations of bone marrow from patients with sideroblastic anemia. *Amer. J. Path.*, **40**, 297.

SPITZER, N. NEWCOMB, T. F. and NOYES, W. D. (1966). Pyridoxine-responsive hypolipidemia and hypocholesterolemia in a patient with pyridoxine-responsive anemia. *New Engl. J. Med.*, **274**, 772.

VAVRA, J. D. and POFF, S. A. (1967). Heme and porphyrin synthesis in sideroblastic anaemia. *J. lab. clin. Med.*, **69**, 904.

VERLOOP, M. C. (1967). Anémies hypochromes hypersidérémiques. In *Progrès en Hématologie*, Editions Médicales Flammarion, Paris, ed. B. Dreyfus, p. 133.

VERLOOP, M. C., BIERENGA, M. and DIEZERAAD-NJOO, A. (1962). Primary or essential sideroachrestic anaemias. Pathogenesis and therapy. *Acta haemat. (Basel)*, **27**, 129.

VERLOOP, M. C., PLOEM, W. and LEUNIS, J. (1964). Hereditary hypochromic hypersideraemic anaemia. In *Iron Metabolism: an International Symposium sponsored by CIBA, Aix-en Provence*, 1963, p. 376. Chairmen, Dreyfus, J-C. and Schapira, G. Berlin: Springer-Verlag.

VERLOOP, M. C. and RADEMAKER, W. (1960). Anaemia due to pyridoxine deficiency in man. *Brit. J. Haemat.*, **6**, 66.

VERWILGHEN, R., REYBROUCK, G., CALLENS, L. and COSEMANS, J. (1965). Antituberculous drugs and sideroblastic anaemia. *Brit. J. Haemat.*, **11**, 92.

VOGLER, W. R. and MINGIOLI, E. S. (1965). Heme synthesis in pyridoxine-responsive anemia. *New Engl. J. Med.*, **273**, 347.

VUYLSTEKE, J., VERLOOP, M. C. and DROGENDIJK, A. C. (1961). Favourable effect of pyridoxine and ascorbic acid in a patient with refractory sideroblastic anaemia and haemochromatosis. *Acta med. scand.*, **169**, 113.

WICKRAMASINGHE, S. N., CHALMERS, D. G. and COOPER, E. H. (1968). A study of ineffective erythropoiesis in sideroblastic anaemia and erythraemic myelosis. *Cell and Tissue Kinetics*, **1**, 43.

WISGIRD, J. P., GREENBERG, L. D. and MOON, H. D. (1965). Hepatic lesions in pyridoxine deficient monkeys. *Arch. Path.*, **79**, 317.

SECTION IV

HISTOLOGY

Section Editor

M. S. DUNNILL

M.D.(Bristol), M.R.C.P.(Lond.), M.C.Path.
Director of Clinical Studies, University of Oxford,
Consultant Pathologist, Radcliffe Infirmary, Oxford

Chapter 18

HUMAN CHROMOSOMES

A. I. Spriggs and D. J. Bartlett

INTRODUCTION

UNTIL 1956 *Homo sapiens* did not know his own chromosome count, and this in spite of knowing the correct chromosome numbers of thousands of other species of organism. The sudden flood of investigations concerning the human chromosomes resulted from the discovery of some simple technical tricks, particularly hypotonic pre-treatment before fixation (Tjio and Levan, 1956; Ford and Hamerton, 1956).

The whole subject of human cytogenetics is dealt with in various textbooks, some of which are recommended in the bibliography at the end of this chapter. It would be unreasonable to attempt a balanced summary here, covering even the principal fields of usefulness of chromosome studies in the human species. We believe, however, that there is a need for a practical description of techniques which have been found to work. This is followed by a section on chromosome identification and a simplified list of the cytogenetic abnormalities found in certain recognized syndromes. There follow sections on chromosome breakage and on the chromosome changes in neoplastic diseases, partly because these belong more clearly to the domain of clinical pathology, and also because they have not yet been adequately dealt with in the textbooks.

TECHNIQUES

I. Sex Chromatin

(*a*) **Buccal Smear.** Examination of the nuclei of buccal mucosal cells for the presence or absence of sex chromatin is a rapid and efficient method of obtaining information about the X chromosome complement of an individual. The sex chromatin or Barr body appears typically as a crescent-shaped area of condensed chromatin at the periphery of the nucleus. The presence of one or more Barr bodies indicates that the individual possesses one more X chromosome than the number of visible sex chromatin masses. The absence of a Barr body indicates the presence of only one X chromosome.

In good preparations from normal females, the Barr body is visible in 20–70 per cent of carefully selected buccal cell nuclei. Unselected nuclei may give lower counts if there is much pyknosis. Each laboratory has to determine its normal range.

Technique

(1) With a clean metal or wooden spatula (a sterile throat swab in the case of a very young baby) gently but firmly scrape the inside of the cheek.

298

(2) Transfer a layer of buccal mucosal cells and mucus to the surface of a clean, labelled glass slide by running the surface of the spatula over the slide once from one end to the other.

(3) Place the slide immediately in fixative, ethanol or 50:50 ether-ethanol mixture, for at least 10 minutes.

(4) Rinse in 70 per cent alcohol.

(5) Wash in tap water.

(6) Stain in 0·5 per cent cresyl violet for 5–10 minutes.

(7) Rinse in tap water.

(8) Dehydrate and differentiate through 70 per cent and 95 per cent ethanol.

(9) Clear in xylol and mount in D.P.X.

An alternative method which also gives good results is as follows (Atkin, 1967):

(1) Fix in 95 per cent ethanol.

(2) Dry the slide.

(3) Place in a jar of 2 per cent acetic orcein (G. T. Gurr Ltd.) for 20 minutes.

(4) Drain off excess stain until only a trace remains.

(5) Add one or two drops of glycerol and place a cover-glass in position.

(6) If desired, seal with Kronig's cement.

If speed is important, a drop or two of the orcein solution can be put on the fixed smear and a cover-glass placed on top; examination can then be done almost at once.

(*b*) **Drumsticks in Polymorphonuclears.** The sex chromatin appears in some polymorphs as a pedunculated body (drumstick) about 1 μ in diameter. It is not seen in normal males, and its significance is the same as that of the Barr body, but care has to be taken not to confuse it with other chromatin masses. In a Romanowsky-stained blood film, a count of 200 polymorphs is nearly always enough to distinguish between a normal male (no drumsticks) and a normal female (at least 2 drumsticks).

The technique of preparation is as for ordinary microscopy of a blood film.

II. Preparation of Chromosomes for Analysis

In order to obtain chromosomes for analysis from different tissues, a number of different methods are given below. The first method—blood culture—is described in full, but since the final stages in sections (4) to (10) apply equally to the methods given for obtaining chromosomes from skin, bone marrow and other tissues, they are not described again in full for each method.

(*a*) **Blood Culture.** Preparations suitable for chromosomal analysis are probably most easily obtained from cultures of leucocytes in samples of peripheral blood by the method of Moorhead, Nowell, Mellman, Batipps and Hungerford (1960).

The following method is suitable for very small blood samples.

Solutions

(1) Heparin B.P. sterile ampoules of 20,000 units (Boots Pure Drug Co.). Solution made up to 2,000 U/ml. in distilled water.

(2) Phytohæmagglutinin (in ampoules) (Burroughs Wellcome).

(3) Parker's T.C. 199 medium (Burroughs Wellcome), Eagle's medium (Burroughs Wellcome), or T.C.-medium Ham F10 (DIFCO).

(4) Sterile human AB serum—inactivated by heating at 56°C for 30 minutes.

(5) Fixative—3 : 1 mixture of ethanol (74 O.P. Spirit) and glacial acetic acid.

(6) Colcemid (Ciba)—0·04 per cent solution.

(7) Two per cent lactic acetic orcein—2 g. natural orcein in 50 : 50 glacial acetic acid and 70 per cent lactic acid.

(8) Forty-five per cent acetic acid.

(9) Sodium citrate—0·95 per cent tri-sodium citrate solution.

(10) 2-Ethoxy-ethanol. Euparal Essence. Euparal.

Culture Medium

AB serum 2·5 ml.
TC 199 medium 2·5 ml. } prepared aseptically
Heparin 0·05 ml.
Phytohæmagglutinin 0·3 ml.
Gas with 5 per cent CO_2 in air

Technique

(1) Eight to ten drops (0·2 ml.) blood are added to 5 ml. culture medium in a universal bottle and incubated in a water bath at 37°C after standing for two hours at room temperature. (Successful preparations have been obtained from specimens which have not been incubated until 48 hours after collection.)

(2) After three days' incubation, 0·5 ml. Colcemid solution pre-warmed to 37°C is added to inhibit spindle formation and arrest cell division at metaphase.

(3) After a further three hours the culture is removed from the water bath, transferred to a conical centrifuge tube and centrifuged at 1,000 r.p.m. (R.C.F. 240) for 10 minutes. The clear supernatant fluid is discarded.

(4) The cells are carefully resuspended in 4–5 ml. *freshly prepared*, pre-warmed sodium citrate solution, in order to swell the cells and disperse the chromosomes, and left for 15–30 minutes at 37°C.

(5) The suspension is again centrifuged at 1,000 r.p.m. for five minutes and most of the supernatant fluid discarded.

(6) The cell mass is again carefully resuspended in the remaining supernatant fluid and *freshly prepared* fixative is gently added drop by drop down the side of the tube while mixing continuously. It is important to avoid the formation of a solid mass of insoluble hæmatin which will enmesh the leucocytes.

(7) The tubes are allowed to stand for 5–15 minutes at room temperature before the cells are again spun down and further changes of fixative (2–5) are made in order to eliminate the hæmatin. The cells are resuspended in 45 per cent acetic acid.

(8) After at least one hour preparations may be made (but the suspension at this stage can be stored for long periods at −20°C). The suspension is concentrated to a slight visible turbidity. A large drop is placed on an *absolutely grease-free* slide, and the slide warmed over a Bunsen flame. The drop is allowed to run to and fro over the surface of the hot slide until entirely evaporated.

(9) Wet preparations may be made by placing a drop of lactic-acetic-orcein on a polished coverslip and picking this up on the prepared slide by capillary attraction. The preparation may be examined after a few minutes, but the stain should be allowed to act for at least two hours.

(10) Permanent preparations are made by floating off the coverslip in 45 per cent acetic acid, immersing in two changes of 2-ethoxyethanol and one of Euparal Essence and finally mounting in Euparal.

(*b*) **Skin Culture.** This technique is of particular value where it is difficult to obtain a blood sample, where information is required about the chromosome complement of an individual with suspected mosaicism, or where a method involving long-term cell culture is required. It is a more complex method than that of blood culture, and there is a greater delay before suitable preparations can be obtained. The following description of the technique is based on those of Harnden (1960) and Hsu and Kellogg (1960).

Solutions

(1) Human AB serum. Blood is collected from donors into a dry bottle without anticoagulant and allowed to clot. The serum is removed aseptically and distributed

into aliquots which are incubated for 24 hours to check for sterility. It is then stored at −20°C.

(2) Freeze-dried chicken plasma (DIFCO)—reconstituted as necessary.

(3) Hanks's phosphate buffered saline—

CaCl$_2$ 0·14 g.   MgSO$_4$7H$_2$O 0·2 g.
NaCl 8·0 g.   KH$_2$PO$_4$2H$_2$O 0·054 g.
KCl 0·4 g.   Na$_2$HPO$_4$2H$_2$O 0·058 g.
Glucose 1·0 g.   0·2 per cent Phenol red 10 ml.

Made up to 1 litre with distilled water, and sterilized by autoclaving at 10 lb. p.s.i. for 10 minutes.

If desired, antibiotics may be added:

Penicillin   final conc. 100 I.U./ml.
Streptomycin   final conc. 100 mg/ml.
Mycostatin (Nystatin)   final conc. 50 I.U./ml.

The same solution is also prepared omitting the Ca and Mg salts.

(4) Chicken embryo extract. Ten-day-old chick embryos are removed aseptically from their eggs, placed in a sterile 20 ml. syringe, pulped and mixed with an equal volume of 5 per cent Hanks's phosphate buffered saline. The mixture is centrifuged to remove most of the solid material and the supernatant is frozen and thawed about six times to kill any remaining cells. A final centrifugation is carried out to remove remaining solids and the supernatant extract is incubated for 24 hours to check sterility before storing at −20°C.

(5) Trypsin (1 : 250 Bacto Trypsin) 0·5 per cent solution. in Ca and Mg free phosphate buffered saline. Sterilize by filtering through a sintered glass bacterial filter (No. 5).

(6) E.D.T.A. (Versene) solution. 0·5 per cent disodium ethylene diamine tetra-acetate in Ca and Mg free phosphate buffered saline, sterilized as above.

(7) Trypsin/E.D.T.A. harvesting solution. Trypsin 0·5 per cent solution, E.D.T.A. 0·5 per cent solution and Ca and Mg free phosphate buffered saline are mixed aseptically in the proportions 10 : 10 : 80 respectively.

(8) Harnden Medium A. AB Serum, Chick embryo extract and T.C. 199 are mixed in the proportions 20 : 20 : 60 respectively.

(9) Harnden Medium B. Chick embryo extract, AB serum and T.C. 199 are mixed in the proportions 10 : 20 : 70 respectively.

Technique

(1) A 1–4 sq. mm. skin biopsy specimen (removed by slicing over forceps so that minimal capillary bleeding may occur from the dermis) is collected into a bottle containing T.C. 199. Subsequently it is cut up aseptically into minute pieces with fine scissors in a draught-free cabinet. About five of these pieces are placed separately into a small Carrel flask previously placed in the cabinet and each is then covered by a drop of chicken plasma and a drop of embryo extract. The flasks are stoppered with non-toxic white rubber or silicone rubber bungs.

(2) Sterile air-CO$_2$ mixture (95 per cent air to 5 per cent CO$_2$) is introduced into the flasks which are then left for at least 30 minutes to allow the clots to harden before adding Harnden A medium, 2 ml. to a 50 mm. diameter flask.

(3) Primary culture. The flasks are incubated at 37°C. The medium may be changed every three to four days, or as necessary, during incubation, which is continued until a heavy growth of cells is seen surrounding the tissue fragments.

(4) Harvesting. The culture medium is removed from the flasks, 2 ml. Trypsin/ E.D.T.A. harvesting solution is added and the flask is returned to the incubator for 10–15 minutes. If the cell sheet has not detached from the glass, incubation is continued until this occurs.

(5) Secondary culture. The cell suspension is transferred to a centrifuge tube and spun at 1,000 r.p.m. for five minutes. After pouring off the supernatant fluid, the sedimented cells are resuspended in 5 ml. Harnden Medium B and a large Carrel flask (80 mm. diameter) is inoculated with the total yield of cells. Gassing with the air/CO$_2$ mixture is carried out as before, and the culture is incubated at

37°C with periodic changes of medium as necessary, until a full sheet of cells has grown on the bottom of the flask, at which time the culture is ready to be harvested for chromosome preparations.

(6) Chromosome preparations. Subculturing proceeds as before, but only a proportion (approximately 40 per cent) of the total cell population is used. The rest is divided between a portion (approximately 30 per cent) used to re-subculture the large flask as a stock culture, and a further portion used to subculture a fresh flask for chromosome preparation. Harnden B Medium is used for both flasks, and after re-gassing, the cultures are again incubated at 37°C.

(7) After 22 hours' incubation, 0·5 ml. of 0·04 per cent Colcemid solution is added to the 5 ml. medium in the flask containing cells to be used for chromosome preparation. Incubation is continued for a further six hours. The medium is then removed, the cells harvested with Trypsin/E.D.T.A. as above, and subsequently separated from the harvesting solution by centrifugation.

(8) Chromosome preparations are obtained as by stages (4) to (9) of the method for blood culture.

(c) **Bone Marrow.** Since the examination of chromosomes in bone marrow cells is most commonly carried out in the investigation of leukæmia, it is important to avoid culture methods which may allow normal cells to over-grow the abnormal ones. A "direct" method is therefore preferred, in which cells are examined which were already in mitosis at the time of biopsy. The method is adapted from that of Tjio and Whang (1962), but the hypotonic solution is the one recommended by Yamada et al. (1966).

Solutions

(1) Collecting medium. 5 ml. T.C. 199, 2½ ml. inactivated human AB serum and 300 U heparin.

(2) Hypotonic solution. 0·3 per cent glucose, 0·35 per cent sodium chloride, 0·2 per cent sodium citrate.

(3) Colcemid (Ciba). 100 mg. per cent in saline.

Technique

(1) A few drops of cellular marrow are placed in the collecting medium and dispersed by shaking.

(2) When received in the laboratory, two drops of colcemid solution are added to 7½ ml. cell suspension and incubated for two hours at 37°C.

(3) The suspension is centrifuged, and the cells resuspended in the hypotonic solution. Incubation is continued for a further 10 minutes.

(4) The remainder of the technique is as for a blood culture, from stage (5) onwards.

(d) **Tumours and other Solid Tissues.** A freshly removed fragment, which must not be necrotic, is minced with scissors or teased out with needles or sharp-pointed forceps in hypotonic solution (as given in the section on bone marrow) so as to free the cells mechanically. The cell suspension is pipetted off from remaining fibrous tissue and visible fragments, and incubated at 37°C for 10 minutes. It is then handled as described for blood culture from stage (5).

If the cells are to be exposed to colcemid before processing, the specimen should be teased out in the collecting medium for bone marrow described above, and then handled in exactly the same way. This preliminary colcemid treatment has been thought to improve chromosome contraction and spreading but is not essential.

(e) **Gonad**. Stages of meiotic cell division can be studied by examining cells obtained by testicular (or ovarian) biopsy. The appearance of paired chromosomes (bivalents) at diakinesis and metaphase may help considerably in the interpretation of structural chromosomal aberrations and even in the detection of some abnormality which has not been visible from a study of mitotic preparations (McIlree, Tullock, Newsam and Barclay, 1966). Very fresh specimens are essential to obtain good preparations.

Solutions

(1) Sodium citrate ($Na_3C_6H_5O_7.2H_2O$)—

isotonic 2·2 per cent solution
hypotonic 1·2 per cent solution.

(2) Fixative. 3 : 1 ethanol (74 O.P.) : glacial acetic acid. Chloroform is added, 1 part to 40 parts of above fixative mixture.

(3) Lactic-acetic-orcein. 2 per cent solution.

Technique (Evans, Breckon and Ford, 1964)

(1) A testicular biopsy specimen of 15–20 mm.^{3} is removed under light general anæsthesia (Kjessler, 1966) or local anæsthesia (Rowley and Heller,1966).

(2) The tubules of the specimen are carefully teased out under isotonic citrate solution, and their contents expelled by gentle pressure with curved forceps. When the tubules have been emptied as far as possible, they are allowed to settle, and the supernatant fluid is transferred to a 15 ml. centrifuge tube.

(3) The cell suspension is centrifuged at 500 r.p.m. for five minutes and the supernatant is discarded.

(4) Chromosome preparations are obtained as by stages (4) to (9) of the blood culture method, using a 1·2 per cent solution of sodium citrate and centrifuging at 500 r.p.m. (R.C.F. 60).

(*f*) **Autoradiography.** Certain radioactive substances can be incorporated into the new molecules of deoxyribonucleic acid (DNA) which are produced when chromosomes undergo replication during interphase. The presence of these substances can then be detected by placing a special photographic film in contact with a preparation containing chromosomes which have been so "labelled". When the film is developed the autoradiograph will show a pattern of silver grains over the chromosomes corresponding to the degree and distribution of the incorporated radioactive substance. Since the timing of DNA synthesis varies for different chromosomes and for different areas of chromosomes, the technique of autoradiography is of particular use in helping to characterize certain chromosomes which could not otherwise be differentiated on a morphological basis. The radioactive substance most commonly used for this technique is tritiated thymidine.

Materials

(1) Tritiated thymidine (Radiochemical Centre, Amersham, Bucks). 2·5 Ci/m.Mol. activity. Sterility is important as contamination will neutralize the solution.

(2) Kodak Autoradiographic Stripping Plates (AR-10). Plates $6\frac{1}{2}. \times 4\frac{3}{4}$ in. Store at 4°C.

(3) Kodak D 19b Developer.

(4) Potassium bromide 10 mg/litre solution.

(5) Photographic fixer.

Technique

(1) A blood culture is set up as described.

(2) Continuous labelling. At four hours prior to cell fixation a tritiated thymidine solution, made up with isotonic saline or distilled water and containing 20 μCi/ml. is added to the culture at the rate of 0·01 ml. thymidine solution/1 ml. culture.

(3) At $1\frac{1}{2}$ hours prior to cell fixation, 0·5 ml. of a 0·04 per cent solution of colcemid is added.

(4) The culture is processed as already described for exposure to hypotonic citrate, fixative and stain and the slides are examined for suitable metaphases. Their positions on the slide are noted and the chromosomes photographed. The coverslips are then floated off in euparal essence and the unmounted slides are ready for autoradiographic preparation.

(5) Autoradiographic stripping plates should be warmed to room temperature (21°C) before use. The plates should be handled in a dark room, but a Kodak Wratten Series I safe-light may be used at a distance of not less than 4 ft.

(6) One plate is removed from the box of twelve and $\frac{1}{4}$ in. of the emulsion is cut off with a sharp scalpel from either end of the plate.

(7) The rest of the emulsion is divided by the scalpel into twelve rectangles. At this point the relative humidity of 60–64 is very critical; it is either too low or too high the effect on the pieces of film will be seen.

(8) Each rectangle of film is removed by lifting one corner with the scalpel and then peeling off with the fingers or a pair of forceps.

(9) The rectangles are floated *face down* for 6–8 min. in a bowl of potassium bromide solution at 26°C to minimize fogging, and allow complete expansion of the film to take place.

(10) The pieces of film are then floated carefully on to the slides containing the chromosome preparations so that there is a direct contact between specimen and film.

(11) The slides are dried upright to assist drainage. An electric fan will also help in the drying process which should be complete in $1\frac{1}{2}$ hr. (If the slides will not be exposed for more than 30 days they should be stored at 4°C in light-proof tins containing a drying agent, e.g. silica gel. For storage periods of more than 30 days, an atmosphere of CO_2 is necessary.)

(12) Development. Temperature is extremely critical at this stage. Any change while the film is wet may shift the silver grain images away from their source. The slides should be at room temperature and are then placed in Kodak D 19b developer at 19°C for 6 min., rinsed in distilled water at 17–18°C for 15–30 sec., and placed in fixer at 17–18°C for 10 min. Finally the slides are washed in running tap water (or several changes of tap water) at 17–18°C for 15 min.

(13) After drying, excess film can be trimmed off and the specimen examined. If successful the slide is mounted in euparal; if not, the film can be stripped off and the autoradiographic process repeated (as the isotope has a half-life of 12·3 years) until successful.

A Liquid-emulsion technique (Rogers, 1967) may be substituted for the stripping-film technique described above. This has the advantage of giving a closer contact between emulsion and specimen, and the possibility of achieving an autoradiograph of higher resolution (using Ilford L4 or K2 emulsion) than can be achieved with stripping film. The main disadvantage is the difficulty of producing an emulsion layer of constant thickness.

CHROMOSOME IDENTIFICATION

The normal human somatic cell possesses a diploid ($2n$) complement of 46 chromosomes made up of 23 chromosomes derived from the gametic cells of the father and 23 from the mother, and these reduced, or haploid (n), numbers are found in all the more mature forms of gametic cells beginning with the secondary spermatocytes and secondary oocytes.

The diploid set consists of a pair of sex chromosomes and 22 other pairs known as autosomes. Members of an autosomal pair are alike in appearance. The sex chromosomes are alike in the female (XX) but different in the male (XY).

Morphological differentiation between chromosomes is dependent on four main features—the size of the chromosomes, the position of the centromere, the presence of secondary constrictions and the presence of satellites.

Relative *size* is a distinguishing character, but absolute size is of no importance because the degree of contraction varies from cell to cell.

The *centromere* is the point at which the two chromatids forming the chromosomes are held together. Its position may be described by the ratio of the short arm length to the total length of the chromosome, or by the use of descriptive terms—*metacentric* for a chromosome with arms of equal length, *submetacentric* for a chromosome with one pair of arms noticeably shorter than the other, and *acrocentric* for a chromosome with a nearly terminal centromere, so that the short arms are almost invisible.

Secondary constrictions are areas of diminished staining seen in certain chromosomes (the centromere is regarded as the primary constriction). The presence of a secondary constriction may help to pair two chromosomes which otherwise are difficult to differentiate from another pair of autosomes, but secondary constrictions are not always seen on both members of a chromosome pair, and they vary with the technique of preparation.

Satellites are small, circumscribed areas of chromatin found at the ends of the short arms of acrocentric chromosomes. Their frequent apparent lack of attachment to the short arms may be regarded as an extreme expression of secondary constriction. Satellites have been described in association with all the acrocentric chromosomes with the exception of the male sex chromosome (Y), but they are not invariably seen. When present they may help to differentiate one pair of acrocentric chromosomes from another.

Photographs of cells in metaphase may be cut up to allow arbitrary pairing of the chromosomes, and arrangement of the pairs in the form of a karyotype for the cell concerned. By convention, the chromosome pairs are arranged roughly according to size from the largest to the smallest, 1-22 (Denver system), and further separated into seven groups referred to as A, B, C, D, E, F and G (Patau system). A male and a female cell are shown arranged in this way in Figs. 1 and 2. (On chromosome identification see K. Patau in Yunis (1965), in bibliography.)

Within the A group it is possible to distinguish Nos. 1, 2 and 3. The distinctive metacentric E16 chromosome can be distinguished from the rest of the E group chromosomes. It is doubtful whether the autosomal members within the other groups can be distinguished from one another in ordinary preparations, but some chromosomes have characteristic autoradiographic labelling patterns; this also applies to one of the X pair in the female, which is otherwise indistinguishable from the rest of the C group.

The Y chromosome more or less resembles the autosomes of the G group (Nos. 21 and 22), but can often be distinguished from them. It is characteristically larger than 21 and 22 (although there is much variation in size); its long arms are often more parallel and may possess a secondary constriction, or appear diffuse at their distal ends. The short arms have a sharply cut-off appearance and do not have satellites.

Reliable karyotype analysis demands first-rate preparations. In every preparation there are cells which cannot be used because of excessive overlapping of chromosomes. Some cells are in late prophase or too early in metaphase for chromosome identification. If the chromatids are separating,

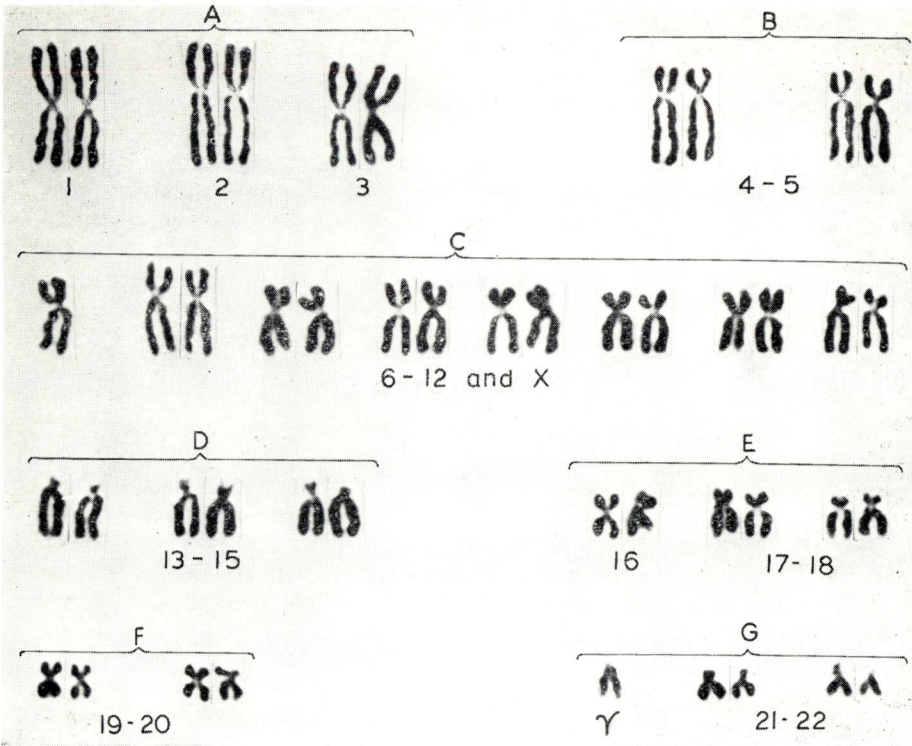

FIG. 1. Chromosomes of a normal male somatic cell. Note dissimilar sex chromosomes —X and Y— the former not certainly distinguishable from the rest of the C group.

or if the chromosomes are over-contracted by colchicine, analysis is made difficult. A few reliable observations are better than a large number of dubious ones, and time is well spent in searching for the finest examples of arrested metaphase.

ABNORMALITIES OF CHROMOSOMAL MORPHOLOGY AND COMPLEMENT

Chromosome abnormalities are conveniently classified as resulting from structural change occurring within one or more chromosomes or from numerical change affecting the normal chromosome complement.

I. Anomalies resulting from Structural Rearrangement

A prerequisite for all forms of structural rearrangement involving either one or more chromosomes is breakage or discontinuity of part of the chromosome. Reunion may follow on some form of incorrect realignment and this may or may not result in a visible chromosomal anomaly. The subject of chromosome breakage is dealt with below (p. 314), but its persistent effects are as follows:

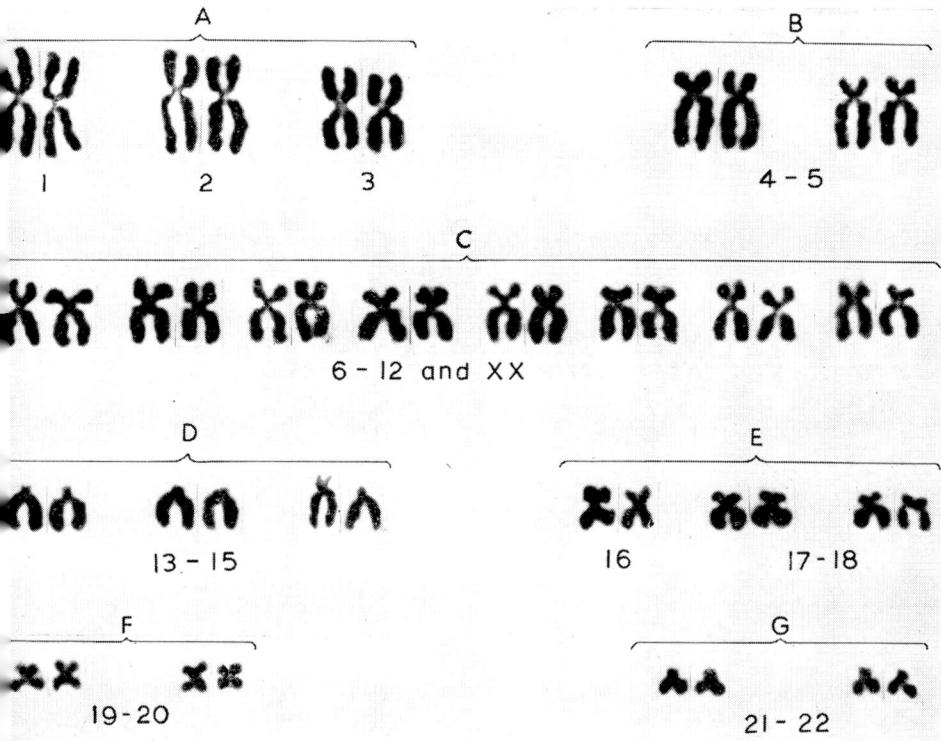

Fig. 2. Chromosomes of a normal female somatic cell. Note similar sex chromosomes—XX —which are not certainly distinguishable from the rest of the C group.

(*a*) **Deletion.** Simple breakage may result in failure of reunion and loss of the fragment (Fig. 3).

(*b*) **Translocation.** Interchange of chromatin material may occur within a single chromosome; or between homologous chromosomes, giving rise to *duplication* of a segment in one chromosome with a corresponding loss in its homologous partner; or between non-homologous chromosomes. Such an interchange between chromosomes may involve the centromere of one of the chromosomes, giving rise to the formation of a *dicentric chromosome* and an *acentric fragment*, which will eventually be lost in the course of subsequent cell divisions, since it will be unable to form a metaphase spindle attachment. Provided, however, that no portion of either chromosome is lost following breakage, a *balanced translocate* will result and there may be no detectable phenotypic effect. But the presence of such a translocation in the gametes may involve transmission of additional chromosomal material to the off-spring, in whom a phenotypic anomaly may give the first indication of the true state in the parent.

(*c*) **Inversion.** Simple reversal of a section of a chromosome may occur following breakage. If the section involved does not include the centromere, i.e. paracentric rather than pericentric, the morphological appearance of the

K

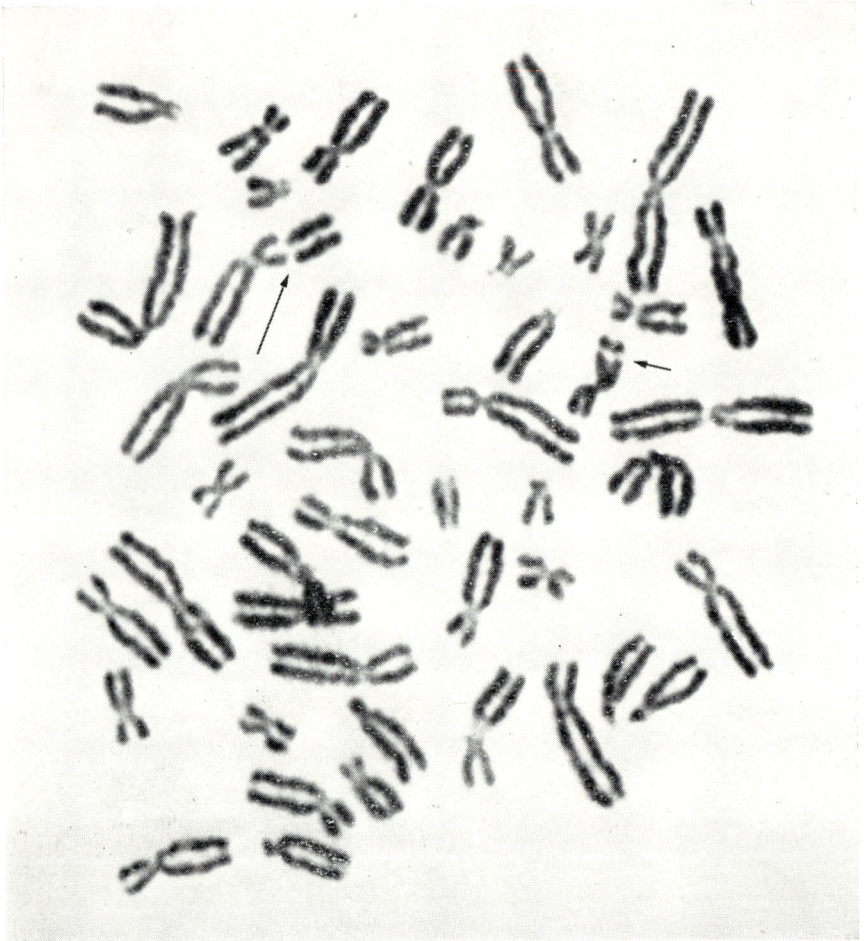

FIG. 3. Cell from blood culture of a patient with psoriasis under treatment with ametho-
pterin. There are two chromosome (isochromatid) defects; the one marked with a short
arrow is a gap with no displacement. That marked with a long arrow is a break, with
visible displacement of the fragment.

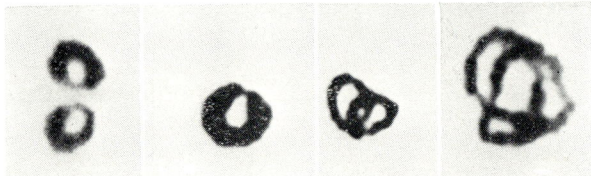

FIG. 4. *a, b, c,* and *d.* Varying appearances of a ring chromosome (probably derived from
a B group chromosome) in a blood culture.

chromosome will probably not be altered, but the rearranged juxtaposition of different genes may show a "position effect" in the phenotype of the individual.

(*d*) **Ring Chromosome.** This form of anomaly may result from the reunion of the broken ends of an incomplete chromosome (Fig. 4). If the centromere is not included, the ring chromosome will be lost as an acentric fragment.

(*e*) **Isochromosome.** This anomaly, of unknown mechanism, is classically explained by a transverse misdivision of the centromere. The homologous chromatids of one arm are realigned on either side of the centromere, and form an exactly metacentric chromosome with both arms genetically identical.

II. Anomalies of Chromosomal Complement

A prerequisite for any departure from the normal chromosome complement is some abnormality of cell division.

(*a*) **Aneuploidy** (abnormal chromosome number, other than multiples of the haploid set). Some aneuploid cells, particularly those with random loss of chromosomes, are often found in cultures and in direct chromosome preparations; they probably do not occur with significant frequency in the living tissues of normal persons.

Loss or gain of chromosomes may result from maldivision at meiosis or mitosis, by two different mechanisms:

(i) *Anaphase lagging* of a chromosome on the spindle with the possible subsequent elimination from the daughter cell.

(ii) *Non-disjunction* occurring at anaphase, so that both members of a chromosome pair are included in the same daughter cell.

The occurrence of one extra chromosome is known as *trisomy*, and several trisomic states are compatible with life, involving autosomes as well as sex chromosomes. *Monosomy* (the loss of one chromosome), on the other hand, is apparently lethal except where a sex chromosome is concerned.

(*b*) **Polyploidy.** Polyploid cells contain multiples of the haploid number and may be triploid (69), tetraploid (92) or some larger multiple. Multiples of the diploid set can occur in small numbers in normal tissues, but triploid and tetraploid embryos do not usually survive.

Triploidy is thought to result from the union of an unreduced diploid gamete with a normal haploid cell. (In theory, a triploid cell could also result from alternate disjunction and non-disjunction of homologous chromosomes at mitosis. Similarly, a tetraploid cell might result from union of two diploid gametes, or one triploid and one haploid gamete, or from non-disjunction of the whole chromosome set at mitosis.)

Polyploidy commonly results from two further abnormal forms of cell division; "endomitosis" and "endoreduplication". In the former no spindle or metaphase plate is formed and the nuclear membrane remains intact, but the chromatids of each chromosome separate from each other and subsequently reduplicate so that the chromosome number of the cell is effectively doubled (Fig. 5). Very large numbers of chromosomes may be found in one cell as a result of repeated endomitotic division. Such cells are frequently seen in malignant tissues.

In endoreduplication, a double DNA replication cycle occurs during interphase so that in such a cell, arrested with colcemid at metaphase, 92 chromosomes appear to be already arranged in homologous pairs (diplo-chromosomes) (Fig. 6). At present no particular significance is attached to the finding of a few such cells in a culture.

(*c*) **Mosaicism.** Non-disjunction occurring immediately after the formation of the zygote will give rise to two cells with abnormal chromosome complements and the persistence of those cell lines at subsequent mitotic divisions

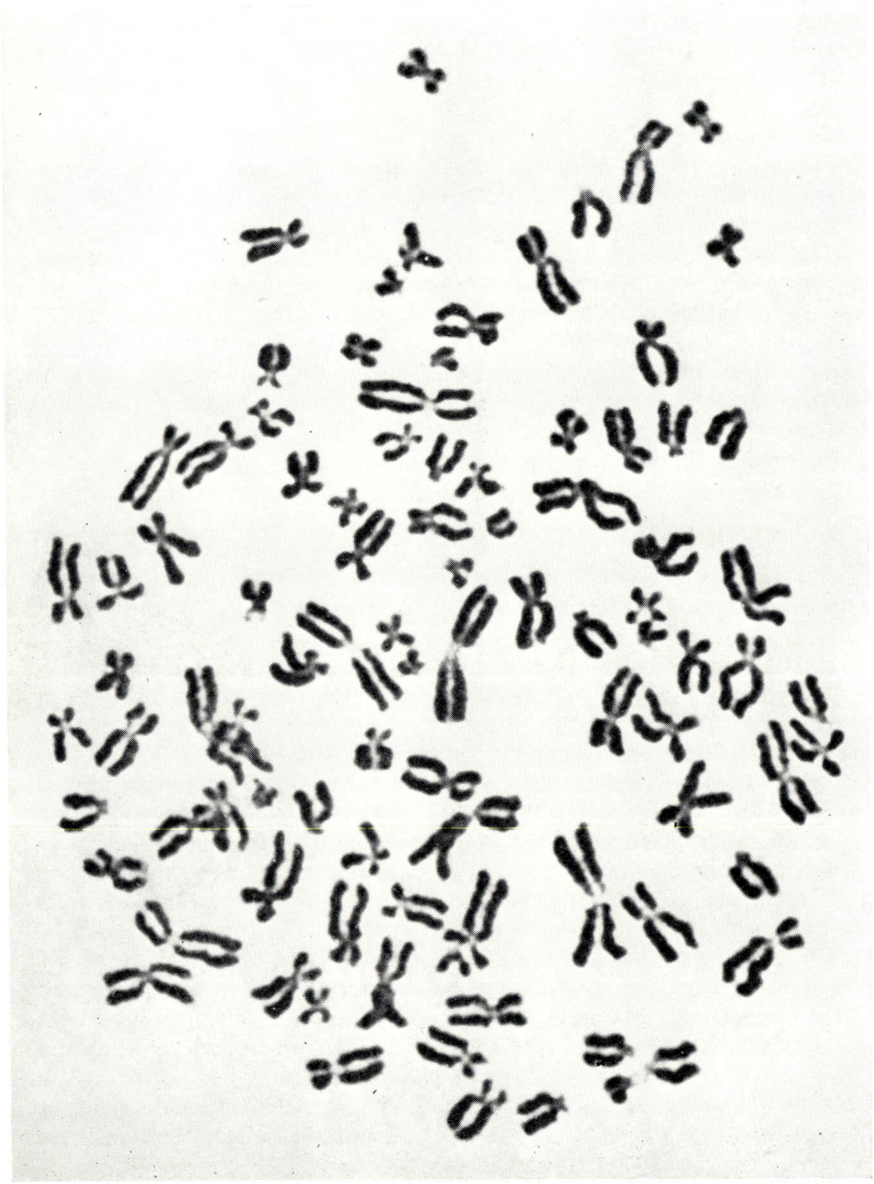

FIG. 5. Chromosomes of a tetraploid (92) female fibroblast which has probably undergone endomitosis in culture.

will result in the formation of a "mosaic" individual. A normal first post-zygotic division followed by non-disjunction occurring in only one of the daughter cells would result in a mosaic individual with three cell lines—one

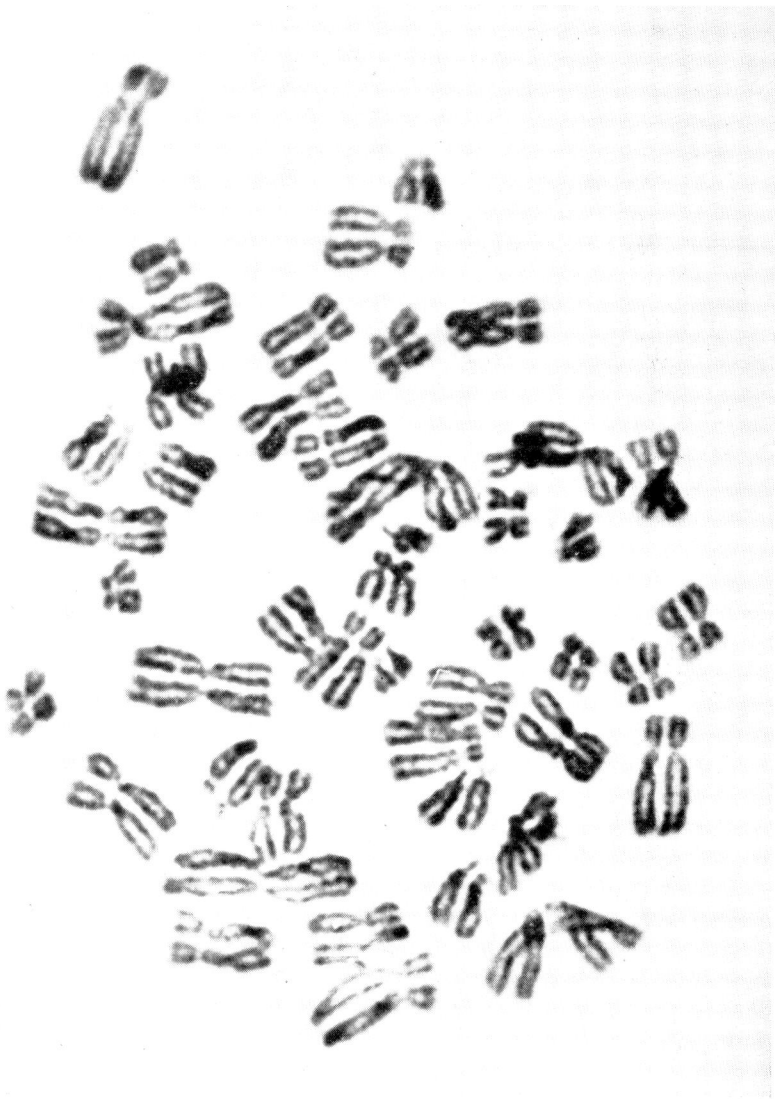

FIG. 6. Chromosomes of a cell from the same culture which has undergone endoreduplication.

with a normal chromosome complement and two with abnormal complements. The further from the early post-zygotic mitoses that an abnormal cell division occurs, the less likely it is that the resulting mosaic state will be detected, and since only one tissue in the body may be affected, it is not known how widespread the phenomenon may be. In practice, the demonstration of an abnormal chromosome complement in a proportion of the cells is only regarded as evidence for mosaicism if the abnormality can be shown to be consistent within the abnormal cell population. The presence of an abnormal phenotype may contribute to this evidence.

Nomenclature Symbols

It has been proposed by the Chicago Conference of 1966 (Standardization in Human Cytogenetics; see Bergsma (1966) in Bibliography) that the following symbols should be used in giving brief descriptions of cytogenetic findings:

A-G	the chromosome groups
1–22	the autosome numbers (Denver System)
X, Y	the sex chromosomes
diagonal (/)	separates cell lines in describing mosaicism
plus sign (+) or minus sign (−)	when placed immediately after the *autosome number or group letter designation* indicates that the particular chromosome is extra or missing; when placed immediately after the *arm or structural designation* indicates that the particular arm or structure is larger or smaller than normal
question mark (?)	indicates questionable identification of chromosome or chromosome structure
asterisk (*)	designates a chromosome or chromosome structure explained in text or footnote
ace	acentric
cen	centromere
dic	dicentric
end	endoreduplication
h	secondary constriction or negatively staining region
i	isochromosome
inv	inversion
inv (p+q−) or inv (p−q+)	pericentric inversion
mar	marker chromosome
mat	maternal origin
pat	paternal origin
p	short arm of chromosome
q	long arm of chromosome
r	ring chromosome
s	satellite
t	translocation
tri	tricentric
repeated symbols	duplication of chromosome structure

INBORN DISORDERS ASSOCIATED WITH CHROMOSOMAL ANOMALIES

It has been estimated that some form of chromosomal anomaly will be found in approximately one out of every hundred live-born children in a "white" population (UNSCEAR, 1966). After ten years of intensive study of persons with congenital abnormalities, there is a massive body of knowledge, relating chromosome changes to recognizable syndromes; a list of the important conditions with positive findings is given here for quick reference.

I. Sex Chromosome Anomalies

(a) In the Apparent Female

Turner's Syndrome (1 in 2,500 live births). Affected babies are usually small, have a low neck hair-line, loose skin and transient lymphœdema of the extremities. The chest is broad ("shield-chest") and the nipples widely spaced. Congenital cardiovascular defects, e.g. coarctation of the aorta and telangiectases, may occur. In later life, primary amenorrhœa, short stature, neck webbing, cubitus valgus and generalized osteoporosis may be additional features of the condition. Ovaries are usually vestigial, but ovarian stroma and atretic follicles may be present.

Chromosome constitution 45, XO. There are many examples of mosaics in which other cell lines are present as well (XO/XX, XO/XY, XO/XXX, XO/XX/XXX, XO/XYY). In other cases with 46 chromosomes, one of the X chromosomes has a deletion, or is represented by an isochromosome or a ring.

Ovarian Dysgenesis without Stigmata of Turner's Syndrome. Affected individuals usually present with primary amenorrhœa. They may be tall, have poor breast development, scanty axillary and pubic hair and have normal or infantile external and internal genitalia, but the clitoris may be enlarged. The gonads are small, contain no follicles, and are subject to an increased risk of tumour formation.

Various findings: XO, XX, XXX/XO, XO/XYY, structural aberrations of an X.

Pure Gonadal Dysgenesis. Similar clinical picture to above. Streak gonads may show ovarian rudiments. Chromosome constitution 46, XY.

Overzier's Syndrome (true agonadism). Similar clinical picture to above but external genitalia may be rudimentary and only evidence of internal genitalia may be some persistence of vestigial remains of Mullerian and Woolfian ducts. Gonads are absent. Chromosome constitution 46, XY.

In all the above conditions, 17-ketosteroid excretion levels are usually normal (4·5–17·0 mg./24 hr.) or lowered, and the pituitary gonadotrophin levels are normal (4–40 M.U./24 hr.) or increased.

Testicular Feminization. Affected individuals are female in appearance with good breast development and normal external genitalia, but present with primary amenorrhœa and have absent axillary and pubic hair. The vagina may be absent or end blindly and the uterus is typically absent. Gonads are testes and may present as inguinal herniæ, or be found in the labia majora or abdomen. There is an increased risk of tumour formation. 17-ketosteroid excretion levels are variable and gonadotrophin levels may be raised. There is a marked familial tendency.

Chromosome constitution 46, XY.

Multiple X Females. Individuals are of normal female appearance and are usually fertile, but may be intellectually retarded or psychotic.

Chromosome constitution XXX, XXXX, or XXXXX.

(b) In the Apparent Male

Klinefelter's Syndrome (1 in 400–1,000 live births). Individuals are of typically asthenic appearance, tall with long limbs, large extremities and gynæcomastia, but may be of normal or sthenic build. Facial hair is slow to develop and the pubic hair sparse and of female distribution. External genitalia are normal or reduced in size and the testes, after puberty, are small. There may be mental retardation and behavioural difficulties. 17-ketosteroid excretion levels are low and gonadotrophin levels are raised.

Chromosome count 47, XXY. There are also mosaics (XXY/XX XXY/XY) as well as cases in which further sex chromosomes are present, but always including a Y (XXXY, XXXXY, XXYY).

Multiple Y. Affected individuals may be tall, but otherwise appear normal. There may be early manifestation of instability and anti-social behaviour (Editorial, 1967).

Chromosome constitution XYY, XYYY, XY/XYY.

(c) True Hermaphroditism

No consistent finding; some are mosaics, but a number of cases have shown only XX cells.

II. Autosomal Anomalies

Mongolism (Down's Syndrome) (1 in 500 live births). Chromosome count 47. Trisomy of G21. In some cases, particularly those born to younger mothers, the count is 46 and the additional chromosomal material is translocated on to the short arms of another G or D group chromosome, producing a compound structure which may be inherited. In this case those relatives with 46 chromosomes including the abnormal one will be mongols, while those with 45, apparently having only one No. 21 chromosome, will be phenotypically normal "carriers".

Patau's Syndrome (1 in 14,500 live births). A rare condition recognizable at birth. Affected baby has microcephaly, cranial and cerebral defects, narrow palpebral fissures, microphthalmos, coloboma, hare lip, cleft palate, polydactyly and fixed flexion deformities of the fingers. Telangiectasia and congenital heart deformities are common.

Chromosome count 47, with trisomy of one of the D group chromosomes. In this condition there are also unusual numbers of hook-like appendages on the neutrophils, as seen in blood films (Huehns *et al.*, 1964) (Fig. 7).

Edwards's Syndrome. Commoner than above (1 in 3,500–4,500 live births). Affected baby has malformed skull with prominent occiput, slight exophthalmia, low set and malformed ears, micrognathia and neck-webbing. Flexion deformities of the fingers with the index finger deviated to the ulnar side, and "rocker-bottom" feet with convex soles are characteristic.

Chromosome count 47, with trisomy of No. 18.

Cri-du-chat or Lejeune's Syndrome. Affected baby has a characteristic weak, shrill cry and shows failure to thrive. There is microcephaly, a round-moon face, oblique palpebral fissures, epicanthic folds, hypertelorism, low-set ears, beaked nose and micrognathia.

Chromosome count 46. Deletion of the short arm of one of the B group chromosomes (4–5). An example is shown in Figure 8.

CHROMOSOME BREAKAGE

The "condensed" chromosomes seen at metaphase are produced by folding or twisting of strands of DNA, which are more or less unravelled in

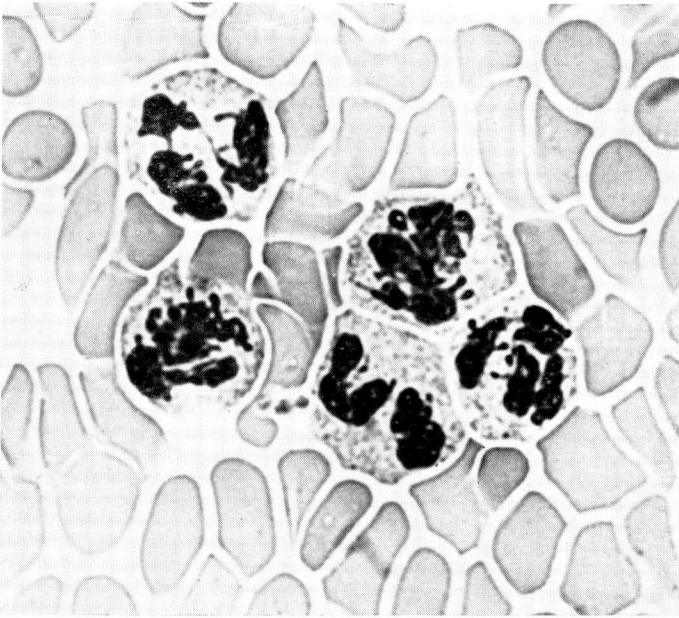

Fig. 7. Group of polymorphonuclear leucocytes from the blood film of an infant with Patau's syndrome. Note the multiple nuclear projections. (May-Grünwald-Giemsa ×1400).

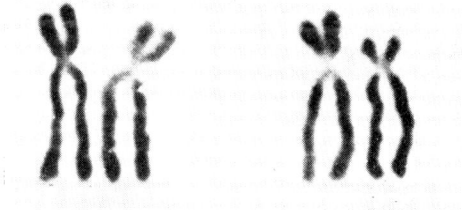

Fig. 8. B group chromosomes from two cells obtained from blood cultures of a 3 month-old baby with "cri-du-chat" syndrome. One of the chromosomes in each cell has a deletion of the short arms.

interphase. Anything that breaks a DNA molecule can probably break a whole chromosome. If a metaphase chromosome is shown to have a defect at the same level in both chromatids, it may be assumed that the damage occurred before replication. If, on the other hand, only one chromatid is affected, the damage presumably occurred after the synthetic period. Because of the crudeness of the picture obtained by ordinary microscopy, it is often difficult to be sure whether an apparent defect reflects a complete loss of continuity. It is therefore usual to speak of a "break" where the fragment is actually separated—("isochromatid break", if it occurs at the same level in both chromatids), and a "gap" if the apparent fragment is still correctly aligned (Fig. 3).

Broken ends of chromatin threads may join as described above (p. 306), producing abnormal chromosomes—translocations, dicentrics, rings. Most of these are "two-hit" aberrations which (if determined by ionizing radiations) increase with the square of the dose and are therefore characteristic of a high rate of damage (Fig. 9). Some abnormal chromosomes, and particularly acentric fragments, are apt to be lost in successive cell divisions, and it is important to study cells in the first division after a possible injury,

Buckton *et al.* (1962) have used a notation to represent the different types of damage by radiation, but it would be applicable to damage from other agents as well:

A cells   cells with no apparent structural abnormality;
B cells   cells with only a chromatid gap or break, or an isochromatid gap;
C_u cells   cells with unstable aberrations, i.e. dicentrics, rings or acentric fragments;
C_s cells   cells with stable aberrations, i.e. abnormal monocentric chromosomes, produced by deletion, inversion or translocation.

Chromosome breakage occurs to a small extent in the cells of normal persons studied by culture techniques, and before regarding any particular level of breakage as pathological it is essential to examine controls in the same way at the same time. Unknown factors cause variations in different laboratories. Court Brown *et al.* (1966) found about 3 per cent of cells to have B aberrations and about 3 per cent to have C aberrations in normal subjects.

Chromosome breakage can be produced by a number of different agencies, but the following are the most important:

(*a*) **Ionizing Radiations.** Patients who have had therapeutic doses usually have persistent chromosome aberrations—persistent because some of the lymphocytes, which are usually used for culture, have a long life and may be induced to go into their first post-treatment division many years after the date of irradiation. Soon after high doses there may be very severe abnormalities (Fig. 9); at the opposite extreme it is possible that even diagnostic X-rays may produce statistically significant increases (Bloom and Tjio, 1964), though below doses of 10 rads this becomes very difficult to demonstrate. Obviously, the smaller the effect the larger the number of cells that have to be analysed to show it, and at present the use of this method to estimate occupational exposure is impracticable.

(*b*) **Chemical Damage.** Chromosome breakage and sometimes recombination have been reported in patients having certain cytotoxic drugs, for instance nitrogen mustard (Nasjleti and Spencer, 1966) and folic acid antagonists (see Fig. 3). Benzene causes chromosome aberrations from industrial exposure (Tough and Court Brown, 1965); this may be important in view of the effect of benzene in producing marrow aplasia and leukæmia.

(*c*) **Viruses.** In experimental virus-induced tumours the possibility that chromosome damage may play a part in their production has led to the

FIG. 9. Karyotype of a dividing cell from the blood culture of a leukaemic child with a thymoma, which had been treated with large doses of X-rays. There are 16 dicentrics, and at least four rings (bottom right). At bottom left are a series of acentric fragments. The presence of certain abnormal chromosomes in pairs shows that this cell is not in its first division after injury.

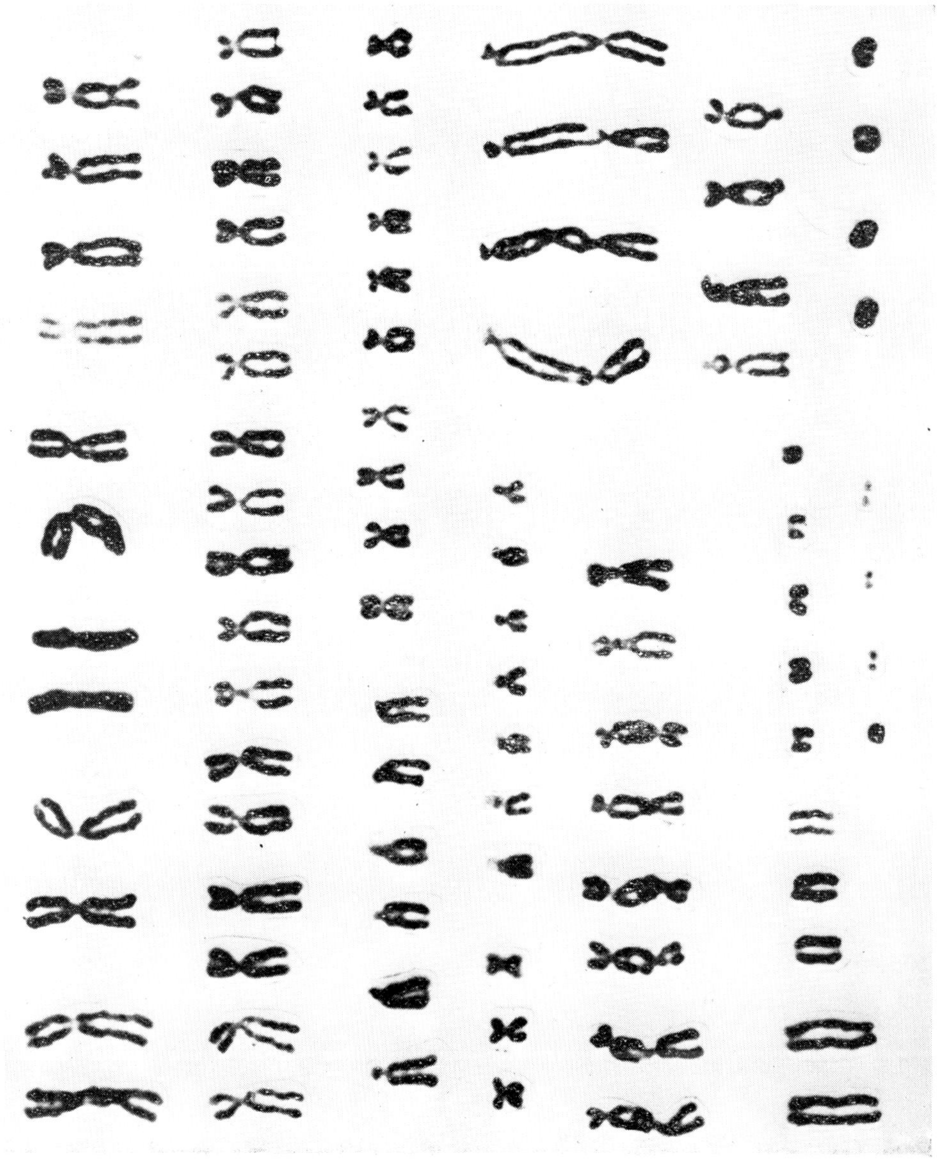

search for chromosome damage in infected cells; this has now been repeatedly demonstrated *in vitro*, using many different viruses. Nichols *et al.* (1965) have described an extreme degree of chromosome fragmentation ("pulverization") in human cells in culture infected with measles virus, and this is also known from herpes simplex infection. It is of great interest to know whether any effect can be shown in naturally occurring human infections. This has been reported from cases of measles and chicken-pox, but has not been found by all observers.

If a variety of common infections can damage chromosomes, in much the same way as ionizing radiations, this may well be a common path in the production of certain malignant diseases.

(*d*) **Syndromes associated with Chromosome Breakage.** At least two congenital diseases, believed to be inherited as autosomal recessives, are characterized by a high rate of chromosome breakage and recombination.

(1) Fanconi's anæmia (Bloom *et al.*, 1966).
(2) Bloom's Syndrome—congenital telangiectatic erythema with stunted growth (German *et al.*, 1965).

In both these conditions, aberrations of the chromosomes are common in cultured lymphocytes, and take the form of breaks, fragments, tri- or quadriradiate figures, dicentrics and rings—similar in fact to the changes which follow irradiation. Cells of other cultured tissues and of bone marrow have also been found to be affected. In both of the syndromes referred to, there is an increased risk of leukæmia (Sawitsky *et al.*, 1966).

CHROMOSOMES AND NEOPLASIA

So far as is known, the normal tissues are composed of cells with the regular $2n$ chromosome set of the zygote, apart from perhaps a few polyploids, and the haploid gametes. It is unlikely that there is any significant departure of cells from this ideal state (Bowey and Spriggs, 1967, 1968), and it is certain that systematic departure from it sometimes has disastrous consequences. Most malignant tumours are known to consist of clones with a new and abnormal karyotype, which can hardly be an irrelevant epiphenomenon.

From the diagnostic standpoint, it would be useful to have a dividing-line between tissues which are neoplastic and those which are not, and the question arises whether a study of the chromosomes could serve this purpose. As a generalization, it certainly cannot. Highly malignant tumours have been described which have no visible chromosome anomaly, for instance, certain malignant tumours of children (Cox. 1966); and mosaicism might well introduce errors, as would exposure to irradiation. But in a clinical situation the demonstration that a suspected specimen has a stemline visibly different from the normal must constitute strong evidence of neoplasia.

I. Serous Fluids

Following the experimental work on malignant stemlines in "ascites tumours" (Makino, 1957; Hauschka, 1958), it was soon confirmed that human malignant effusions regularly contained cells with abnormal karyotypes (Makino *et al.*, 1959; Ishihara *et al.*, 1961; Spriggs *et al.*, 1962; Ishihara *et al.*, 1963; Makino *et al.*, 1964). Pleural and peritoneal fluids also may contain benign cells in mitosis, most of which are mesothelial cells or plasma cells, and these have normal chromosome sets. Some malignant effusions contain few or no tumour cells in division, and in this case only cells with normal karyotypes will be found; but when malignant cells are actively dividing they show some or all of the following characteristics: (1) An abnormal chromosome count, sometimes below but more commonly above 46. (2) Variation of counts above and below the mode, and often secondary peaks at multiples of the modal number. (3) Marker chromosomes, that is, chromosomes which are recognizably different from any in the normal human set.

An example is shown here from a pleural effusion due to carcinoma of the breast with abundant free mucus-secreting malignant cells. The histogram (Fig. 10) shows the distribution of counts and Figures 11 and 12 two cut-out karyotypes of typical cells.

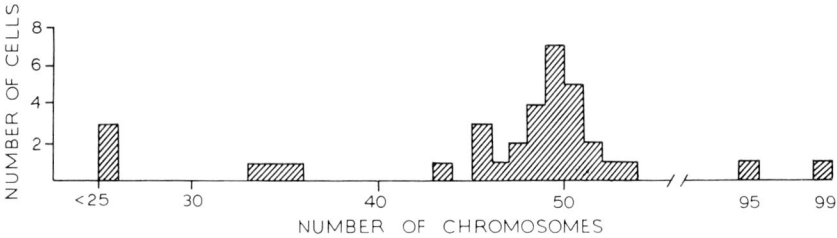

FIG. 10. Histogram showing distribution of chromosome counts in the cells of a malignant pleural effusion due to carcinoma of the breast. Note the distribution of values around an abnormal modal value, in this case 49.

The chromosome abnormality has been different in every case; the diagnostic feature is the identification of a number of cells with a similar abnormal karyotype from the same fluid.

II. Solid Tumours

Primary carcinomas almost always consist of cells with altered karyotypes (Fig. 13) (Lubs and Clark, 1963; Atkin and Baker, 1966). This has not yet been found useful in diagnosis because of the technical difficulties involved. Since the change occurs before the onset of invasion, at least in the case of carcinoma of the cervix (Boddington *et al.*, 1965; Wakonig-Vaartaja and Kirkland, 1965), it is possible that this type of investigation may prove useful in determining which epithelial abnormalities are irreversible (Fig. 14).

All malignant tumours are not alike in the degree of abnormality shown. Carcinomas usually show very striking deviations from normal; their modal numbers are generally just above 46 or else in the 60–80 region. Certain tumours of childhood, however, have shown smaller deviations or else no visible abnormality at all (Cox, 1966).

A unique example of what seems to be a specific marker chromosome for a tumour type has been reported by Martineau (1966). In five cases of testicular seminoma or teratoma, a long dicentric chromosome was observed as well as other karyotypic anomalies; a similar chromosome has subsequently been found in other cases (Martineau, 1967).

320   HISTOLOGY

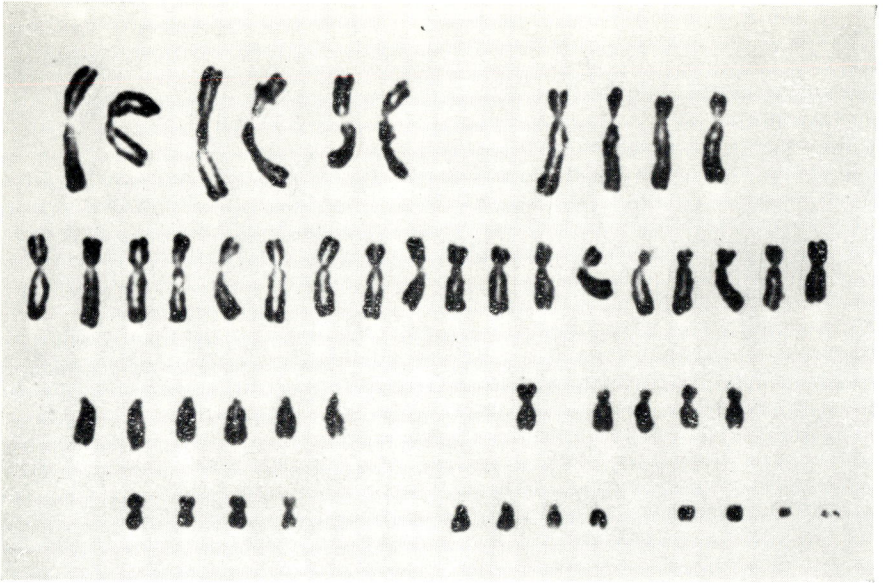

FIG. 11. Karyotype of a malignant cell from the same case as Fig. 10. It has 51 chromosomes including a "double minute" and three structures which are probably small ring chromosomes.

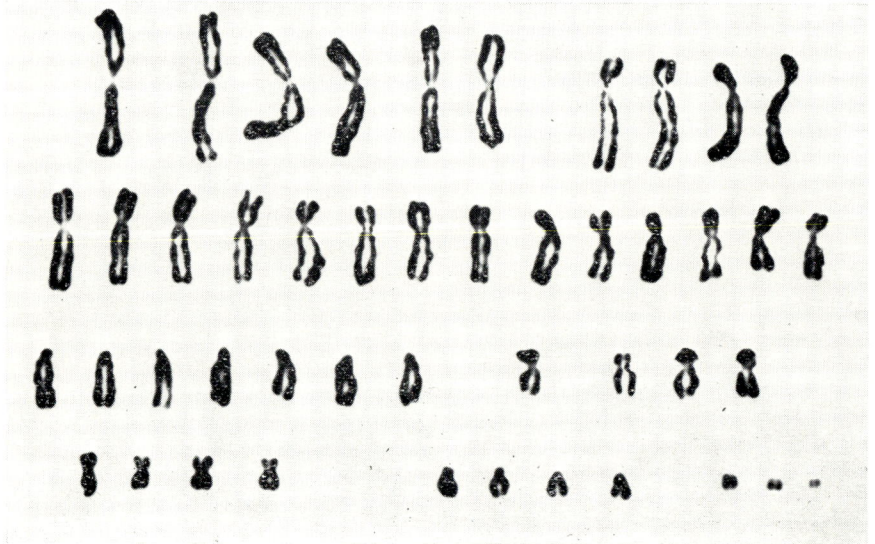

FIG. 12. Karyotype of another malignant cell from the same effusion as Fig 11. It has 46 chromosomes including the minute rings. Note that the distribution in chromsome groups is similar enough to demonstrate that the two cells have a common origin from a single ancestral malignant cell.

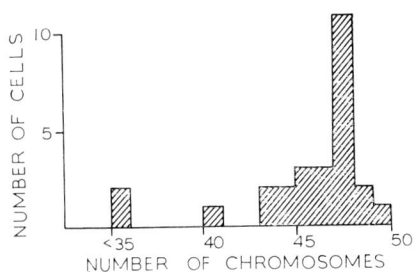

FIG. 13. Histogram of chromosome counts from a direct preparation of curettings from a carcinoma of the endometrium. The distribution around an abnormal modal number, with some scatter to the left, is similar to that found with malignant cell populations in effusions (Fig. 10).

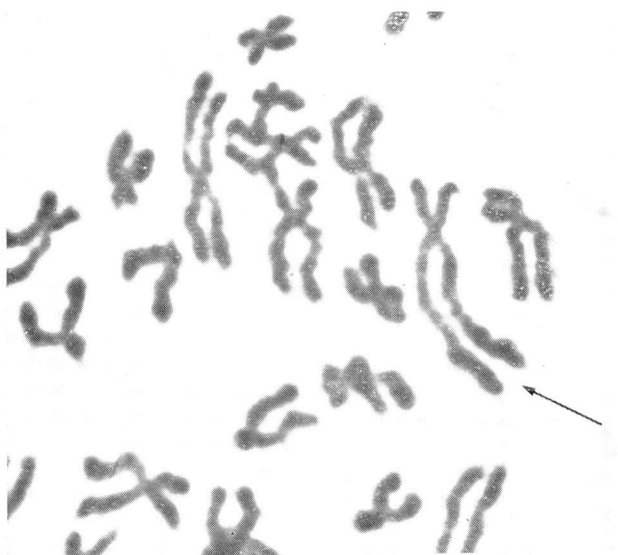

FIG. 14. Part of a metaphase from a direct preparation made from a cervical biopsy showing carcinoma *in situ*. The cells were near-diploid. The arrow shows a long abnormal marker chromosome, present in other cells from the same piece of tissue.

As for benign tumours, very little is known about their karyotypes; the evidence from DNA estimations (Stich *et al.*, 1960; Stich, 1963) and from a small number of cytogenetically studied tumours (Lubs and Clark, 1963; Socolow *et al.*, 1964; Enterline and Arvan, 1967) suggests that they either show no recognisable abnormality at all, or small numerical changes such as one or two extra chromosomes. The scarcity of mitoses and the difficulty of separating the cells makes these tumours almost inaccessible at the moment.

III. Acute Leukæmia

In some of the literature of cancer research it seems to be assumed that leukæmias are models for "cancer" in general. Chromosome studies do not entirely support this. The "blast cells" found in marrow and circulating blood in acute leukæmia frequently show no recognizable chromosomal abnormality at all, and when they do it is usually less in degree than occurs in carcinomas. (It is of course difficult to prove that cells found in division with normal karyotypes are actually blast cells and not associated normal ones. Even when they obviously are blast cells, undetectable chromosome changes may well be present.) The commonest changes are loss or gain of a C or G group chromosome. The next commonest groups to be affected are D, E and F, but there is great diversity and markers may be found as well. Usually a single stemline has been described, but cases are known with more (Ford and Clarke, 1963; Sandberg et al., 1964a).

The blast cells of acute myeloid leukæmia show smaller deviations than those of the lymphoid type. According to Sandberg et al. (1964a) there is a different distribution of modal counts between the two diseases; acute lymphoid leukæmia always showed modal numbers of 46 or above (sometimes even 92 or more) while acute myeloid leukæmia showed modal counts of 46 or below, with a few inconstant ones at 47. The modal range of 70–85 which is so common in carcinoma is practically unknown in leukæmic cells, though it occurs in reticulosarcoma. However, Reisman et al. (1964) refer to two cases of acute childhood leukæmia where the modal number was 65.

Leukæmic cells, in common with other neoplastic cells, often show fuzzy metaphase chromosomes, as if fixation was incomplete. Since normal cells in the same material have well-condensed chromosomes this can be of diagnostic use, and in any case must have some significance concerning the folding of DNA strands, the protein coating of the DNA, or activity of DNase.

The most convincing results are obtained from direct preparations of leukæmic marrow, where the blast cells are in a large majority. Cultures may also sometimes reveal the abnormal cells, but if phytohæmagglutinin (PHA) is used they will usually be diluted by many normal transformed lymphocytes, and a normal finding gives no diagnostic information. In all cytogenetic studies of leukæmic cells, it is essential to make good stained films of the material before hypotonic treatment, so that an opinion can be given whether it is really the leukæmic cells that are in division.

In complete remissions of acute leukæmia, the blast cells disappear from the blood and marrow, and the cytogenetic findings therefore return to normal. Only the blast cells constitute the malignant clone, while the erythroid, myeloid and platelet precursors as well as circulating lymphocytes are normal.

Chromosomal abnormalities have sometimes been found in patients with myeloproliferative diseases or pancytopenia before the onset of acute myeloid leukæmia (Nowell, 1965). This group of diseases is referred to below (p. 324).

IV. Chronic Myeloid Leukæmia

This disease is associated with a specific chromosomal defect in the hæmopoietic cells, consisting of a loss of material from the long arm of one of the G chromosomes. Whether this is a deletion or a translocation on to another larger chromosome is not known. The shortened chromosome is known as the Ph[1] chromosome (Nowell and Hungerford, 1960). The typical appearance of the Ph[1] chromosome is shown in Figure 15. Because of the reduction in the long arm, it is more metacentric than the other G group chromosomes, and this together with its small size is very distinctive in good preparations.

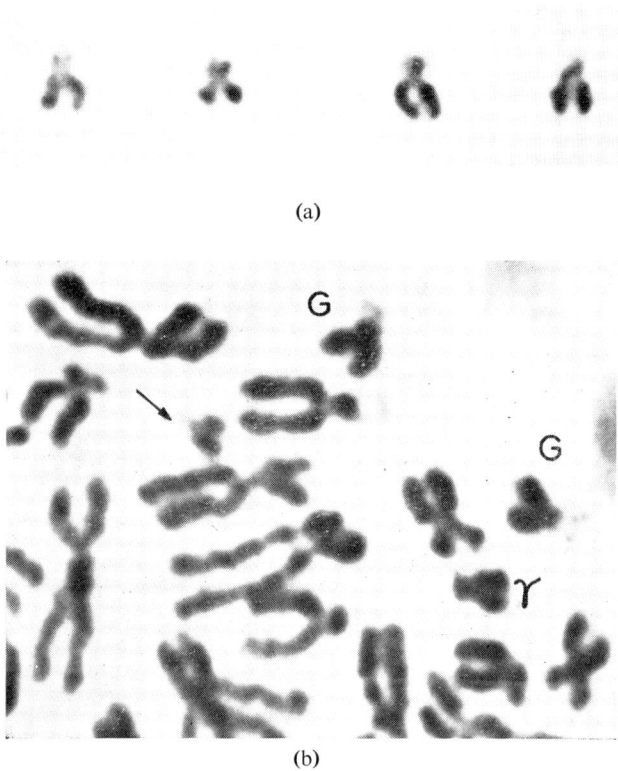

(a)

(b)

FIG. 15. Chronic myeloid leukæmia.

(a) The four G-group chromosomes from a cell from cultured peripheral blood, showing the small Ph[1] chromosome placed second in the row.

(b) Part of a metaphase from a leukocyte culture of another case, showing the Ph[1] chromosome (arrow), two other G group chromosomes and the Y.

The erythroid, myeloid and thrombopoietic cells are all affected. As myeloid tissue cannot be safely eliminated by treatment, the defect persists in the marrow in treated patients.

The lymphocytes are not affected and cultures with PHA therefore produce cells with normal karyotypes. Blood cultures can be used, but success in finding the Ph[1] chromosome depends on obtaining myeloblasts or myelocytes in mitosis; for this reason one- or two-day cultures without PHA or direct marrow preparations are preferable.

In some cases other abnormalities are found besides the Ph[1] chromosome, either an extra Ph[1] (Kiossoglou et al., 1965) or other numerical or structural alterations. These represent new leukæmic clones and often presage an acute terminal stage of the disease, though this has not always been the case.

There have been interesting examples of clonal evolution in this group in which it has been possible to trace a succession of cumulative changes (Ford and Clarke, 1963; de Grouchy *et al.*, 1966a).

There is a form of the disease in which the chromosomes appear entirely normal. The patients are on the average younger and the prognosis is worse (Tjio *et al.*, 1966).

V. Other Myeloproliferative Diseases and Myelosclerosis

In most cases of myeloid metaplasia, myelosclerosis and polycythæmia vera the chromosomes have been reported to be normal (Sandberg *et al.*, 1962; Kiossoglou *et al.*, 1966). There has, however, been a remarkable observation by Kay *et al.* (1966) of an unusually small F group chromosome in the bone marrow of five cases of polycythemia vera (four following treatment), as well as aneuploidy in seven out of eleven untreated cases, including clear evidence of abnormal clones. Those with a consistent abnormality showed an extra C chromosome (two cases) and a missing Y (one case). Abnormalities in one of the F chromosomes have also been reported by de Grouchy *et al.* (1966b) in five out of six cases of sideroblastic anæmia.

VI. Chronic Lymphocytic Leukæmia

The lymphocytes in this disease apparently do not go into mitosis *in vivo*, nor *in vitro* with brief PHA stimulation. With longer stimulation, inconstant abnormalities are now being reported (Goh, 1967). A familial form described by Gunz *et al.* (1962) was associated with a deletion of the short arms of a G group chromosome, but this is not accepted as bearing more than a chance association with the disease.

VII. Malignant Reticuloses (Lymphomas)

This group of diseases is not associated with any chromosomal anomaly of the lymphocytes as studied in cultures with PHA. In the highly malignant forms (reticulosarcoma, lymphosarcoma), the tumour cells have abnormalities unique to each case, as is found in carcinoma (Sandberg *et al.*, 1964b; Spiers and Baikie, 1966). In Burkitt's lymphoma, on the other hand, visible karyotype changes are often absent, though pseudodiploid and aneuploid cells can also occur (Jacobs *et al.*, 1963).

In Hodgkin's disease, direct preparations from lymph nodes have not given a consistent picture in the cases so far described, but the most usual finding is a clone of hypotetraploid cells, corresponding to Sternberg-Reed cells (Fig. 16), and another population with a normal karyotype which corresponds to dividing lymphoid cells (Miles *et al.*, 1966; Seif and Spriggs, 1967). Other changes have been described but are not of agreed significance.

Inconsistent abnormalities have been found in Brill-Symmers' disease (Spiers and Baikie, 1966). Other diseases in this group have not been studied often enough for any picture to emerge.

VIII. Multiple Myeloma

Considering the high concentration of tumour cells frequently found in the bone marrow in this disease, it may seem surprising that so little is

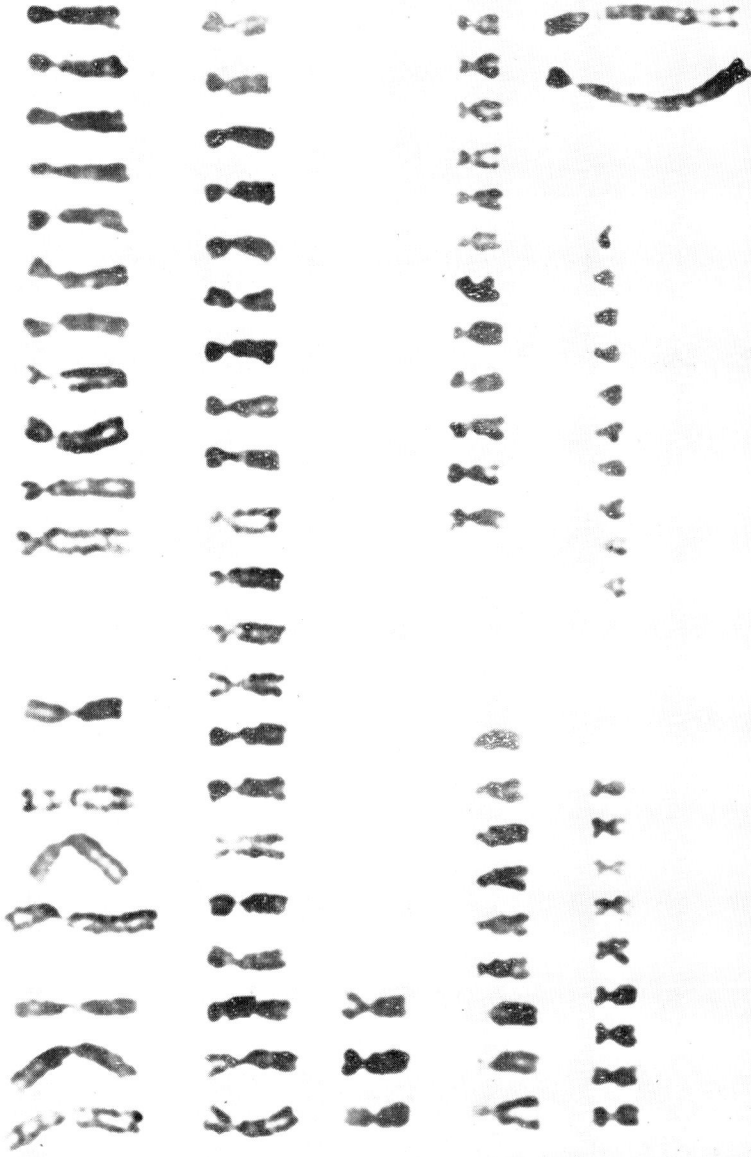

Fig. 16. Karyotype of a cell from a direct preparation of an excised lymph-node in Hodgkin's disease. It has 84 chromosomes including two long markers. Twenty-two cells were found in the 77-86 range, and all of them had the two markers, proving that they were of common descent.

known about their chromosomes. The explanation seems to be that the mitotic rate is usually low, so that only the occasional case can be effectively studied from direct preparations. The finding of a normal karyotype is only relevant if the preparations are made direct from marrow in which the myeloma cells can be seen to be dividing, a detail very seldom mentioned. Some of the reported cases have had karyotype changes in the tumour cells, the modal number being either near-diploid (Castoldi *et al.*, 1963; Bottura, 1963) or hypotetraploid (Lewis *et al.*, 1963). In the series of Tassoni *et al.* (1967), five cases out of fourteen had a long acrocentric marker.

IX. Waldenström's Disease

In 1961, Bottura and his colleagues observed an extra abnormal chromosome in the colchininized bone marrow of a man of 71 with macroglobulinæmia. There was some variation round the modal number of 47. The supernumerary chromosome was the length of a No. 1 but had a subterminal centromere.

Since that time a number of other cases have been examined. Some have had no detectable abnormality, but others have been shown to have chromosomal abnormalities both in marrow and in blood cultured with PHA. Usually the abnormality has been the presence of an extra large chromosome, but not necessarily with the same relative size or centromere position as in Bottura's case; it may be a very long metacentric (German *et al.*, 1961; Benirschke *et al.*, 1962) or submetacentric (Elves and Israels, 1963; Ferguson and Mackay, 1963) and other forms are known (Spengler *et al.*, 1966). These findings have an interest beyond any application to clinical diagnosis, because they are a direct demonstration that a unique immunoglobulin marks the presence of a clone of lymphoid cells with an irreversible alteration of the genome. Whether to call these cells neoplastic is a matter of semantics and not of biology.

Bibliography
(Books suggested for further reading)

BERGSMA, D. (Ed.) (1966). "Chicago Conference: Standardization in Human Cytogenetics." *Birth Defects: Original Article Series*, Vol. II, No. 2.
COURT BROWN, W. M. (1967). *Human Population Cytogenetics.* North Holland Publishing Co., Amsterdam.
EVANS, H. J., COURT BROWN, W. M. and MCLEAN, A. S. (Eds.) (1967). *Human Radiation Cytogenetics.* North Holland Publishing Co., Amsterdam.
LENNOX, B. (1966). "Chromosomal Abnormalities in Man." In *Recent Advances in Pathology*, 8th ed. (Ed. C. V. Harrison). J. & A. Churchill, London.
MITTWOCH, U. (1967). *Sex Chromosomes.* Academic Press, London.
MOORE, K. L. (Ed.) (1966). *The Sex Chromatin.* W. B. Saunders Co., Philadelphia and London.
STEVENSON, A. C. (1966). "Applications of Chromosome Studies in Obstetrics and Gynæcology." In *Recent Advances in Obstetrics and Gynaecology*, by J. Stallworthy and G. Bourne. J. & A. Churchill Ltd., London.
TURPIN, R. and LEJEUNE, J. (1965). *Les Chromosomes Humains.* Gauthier-Villars, Paris.
VALENTINE, G. H. (1966). *The Chromosome Disorders. An Introduction for Clinicians.* Heinemann Medical Books Ltd., London.
YUNIS, J. J. (Ed.) (1965). *Human Chromosome Methodology.* Academic Press, New York and London.

References

ATKIN, N. B. (1967). Personal communication.
ATKIN, N. B. and BAKER, M. C. (1966). *J. Nat. Cancer Inst.* **36**, 539.
BENIRSCHKE, K., BROWNHILL, L. and EBAUGH, F. G. (1962). *Lancet*, **i**, 594.
BLOOM, A. D. and TJIO, J. H. (1964). *New Engl. J. Med.* **270**, 1341.
BLOOM, G. E., WARNER, S, GERALD, P. S. and DIAMOND, L. K. (1966). *New Engl. J. Med.* **274**, 8.
BODDINGTON, M. M., SPRIGGS, A. I. and WOLFENDALE, M. R. (1965). *Brit. med. J.* **i**, 154.
BOTTURA, C. (1963), *Acta Haemat.* **30**, 274.
BOTTURA, C., FERRARI, I. and VEIGA, A. A. (1961). *Lancet* **i**, 1170.
BOWEY, C. E. and SPRIGGS, A. I. (1967). *J. med. Genet.* **4**, 91.
BOWEY, C. E. and SPRIGGS, A. I. (1968). *J. med Genet.* **5**, 58.
BUCKTON, K. E., JACOBS, P. A., COURT BROWN, W. M. and DOLL, R. (1962. *Lancet* **2**, 676.
CASTOLDI, G. L., RICCI, N., PUNTURIERI, E. and BOSI, L. (1963). *Lancet* **i**, 829.
COURT BROWN, W. M., BUCKTON, K. E., JACOBS, P. A., TOUGH, I. M., KUENSSBERG, E. V. and KNOX, J. D. E. (1966). Chromosome studies on adults. Cambridge. Eugenics Laboratory Memoirs XLII.
COX, D. (1966). *Cancer, Philad.* **19**, 1217.
EDITORIAL (1967), *Brit. med. J.* **i**, 64.
ELVES, M. W. and ISRAËLS, M. C. G. (1963). *Brit. med. J.* **ii**, 1024
ENTERLINE, H. T. and ARVAN, D. A. (1967). *Cancer, Philad.* **20**, 1746.
EVANS, E. P., BRECKON, G. and FORD, C. E. (1964). *Cytogenetics* **3**, 289.
FERGUSON, J. and MACKAY, I. R. (1963). *Austral. Ann. Med.* **12**, 197.
FORD, C. E. and CLARKE, C. M. (1963). *Canad. Cancer Conf.* **5**, 129.
FORD, C. E. and HAMERTON, J. L. (1956). *Nature. Lond.* **178**, 1020.
GERMAN, J., ARCHIBALD, R. and BLOOM, D. (1956). *Science* **148**, 506.
GERMAN, J. L., BIRO, C. E. and BEARN, A. G. (1961). *Lancet* **ii**, 48.
GOH, K-O. (1967). *J. Lab. Clin. Med.* **69**, 938.
DE GROUCHY, J., DE NAVA, C., CANTU, J. M., BILSKI-PASQUIER, G. and BOUSSER, J. (1966a). *Am. J. Hum. Genet.* **18**, 485.
DE GROUCHY, J., DE NAVA, C., ZITTOUN, R. and BOUSSER, J. (1966b). *Nouv. Rev. franç. Hémat.*, **6**, 367.
GUNZ, F. W., FITZGERALD, P. H. and ADAMS, A. (1962). *Brit. med. J.* **ii**, 1097.
HARNDEN, D. G. (1960). *Brit. J. exp. Path.* **41**, 31.
HAUSCHKA, T. S. (1958). *J. Cell Comp. Physiol.* **52**, Suppl. 1. 197.
HSU, T. C. and KELLOGG, D. S. (1960). *J Nat. Cancer Inst.* **25**, 221.
HUEHNS, E. R., LUTZNER, M. and HECHT, F. (1964). *Lancet.* **i**, 589.
ISHIHARA, T., KIKUCHI, Y. and SANDBERG, A. A. (1963). *J .Nat. Cancer Inst.* **30**, 1303.
ISHIHARA, T., MOORE, G. E. and SANDBERG, A. A. (1961). *J. Nat. Cancer Inst.* **27**, 893.
JACOBS, P. A., TOUGH, I. M. and WRIGHT, D. H. (1963). *Lancet.* **ii**, 1144.
KAY, H. E. M., LAWLER, S. D. and MILLARD, R. E. (1966). *Brit. J. Haematol.*, **12**, 507.
KIOSSOGLOU, K. A., MITUS, W. J. and DAMASHEK, W. (1965). *Lancet* **i**, 665.
KIOSSOGLOU, K. A., MITUS, W. J. and DAMASHEK, W. (1966). *Blood* **28**, 241.
LEWIS, F. J. W., MacTAGGART, M., CROW, R. S. and WILLS, M. R. (1963). *Lancet* **i**, 1183.
LUBS, H. A. and CLARK, R. (1963). *New Engl. J. Med.* **268**, 907.
McILREE, M. E., TULLOCH, W. S., NEWSAM, J. E. and BARCLAY, J. (1966). *Lancet* **i**, 679.
MAKINO, S. (1957). *Intern. Rev. Cytol.* **6**, 25.
MAKINO, S., ISHIHARA, T. and TONOMURA, A. (1959). *Z. Krebsforsch.* **63**, 184.
MAKINO, S., SASAKI, M. S. and TONOMURA, A. (1964). *J. Nat. Cancer Inst.* **32**, 741.
MARTINEAU, M. (1966). *Lancet* **i**, 839.
MARTINEAU, M. (1967). *Lancet.* **i**, 386.
MILES, C. P., GELLER, W. and O'NEILL, F. (1966). *Cancer, Philad.* **19**, 1103.
MOORHEAD, P. S., NOWELL, P. C., MELLMAN, W. J., BATTIPS, D. M. and HUNGERFORD, D. A. (1960). *Exp. Cell Res.* **20**, 613.
NASJLETI, C. E. and SPENCER, H. H. (1966). *Cancer Res.* **26**, 2437.
NICHOLS, W. W., LEVAN, A., AULA, P. and NORRBY, E. (1965). *Hereditas* **54**, 101.
NOWELL, P. C. (1965). *Arch. Path.* **80**, 205.
NOWELL, P. C. and HUNGERFORD, D. A. (1960). *Science* **132**, 1497.
REISMAN, L. E., MITANI, M. and ZUELZER, W. W. (1964). *New Engl. J. Med.* **270**, 591.
ROGERS, A. W. (1967). "Techniques of Autoradiography". Amsterdam, London and New York. Elsevier.
ROWLEY, M. J. and HELLER, C. G. (1966). *Fertil. Steril.* **17**, 177.
SANDBERG, A. A., ISHIHARA, T., CROSSWHITE, L. H. and HAUSCHKA, T. S. (1962) *Blood* **20**, 393.

SANDBERG, A. A., ISHIHARA, T., KIKUCHI, Y. and CROSSWHITE, L. H. (1964a). *Ann. N. Y. Acad. Sci.* **113**, 663.

SANDBERG, A. A., ISHIHARA, T., KIKUCHI, Y. and CROSSWHITE, L. H. (1964b). *Cancer, Philad.* **17**, 738.

SAWITSKY, A., BLOOM, D. and GERMAN, J. (1966). *Ann. int. Med.* **65**, 487.

SEIF, G. S. F. and SPRIGGS, A. I. (1967). *J. Nat. Canc. Inst.* **39**, 557.

SOCOLOW, E. L., ENGEL, E., MANTOOTH, L. and STANBURY, J. B. (1964). *Cytogenetics* **3**, 394.

SPENGLER, A. G., SIEBNER, H. and RIVA, G. (1966). *Acta Med. Scand. Suppl.* **445**, 132.

SPIERS, A. S. D., and BAIKIE, A. G. (1966). *Lancet* **i**, 506.

SPRIGGS, A. I., BODDINGTON, M. M. and CLARKE, C. M. (1962). *Brit. med. J.* **ii**, 1431.

STICH, H. F. (1963). Chromosomes and Carcinogenesis. *In. Canad. Cancer Conf.* **5**, 99.

STICH, H. F., FLORIAN, S. F. and EMSON, H. E. (1960). *J. Nat. Cancer Inst.* **24**, 471.

TASSONI, E. M., DURANT, J. R. BECKER, S. and KRAVITZ, B. (1967). *Cancer Res.* **27**, 806.

TJIO, J. H., CARBONE, P. P., WHANG, J. and FREI, E. (1966). *J. Nat. Cancer Inst.* **36**, 567.

TJIO, J. H. and LEVAN, A. (1956). *Hereditas (Lund)* **42**, 1.

TJIO, J. H. and WHANG, J. (1962). *Stain Tech.* **37**, 17.

TOUGH, I. M. and COURT BROWN, W. M. (1965). *Lancet* **i**, 684.

UNSCEAR (United Nations Scientific Committee on the Effects of Atomic Radiation) (1966). Report to the General Assembly Official Records Twenty-first Session. Suppl. No. 14 (A/6314). New York: United Nations, p. 103.

WAKONIG-VAARTAJA, R. and KIRKLAND, J. A. (1965). *Cancer, Philad.* **18**, 1101.

YAMADA, K., TAKAGI, N. and SANDBERG, A. A. (1966). *Cancer, Philad.* **19**, 1879.

Chapter 19

CATECHOLAMINE-SECRETING TUMOURS

G. WALTERS

THE adrenal medulla and the sympathetic nervous system both develop from the neural crest, so that the phæochromocytoma, neuroblastoma and ganglioneuroma are embryologically related. This common histogenetic origin is supported by the occurrence of the ganglioneuroblastoma containing both primitive neuroblasts and ganglion cells, and very rarely, also phæochromocytoma elements. The close relationship of this group has been further emphasized by the discovery that tumours of the neuroblastoma-ganglioneuroma group have secretory properties similar to the phæochromocytoma. Recent reports of noradrenaline-secreting glomus tumours suggest that these also are of neural crest origin.

Normally, the adrenal medulla secretes both adrenaline and noradrenaline. The relative amount of each in the gland varies with age, noradrenaline predominating at birth, and adrenaline in the adult. Noradrenaline is also the chemical mediator of the sympathetic nervous system and, in addition, it is found together with its precursor dopamine in some parts of the central nervous system; only very small amounts of adrenaline have been found in sympathetic tissue. All three compounds are excreted in the urine, dopamine usually being the most abundant. The main synthetic pathway is:

phenylalanine→tyrosine→dopa→dopamine→noradrenaline→adrenaline

The enzymes concerned in this pathway are all known and their properties are reviewed by Goldstein (1966). The various reactions occur in different fractions of the cell, dopamine, for example, being formed in the soluble fraction but converted to noradrenaline inside fine intracytoplasmic granules. Noradrenaline migrates into the soluble fraction where adrenaline is formed, but both adrenaline and noradrenaline are stored in the granules. There is evidence that there are two types of medullary cell, one of which synthesizes only noradrenaline, the other being capable of the final conversion to adrenaline (Hillarp and Hökfelt, 1953; Eränkö, 1955).

PHÆOCHROMOCYTOMA

The phæochromocytoma and its striking clinical manifestations have been known for many years. The majority occur in the abdomen, but they have also been found in the neck, thorax and bladder. These tumours have the capacity to store large amounts of adrenaline and noradrenaline, and have been shown by centrifugation studies and electron microscopy to contain fine intracytoplasmic granules like the storage granules of the adrenal medulla. But the binding of catecholamines in the tumour cell appears to be abnormal, and unlike the normal medulla, varying amounts have been found in the soluble fraction of the cell suggesting that, in tumours, storage is not confined to the granules (Hillarp *et al.*, 1961).

Abnormalities found in the neuroblastoma group and some malignant phaeochromocytomata

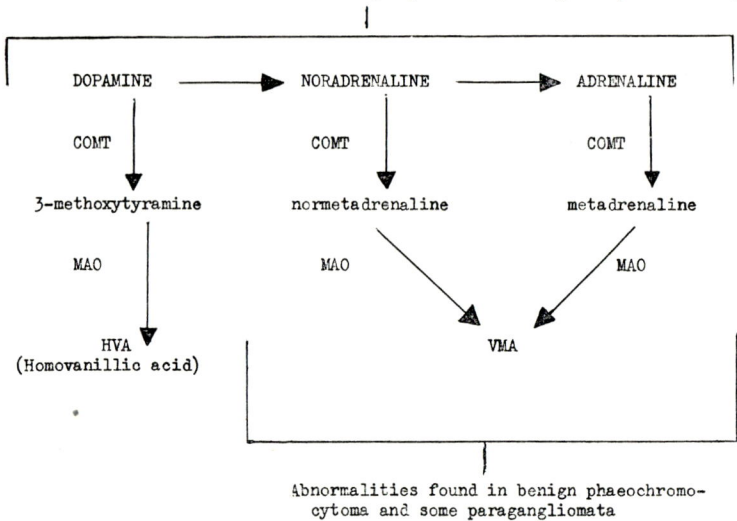

COMT = Catechol-O-methyltransferase   MAO = Monoamine oxidase

FIG. 1. Catecholamine metabolism showing main pathways of clinical importance. For review of less frequent abnormalities see von Studnitz (1966).

Laboratory Diagnosis

A great advance in the diagnosis of phæochromocytoma was made in 1950 when Engel and von Euler found increased catecholamines in the urine of two patients, and this was soon confirmed by others (von Euler and Ström, 1957). Subsequently, the identification by Armstrong *et al.* (1957) and Axelrod (1957) respectively of 4-hydroxy-3-methoxymandelic acid (VMA)[1] and the 3-0-methyl derivatives of adrenaline and noradrenaline (metadrenalines) as the major metabolites, led to the discovery that the excretion of these compounds is also increased in phæochromocytoma. Estimation of catecholamines and their metabolites in urine is now firmly established as the main method of diagnosis.

As experience accumulates it has become apparent that increased excretion is sometimes found in the absence of a tumour, and that in phæochromocytoma, the relative increase in the excretion of catecholamines and the different metabolites is variable (Kelleher *et al.*, 1964). Nevertheless, it is usual in phæochromocytoma for the excretion of all these substances to be increased to diagnostic levels, and the choice of routine method is largely one of convenience. In a minority of cases, however, the excretion of one

---

[1] This compound is designated by various abbreviations. HMMA is correct, but VMA, taken from vanilmandelic acid which it was called by Armstrong, is more often used. MHMA has also been used.

compound is increased proportionately much more than the others. Sometimes a relatively large increase in urinary catecholamines is accompanied by
a much smaller increase in the excretion of metabolites (Fig. 2). The converse
also occurs (Fig. 3), probably due to metabolism of the catecholamines in
the tumour itself (Crout and Sjoerdsma, 1964). In the latter case, if the
tumour secretes metabolites continually while releasing catecholamines
intermittently, it is possible for increased excretion of metabolites to be found

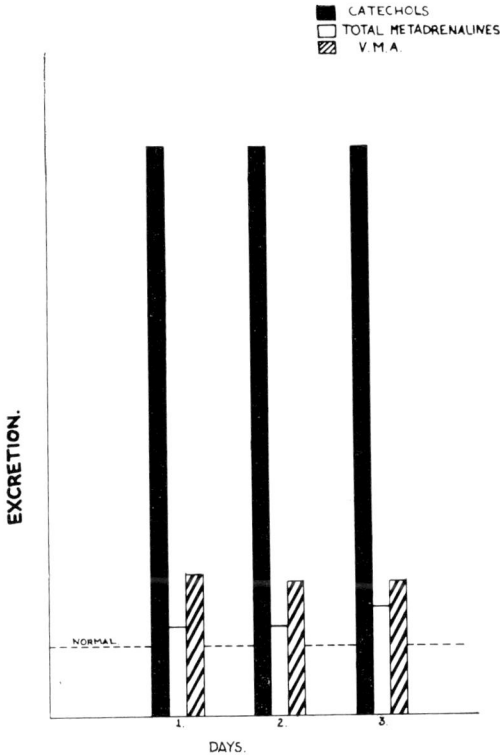

FIG. 2. Urinary catecholamines and metabolites in phæochromocytoma, showing
greatly increased excretion of catecholamines with a relatively slight increase of
metabolites.

in the presence of normal excretion of catecholamines. In one such case
described by Brown *et al.* (1966), the excretion of metabolites was persistently
raised to diagnostic levels, although catecholamine excretion remained
within the normal range even after an attack of symptoms.

Proving the diagnosis when increased excretion of both metabolites and
catecholamines occurs intermittently may occasionally be difficult, despite the
clear indication of secretion given by the paroxysmal symptoms. If attacks are
sufficiently brief, the 24-hour excretion of both catecholamines and the
metabolites may fail to rise to diagnostic levels, and may not even exceed
normal limits (Fig. 4a). Routine urine collections will often not coincide
with attacks, and in the case illustrated in Figure 4a, the diagnosis was
finally established by collecting every urine specimen separately and analysing

those preceded by an attack; a diagnostic increase in the excretion of catecholamines, but not of metabolites, was then found during a short period immediately after an attack (Fig. 4b). When this increase was diluted by the remainder of the 24-hour urine collection its diagnostic significance was very much less, a sixfold increase in excretion being reduced to less than twofold.

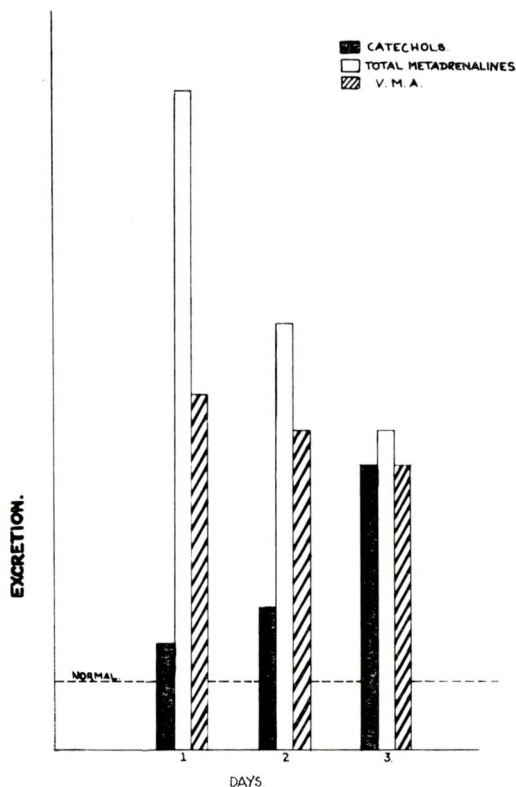

FIG. 3. Urinary catecholamines and metabolites in phæochromocytoma, showing preponderance of metabolites on the first two days.

These diagnostic difficulties are fortunately uncommon and measurement of the excretion of free catecholamines alone or of one of the metabolites is usually adequate for diagnostic purposes. But, it must be stressed that occasionally, some thought may be required as to the best diagnostic approach.

Appearance of the Tumour

The tumours are typically smooth, soft and often feel cystic. They vary enormously in size and may, in the adrenal medulla, be so small as not to distort the gland. Such small tumours may be difficult to distinguish from hyperplasia as even larger tumours may not be separated from the cortex by a fibrous capsule (Fig. 5). The cut surface often presents a variegated

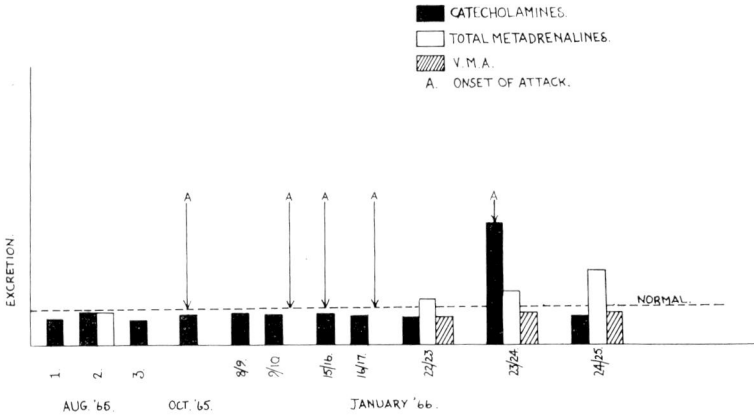

FIG. 4a. Urinary catecholamines and metabolites in phæochromocytoma, illustrating the difficulty of synchronising 24-hour urine collections with attacks of symptoms. On some occasions, the attacks were too brief to increase the excretion above normal.

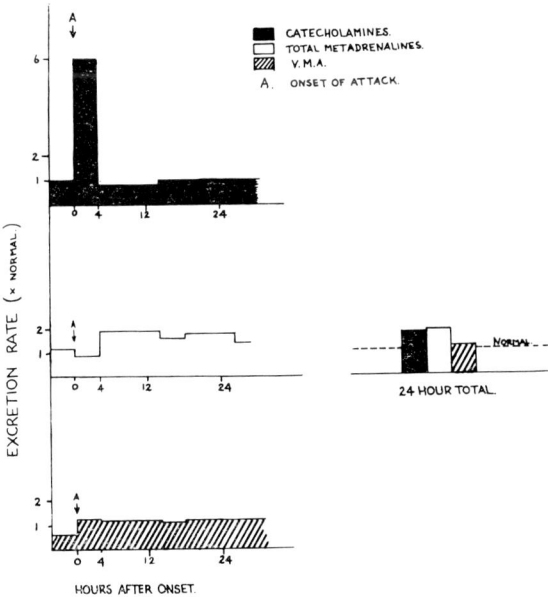

FIG. 4b. Same case as Figure 4a—after an attack. A brief but large increase in excretion of catecholamines was not accompanied by a corresponding increase in the excretion of metabolites. The diagnostic significance of the increase would have been lost if only a 24-hour collection had been examined.

appearance with grey or yellowish brown areas set against a general dusky reddish grey. Cavities containing blood or blood clot are not uncommon, and areas of necrosis, fibrosis or calcification may be seen.

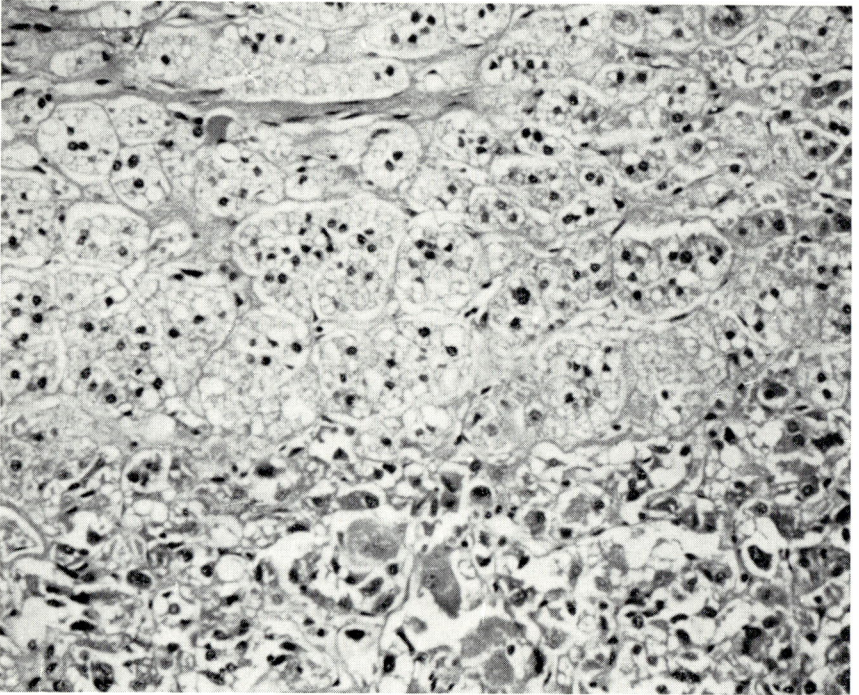

Fig. 5. Phæochromocytoma showing the absence of a capsule between the cells of a tumour 5 cm. diameter and the adrenal cortex. (× 160.(

Histologically, the appearance is very variable, even within the same tumour (Figs. 6 to 8). Usually, the majority of the cells resemble those of the adrenal medulla, and are disposed in sheets or divided into smaller collections by thin or coarse fibrous septa. Numerous thin-walled, dilated blood vessels are often intimately related to the tumour cells which may appear to line the lumen or to lie free within it. The cytoplasm of the cells may be scanty and vacuolated, or possess granules with variable staining properties (Sherwin, 1959). Some cells reach large dimensions with densely granular eosinophilic cytoplasm, and contain one or more nuclei which may be bizarre and hyperchromatic. Mitoses are usually scanty. Differentiation towards ganglion cells may, infrequently, be sufficient to warrant description as a mixed tumour, and there have been rare cases which have shown neuroblastomatous elements as well (Wahl and Robinson, 1943).

Recognition of Malignancy

Malignant change in phæochromocytoma is rare, occurring only in about 10 per cent of cases, and its recognition is extremely difficult in the absence

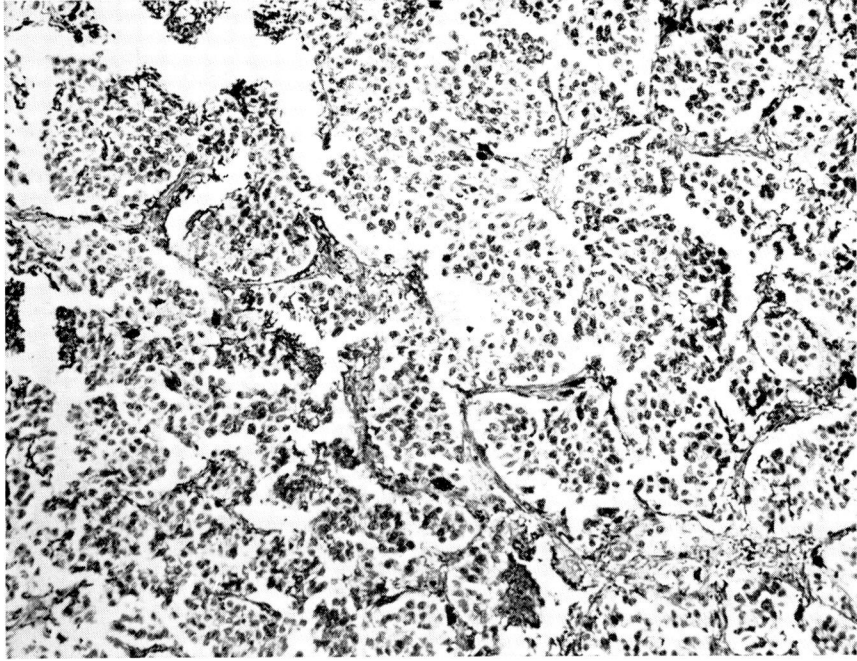

FIG. 6. Phæochromocytoma showing general alveolar-like arrangement. ($\times$ 30.)

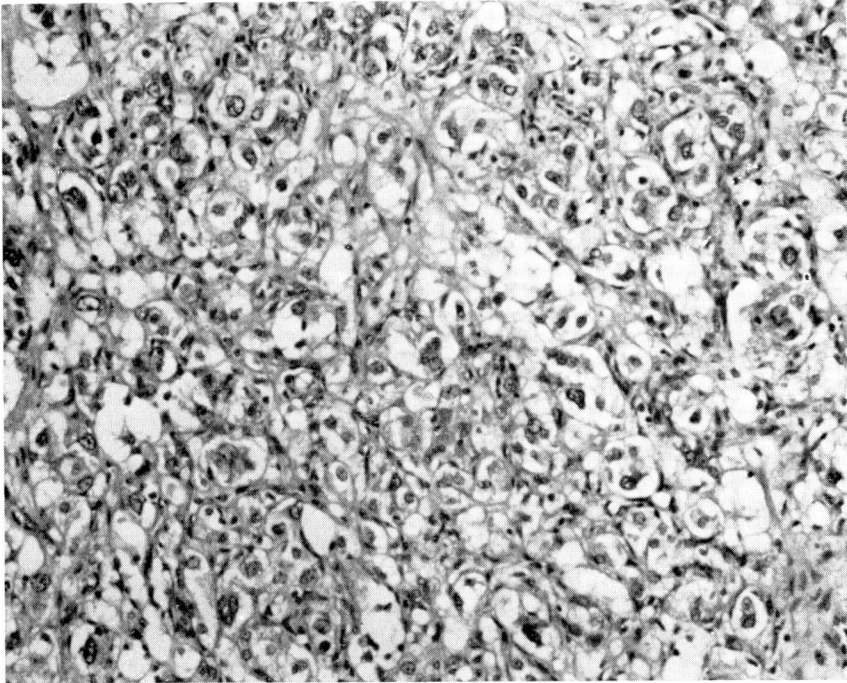

FIG. 7. Phæochromocytoma showing cells with scanty vacuolated cytoplasm. ($\times$ 160.)

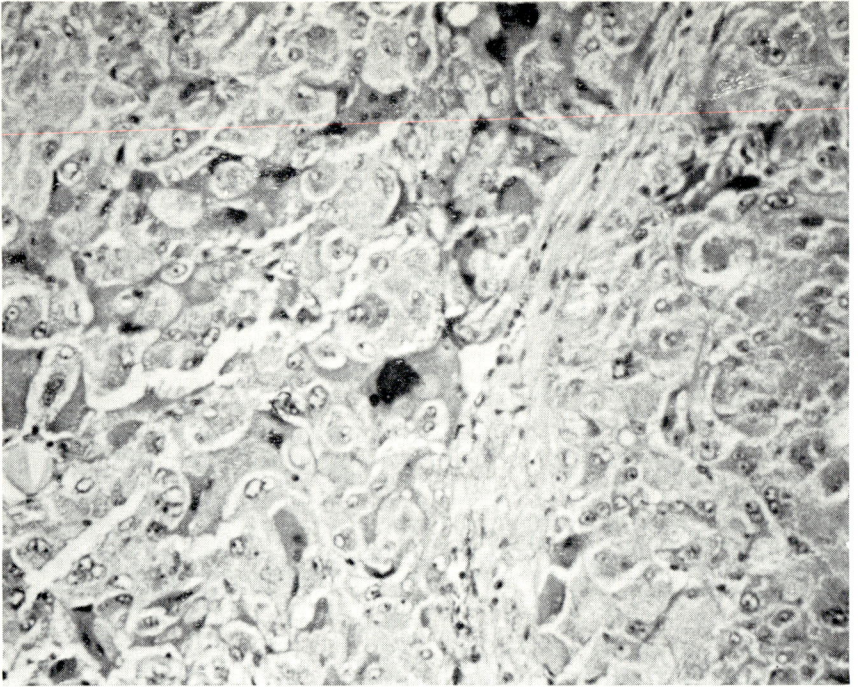

FIG. 8. Phæochromocytoma showing cells with abundant granular cytoplasm, some of which are very large with bizarre hyperchromatic nuclei. (× 160.)

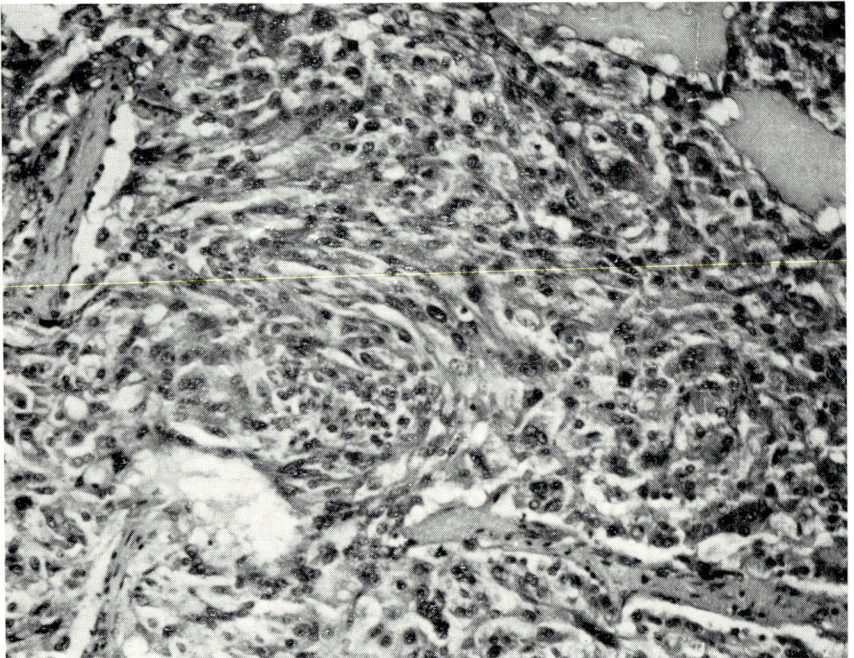

FIG. 9. Metastasising phæochromocytoma showing spindle cell formation. (× 160.)

of metastases. Cellular pleomorphism and bizarre hyperchromatic nuclei are seen frequently in benign tumours, while even capsular invasion does not necessarily signify the ability to metastasise (Symington and Goodall, 1953). Conversely, tumours with a uniform "benign" appearance and showing no evidence of local spread have given rise to distant metastases (Kennedy et al., 1961). A feature of some of the reported malignant cases has been a tendency to spindle cell formation (Fig. 9), but this too has occasionally been seen in tumours which did not metastasize (Sherwin, 1959).

The observation of McMillan (1956), that a locally invasive phæochromocytoma contained a very large amount of dopamine associated with an increase in the urinary excretion, led her to suggest that increased dopamine secretion might be related to malignancy. There have since been reports of several malignant phæochromocytomata with increased urinary excretion of dopamine or its major metabolite homovanillic acid (Sankoff and Sourkes, 1963; Robinson et al., 1964; Käser, 1966; Moloney et al., 1966). It would appear that a large increase in either of these substances in the urine is strong evidence of the ability to metastasize. However, it must not be assumed that the absence of increased dopamine production excludes malignancy, as several cases with metastases have been reported either with no increase of dopamine in the tumour (Manger et al., 1954; Kennedy et al., 1961) or with normal urinary dopamine and homovanillic acid (Sato and Sjoerdsma, 1965; Tressider and Higgins, 1966).

NEUROBLASTOMA-GANGLIONEUROMA GROUP

Secretory Properties

Despite the known histogenetic relationship of this group to the phæochromocytoma, their secretory properties were not recognized until comparatively recently. In 1957, Mason et al. described a case of neuroblastoma with hypertension and increased excretion of pressor amines in the urine. Some cells gave a weakly positive chromaffin reaction and pressor amines were found in an extract assayed biologically. Confirmatory reports soon followed, and intracytoplasmic storage granules like those in phæochromocytoma have been demonstrated (Page and Jacoby, 1964). The overall excretory pattern is, however, more complex than in phæochromocytoma. Not only is the excretion of noradrenaline and the metabolites VMA and normetadrenaline increased, but, in contrast to phæochromocytoma, the excretion of dopamine and its metabolites is also frequently raised. The detailed excretory pattern is inconstant from case to case, and sometimes increased excretion of dopa and dopa metabolites has also been found. The most consistent abnormality appears to be increased excretion of VMA, but as this does not always occur, estimation of both VMA and HVA is recommended for diagnosis. The now extensive literature on this subject has been reviewed by von Studnitz (1966) and Käser (1966).

Fewer data are available for the well-differentiated ganglioneuroma, but it is apparent that while many are non-secretory, others are, and may even be associated with increased excretion of homovanillic acid. The prognostic significance of this is discussed below.

An interesting feature of some cases, not encountered in phæochromo-cytoma, is the occurrence of a syndrome of chronic diarrhœa, abdominal pain and flushing (Rosenstein and Engelman, 1963). It is seen more often with ganglioneuroma than with neuroblastoma, and disappears after excision of the tumour. This suggests a humoral mechanism, which remains obscure. The clinical picture may be similar to the carcinoid syndrome, but no abnormality of serotonin metabolism has been described. This similarity should be borne in mind when investigating patients with this symptom complex.

Appearance of the Tumour

Neuroblastomata are usually smooth or lobulated tumours, which often attain much greater size than the phæochromocytoma. The cut surface is not dissimilar in colour, but the tissue tends to be softer and more friable; calcification is commonly present. More differentiated forms are firmer and tend to be grey or yellowish on the cut surface.

Microscopically the appearance is very variable. The completely undifferentiated tumours consist of sheets of sympathogonia, divided by connective tissue septa; these are small cells with very darkly staining nuclei and hardly any visible cytoplasm. Maturation proceeds through the sympathoblast, a larger cell with vesicular nucleus and more cytoplasm which may sometimes appear to be syncytial; nucleoli become prominent. These two cells are often present together, though one or other type may predominate. The appearance of nerve fibrils may give rise to the well-known rosettes, which are, however, often absent. Sometimes partial maturation of the sympathoblasts to ganglion cells results in a mixed picture containing all three cellular elements and many nerve fibres, namely the ganglioneuro-blastoma (Figs. 10 and 11).

In the fully differentiated ganglioneuroma (Fig. 12), the picture is one of profuse neurofibrillary material intermingled with ganglion cells. The latter vary in size, shape and fibril formation; most contain a single vesicular nucleus with a prominent nucleolus, but cells containing two or three nuclei are not uncommon. In view of the variable appearance of different parts of the mixed tumours, several regions of the tumour should be examined before pronouncing it to be a pure ganglioneuroma.

The difficulties that arise over the histological identification of the small cell tumours are well known, and opinions vary widely on the nature of Ewing's tumour, most of which Willis (1960) believes to be examples of metastatic neuroblastoma. According to Marsden and Steward (1964), differences in age incidence, progress, metastatic spread and gross and microscopical appearance enable these two tumours to be distinguished, but the differences they describe are inadequate for certain differentiation always to be made in biopsy material. Since it is now clear that the great majority of neuroblastomata secrete catecholamines, many of the histological difficulties might be resolved by appropriate examination of the urine. It must be stressed, however, that if only catecholamines or a single metabolite are sought, the tumour might incorrectly be assessed as non-secretory. This should only be accepted when the excretion, not only of catecholamines, but

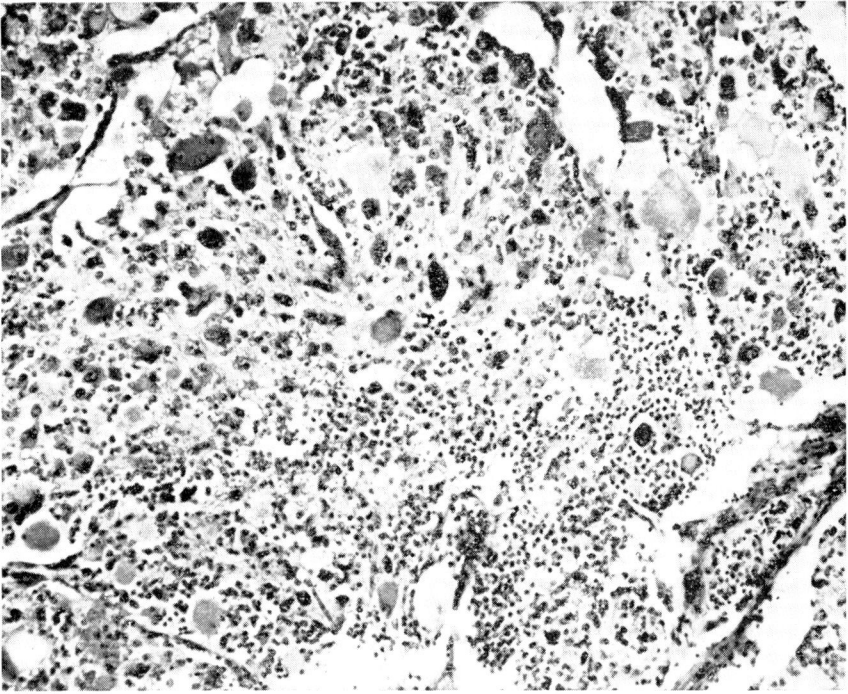

FIG. 10. Ganglioneuroblastoma showing sympathogonia, sympathoblasts and immature ganglion cells. (× 160.)

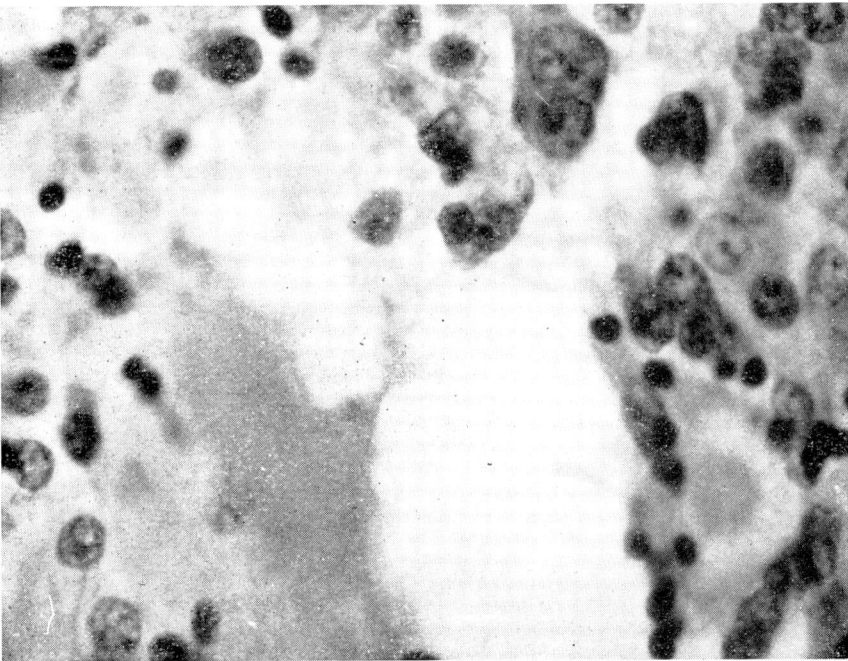

FIG. 11. Ganglioneuroblastoma. High power view of Figure 10. (× 640.)

L

also of the whole gamut of its metabolites, has been shown to be normal.[1] Demonstration of secretion is most helpful in these circumstances, but whether the absence of secretion excludes a neuroblastoma is not yet agreed. Examples of non-secretory neuroblastoma have been described, but Bell (1966) believes they rest on faulty diagnosis, and that non-secretory neuroblastomata do not exist.

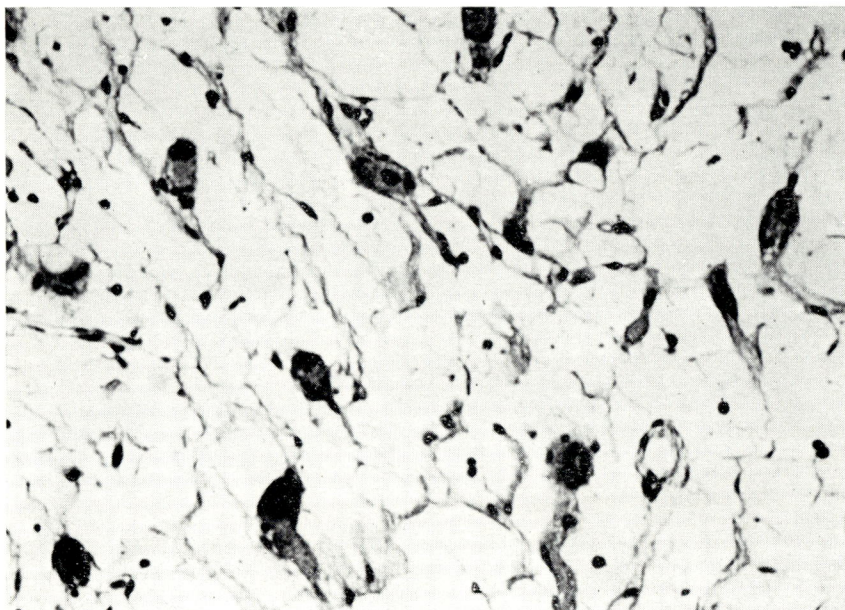

FIG. 12. Ganglioneuroma. Typical appearance of ganglion cells intermingled with fibrillary material. ($\times$ 160.)

This divergence of opinion is unlikely to be resolved by histological methods, but the issue might be clarified by studying such tumours in tissue culture. Grant and Pulvertaft (1966) have recently discussed the value of this technique for studying neuroblastomata, and how it enabled them to identify a neuroblastoma that was histologically indistinguishable from Burkitt's tumour (Fig. 14).

Secretory Properties and Prognosis

The neuroblastoma is usually highly malignant and the ganglioneuroma benign, but the prognosis is variable. Voorhess and Gardner (1962) first pointed out that the excretory patterns in this group were inconstant, and that the variations bore no relation to the histological appearance of the

[1] The widely used screening method of Hingerty (1957) for increased urinary catecholamines is not entirely suitable in these circumstances. It does not estimate dopamine, which is often the catecholamine showing the greatest increase. If it is used, the amount of urine taken and the range of standards included, should be modified to allow for the much smaller excretion in children than in adults. In neuroblastoma, the method of Bell et al. (1958) is to be preferred.

tumour. They therefore suggested a classification based on biochemical characteristics, and since then, other attempts have been made to relate the excretory pattern in the urine to prognosis (Bell, 1966; Gjessing, 1966). It is too soon for full evaluation of this aspect, but so far no clear-cut correlation has emerged. For example, Bell has suggested that prognosis might be better if there is no increase in excretion of dopamine and homovanillic acid. This implies a poor prognosis for ganglioneuromata with increased excretion of homovanillic acid, and the question arises are such tumours really ganglio-neuroblastomata? The prominence of neuroblastomatous elements in mixed tumours is variable, as illustrated in Figures 10 to 13. Figure 10 shows a typical field from a ganglioneuroblastoma removed from a boy aged 11 years who excreted very large amounts of VMA and homovanillic acid. Despite

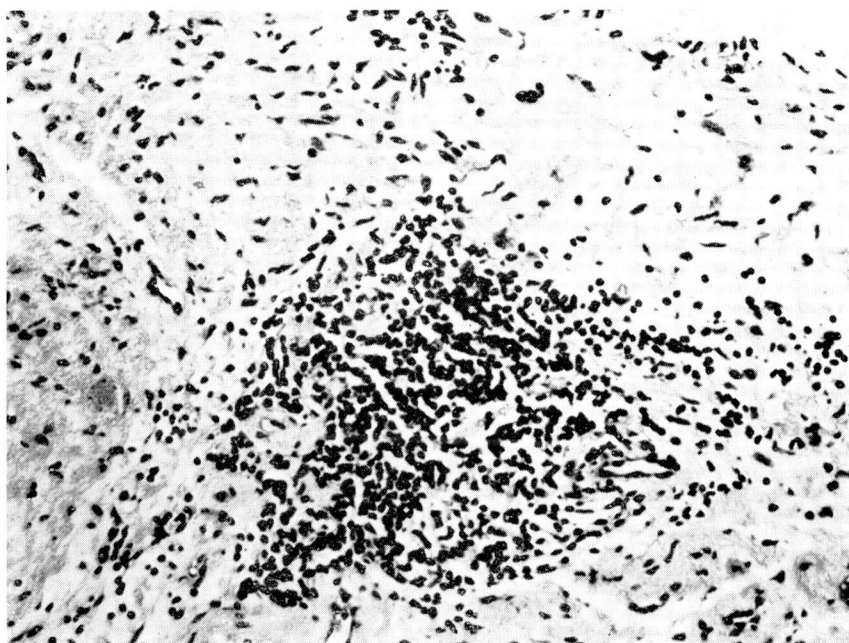

FIG. 13. Ganglioneuroma showing a focus of small, darkly staining cells. Same case as Figure 12. (× 160.)

this he is alive and well with normal excretion of these compounds three years after the operation. Figure 12 illustrates a typical field from another tumour with the same excretory pattern, which was classified as a ganglio-neuroma because the two sections examined first showed only this picture. When six more blocks were taken from different parts of the tumour, one or two small foci of small darkly staining round cells were seen in each section (Fig. 13). Whether these are sufficient to explain the high excretion of homovanillic acid, or warrant reclassifying the tumour as a ganglioneuro-blastomata with its prognostic implications, is debatable, and time alone will tell whether the prognosis in this case is better related to the excretion of homovanillic acid or to the histological appearance. Eighteen months after

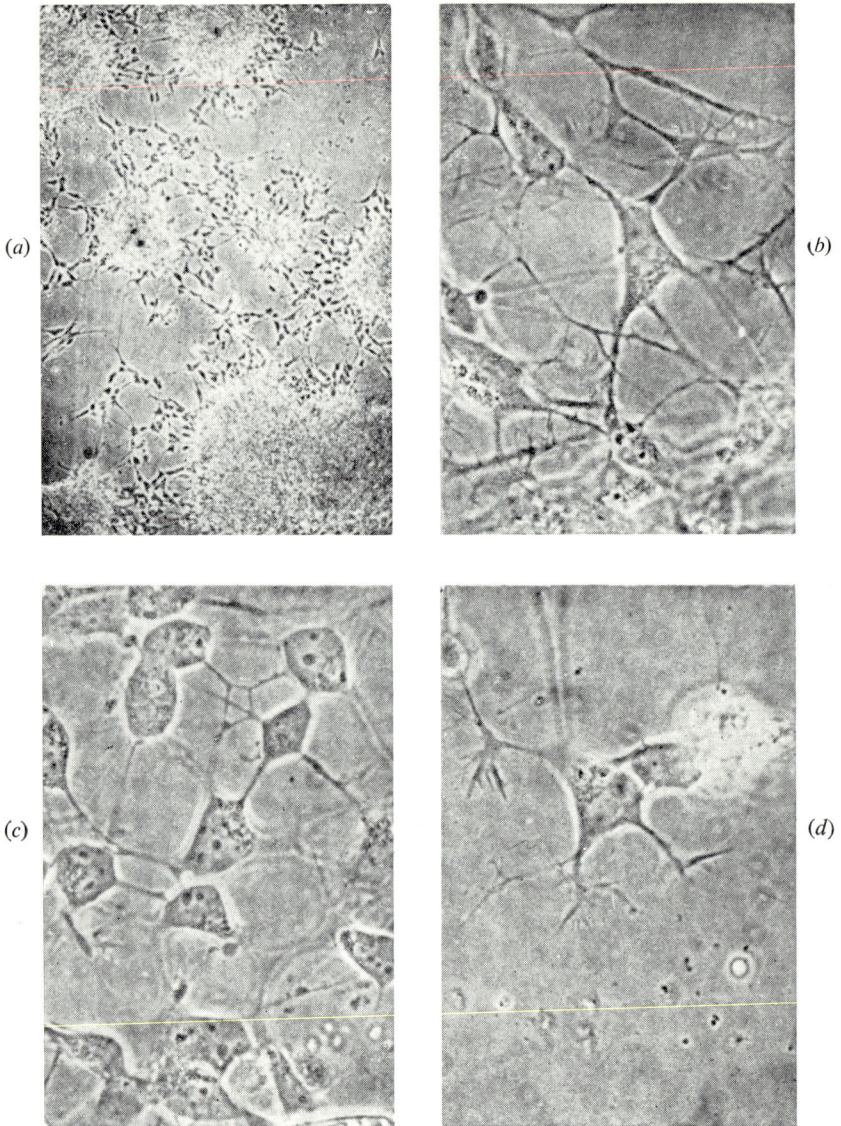

FIG. 14. Developing neuroblasts in tissue culture (a) Tissue Culture ($\times 100$); (b) and (c) fibril formation ($\times 1000$); and (d) end-plates ($\times 1000$) (from Grant and Pulvertaft, 1960).

operation the patient is well, with normal excretion of catecholamines and metabolites.

Most authors have found that successful treatment of these tumours is accompanied by a return of urinary catecholamine excretion towards normal. This has been complete in "cured" cases, while persistent abnormality has indicated the presence of residual disease. Likewise, reappearance of an abnormal pattern in an apparently cured case may be the first indication of recurrence, a point of therapeutic importance.

PARAGANGLIOMA

Tumours of the Carotid Body and Glomus Jugulare (Chemodectoma). The carotid body and glomus jugulare have been included among the so-called "non-chromaffin paraganglia". But Lever *et al.* (1959) have shown that a positive chromaffin reaction is given by the glomus cells of the cat and rabbit if an appropriate technique is used. There have since been reports of several tumours of the carotid body (Glenner *et al.*, 1962; Berdal *et al.*, 1962) or glomus jugulare (Duke *et al.*, 1964) associated with increased excretion of catecholamines. The tumours contained large amounts of noradrenaline with smaller amounts of adrenaline, thus supporting the view that at least some of the cells of these chemoreceptor sites are of neuroectodermal origin. In all but one of them the chromaffin reaction was negative, but this can be attributed to the use of unsatisfactory methods; the reaction was attempted on tissue fixed in formalin or Zenker's solution, both of which are unreliable (see below). Electron microscopy has shown the presence of granules similar to those in other catecholamine containing-tissues (Gejrot *et al.*, 1964).

The above-mentioned tumours resembled the phæochromocytoma in hormone content and produced similar circulatory changes. An example resembling the ganglioneuroma has also been described (Chamberlain, 1961). In the latter, urinary catecholamines were normal, but abdominal pain and diarrhœa were prominent symptoms which were relieved by the removal of the tumour; the excretion of metabolites was not described.

These tumours are usually comparatively small and of firm consistency. They may be attached to surrounding tissue, and may surround the carotid artery. As in the tumours discussed previously, the microscopic appearance is variable. The cells are usually arranged in small groups separated by bands of vascular connective tissue (Fig. 15), but may be arranged in sheets. They are intimately related to blood vessels. The cytoplasm may be granular or clear, and the cellular outline may be so indistinct as to suggest a syncytium. The nuclei may be vesicular or hyperchromatic, and multinuclear cells occur.

Histological recognition of malignancy is again difficult. As with the phæochromocytoma, the cellular appearance and apparent invasion of blood vessels are not reliable criteria (Le Compte, 1951), and it is to be hoped that biochemical analysis of the urine will prove to be useful in this respect; in a case of metastasizing carotid body tumour mentioned by Robinson (1966) the urinary excretion of homovanillic acid was increased.

Other "Non-chromaffin" Paragangliomata. Tumours which closely resemble the glomus tumours histologically may arise in other parts of the body, and are well recognized in the retroperitoneal tissue, the thorax and the neck, and have occasionally been found in the lung (Fawcett and Husband, 1967). Histologically they resemble the carotid body tumour (Fig. 16). Smetana and Scott (1951) reviewed a group of tumours arising in the thigh and usually diagnosed as granular myoblastoma or mistaken for metastases. Microscopically, the similarity of the cellular components and organoid structure to the glomus tumour led Smetana and Scott to suggest that they

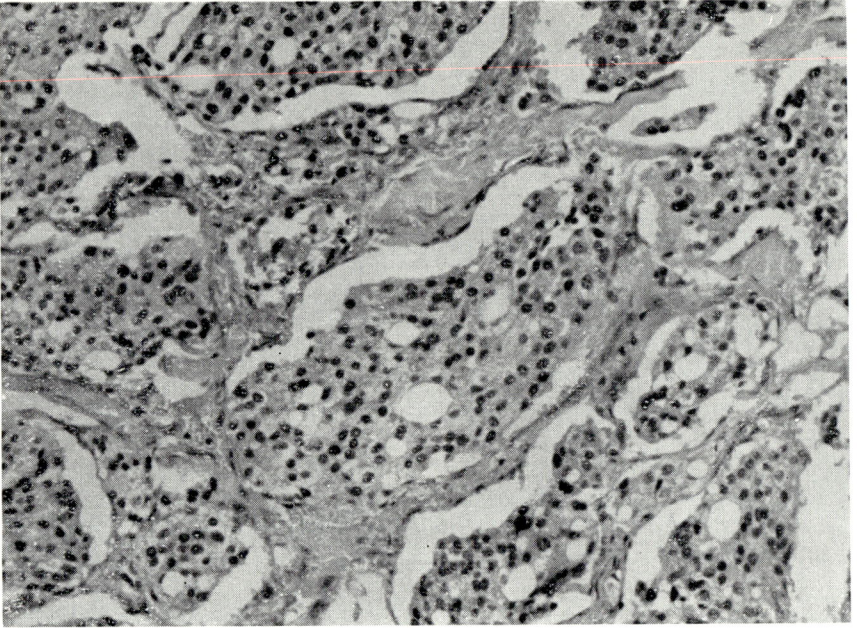

FIG. 15. Carotid body tumour. Clumps of cells are separated by fibrous septa. In places there are numerous dilated, thin-walled blood vessels. (×160.)

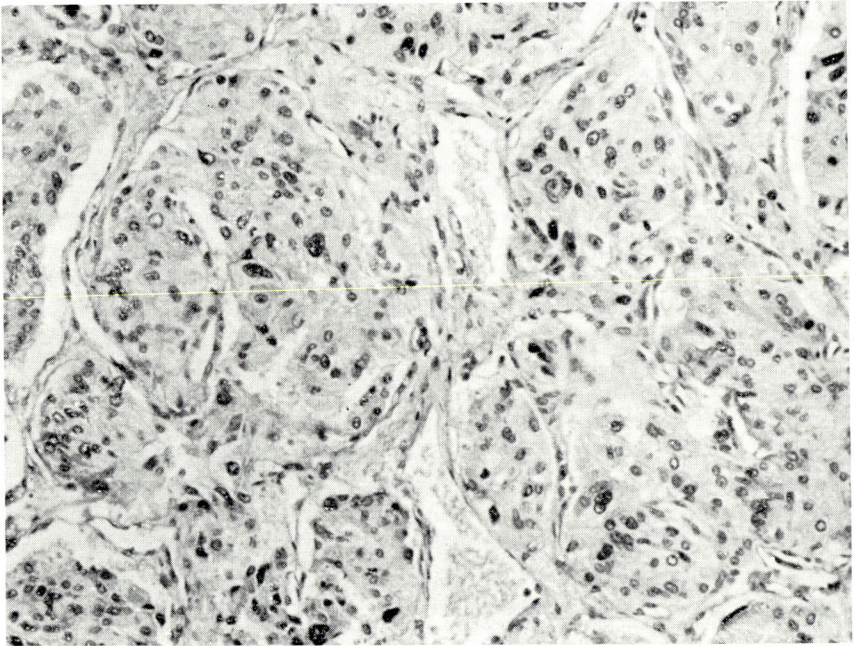

FIG. 16. Abdominal paraganglioma (noradrenaline secreting). The alveolar appearance and blood vessels resemble some glomus tumours and adrenal phæochromocytoma. (×160.)

should be included with the paragangliomata, and that they arise in structures resembling the carotid body located around the large femoral vessels. The chromaffin reaction was negative, but again was often performed on formalin or Zenker fixed tissue.

Hypertension and circulatory crises during operation are usually absent in these paragangliomata, but this does not necessarily exclude secretory properties. Hypertension is often absent in patients with secretory tumours of the neuroblastoma group, for reasons not yet fully explained, and that some paragangliomata may behave similarly is suggested by the carotid body tumour with the diarrhœa syndrome quoted above. Conclusions as to secretory properties drawn from the negative chromaffin reaction in the past must be treated with caution in view of the negative results reported with glomus tumours shown by chemical analysis to contain large quantities of catecholamines.

The glomus tumour, paraganglioma and adrenal phæochromocytoma are histologically similar, so that classification of a tumour is often based on its anatomical location. The relationship of these tumours to each other needs to be reassessed by means of biochemical studies on the urine and tumour tissue. The secretory chemodectomata may form only a small proportion of the total, and warrant separate classification with the phæo-chromocytoma.

EXAMINATION OF THE TUMOUR

Despite the advances in laboratory methods of diagnosis, these tumours are sometimes found more or less unexpectedly at operation or at autopsy. Two problems then face the pathologist, namely histological identification of the tumour and elucidation of its functional activity. The former is a matter of microscopy; the latter, which may be of great value in proving the identity, requires some form of chemical examination. This should always be done, for such tumours may contain large amounts of hormone despite the apparent absence of clinical manifestations. The tumour and any metastases must therefore be divided into several parts for the following examinations, and any urine found in the bladder at autopsy should be acidified to pH 2–3 and retained for chemical analysis.

1. Histology. Place a portion into a routine fixative.

It should be noted that Zenker's fluid cannot be relied upon to give consistent results for the chromaffin reaction, and a dichromate solution such as the one mentioned below must be used for the chromaffin reaction.

The histology has been described briefly above. For a detailed account, the reader is referred to standard works (Willis, 1960; Winston Evans, 1966).

2. Chemical Analysis. Place a portion in the deep freeze as soon as possible. Alternatively a piece of tumour may be placed in several times its volume of 0·01 N hydrochloric acid; the latter is preferable if the tumour is to be sent through the post.

The catecholamines are extracted from part of the tumour with several times its volume of 0·01 N hydrochloric acid or acidified ethanol, then purified by passage through a column of alumina or ion exchange resin, and estimated fluorimetrically.

An alternative and less elaborate procedure is to examine the extract directly by chromatography on Whatman No. 1 or 3 MM paper, with water-saturated phenol as solvent. The equivalent of 20 mg. of tumour is a convenient amount to apply to the paper initially. After developing overnight, the phenol is removed by washing with Analar benzene and drying in cold air. A suitable location reagent (McMillan, 1957) is applied and the extract compared with known amounts of the pure catecholamines. It is possible with this method to detect as little as 20 μg. of adrenaline, noradrenaline and dopamine per gram of tumour, but the method is not suitable for the very small amounts found in many neuroblastomata.

The amount of catecholamines found in tumour tissue varies with the nature of the tumour. In most phæochromocytomata, noradrenaline is present in amounts ranging from several hundred to several thousand micrograms per gram of tumour. Adrenaline in similar amounts often accompanies noradrenaline in tumours arising in the adrenal medulla, but is absent from tumours of extra-adrenal origin or present only in minute amounts. Dopamine is either undetectable or present in small quantities up to about 20 μg. per gram in benign tumours, but may be present in milligram amounts in malignant variants.

In the neuroblastoma-ganglioneuroma group, the findings are strikingly different. Most authors have found less than 10 micrograms of catecholamines per gram of tissue, and even in known dopamine secretors, the amount of dopamine found in the tumour has been less than in some benign phæo-chromocytomata. Adrenaline has been found only in minute amounts when estimated by chemical methods.

The chemodectomata so far reported with clinically manifest secretory properties contained noradrenaline in amounts similar to the phæochromo-cytoma, and, interestingly in view of their extra-adrenal origin, some also contained significant amounts of adrenaline. Smaller amounts of noradrena-line have been found in several others (Pryse-Davies et al., 1964).

3. Chromaffin Reaction. (a) Fix thin slices in a solution consisting of 100 parts of 5 per cent potassium dichromate and 7 parts of 5 per cent potassium chromate. Paraffin sections may be examined unstained or with light nuclear staining.

(b) A useful technique for gross specimens (Sherwin, 1959) is to place two slices of tumour each about 2 cm. square and 1–2 mm. thick, side by side on a glass plate, or in separate jars. Just cover one with the dichromate solution, leave exposed to the air and inspect at intervals. The slice in dichromate solution turns dark brown, usually within a few hours, if the tumour contains an appreciable amount of catecholamines. Adrenaline-containing tumours seem to give the darkest colours. This technique works well with frozen tissue, so that if the dichromate solution is not readily available, unfixed tissue may be frozen and the test performed within a day or two (Fig. 17).

The chromaffin reaction is still of great value in the histological diagnosis of phæochromocytoma, but it is generally unhelpful in the investigation of tumours of the neuroblastoma group, due no doubt to the relatively minute amounts of catecholamines usually present.

Although it has been categorically stated that the diagnosis of phæo-chromocytoma cannot be made with certainty in the absence of a positive chromaffin reaction (Karsner, 1950), the reaction is still widely regarded as being somewhat capricious. This is probably due to the lack of uniformity in technique. Some recommended dichromate fixatives have an unsuitable pH (see below), and the other staining procedures of Schmorl, Sevki and Gomori are non-specific and may give false positive results (Sherwin, 1959). The well-known failure of the chromaffin reaction to work with formalin-fixed tissue is readily explained by the fact that adrenaline and noradrenaline rapidly disappear from such tissue, and can barely be detected in extracts of tumour fixed in formol-saline for 24 hours.

Despite these objections, the chromaffin reaction remains the most useful histochemical test for catecholamines, provided that it is properly performed. The detailed studies of Hillarp and Hökfelt (1953) established the importance of the pH of the dichromate solution, which should lie within the range of 5 to 6; outside this range the reaction becomes weaker and ultimately negative. This was confirmed by Kennedy *et al.* (1961), who went so far as to suggest that failure to use a dichromate solution of the correct pH is the most important cause of false negative results with phæochromocytomata, a criticism equally applicable to many of the negative results obtained with paragangliomata.

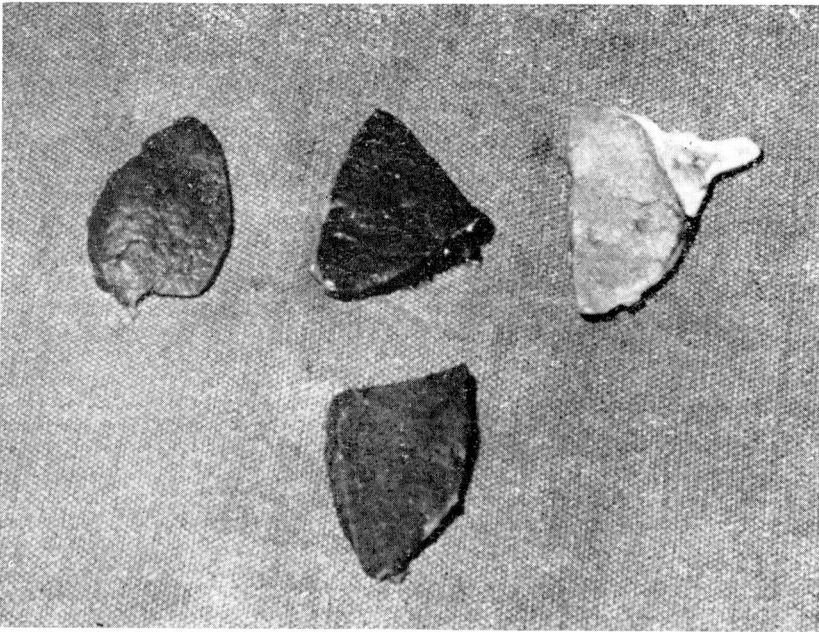

FIG. 17. Slices of phæochromocytoma covered with different dichromate solutions and left exposed to the air.

Top Left to Right—Müller's fluid (pH 4·1), Hillarp and Hökfelt (pH 5·7), Zenker, without acetic acid (pH 4·0).

Bottom—Régaud's fluid (pH 4·8).
     The tumour contained 1·2 mg. noradrenaline and 7·0 mg. adrenaline per gram of tissue

It is conceivable that, in some cases, the reaction may be negative because the tumour contains insufficient catecholamines for histochemical demonstration. While this appears to be the rule for the neuroblastoma, thus necessitating chemical analysis, it probably never occurs in the case of the phæochromocytoma. Hillarp and Hökfelt (1955) and Kennedy *et al.* (1961) both recommend a solution containing a mixture of potassium dichromate and potassium chromate to give a pH of 5·6 and 5·8 respectively. These solutions appear to be very reliable and a positive reaction has been obtained with one or other in 14 consecutive phæochromocytomata, shown by chemical analysis to contain catecholamines (Fig. 18). Insistence on demonstrating chromaffin granules, however, can lead to misinterpretation. In tumours, the catecholamines are not confined to the storage granules, and a diffuse brown staining, which may be very intense, is often seen without convincing granules, even when thin slices are cut and placed in the recommended solution immediately after removing the tumour.

The dichromate-chromate mixture recommended also gives excellent results with the macro-technique. Sherwin (1959) originally found Zenker's solution, made up without acetic acid, to be the best of the dichromate solutions he examined, which did not however include that recommended by Hillarp and Hökfelt. In fact, even without acetic acid, the pH of Zenker's solution is too low, and though it will work with tumours which contain large amounts of catecholamines, the results are likely to be erratic, especially with those containing only noradrenaline which is oxidized slowly at pH 4. Figure 17 shows the variation in intensity of the brown colour of tumour slices placed in several dichromate solutions. That of Hillarp and Hökfelt has given the best results, and Zenker's the worst; this also applies to histological evaluation of the reaction.

Cells containing adrenaline stain brown at pH 5·6, and those containing noradrenaline stain yellow, but, as many phæochromocytomata contain both in very variable proportions, too much significance should not be attached to the colour of the staining. The presence of noradrenaline is better inferred from the iodate reaction.

4. Iodate Reaction. (a) Place slices about 0·5 mm. thick into saturated potassium iodate solution with a little glass-wool at the bottom. After 24 or 48 hours, transfer to formol saline, and after a further 24 hours examine frozen sections unstained or with light nuclear staining. Noradrenaline-containing cells stain brown, adrenaline-containing cells remaining unstained. When only relatively small amounts of noradrenaline are present, the staining may be pale and yellow.

(b) It is convenient to inspect the slices in the iodate solution at the same time as that covered with dichromate; those in iodate also turn dark brown rapidly if the tumour contains noradrenaline. Even more striking with phæochromocytoma tissue is the red coloration which rapidly appears, often within 10 minutes, and slowly diffuses throughout the solution which ultimately becomes deep red. After several days on the bench the solution turns brown. The red coloration is probably not specific for noradrenaline, as both adrenaline and noradrenaline form water-soluble, red intermediate products on oxidation with iodate.

Adrenaline and noradrenaline are both converted to a brown pigment by oxidation with iodate but the pigment differs from that formed by dichromate. The reaction was studied histochemically by Hillarp and Hökfelt (1953, 1955), who found that with a saturated solution of iodate, only the noradrenaline-containing cells of the adrenal medulla are stained. Dopamine and dopa also behave like noradrenaline, and though unimportant in the adrenal medulla, these compounds may be found in histochemically demonstrable amounts in some malignant phæochromocytomata. The discrete staining of individual cells obtained under experimental conditions is much less likely to be achieved with clinical material, as some diffusion out of the cells will almost certainly have occurred before it can be processed. Sections of iodate treated phæochromocytoma usually show diffuse brown or yellow staining which may be patchy or may vary in intensity in different parts of the section (Fig. 19), but

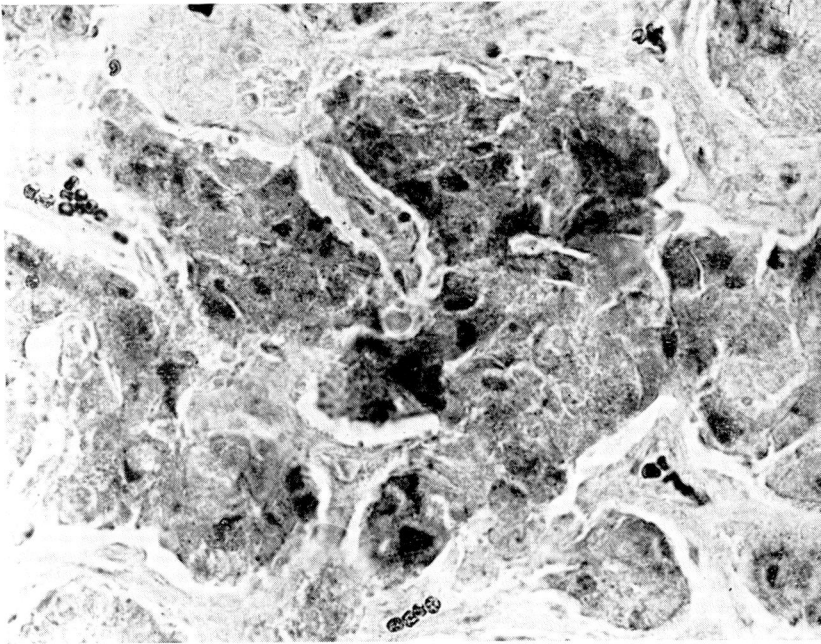

FIG. 18. Chromaffin reaction at pH 5·6. Although well marked granules are visible, other parts of the same section showed diffuse staining.

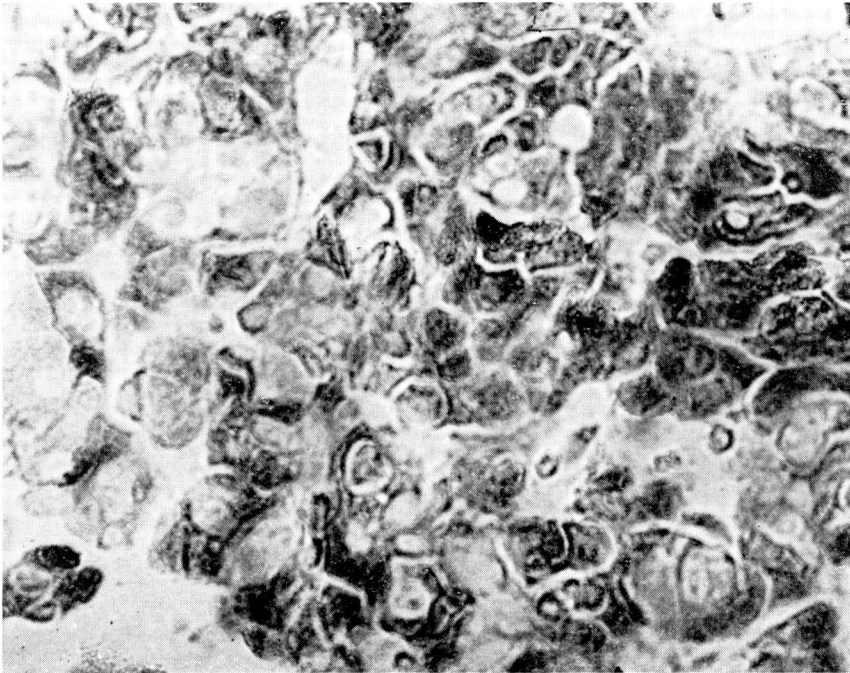

FIG. 19. Phæochromocytoma treated with saturated potassium iodate. Note the uneven staining of the cells. The tumour contained 2.0 mg. of noradrenaline and 2.1 mg. adrenaline per gram of tissue.

negative results were reported by Kennedy *et al.* with two tumours which contained relatively small amounts of noradrenaline. Experience with the neuroblastoma is limited, but as might be expected, so far the histochemical results have been negative though the iodate solution may turn pink if allowed to stand with an equal volume of minced tumour.

5. Fluorescence Microscopy. Cells containing catecholamines can also be identified by fluorescence microscopy of formalin fixed tissues. The catecholamines condense with formaldehyde to form dihydroisoquinoline derivatives which fluoresce green to yellow-green when excited with light of wavelength 410 mμ. Conditions can be chosen so that only dopamine and noradrenaline react to any significant extent. The method is very sensitive and has been used to study the localization of noradrenaline in adrenergic neurones and nerve endings.

According to Falck (1962), the best results are obtained by immediately freezing the tissue and drying *in vacuo* at $-35°$C for 8–10 days, followed by vacuum embedding in paraffin; sections, deparaffinized in xylene, are then exposed to the vapour from paraformaldehyde for one hour at 80°C. The water content of the formaldehyde vapour is somewhat critical; too little inhibits the reaction and too much allows diffusion from the storage sites and may quench the fluorescence (Hamberger *et al.*, 1965). Increased specificity is achieved by subsequent treatment of the sections with sodium borohydride (Corrodi *et al.*, 1964). This reduces the fluorescent compounds to the corresponding non-fluorescent tetrahydro derivatives, the dull-green background fluorescence remaining unchanged; re-exposure to formaldehyde vapour restores the fluorescence. With prolonged exposure to formaldehyde, adrenaline also reacts, but fluorescence derived from adrenaline or dopamine can be distinguished from that due to noradrenaline by following the borohydride treatment with potassium periodate; the tetrahydro derivative from noradrenaline is selectively oxidized so that regeneration of the fluorescence by formaldehyde cannot occur (Mukherji *et al.*, 1966).

Given the experimental conditions outlined above, fluorescence microscopy may prove useful for studying the tumours which contain only very small amounts of catecholamines, but routine fixation in formalin is clearly far from ideal and cannot be expected to give good results. When only formalin fixed material is available from tumours which usually contain large amounts of catecholamines, fluorescence microscopy might be the means whereby secretory activity can be determined, but has not been fully evaluated. In such cases, fluorescence in routine sections deparaffinized in xylene tends to be diffuse and may be of low intensity and appear non-specific, so that the effect of borohydride should always be ascertained. Prolonged fixation is undesirable as the progressive brown discoloration of the formalin in these cases indicates accumulation of fluorescent compounds in the solution.

ACKNOWLEDGMENTS

I wish to thank Dr. A. G. Marshall who kindly gave me the facilities of his department; the editor of the Archives of Diseases of Childhood for permission to publish Figure 14; Dr. M. K. Alexander for the sections of the malignant phæochromocytoma (Fig. 9) and Dr. M. Symons for the sections of the ganglioneuroblastoma (Fig. 10).

References

ARMSTRONG, M. D., McMILLAN, A. and SHAW, K. N. F. (1957). *Biochm. Biophys. Acta*, **25**, 422.
AXELROD, J. (1957). *Science*, **126**, 400.
BELL, M. (1966). In *Recent Results in Cancer Research*, Vol. 2. "Neuroblastomas—Biochemical Studies" p. 42, Berlin, Heidelberg, New York: Springer-Verlag.
BELL, M., HORROCKS, R. H. and VARLEY, H. (1958). In *Pract. Clinical Biochem.* (Varley) 2nd Ed., 1958, p. 527, Heinemann.
BERDAL, P., BRAATEN, M. CAPPELEN, C., Jr., MYLIUS, E. A. and WALAAS, O. (1962). *Acta Med. Scand.* **172**, fasc. 2, 249.
BROWN, J. J., RUTHVEN, C. R. J. and SANDLER, M. (1966). *J. Clin. Path.* **19**, 482.
CHAMBERLAIN, Z. D. (1961). *Proc. Roy. Soc. Med.* **54**, 227.
CORRODI, H., HILLARP, N-Å and JONSSON, G. (1964). *J. Histochem. Cytochem.* **12**, 582.
CROUT, J. R. and SJOERDSMA, A. (1964). *J. Clin. Invest.* **43**, 94.
DUKE, W. M., BOSHELL, B. R., SOTERES, P. and CARR, J. H. (1964). *Ann. intern med.* **60**, 1040.
ENGEL, A. and EULER, U. S. von (1950), *Lancet*, **ii**, 387.
ERÄNKÖ (1955). *Nature*, **175**, 88.
EULER, U.S. von and STRÖM, G. (1957). *Circulation*, **15**, 5.
EVANS, W. (1966). Histology of Tumours.
FALCK, B. (1962). *Acta Physiol. Scand.* **56**, Suppl. 197.
FAWCETT, F. J. and HUSBAND, E. M. (1967). *J .Clin. Path.* **20**, 260.
GEJROT, T., LAGERLÖF, B. and WERSALL, J. (1964). *Acta oto-laryng.* Suppl. 188, p. 220.
GJESSING, L. R. (1966). In Recent Results in Cancer Research, vol. 2. "Neuroblastomas—Biochemical Studies" p. 26, Berlin, Heidelberg, New York: Springer-Verlag.
GLENNER, G. G., CROUT, J. R. and ROBERTS, W. C. (1962). *Arch. path.* **73**, 66.
GOLDSTEIN, (1966). In *Recent Results in Cancer Research*, vol. 2. "Neuroblastomas—Biochemical Studies" p. 66, Berlin, Heidelberg, New York: Springer-Verlag.
GRANT, H. and PULVERTAFT, R. J. V. (1966). *Arch. Dis. Childh.* **41**, 193.
HAMBERGER, B., MALMFORS, T., and Sachs, C., (1965). *J. Histochem. Cytochem.* **13**, 147.
HILLARP, N-Å. and HÖKFELT, B. (1953). *Acta. Physiol. Scand.* **30**, 55.
HILLARP, N-Å. and HÖKFELT, B. (1955). *J. Histochem. Cytochem.* **3**, 1.
HILLARP, N-Å., LINDQVIST, M. and VENDSALU, A. (1961). *Exper. Cell. Res.* **22**, 40.
HINGERTY, D. (1957). *Lancet*. **1**, 766.
KARSNER, H. T. (1950). *Tumours of the Adrenal*, A.F.I.P. Atlas of Tumour Pathology Section VIII, Fascicle 29.
KÄSER, H. (1966). *Pharmacol. Rev.* **18**, 659.
KELLEHER, J., WALTERS, G., ROBINSON, R. and SMITH, P. (1964). *J. Clin. Path.* **17**, 399.
KENNEDY, J. S., SYMINGTON, T. and WOODGER, B. A. (1961). *J. Path. & Bact.* **81**, 409.
LE COMPTE, P. M. (1951). *Tumours of the carotid body and related structures* (*chemoreceptor system*) A.F.I.P. Atlas of Tumour Pathology, Section IV, Fascicle 16.
LEVER, J. D., LEWIS, P. R. and BOYD, J. D. (1959). *J. Anat.* **93**, 478.
McMILLAN, M. (1956). *Lancet*, **ii**, 284.
McMILLAN, M. (1957). *Lancet*, **i**, 715.
MANGER, W. M., FLOCK, E. V., BERKSON, J., BOLLMAN, J. I., ROTH, G. M., BALDES, E. J. and JACOBS, M. (1954). *Circulation* **10**, 641.
MARSDEN, H. B. and STEWARD, J. K. (1964). *J. Clin. Path.* **17**, 411.
MASON, G. A., HART-MERCER, J., MILLAR, E. J., STRANG, L. B. and WYNNE, N. A. (1957). *Lancet*, **ii**, 322.
MALONEY, G. E., COWDELL, R. H. and LEWIS, C. L. (1966). *Brit. J. Urol.* **38**, 461.
MUKHERJI, M., RAY, A. K. and SEN, P. B. (1966). *J. Histochem. Cytochem.* **14**, 479.
PAGE, L. B. and JACOBY, G. A. (1964). *Medicine*, 43, 379.
PRYSE-DAVIES, J., DAWSON, I. M. P. and WESBTURY, G. (1964). *Cancer*, **17**, 185.
ROBINSON, R. (1966). *In Recent Results in Cancer Research*, vol. 2. "Neuroblastomas—Biochemical Studies" p. 37, Berlin, Heidelberg, New York: Springer-Verlag.
ROBINSON, R., SMITH, P. and WHITTAKER, S. R. F. (1964). *Brit. Med.J.* **1**, 1422.
ROSENSTEIN, B. J. and ENGELMAN, K. (1963). *J. Paed.* **63**, 217.
SANKOFF, I. and SOURKES, T. L. (1963). *Canad. J. Biochem. Physiol.* **41**, 1381.
SATO, T. L. and SJOERDSMA, A. (1965). *Brit. Med. J.* **2**, 1472.
SHERWIN, R. P. (1959). *Cancer*, **12**, 851.
SMETANA, H. F. and SCOTT, W. F., Jnr. (1951). *Milit. Surg.* **109**, 330.

STUDNITZ, W. von (1966). *Pharmacol. Rev.* **18**, 645.
SYMINGTON, T. and GOODALL, A. L. (1953). *Glas. Med. J.* **34**, 75.
TRESSIDER, G. C. and HIGGINS, P. McR. (1966). *Brit. Med. J.* **ii**, 1073.
VOORHESS, M. L. and GARDNER, L. I. (1962). *J. Clin. Endocrinol.* **22**, 126.
WAHL, H. R. and ROBINSON, D. (1943). *Arch. Path.* **35**, 571.
WILLIS, R. A. (1960). Pathology of Tumours.

Chapter 20

MUSCLE BIOPSY IN THE DIAGNOSIS OF NEUROLOGICAL AND MUSCLE DISEASE

J. Trevor Hughes and Betty Brownell

This account deals with the technique of muscle biopsy and the interpretation of the histological changes in denervation and primary muscle disease.

TECHNIQUE OF MUSCLE BIOPSY

Choice of Patient and Muscle

The type of diagnostic problem most likely to be assisted by muscle biopsy is a progressive muscular wasting, and the investigation is particularly useful in distinguishing diseases centred in the nervous system from those in the muscle itself (Greenfield, Cornman and Shy, 1958). In certain other conditions, such as the collagen diseases, muscle biopsy may establish the diagnosis, and in familial diseases a muscle biopsy of a relative of a patient may show a subclinical disorder or the minor changes of a carrier state.

In choosing a site for biopsy, electromyography is useful in assessing the severity of involvement of a particular muscle, but the biopsy should not be taken from a site actually needled at electromyography. The muscle chosen should be affected by the disease but should not be completely atrophic as then it may consist largely of fat and connective tissue. It is desirable to choose a muscle with parallel fascicles so that sections may be cut transverse and longitudinal to the muscle's fibres. Suitable muscles are as follows: deltoid, palmaris longus, biceps brachii, brachioradialis, rectus abdominis, pectoralis major, peroneus longus, peroneus brevis, vastus medialis, tibialis anterior. These examples are of convenient muscles but many others technically suitable could be cited. The intrinsic muscles of the hands and feet, digastric muscle and ocular muscles are not suitable for biopsy because of the disability which might be caused, but they yield excellent sections when, as at necropsy, they can be examined. In localized muscle diseases the choice is limited but the same principles apply. In some generalized diseases such as polyarteritis nodosa there may be local tenderness to guide the physician to an appropriate muscle.

In all biopsies it is of great advantage to examine a portion of muscle which includes the terminal innervation and this becomes essential in diseases such as myasthenia gravis and the peripheral neuropathies. In the recommended muscles the motor point area will usually be situated half-way between the origin and the insertion of the muscle. The localization of this motor point area can be accurately determined by surface electrical stimulation; it is recommended that this should precede the biopsy and that the motor point area should be marked on the skin as a guide to the surgeon.

Obtaining the Biopsy

While it may be possible in special clinics to perform biopsies as a side-room procedure, we advise that muscle biopsy should be carried out in the operating theatre with the normal aseptic precautions. The actual biopsy requires some surgical expertise, and in our experience a sympathetic and practised surgeon is of the greatest help in this work.

To perform a full examination on a muscle biopsy in an adult, a minimum size of $3 \times 2 \times 1$ cm. is required although naturally in the case of a child one may have to accept a smaller specimen. This size of specimen refers to an undamaged single portion of muscle and the skin incision should be larger than the maximum longitudinal length of 3 cm. so that good exposure is obtained. The muscle should be excised with a very sharp scalpel and with the minimum of handling by forceps, which should not touch the muscle fibres themselves but may conveniently grasp the surrounding aponeurosis. The excised tissue should be immediately laid on a clean white card and allowed to adhere. At this point small portions can be removed and minced into an osmium or glutaraldehyde fixative for electron microscopy and further portions are rapidly frozen in solid carbon dioxide for histochemistry. The major part of the specimen is left on the card for 10–20 minutes and during this period the muscle relaxes and adheres firmly to the card. The card and muscle are then transferred to fixative. Many varieties of fixatives have been recommended, but we have had excellent results using 10 per cent neutralized formalin.

Processing the Biopsy

A full histological examination of a muscle biopsy requires: (1) satisfactory paraffin-embedded sections stained by conventional tissue stains, (2) the demonstration, by silver impregnation techniques, of the innervation of the muscle, (3) special techniques appropriate to the individual case. In the following account we describe the procedure in our laboratory.

(1) *Paraffin-embedded Sections*. The specimen of muscle, still on its card, is allowed to remain in its original formalin-fixing fluid for at least 24 hours, after which tissue blocks are taken. A complete transverse section of the muscle specimen, approximately 0·5 cm. in thickness, is first taken and then the remainder of the specimen is split longitudinally into two equal halves, one of which is examined by frozen section techniques. The T.S. and L.S. specimens are dehydrated in alcohol cleared with chloroform and embedded in paraffin. Sections, 7 μ thick, are stained with hæmatoxylin and eosin, and hæmatoxylin and Van Gieson stains. A useful addition to these two routine stains is phosphotungstic acid hæmatoxylin and in appropriate cases further special stains may be used. In our experience it is not satisfactory to attempt silver impregnation techniques on paraffin sections.

(2) *Silver Impregnation Techniques on Frozen Sections*. We have obtained consistently satisfactory results from the use of Schofield's modification of Bielschowsky's method for nerve axons (Schofield, 1960) and this is the technique described here. It has the advantage that it is also suitable for the examination of tissues removed at necropsy. Frozen sections, cut at 50 μ, are stained and mounted serially so that a large volume of muscle can be examined. An alternative method is the intravital staining of nerve endings in muscle by the injection of methylene blue prior to the muscle biopsy (Coërs and Woolf, 1959).

(3) *Special Techniques*. Examination for glycogen may be carried out on paraffin-embedded sections or, preferably, on frozen sections. The subneural apparatus of the motor end-plate can be elegantly stained by a histochemical method for cholinesterase activity; the technique of Koelle and Friedenwald can be applied to frozen sections of formalin-fixed tissue. For modifications of this method, and for the use of fresh frozen tissue, see Pearse (1960), who also deals with the other enzymes, over 50 in number, which can be assessed by histochemical

methods. These techniques demand fresh rapidly frozen cryostat sections and it is important that parallel observations be made on similar control normal muscle taken under approximately similar conditions.

Microscopical Examination

The various constituents to be observed may be divided into the muscle fibres themselves, the supportive connective tissue, and the innervation within the muscle. In transverse sections the size of the muscle fibres is noted and if there are atrophic fibres their distribution should be considered. In addition to fibres whose size is abnormal there may be fibres which are undergoing degeneration or regeneration. The changes of degenerating fibres are varied in type, but those accepted as due to regeneration are small size, basophilia of the sarcoplasm, and large vesicular nuclei (Greenfield, Shy, Alvord and Berg, 1957). There may be particular changes to be observed in the sarco-lemmal nuclei which normally are few in number (four to eight per muscle fibre), elongated in the direction of the muscle myofibrils, and situated at the periphery of the sarcoplasm immediately under the sarcolemma. In diseased states the sarcolemmal nuclei may be increased in number, abnormal in size and shape, or centrally situated.

In most muscular atrophies there is a replacement by connective and fatty tissue. In some conditions, such as muscular dystrophy, there is extensive fatty replacement. In scleroderma, lupus erythematosus, rheumatoid arthritis and polymyositis there are significant changes in connective tissue, and in diseases such as polyarteritis nodosa the changes in the medium-sized arteries are diagnostic. In addition, there may be accumulations of inflam-matory cells both in the interstitial spaces between the muscle fibres and occasionally in the muscle fibres themselves. These inflammatory cells may be lymphocytes, polymorphonuclear leucocytes, monocytes or plasma cells. The inflammatory cells most often within the muscle fibre are mononuclear phagocytes and this process of break-up of the muscle fibre and its engulfment by phagocytes is an important diagnostic observation.

The state of the innervation of the muscle can be seen directly in the frozen sections stained by Schofield's method, which will show the amount of nerve present in the muscle and whether this nerve is composed of compact nerve bundles containing axons with a normal covering of Schwann cells. Near the motor point (Fig. 1) there is branching into numerous subdivisions of nerve bundles, and as the motor end plates are approached there is the final branching into individual fine nerve fibres. Normally a single nerve fibre has a terminal arborization which innervates a single muscle fibre and this part of the terminal innervation may show abnormalities which are of diagnostic significance. In degeneration of axons, their course is seen to be interrupted and they may be swollen or beaded. Regenerating fibres can be recognized as fine fibres having regular oval beadlike thickenings and these are often abnormally branched. The other important abnormality is a spread of innervation outside the normal relation of one terminal arborization to one muscle fibre. The silver stains also show the motor end-plates which may be abnormal in being elongated, clubbed or unduly branched. The muscle spindles should be examined, but these are best seen in the transverse section of paraffin-embedded material. The intrafusal muscle fibres of the muscle spindles form a valuable comparison with the much larger extrafusal muscle fibres and in one condition, dystrophia myotonica, they are specifically abnormal.

HISTOPATHOLOGY OF NEUROLOGICAL AND MUSCLE DISEASES

In this account the common disease processes encountered are dealt with, but no mention is made of very rare conditions which are fully described elsewhere (Adams, Denny-Brown and Pearson, 1962; Walton, 1964). It will be convenient to consider the changes in two groups according to whether they are due to denervation or occur in a disease process in which denervation plays no part.

Pathological Changes of Denervation

The changes in the individual muscle fibre when it is deprived of its nerve supply have been studied extensively in the experimental animal. In human material these changes can best be studied in necropsy cases of anterior poliomyelitis graded so as to examine muscles which have been denervated for different periods of time.

The first change, which is seen at about one week, is an enlargement and a rounding of the sarcolemmal nucleus which may be displaced towards the centre of the muscle fibre. These nuclear changes are then followed at about one month after denervation by a reduction in size of the muscle fibres. From the time that the atrophy is noticeable, it progresses rapidly and by two months the fibres may be half their original size. There are further changes in the sarcolemmal nuclei which become shrunken, pyknotic, and arranged in clumps. The sarcolemmal nuclei, which are not diminished in number, often form large groups giving the false impression of nuclear proliferation. The normal striations become unrecognizable and the final stage is that of an extremely thin fibre containing pyknotic sarcolemmal nuclei but without any apparent transverse striations. These denervated atrophic muscle fibres persist unchanged for many years. Whilst these features are common to all the human diseases of the lower motor neurone there are differences according to the site and progression of the disease process.

Acute Spinal Cord Diseases

Acute massive denervation due to destruction of the motor neurones of the anterior grey horn may have various causes such as trauma, hæmatomyelia or acute necrotic myelopathy (transverse myelitis), but the best known example is acute anterior poliomyelitis. In the first few days the changes of axon degeneration can be seen in silver preparations. Within a few days the paraffin-embedded sections show atrophic muscle fibres whose distribution is dependent on the degree of central neuronal destruction. Typically the denervation atrophy affects large numbers of adjacent muscle fibres, but where the denervation is more localized one may see a small scatter of atrophying muscle fibres corresponding to the innervation of a single motor neurone.

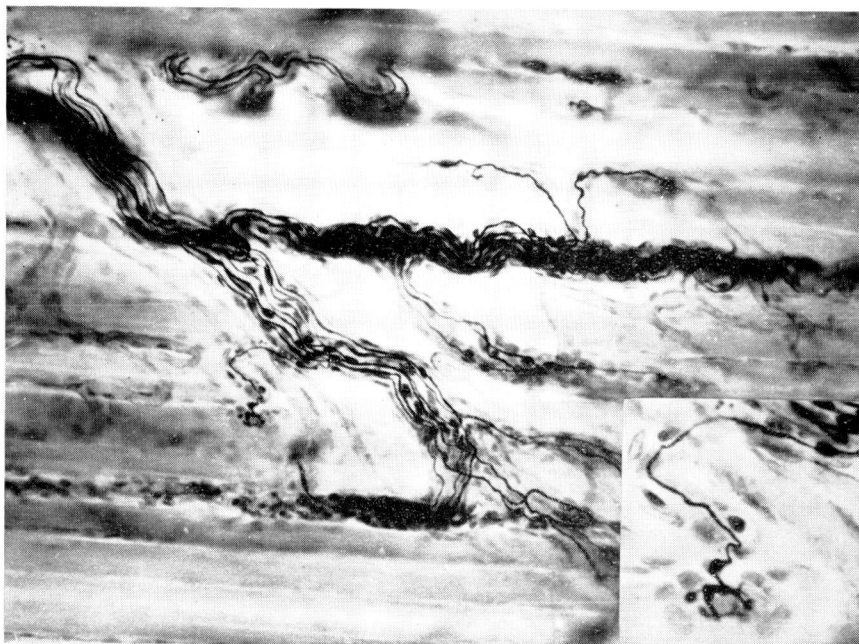

FIG. 1. Normal lumbrical muscle stained by silver impregnation technique to show intra-muscular nerve bundles. The inset picture shows an enlarged view of the motor end plate. (Schofield's stain × 160, inset × 400.)

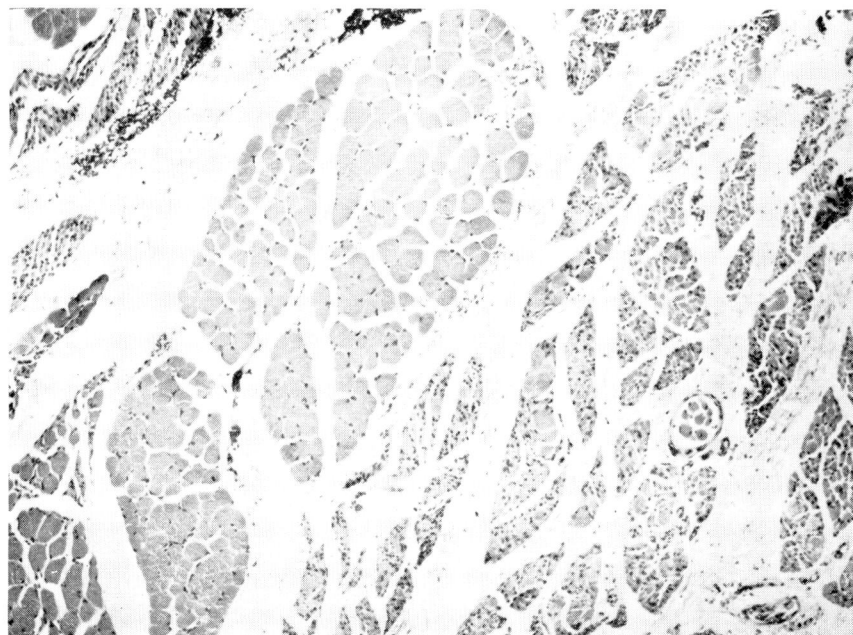

FIG. 2. Werdnig-Hoffman disease. Transverse section of deltoid muscle showing groups of atrophied muscle fibres. Note the normal muscle spindle, lower right. (Hæmatoxylin and eosin × 64.)

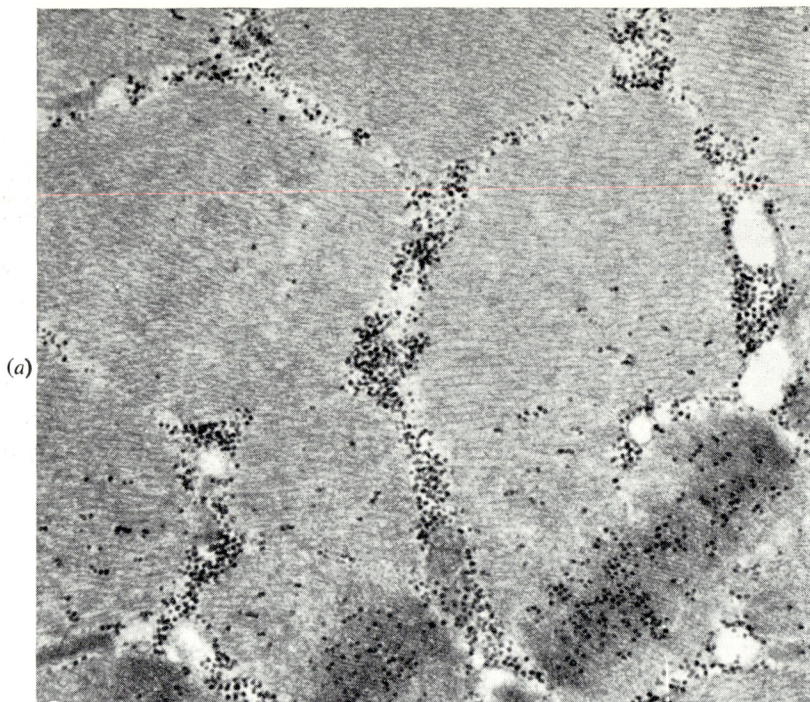

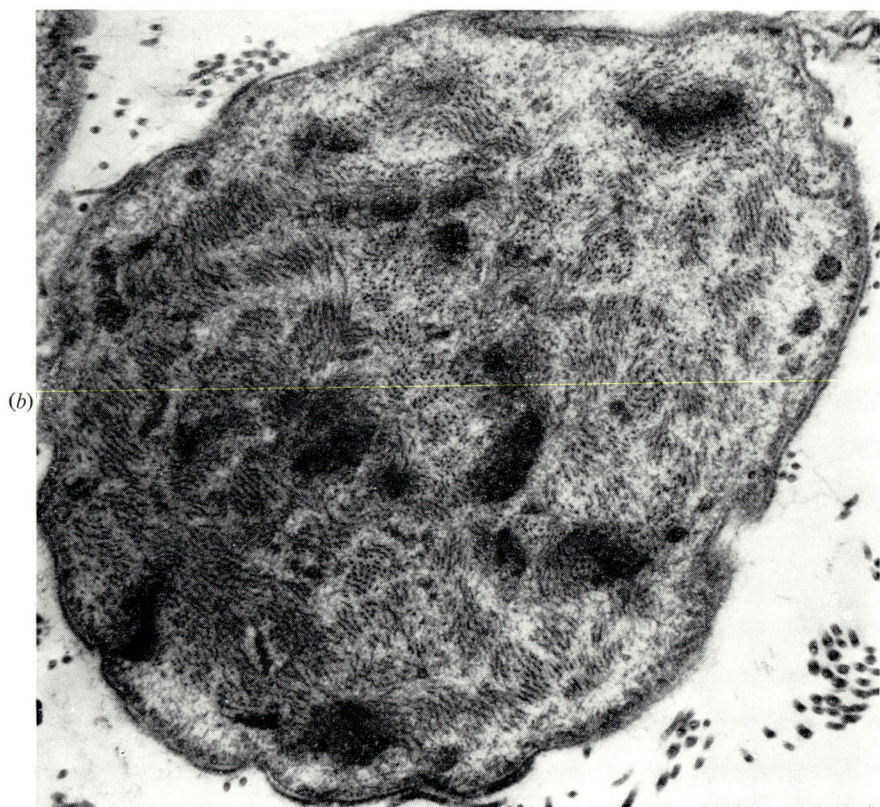

(a)

(b)

Chronic Spinal Cord Disease

Intramedullary tumours, syringomyelia and cervical spondylosis provide occasional examples, but muscle biopsies are more commonly encountered from motor neurone disease and, in infancy, the similar but inherited congenital disorder known as Werdnig-Hoffmann disease. Recently a further inherited denervation disease has been described (Kugelberg and Welander, 1956). In the silver stains it is apparent that the bundles of nerve fibres contain fewer axons than normal with a proportionate diminution in motor end-plates. Evidence of axon sprouting may be seen in the form of repeated branching into fine axons which are beaded and may end in a growth cone. In the paraffin-embedded sections the pattern of the muscle fibre atrophy is very striking (Fig. 2) with fascicles of atrophic fibres contrasting with neighbouring groups of muscle fibres of normal size. This pattern is very well seen both in motor neurone disease and in Werdnig-Hoffmann disease. With electron microscopy the complete disorder of the band structure is apparent (Figs. 3a and 3b).

Acute Peripheral Nerve Diseases

In muscle biopsies from cases of acute polyneuritis the silver stains provide the most information, whilst the paraffin-embedded sections may, in a very acute case, be normal. The axons are undergoing active degeneration with break-up of the axon into droplets (Figs. 4a and 4b). These changes occur in cases of only a few weeks' duration but persist for a long period, particularly if recovery is delayed. These changes of axonic degeneration are often accompanied by regenerative changes, which may be present at an early stage. The most characteristic feature of regeneration in this condition is the presence of a relatively large number of very fine branched and beaded axons.

Chronic Peripheral Nerve Diseases

Examples of this group are alcoholic and diabetic neuropathy, and the neuropathies of porphyria, Déjerine-Sottas's disease and Charcot-Marie-Tooth disease. In these chronic neuropathies the silver stains show marked degenerative and regenerative changes (Figs. 5 and 6). The paraffin-embedded sections show atrophy of the muscle fibres appropriate to the severity of the neuropathy.

In myasthenia gravis a rather different disorder of the terminal axon and end-plates is seen (MacDermot, 1960). The terminal branches of the axon are exceptionally long. The end-plate is distributed along the terminal part of the axon with arborizations arising from it at intervals (Fig. 7), forming a much longer structure than the normal. Sometimes the terminal arborizations branch more frequently than is normal, and finish up in end-plates which similarly show excessive branching. In our experience these abnormalities in motor nerve endings are the most specific changes in myas-

---

FIG. 3a and 3b. Electron micrographs of ultra thin sections, transverse to the muscle fibres. 3a., normal muscle. 3b, denervated muscle from a case of Werdnig-Hoffmann disease. Note the absence of band structure and the disarray of the myofibrils which are cut both transversely and longitudinally. Both these preparations were fixed in osmium tetroxide, embedded, and cut in araldite, and stained with phosphotungstic acid hæmatoxylin. Magnifications × 33,000.

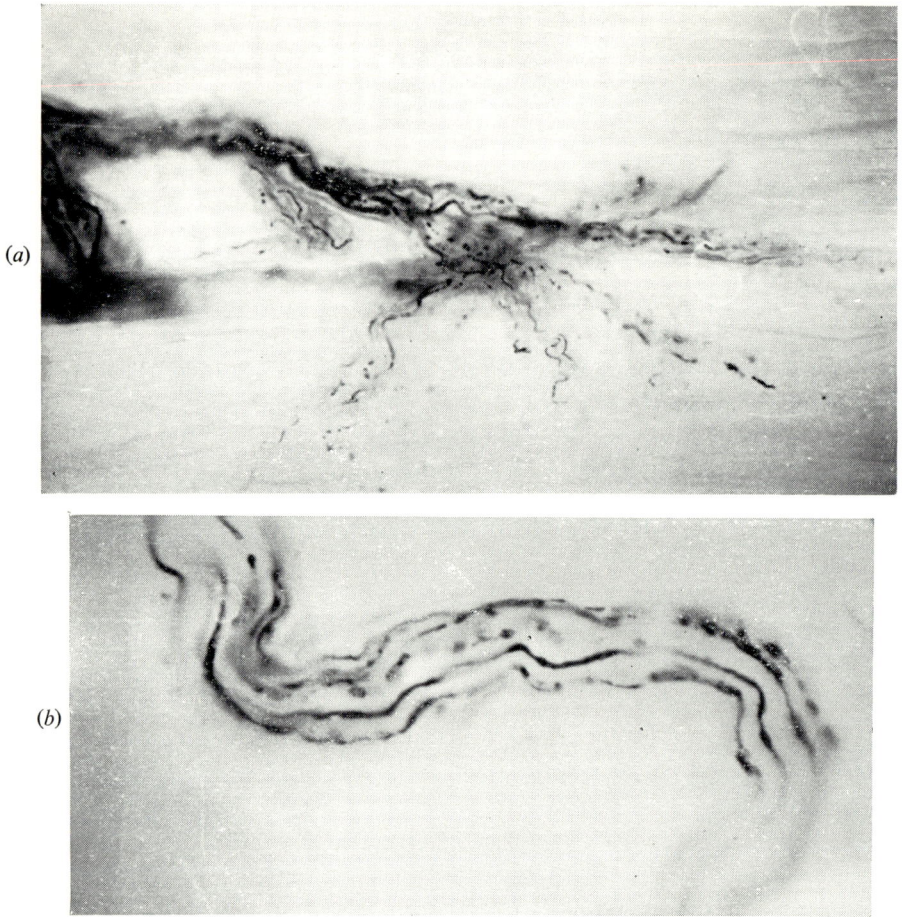

FIG. 4a and 4b. Acute polyneuritis. Intramuscular motor nerve showing fragmentation and droplet formation of the nerve fibres. (Schofield's technique, Fig. 4a × 160, Fig. 4b × 400.)

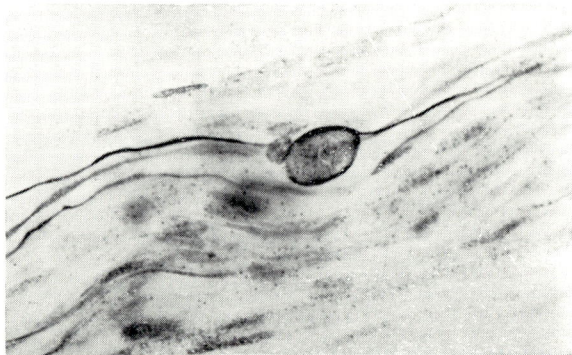

FIG. 5. Chronic neuropathy. Axonic swelling on an intramuscular nerve. (Schofield's technique × 700.)

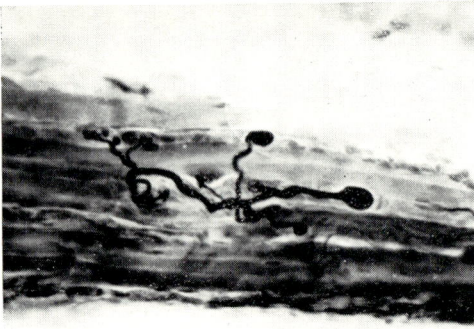

FIG. 6. Chronic neuropathy. Thenar muscle (necropsy specimen) from a case of Charcot-Marie-Tooth disease. There is branching and thickening of the terminal arborisation with growth cones. (Schofield's technique × 160.)

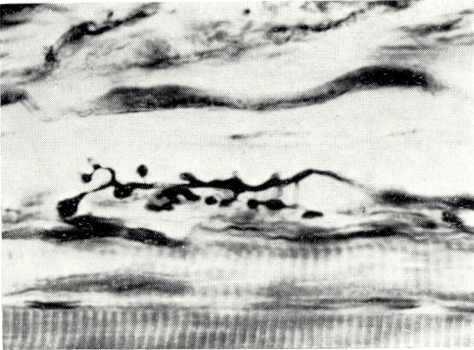

FIG. 7. Myasthenia gravis. Posterior crico-arytenoid muscle (laryngectomy specimen) showing elongation of motor end plate. (Schofield's technique × 500.)

thenia, but lymphorrhages are often present, and there may be degenerative changes in the muscle fibres, as described by Russell (1953). We have seen denervated muscle in chronic myasthenia gravis, and this has also been described by Brody and Engel (1964).

Diseases without a Disorder of Innervation

The classification of many of these disorders according to ætiology is not possible, and for this reason we propose to divide these conditions into three groups, the first being inherited dystrophic conditions, the second polymyositis and allied conditions, and a third miscellaneous group termed myopathies.

Muscular Dystrophy

The inherited dystrophic conditions of voluntary muscle differ in their clinical course. These dystrophies are classified into different types according to the age of involvement, the pattern of voluntary muscles implicated, and the type of genetic inheritance. The commonest is the Duchenne type, which is a severe generalized dystrophy of children inherited by either a sex-linked or an autosomal recessive gene and giving rise to the familiar pseudo-

hypertrophy. The facio-scapulo-humeral muscular dystrophy has a dominant inheritance occurring in either sex in adult life with involvement first of the face and shoulder girdle muscles. These traditional types of dystrophy have been recently added to in various classifications, but as the pathological process is often similar these divisions will not be discussed here. The other inherited condition differing clinically and pathologically is dystrophia myotonica. The pathological features found in the muscular dystrophies may be discussed under the following headings:

(1) *Variation in Size of the Muscle Fibres.* This finding is usually present in every muscle affected clinically and may be apparent in muscles which are

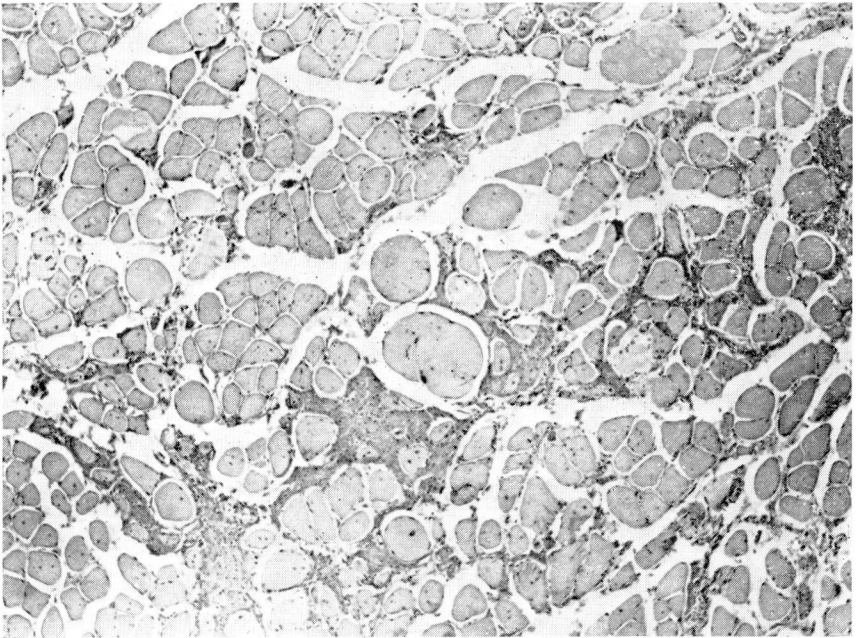

FIG. 8. Muscular dystrophy. Sternomastoid muscle cut in transverse section and showing variation in fibre size and proliferation of sarcolemmal nuclei which are often centrally placed. (Hæmatoxylin and van Gieson × 64.)

clinically normal. Furthermore, it may be found in muscle biopsies of close relatives showing a subclinical carrier state. The typical finding is a random distribution of fibres which are unusually small or unusually large (Fig. 8). Usually the small fibres are in excess, but it is the large fibres that attract attention as they may be up to 250 μ in diameter, whilst the small fibres may be as small as 10 μ in diameter. The large fibres are abnormal in being much rounder than normal muscle fibres and may be split longitudinally into three, four or five daughter fibres.

(2) *Atrophy.* The muscles in these cases may be severely atrophied, but this may be concealed in the pseudo-hypertrophic cases by replacement with adipose tissue. The atrophy of the muscle belly arises from a combination of wasting, degeneration, and loss of the individual fibres (Fig. 9). It often

proceeds to a marked degree when the biopsy may be found to consist of fat and fibrous tissue in which only a few surviving muscle fibres can be found (Fig. 10).

(3) *Nuclear Abnormalities.* The sarcolemmal nuclei are genuinely increased in numbers in contrast to denervation, where there is merely an aggregation of nuclei previously present. The large round nuclei may be abnormally situated, forming chains in the centre of the muscle fibre (Fig. 11). These chains are usually formed of large nuclei in abnormally large muscle fibres

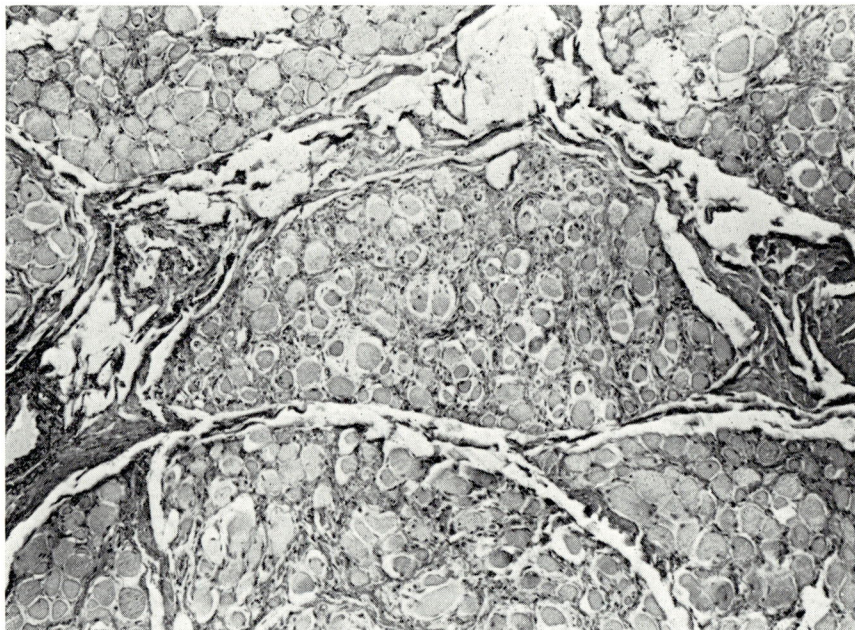

FIG 9. Muscular dystrophy. Transverse section of deltoid muscle showing atrophy and fibrosis. (Hæmatoxylin and van Gieson × 64.)

but may also take the form of chains of small pyknotic nuclei in small muscle fibres. Central nuclei may be found in many disorders, but they are most consistently present in all the inherited dystrophic states of voluntary muscle. They occur prominently in dystrophia myotonica.

(4) *Degenerative Changes.* In all the dystrophic muscle states there are degenerative changes in a small proportion of the muscle fibres. The cytoplasm of the muscle fibre becomes granular (Fig. 12) and may be vacuolated, the normal striations are lost and the myofibrils become completely disorganized. The final stage is the break-up and disappearance of the degenerating fibre. These changes are not associated with much inflammatory reaction or phagocytosis, and regenerating changes are not prominent although they may be present. These findings are consistent with a slowly developing disease process causing degeneration and death of the muscle fibres. When the process is more rapid there may be some cellular reaction with phagocytosis (Fig. 13) and in these circumstances confusion with myositis is possible.

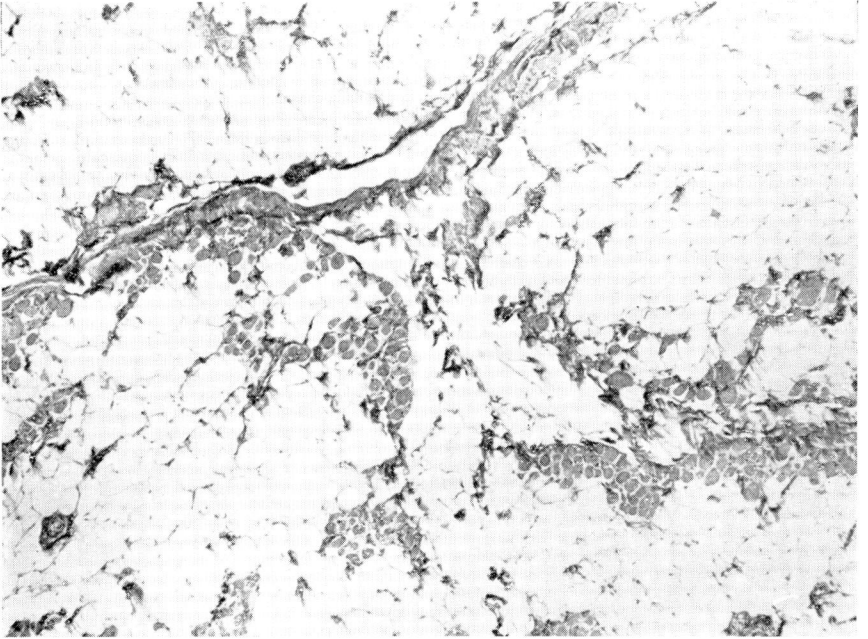

FIG. 10. Muscular dystrophy. Transverse section of *biceps brachii* showing extreme atrophy with fatty replacement. (Hæmatoxylin and van Gieson × 64.)

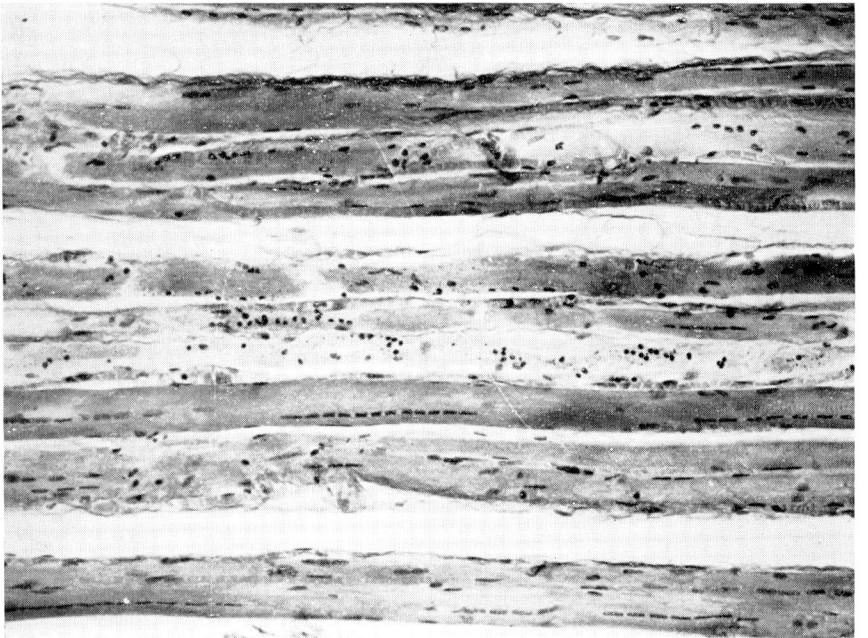

FIG. 11. Muscular dystrophy. Longitudinal section of sartorius muscle, showing degenerating fibres and nuclear chains. (Hæmatoxylin and van Gieson × 60.)

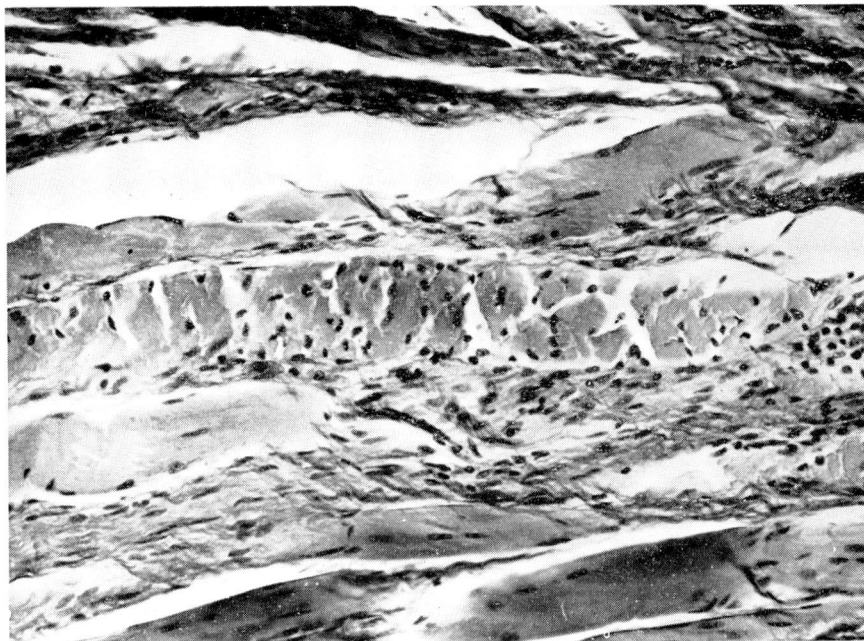

FIG. 12. Muscular dystrophy. Longitudinal section of sternomastoid muscle showing granular degeneration with many phagocytes within muscle fibres. (Hæmatoxylin and van Gieson × 160)

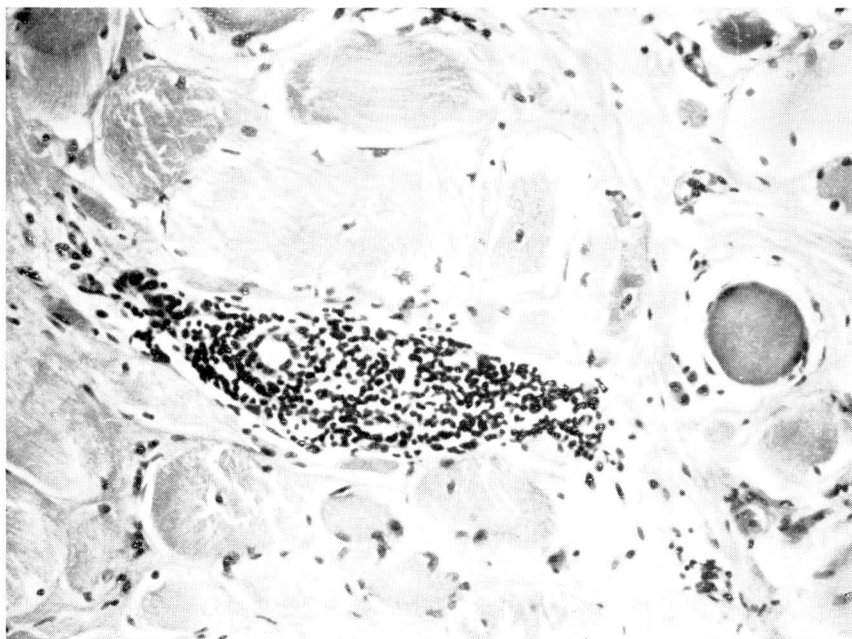

FIG. 13. Muscular dystrophy. Transverse section of deltoid muscle showing infiltration by inflammatory cells (Hæmatoxylin and eosin × 160.)

(5) *Fatty and Fibrous Tissue*. In a severe case of muscular dystrophy the muscle belly becomes converted largely into fatty and fibrous tissue (Fig. 10). This increase in fat is characteristic of muscular dystrophy and may be related to the long duration of the dystrophic process. The connective tissue increase is partly a reaction to, and a replacement of, the degenerating muscle fibres, but there may be an apparent increase due to condensation of the former connective tissue framework.

(6) *Innervation of the Muscle*. In our experience the innervation of the muscle, as seen in the Schofield's stain, is usually normal in these dystrophic conditions. The major nerve trunks have a normal complement of axons and show no evidence of degeneration or regeneration. The terminal expansions of the motor end-plates sometimes show thickening and this may be due to the neuromuscular apparatus making contact with a dying muscle fibre.

Some special features of dystrophia myotonica require mention. Histologically the unusual features are the prominence of central nuclei arranged in longitudinal rows in the muscle fibres, and the presence of ring fibres produced by an altered orientation of the peripheral myofibrils. The other change which may be seen in dystrophia myotonica is an increase in number of the intrafusal fibres of the muscle spindles (Daniel and Strich, 1964). In the other forms of muscle dystrophy no abnormality of the muscle spindles has been detected and they are usually remarkably well preserved amongst the other degenerating muscle fibres.

Polymyositis

The pathology of polymyositis is a degeneration of muscle fibres associated with an acute inflammatory reaction, resulting in destruction and leading to a fibrotic atrophic muscle. The histological features are as follows:

(1) *Degeneration*. Degeneration is seen in the muscle fibres whose cytoplasm loses its detail and normal staining characteristics, becoming hyaline, granular or vacuolar. The sarcolemmal nuclei become shrunken and pyknotic. These muscle fibres are dead or dying and frequently are surrounded by histiocytes and are undergoing phagocytosis (Fig. 14).

(2) *Regeneration*. Amongst the muscle fibres which are degenerating may be seen others which have appearances suggestive of regeneration. These are small fibres with basophilic cytoplasm and a large vesicular nucleus in the centre of the muscle fibre. These regenerating muscle fibres are very prominent in myositis and are seen more often in this condition than in any other muscle disease.

(3) *Inflammatory Changes*. The amount of inflammation varies in individual cases and depends on the stage of the disease. The inflammatory changes are seen both in the connective tissue septa and around the muscle fibres themselves (Figs. 15 and 16). The type of cell varies, but there is always a preponderance of lymphocytes with some plasma cells, monocytes and polymorphs. Some of the inflammatory cells are histiocytes which are engaged in phagocytosis of degenerating muscle fibres and occasionally a whole sarcolemmal tube is filled with phagocytes (Fig. 14).

(4) *Fibrotic Changes*. When the acute inflammation has subsided the degenerated muscle may be partially replaced by fibrous tissue. There is no

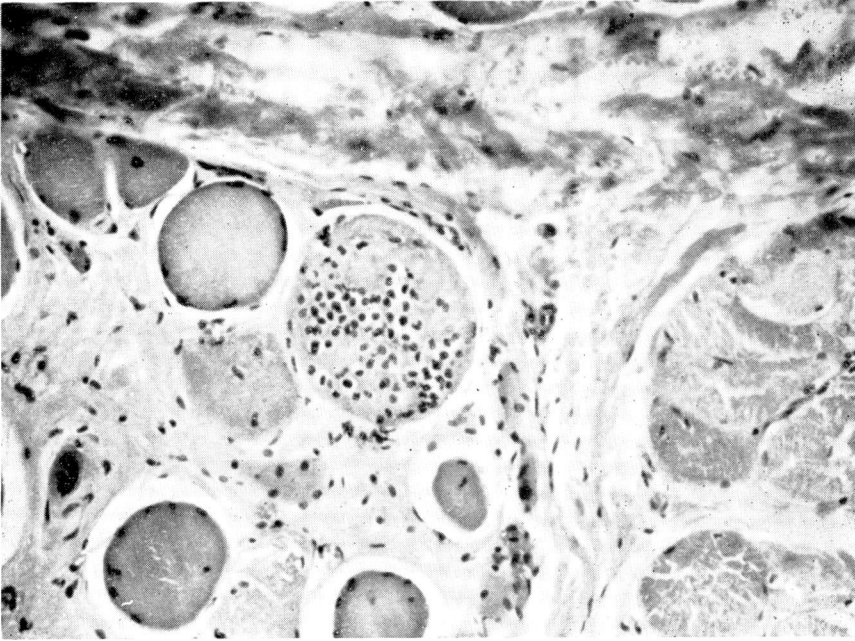

Fig. 14. Polymyositis. Transverse section of deltoid muscle showing phagocytosis of a degenerating fibre. (Hæmatoxylin and eosin × 160.)

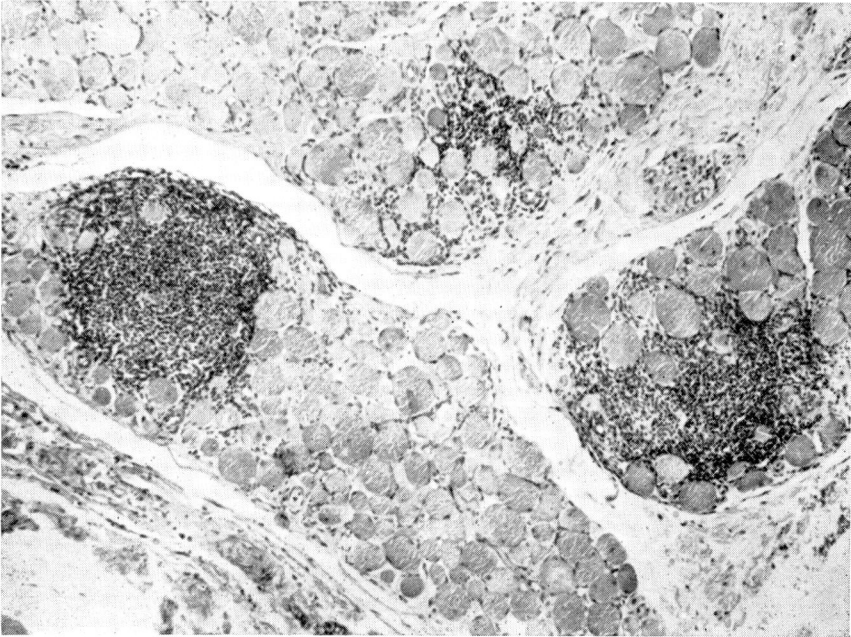

Fig. 15. Polymyositis. Transverse section of deltoid muscle showing widespread inflammatory infiltration. (Hæmatoxylin and eosin × 64.)

evidence of fat deposition and in this respect the appearances in polymyositis differ from those in dystrophy.

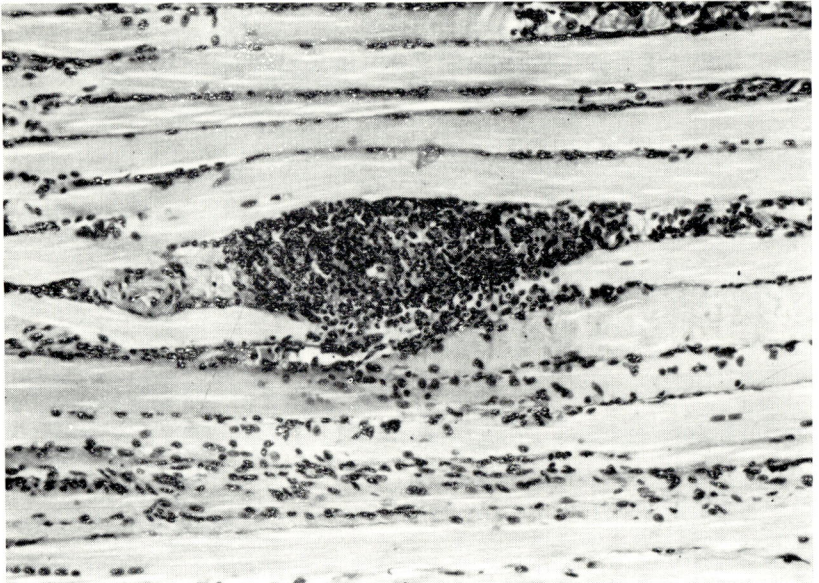

FIG. 16. Polymyositis. Longitudinal section of deltoid muscle showing inflammatory re-action to degenerating muscle fibres. (Hæmatoxylin and eosin × 130.)

Related Conditions

In disorders such as disseminated lupus erythematosus, polyarteritis nodosa, scleroderma and rheumatoid arthritis there may be pathological features similar to myositis but with additional changes. In lupus erythemato-sus hydropic vacuolation of muscle fibres has been described. In polyarteritis nodosa there is an acute inflammation of the whole vessel wall (Fig. 17) and the appearances in the muscle may suggest infarction. A muscle biopsy from polyarteritis nodosa may also show denervation atrophy due to an associated peripheral nerve lesion. In scleroderma the inflammation is particularly distributed among the interstitial connective tissue and there may be recognizable differences in the staining of the collagen. These features may be present in rheumatoid arthritis, which is sometimes accompanied by denerva-tion atrophy due to a neuropathy.

Myopathies

The word myopathy implies a pathological condition of muscle and should be reserved for diseases of the muscle fibres which are not dystrophic, myositic or caused by denervation. In clinical practice myopathies have been described in association with a very large number of diseases. There are no constant histological features and in some instances the muscle has been structurally normal. In the majority of cases the individual muscle fibres show degeneration which may take varying forms and may be accompanied

by some of the features seen in dystrophy and myositis. The diagnosis frequently depends on the recognition of the primary systemic disease or the
specific metabolic defect in the muscle. Most of the myopathies can be
grouped under the headings, toxic, endocrine and metabolic:

(1) *Toxic Myopathies.* From animal experiments it is known that a
number of drugs and poisons cause degeneration of skeletal muscle, but very
few clinical cases have arisen. An example of a drug-induced myopathy is
that due to chloroquin medication in which there is necrosis of muscle fibres
which show conspicuous vacuolation (Fig. 18). Haff disease is an example
of a poison (contained in fish poisoned by factory waste) which causes
muscle necrosis.

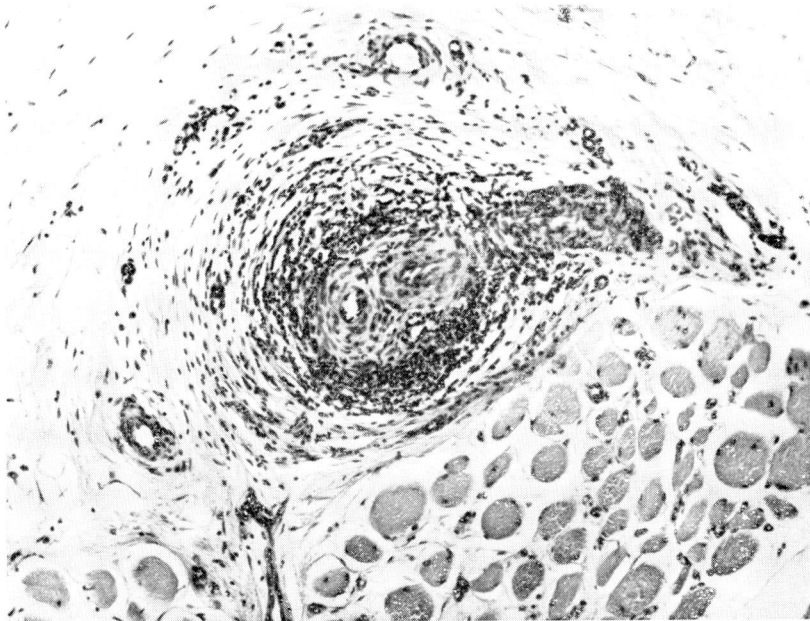

FIG. 17. Polyarteritis nodosa. Transverse section of deltoid muscle showing inflammatory
reaction in relation to an intramuscular artery. (Hæmatoxylin and eosin × 120.)

The diagnosis of carcinomatous myopathy is sometimes made, but in our
experience most cases of muscle weakness associated with carcinoma prove
at necropsy to have growth of tumour into the spinal nerve roots, the
peripheral nerve trunks or the muscles themselves (Fig. 19). What has been
described (Walton and Adams, 1958) is a myositis, but there may be additional features of denervation due to an associated neuropathy.

(2) *Endocrine Myopathies.* Muscle weakness has been described in
thyrotoxicosis, myxœdema and Cushing's disease. There is also a myopathy
associated with cortisone therapy which is comparable to that of Cushing's
disease.

Whilst the clinical syndrome of thyrotoxic myopathy is common, cases
do not always show histological changes in the muscles and in five cases we
found either normal appearances or minimal changes such as a wide range

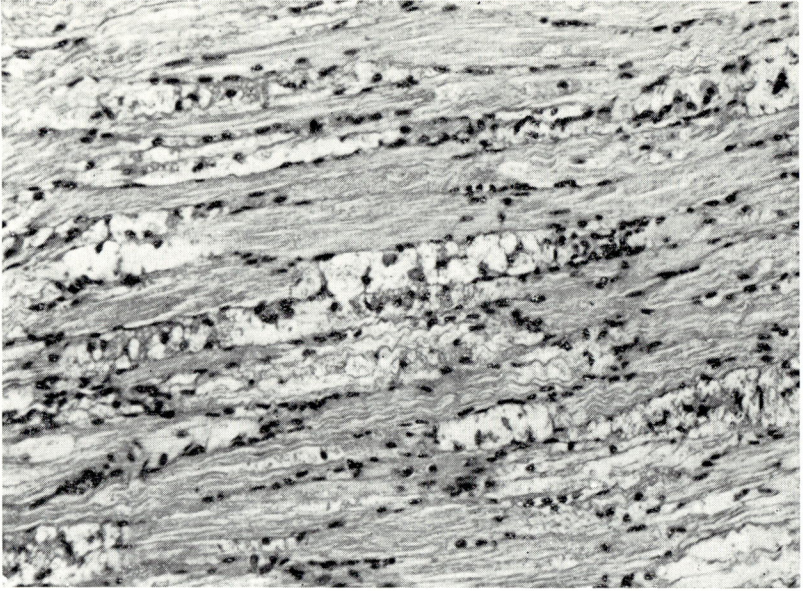

FIG. 18. Chloroquin myopathy. Longitudinal section of deltoid muscle showing vacuolar degeneration. (Hæmatoxylin and eosin × 130.)

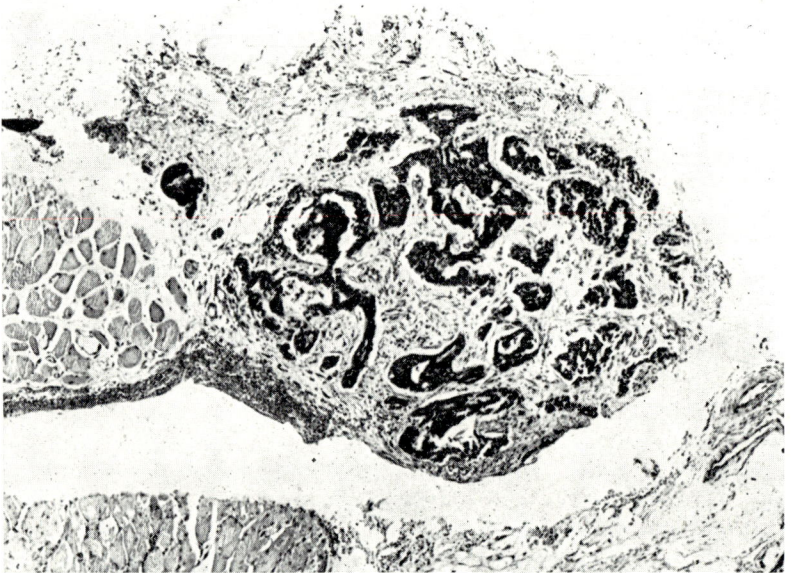

FIG. 19. Secondary carcinoma, metastatic in deltoid muscle. (Hæmatoxylin and eosin × 50.)

of muscle fibre size. A widespread necrotizing myopathy, sarcolemmal crescent formations (Asbøe-Hansen, Iversen and Wickman, 1952) and abnormalities of innervation such as axonic swellings (Havard, Campbell, Ross and Spence, 1963), axon sprouting and multiplicity of end-plates have been described in this condition.

In myxœdema a syndrome of proximal muscle weakness is described but the histological appearances have either been normal or have shown minimal changes of the myopathic type such as scattered small fibres and variation in fibre size.

We have no experience of the myopathy in Cushing's disease but in cortisone myopathy have found a severe degeneration of many muscle fibres with prominent vacuoles. There is often a moderate inflammatory reaction to the severe muscle necrosis. One difficulty in the interpretation of these cases is that the primary condition for which the cortisone is given may itself give rise to changes in muscle.

(3) *Metabolic Myopathies* (often inherited). These conditions are an interesting group of muscle diseases, the investigation of which is yielding information on normal muscle chemistry and enzymatic activity. The best understood are the myopathies associated with a defect of glycogen metabolism and the periodic paralysis associated with hypokalæmia.

There are several inherited disorders of glycogen metabolism, but in some of these, e.g. *von Gierke's disease* and *cardiomuscular glycogen disease*, the effect on the liver and heart outweighs that on skeletal muscle. In the condition called *McArdle's myopathy* (McArdle, 1951), the only defect is in the skeletal muscle which lacks the enzyme phosphorylase concerned in glycogen metabolism. The condition is now known to be inherited as a single recessive autosomal gene. The clinical syndrome is that of pain, stiffness and weakness, all of which appear after exercise, when the diagnosis can be made by demonstrating that the blood lactate does not rise. There is an excess of glycogen which is stored under the sarcolemma in vesicles and can be detected by the use of the PAS or Best's carmine stains. Histochemical methods, carried out on sections from fresh frozen tissue, show an absence or depletion of the enzyme phosphorylase as compared with a normal control muscle. A biopsy examined in our department from a case of this disease showed in addition a number of fibres undergoing granular degeneration with little or no cellular reaction.

Familial periodic paralysis is an inherited disease in which a tendency to intermittent attacks of paralysis is related to a metabolic disorder. In the earliest cases described the attacks of paralysis coincided with a lowered serum potassium, but more recently normokalæmic and hyperkalæmic forms have been described. Muscle biopsies taken during an attack (Shy, Wanko, Rowley and Engel, 1961) have shown vacuolation of the sarcoplasm with little or no cellular reaction.

The muscular weakness associated with *porphyria* is generally considered to be due to a polyneuropathy, but in our experience of three cases (two autopsies and one biopsy) histological changes strongly suggestive of a myopathy were present, in addition to the expected lesions found in peripheral nerves. The muscle lesions consisted of variation in fibre size, nuclear abnormalities, and necrosis of the fibres which frequently showed very

M

striking vacuolation (Fig. 20). A remarkable disorder of the muscle fibre was observed with the electron microscope (Figs. 21a and 21b).

Amyotonia congenita is a rare familial disease, characterized clinically by muscle weakness with extreme hypotonia. The muscles from some cases have shown the typical histological changes of muscular dystrophy, while in other cases the only abnormality has been uniform smallness of muscle fibres. This form has been named *benign congenital hypotonia* by Walton (1956). Yet another group of cases with congenital myotonia has shown the histological changes of "central core disease" (Shy and Magee, 1956). This muscle lesion consists of a central abnormality in many of the muscle fibres, appearing as a dark homogeneous area, which, in histochemical stains, shows an absence of enzyme activity (Dubowitz and Pearse, 1960). This again seems to be an example of a disease in which the metabolism of muscle is at fault though the actual defect has not yet been established.

It is clear that, in the future, biochemical and histochemical investigations used in conjunction will help to identify many more metabolic defects in diseases of muscle.

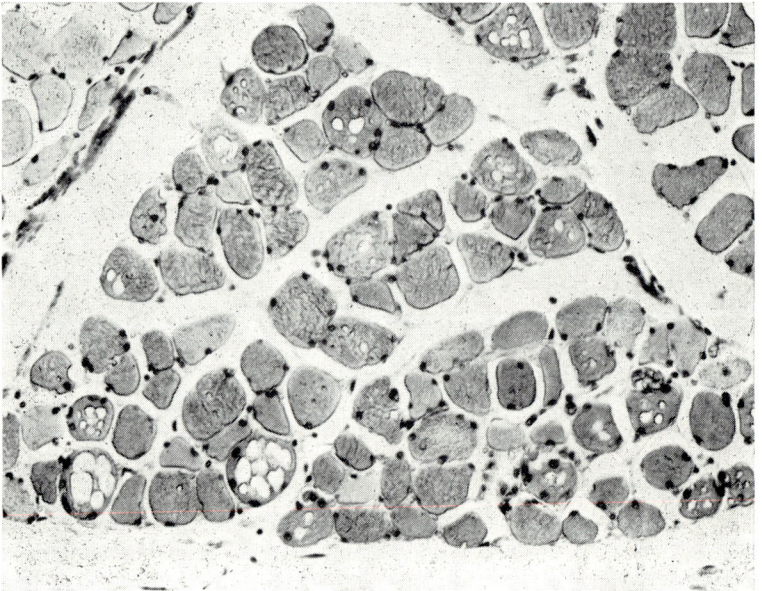

FIG 20. Case of acute porphyria. Transverse section of deltoid muscle showing vacuolation of fibres. (Hæmatoxylin and van Gieson × 120).

FIG. 21a and 21b. Electron micrographs of deltoid muscle cut transversely. Fixed in osmium tetroxide, embedded and cut in araldite stained with phosphotungstic acid hæmatoxylin. Fig. 21a, normal muscle. Fig. 21b, case of acute porphyria. There is disorganisation of the band structure with other degenerative changes. Magnification × 14,000.

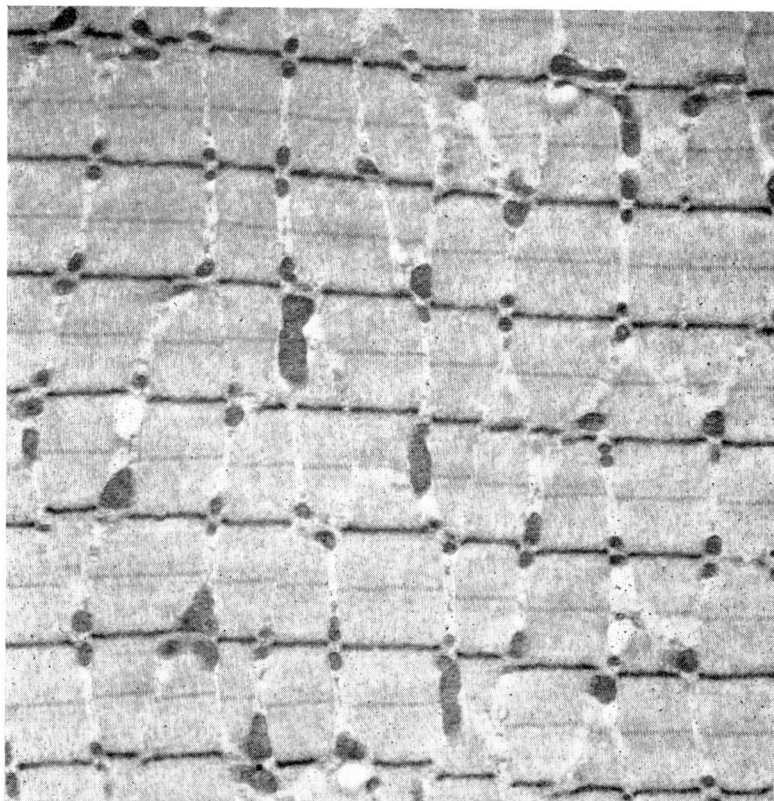

(a)

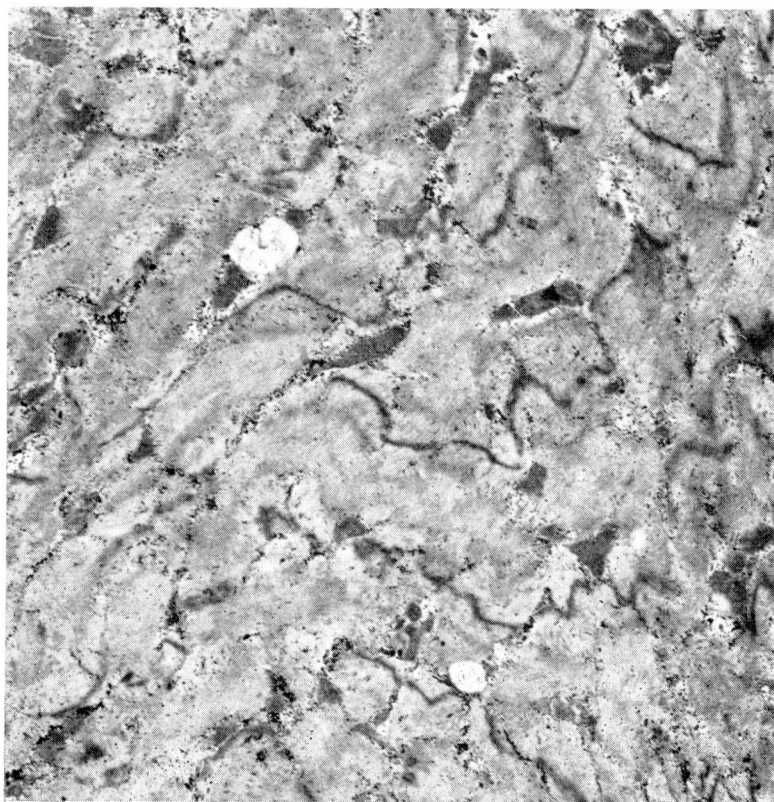

(b)

References

ADAMS, R. D., DENNY-BROWN, D. and PEARSON, C. M. (1962). *Diseases of Muscle* Second Edition. London: Henry Kimpton.

ASBØE-HANSEN, G., IVERSEN, K. and WICKMAN, R. (1952). *Acta endocr. (Kbh.)*, **11**, 376.

BRODY, I. A. and ENGEL, W. K. (1964). *Arch. Neurol. (Chic.)*, **11**, 350.

COËRS, C. and WOOLF, A. L. (1959). *The innervation of muscle*. Oxford: Blackwell.

DANIEL, P. M. and STRICH, S. J. (1964). *Neurology (Minneap.)*, **14**, 310.

DUBOWITZ, V. and PEARSE, A. G. E. (1960). *Lancet*, **2**, 23.

GREENFIELD, J. G., CORNMAN, T. and SHY, G. M. (1958). *Brain*, **81**, 461.

GREENFIELD, J. G., SHY, G. M., ALVORD, E. C. and BERG, L. (1957). *An Atlas of Muscle Pathology in Neuromuscular Diseases*. London and Edinburgh: Livingstone.

HAVARD, C. W. H., CAMPBELL, E. D. R., ROSS, H. B. and SPENCE, A. W. (1963). *Quart. J. Med.*, **33**, 145.

KUGELBERG, E. and WELANDER, L. (1956). *A. M. A. Arch. Neurol. and Psychiat.*, **75**, 500

MCARDLE, B. (1951). *Clin. Sci.*, **10**, 13.

MACDERMOT, V. (1960). *Brain*, **83**, 24.

PEARCE, A. G. E. (1960). *Histochemistry, Theoretical and Applied*, Second Edition. London: Churchill.

RUSSELL, D. S. (1953). *J. Path. Bact.*, **65**, 279.

SCHOFIELD, G. C. (1960). *Brain*, **83**, 490.

SHY, G. M. and MAGEE, K. R. (1956). *Brain*, **79**, 610.

SHY, G. M., WANKO, T., ROWLEY, P. T. and ENGEL, A. G. (1961). *Exper. Neurol.*, **3**, 53.

WALTON, J. N. (1956). *Lancet*. **i**, 1023.

WALTON, J. N. (Ed) (1964). *Disorders of Voluntary Muscle*. London: Churchill.

WALTON, J. N. and ADAMS, R. D. (1958). *Polymyositis*. London and Edinburgh: Livingstone.

Chapter 21

INTERPRETATION OF MUCOSAL BIOPSIES FROM THE GASTRO-INTESTINAL TRACT

R. WHITEHEAD

WITH the development of suction biopsy techniques it is now possible to obtain mucosal biopsies from the stomach, duodenum, jejunum, and the recto-sigmoid region of the large bowel without subjecting the patient to laparotomy. The specimens secured are small but are free from autolytic changes and serious artefacts. They usually include the full thickness of the mucosa and the muscularis mucosa. In addition to providing suitable material for routine histological study the biopsy may be used for electron microscopy, histochemical work and enzyme studies. Special methods of fixation and processing are needed for electron microscopy and histochemical work, but much information may be obtained by examination of the specimen under the dissecting microscope and by light microscopy, and it is with this aspect of the work that we are concerned.

Comments on Procedure

Fresh tissue for electron microscopy or for histochemical methods requiring cryostat sections should be removed immediately the biopsy is obtained. The remainder should then be placed in formol-saline without delay and examined under the dissecting microscope whilst in the fixative. The appearances should ideally be photographed and the tissue subsequently processed and embedded in paraffin, taking care during blocking that sections can be cut perpendicular to the luminal surface.

As a routine sections should be stained by hæmatoxylin and eosin (H. and E.), periodic acid Schiff (PAS) and by Perl's method for iron. There are numerous special procedures which may be employed and these include the phospho-tungstic acid hæmatoxylin (PTAH) or the phloxine tartrazine methods for Paneth cells, the Masson Fontana or diazo methods for argentaffin cells, and the methyl violet and Congo red methods for amyloid. Deparaffinized rehydrated sections can be examined under ultraviolet light for the fluorescence of lipofuscins and after staining with thioflavine T as a further method for amyloid.

THE GASTRIC BIOPSY

The gastric mucosa undergoes extremely rapid post-mortem autolysis and the advent of gastric biopsy via a flexible tube therefore marked the beginning of a new era in the study of its pathology. As a result it is now possible to obtain adequately fresh specimens in conditions hitherto not satisfactorily investigated.

Normal

The body mucosa (Fig. 1) occupies the upper two-thirds of the stomach and contains the gastric glands. At the cardiœsophageal junction and for about one centimetre distally the cardiac glands (Fig. 2) are found. These

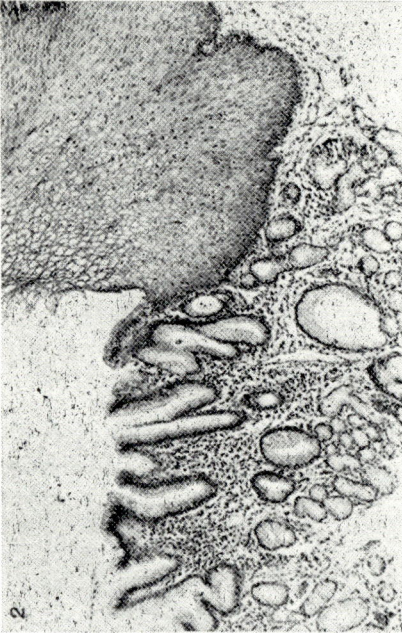

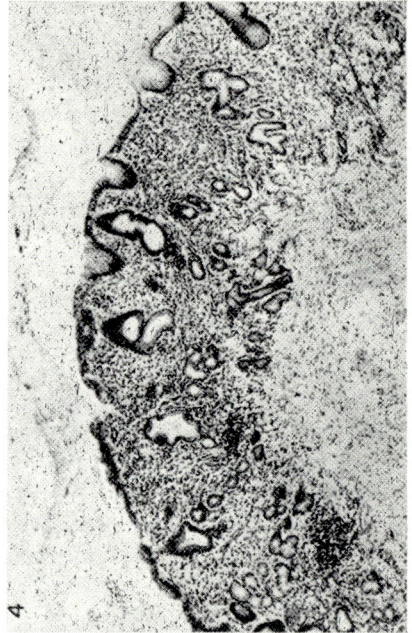

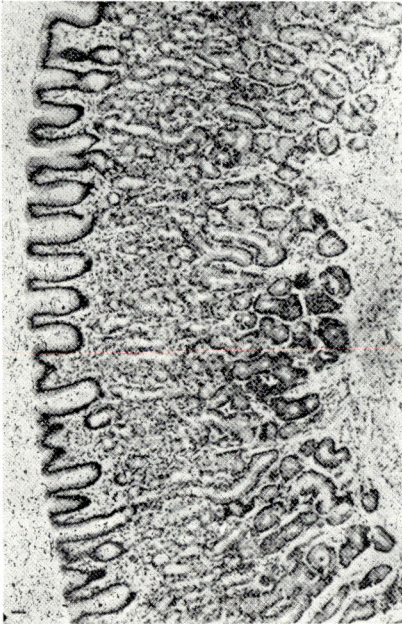

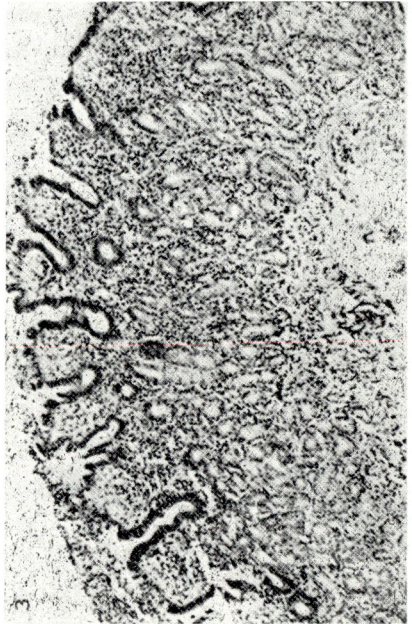

are similar in type and appearance to the pyloric glands. The latter occupy a triangular area in the lower-third of the stomach (Magnus, 1958) extending further along the lesser curve than the greater curve. Usually they reach the incisura angularis on the lesser curve but rarely they extend to the œsophagus as a narrow, continuous or incomplete band. Along the greater curve the glands are found only in the immediate pyloric region. Between the cardia and body and between the body and pyloric areas transition zones occur.

The surface epithelium of the gastric mucosa is PAS-positive and is the same everywhere. It is comprised of tall columnar cells with a basal nucleus and a typically cup-shaped clear or faintly granular mucoid cytoplasm. In the body of the stomach the surface epithelium dips down to form shallow gastric pits into the bottom of which open the long, tightly packed gastric glands. These are simple, straight, but branched tubules, with mucin-producing PAS-positive columnar cells seen in their upper narrower or neck parts. These cells are called the neck mucous cells and may be somewhat inconspicuous if packed between parietal cells which can be numerous and closely placed in the upper part of the gland. Elsewhere the acid-producing parietal cells are scattered singly in the gland tubule, often appearing triangular in appearance with their longest side applied to the basement membrane. The remainder of the gland lining is composed of the pepsin-secreting chief cells. When their secretion is not discharged, these cells contain granules which normally appear basophilic in H. and E. preparations. Towards the bases of the tubules there are occasional argentaffin cells.

In the pyloric region the gastric pits are relatively much deeper and the glands shorter. The glands are simple, branched, coiled tubules composed of mucous-secreting cells, together with an occasional argentaffin cell. The cardiac glands are essentially similar in type to the pyloric glands; they tend, however, to be less tightly packed together and they frequently show slight cystic dilatation. Mitotic figures in normal gastric glands are limited to the base of the pits. The glands throughout the stomach are separated by a scanty vascular connective tissue containing scattered lymphocytes, an occasional eosinophil leucocyte, and plasma cells. In the pyloric region especially an occasional lymphoid follicle may be present.

Acute Gastritis

Because of its nature, acute gastritis has been little studied. It is known to occur in viral infections, anæmia, after dietary indiscretions, excess of alcohol, following ingestion of drugs and a variety of other chemicals and corrosives. Histologically the mucosa shows œdema and an acute inflammatory infiltrate of the lamina propria. There is congestion of vessels and

FIG. 1. Gastric body mucosa. (H. and E. × 80.)

FIG. 2. Cardio-oesophageal junction showing cardiac glands with long pits and short gland tubules; note dilated gland. (H. and E × 80.)

FIG. 3. Chronic superficial gastritis showing distortion of pits and changes in the superficial epithelium. (H. and E × 80.)

FIG. 4. Chronic atrophic gastritis. Note inflammatory infiltrate and loss of specialised gland tubules. (H. and E. × 80.)

mucosal necrosis varying from superficial erosion to complete sloughing, as may occur with some corrosive substances.

Although in most cases of acute gastritis a return to normal is the usual, it seems probable that repeated attacks can lead to chronic gastritis.

Chronic Gastritis

It is the group of histological entities embraced by the term chronic gastritis upon which most attention has been focused since gastric biopsy became a safe and easy procedure. Although the precise definitions vary from author to author, three types or grades are generally recognized: superficial gastritis, atrophic gastritis, and gastric atrophy. It should always be remembered that these are not distinct and separate entities, intermediate appearances are not infrequent, and that progression can occur from one category to another. It is also well to bear in mind that the appearances in a single gastric biopsy may not necessarily reflect the state of the mucosa as a whole.

Chronic Superficial Gastritis. In this (Fig. 3) there is a plasma cell and lymphocytic infiltrate in the superficial layer of the gastric mucosa. Eosinophils and neutrophils in varying number are also seen, and any lymphoid follicles present will show reactive hyperplasia. There are no histological changes in the epithelium of the glands but the superficial epithelium and that lining the pits frequently shows evidence of damage. There is often a loss of power of mucous secretion, the cells becoming flattened and basophilic and their nuclei somewhat pleomorphic and pyknotic, whilst others are clearly dying. In some places regenerative features can be seen and some palisading of the surface cells is present.

Chronic Atrophic Gastritis. When fully developed the gastric mucosa is decreased in thickness (Fig. 4) and there is a chronic inflammatory cell infiltrate involving the whole thickness of the lamina propria. There is also atrophy of glands whether these are gastric or pyloric in type. The superficial epithelium may show changes similar to those in superficial gastritis, together with a variable degree of intestinal metaplasia. Usually of patchy distribution, this may rarely involve the whole stomach. The usual gastric epithelium is replaced by one with a typical striated border and scattered goblet cells. This metaplastic epithelium extends into the atrophic glands where Paneth cells may also be seen. The eosinophilic granules in these cells are larger and more refractile than the granules of chief cells, which can sometimes appear eosinophilic, and in contrast to argentaffin cells the nucleus is placed not nearer the lumen but on the basement membrane of the gland tube. In instances where difficulties in recognition arise, Paneth cells can be clearly demonstrated as containing deeply purple granules in PTAH preparations. The parietal and chief cells largely disappear from the gastric glands, which appear as shorter simple tubes lined by a low columnar epithelium of an apparent simple mucous-secreting type. Such atrophic body mucosa, in the absence of a marked inflammatory, infiltrated and intestinal metaplasia, closely mimics normal cardiac or pyloric mucosa. The change has in fact been termed pyloric gland metaplasia and, although the atrophic glands are more widely separated than the glands in the pylorus or cardiac region, differentiation can be difficult unless other features are present.

In chronic atrophic gastritis the inflammatory infiltrate does not usually extend beyond the muscularis mucosa, but sometimes it is extremely dense and contains numerous lymphoid aggregates. It is unlikely that this represents a special form of chronic gastritis, although it is sometimes referred to as chronic follicular gastritis.

Gastric Atrophy. This is a mucosal appearance essentially similar to chronic atrophic gastritis, except that there is a minimum of inflammatory cells in the lamina propria. It is much more likely to affect the whole of the mucosa, and some authors restrict the term gastric atrophy to mucosæ which show complete intestinal or pyloric metaplasia (Fig. 5) and total loss of chief and parietal cells. There is a consensus of opinion that gastric atrophy is an end-stage in chronic atrophic gastritis.

Significance of Chronic Gastritis. Chronic gastritis may be present in the absence of symptoms and, in contrast, biopsy of patients with persistent dyspepsia may reveal no abnormality (Joske et al., 1955; Shiner and Doniach, 1957; Coghill, 1960). The cause of chronic gastritis is often obscure and its extent and incidence increases with advancing years. Edwards and Coghill (1966) have recently reviewed the evidence suggesting an association with blue eyes, low social class, heavy alcohol consumption, the drinking of hot liquids, heavy cigarette smoking and possibly aspirin taking. Morson (1955) has shown that gastritis is more frequently seen in the gastric canal of Magenstrasse which is formed by the lesser curve and pyloric antrum and is the area most exposed to injury. This is also the common site for gastric ulceration with which chronic gastritis is often associated (Mackay and Hislop, 1966). Chronic gastric ulcers are often sited in alkaline areas in the stomach (Capper et al., 1962) and experimentally induced duodenal reflux in dogs (Lawson, 1964) results in gastritis. Du Plessis (1965) suggests that reflux of alkaline duodenal contents by reducing the barrier effect of gastric mucous induces mucosal damage and gastritis by the action of acid and pepsin. The gastritis would in turn lead to decreased acid production and an increased liability to ulceration. The gastritis so frequently seen in association with carcinoma of the stomach may have a similar cause and be initiated by alterations in mucous production or gastric acidity secondary to the presence of the cancer. The relationship of gastritis to gastric ulcer cannot be regarded as settled.

Much of the other information gained from a study of gastric biopsies has concerned the relationship between the various parameters of gastric function and the histological appearances. In general, it may be said that there is a decreased secretion of acid, pepsin and intrinsic factor which correlates roughly with the degree of atrophy of the gastric mucosa, lowest levels being seen in severe atrophic gastritis and gastric atrophy (Glass et al., 1960; Bock et al., 1963; Ardeman and Chanarin, 1966).

In pernicious anæmia the gastric biopsy always shows either severe atrophic gastritis or, less commonly, gastric atrophy. A commonly held view is that the antrum remains uninvolved, but this needs verification. It is probable that gastric atrophy is the end result of atrophic gastritis but if it is unrelated then clearly pernicious anæmia may result from primary gastric atrophy or from secondary post-gastritic atrophy. In addition there are now several cases on record where there is a selective failure of intrinsic factor secretion. This occurs in children who are anæmic and fail to thrive and who may have neurological manifestations. Although the condition is called juvenile pernicious anæmia, the gastric biopsy is normal and so is acid secretion (Harris-Jones et al., 1957; Lillibridge et al., 1967). A disorder similar to juvenile pernicious anæmia has been described (Imerslund, 1960, Imerslund and Bjornstad, 1963) in which a normal mucosa and a normal intrinsic factor secretion is associated with a defective absorption of vitamin B_{12}.

Between 30 and 60 per cent of patients with iron-deficiency anæmia have an atrophic gastritis (Badenoch et al., 1957; Coghill and Williams, 1958). It remains to be resolved whether iron deficiency precedes the gastritis or whether gastritis causes iron deficiency. It has been shown, nevertheless, that gastritis is much more common in iron-deficiency anæmia of so-called idiopathic type where no other cause of iron deficiency can be found (Coghill, 1960).

Gastric biopsy has also facilitated the study of the immunological aspects of chronic gastritis. Pernicious anæmia is now considered along with certain thyroid diseases as an auto-immune phenomenon. Indeed, there is a considerable immunological overlap between the two (Irvine et al., 1962; Doniach et al., 1963). Antibodies against the microsomal fraction of the gastric parietal cell are rarely found when the gastric mucosa is normal, but their prevalence increases with increasing severity of the histological lesion (Fisher and Taylor, 1965). Wright et al. (1966), however, have shown that it is the disease process in which chronic gastritis occurs, e.g. pernicious anæmia or idiopathic hypochronic anæmia, which determines the presence of parietal cell antibodies rather than the histological abnormality itself.

Antibodies to intrinsic factor are less common than parietal cell antibodies (Fisher and Taylor, 1965) and are associated with the more severe grades of chronic gastritis. Bardhan has investigated most of the parameters of gastric secretion, together with the serum pepsinogen, serum vitamin B_{12}, and gastric parietal cell and intrinsic factor antibody in the same large group of patients. When appraised in correlation with the gastric biopsy (Bardhan and Whitehead) the general tendency for decreasing secretion to follow increasing inflammation and destruction of the mucosa is verified. It has also become clear that, while the presence of gastric parietal cell antibody means that there has been damage to the gastric mucosa, its absence, however, does not mean that the mucosa is normal. Intrinsic factor antibody is rarely if ever found except in patients with pernicious anæmia and latent pernicious anæmia.[1]

Miscellaneous.—Gastric biopsy will reveal iron in the chief cells of most patients with hæmochromatosis (Joske et al., 1955) and provides an alternative to liver biopsy if this is difficult or contraindicated. Uncommonly the biopsy will reveal amyloidosis (Filipe and Correia, 1963), lymphoma or sarcoidosis (Ross, 1965).

Additional evidence for diagnosis may be provided by examination of the gastric biopsy in so-called hypertrophic gastritis (Menetrier's disease), a condition often first suspected radiologically. Ross (1965) describes the mucosa showing increased thickness with elongated pits and branched glands. Butz (1960) also describes a typical disruption of the muscularis mucosa with smooth muscle fibres extending into the lamina propria. An increase in the gland layer might also well be expected in gastric rugal hypertrophy of the Zollinger-Ellison syndrome.

[1] See Chapter 29. p. 497.

Biopsy of the stomach and of the pyloric region especially may reveal the changes of eosinophilic gastritis or granuloma. This is claimed to be allergic in origin and many, if not all, cases may well be due to ingestion of the eggs or larvæ of *Eustoma rotundatum*, a parasite occurring in the peritoneum of the North Sea herring (Kuipers *et al.*, 1960a, b; Ashby *et al.*, 1964). The lesion produced, which is probably a local gastro-intestinal reaction to ingested allergen, is usually diffuse or phlegmonous but can be grossly polypoidal. Histologically there is a character-istic vascularity and œdema of the mucosa. A massive infiltration of eosinophils occurs throughout the lamina propria and may extend through the muscularis mucosa. The surface epithelium is usually intact but ulceration may occur and occasionally the remains of parasites may be seen.

THE SMALL INTESTINAL BIOPSY

Normal

With the dissecting microscope the normal jejunal mucosa (Fig. 6) is characterized by its finger-like villi. Not infrequently, however, leaf- or tongue-shaped structures and short ridges are seen. These features are much more common in the duodenum, where the villi tend to be shorter and have a broader base.

Histologically the villi are covered by a columnar epithelium which has a distinct PAS-positive brush border. This can often be seen in H. and E. sections as a refractile line at the luminal surface if the microscope substage is racked down slightly. The villi are from two to three times as long as the crypt-like glands which take origin from their bases to dip into the lamina propria (Fig. 7). The villous epithelium is continuous with that lining the crypts, but the latter has a much less distinct brush border and, whereas mitotic figures may be seen in the crypt epithelium, they are never present in the surface epithelium. Towards the bottom of the glands both Paneth cells and argentaffin cells are found and scattered about in the surface epithelium, and in the glands there are PAS-positive mucous-secreting goblet cells. In ordinary preparations the core of the villi and the lamina propria, i.e. the area between the crypts bounded externally by the muscularis mucosa, appears as a delicate reticular network infiltrated by a few lympho-cytes with occasional plasma cells, eosinophils and histiocytes. The villi also contain a central blind ending lacteal and an arteriole and venule joined by a capillary plexus. Extending from the muscularis mucosa, there are thin strands of smooth muscle which surround the central lacteal and pass to the tip of the villi. Sometimes a biopsy includes a lymphoid aggregate and, when present, the overlying villi are short or non-existent.

Villous Abnormalities

1. **Partial Villous Atrophy. The Convoluted Mucosa**. This mucosal change shows features which, although distinct from the flat mucosa (see later), are exaggerations of those which are occasionally seen in the normal. When fully developed, the numerous long branching ridges and broad villous leaves produce a distinct brain-like convoluted pattern, as seen by the dissecting microscope, but clearly many intermediate patterns occur (Figs. 8 and 9). Histologically such a mucosa shows a partial villous atrophy

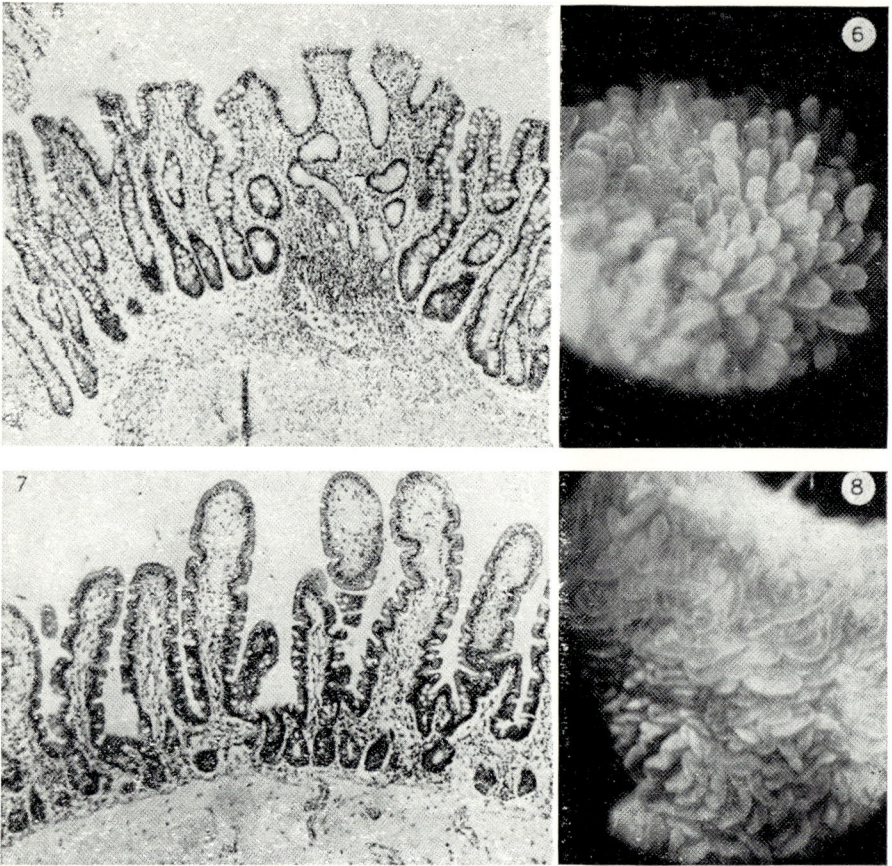

FIG. 5. Gastric atrophy. Cellular infiltrate comparable to that in Fig. 1. There is almost total intestinal metaplasia with prominent goblet cells. (H. and E. × 80.)

FIG. 6. Normal jejunal biopsy as seen with the dissecting microscope. Villi are mainly finger-shaped, but note occasional tongue-shaped forms. (× 16.)

FIG. 7. Normal jejunum corresponding to biopsy seen in Fig. 6. (H. and E. × 90.)

FIG. 8. Jejunal mucosa showing numerous ridges and broad tongue-shaped structures. (× 16.)

(Fig. 10) (Doniach and Shiner, 1957). Some parts of the mucosa may appear normal apart from a thickening of the gland layer. In others broad, irregular and bifid villi with mucosal bridges are seen. The variation depends upon whether the ridges and leaves are cut across their long axis or along it. If the former, fairly normal appearances result, but if the latter the above irregularities occur especially if, as does happen, sections are in an oblique plane through folded ridges and leaf-shaped villi. In tangential cuts, usually seen in sections from towards the end of the blocks, the deeper parts of long anastomosing ridges appear to enclose clefts which represent the intervillous space. There is often a slight excess of inflammatory cells in the lamina propria, but surface epithelial changes similar to those seen in the flat mucosa are usually absent.

No agreement has been reached as to where the line is to be drawn between the lower limit of partial villous atrophy and the normal. This is because a whole range of appearances between the two extremes has been seen and there is evidence that changes in the small bowel mucosa can take place in the space of a few hours in relation to changes in local bowel environment (Rubin *et al.*, 1962; Creamer, 1964a, b; Townley *et al.*, 1964; Watson *et al.*, 1965a). It has recently been suggested that accurate quantitative measurements of villi would overcome some of these delineation difficulties (Shiner, 1965) in that actual figures rather than subjective impressions would be available.

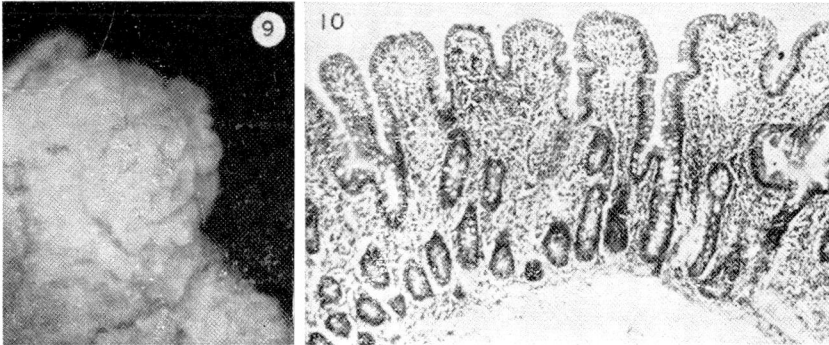

FIG. 9. Fully developed brain-like convoluted pattern of jejunal mucosa. (× 16.)
FIG. 10. Jejunal biopsy showing partial villous atrophy. (H. and E. × 90.)

2. **Subtotal Villous Atrophy. The Flat Mucosa.** Under the dissecting microscope the mucosa is more or less completely flat (Fig. 11) and devoid of villi, but may show a series of low polygonal mounds giving the surface a mosaic pattern (Fig. 12). Histologically the appearances correspond to so-called subtotal villous atrophy (Doniach and Shiner, 1957) (Figs. 13 and 14). The surface epithelium is flattened, appears more basophilic and often the nuclei are stratified and sometimes pyknotic. The brush border is ill-defined and, not infrequently, lymphocytes surrounded by a clear space can be seen migrating through the surface epithelium. An excess of goblet cells is sometimes seen in the crypts, which themselves may be elongated. Paneth cells, usually present in normal numbers, may be absent or diminished (Creamer and Pink, 1967) and the crypt cells show an increased number of mitoses indicating rapid cell turnover. In about a third of cases there is a focal thickening of the basement membrane which is weakly PAS-positive (Schein, 1947; Hourihane, 1963). This must be differentiated from a pink-staining sub-epithelial œdema which is presumed to be an artefact seen also in normal biopsies. It is possibly due to a stronger than usual suction used at biopsy. The lamina propria is infiltrated fairly heavily by a mixture of lymphocytes and plasma cells with some eosinophils and histiocytes. This infiltrate does not extend beyond the muscularis mucosa. The latter structure may occasionally exhibit intracellular lipofuscin pigment deposition (see later).

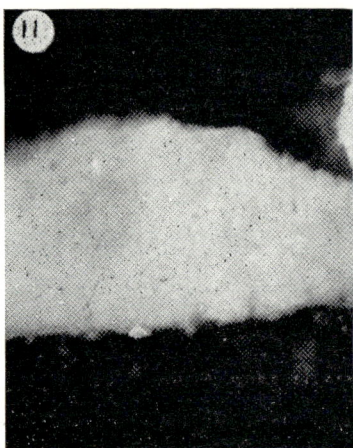
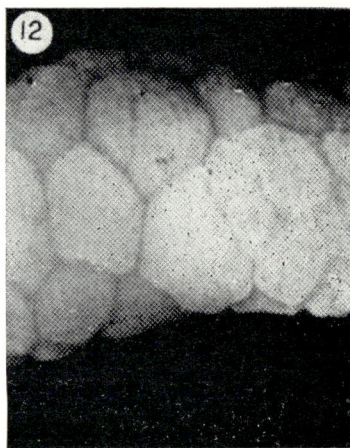
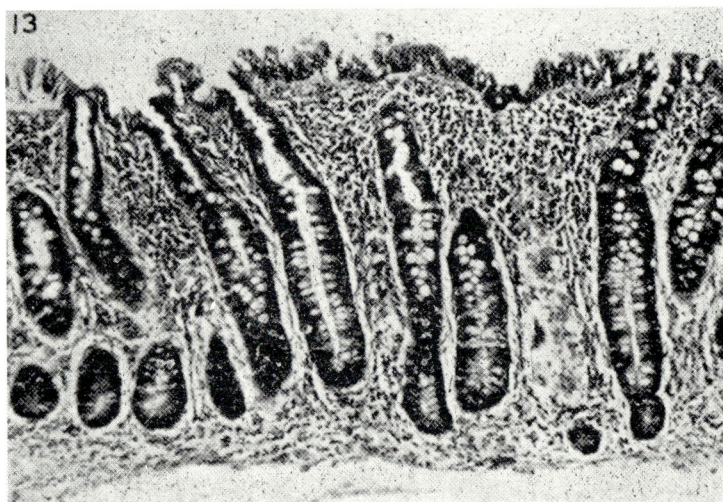
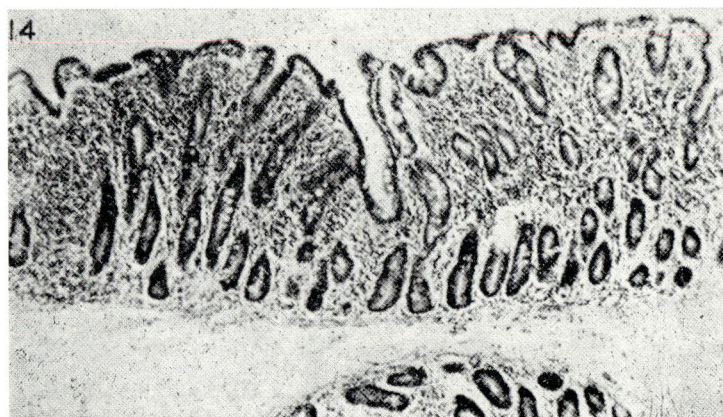

An important histological feature in some biopsies is the presence of meta-plastic simple mucous-secreting glands in the lamina propria (Fig. 15). These are easily distinguishable from Brunner's glands occasionally seen in duodenal biopsies because of their site on the luminal side of the muscularis mucosa. This change has been termed gastric pyloric gland metaplasia and is simply a manifestation of the marked metaplastic potential of the epithelium of the gastrointestinal tract as a whole. The importance of these mucous glands in small intestinal, and especially jejunal, biopsies is that they are invariably present in the vicinity of ulcerating lesions, be these benign (e.g. Crohn's disease) or malignant (e.g. reticulosarcoma). James (1964) and Rhodes (1964) describe gastric epithelium replacing the surface epithelium of villi in a variety of disorders (e.g. duodenal ulcer, the Zollinger-Ellison syndrome) and believe this to be a metaplasia secondary to high acid secretion. It may also accompany pyloric gland metaplasia (Fig. 16).

The Significance of Villous Changes

The flat mucosa, or less commonly the convoluted mucosa, is the lesion usually seen in the *cœliac syndrome* and *idiopathic steatorrhœa*. However, malabsorption, which in all other respects is identical to idiopathic steatorrhœa (Girdwood *et al.*, 1961; Fone *et al.*, 1960) and steatorrhœa secondary to other conditions, e.g. thyrotoxicosis (Cooke *et al.*, 1959; Crane and Evans, 1966) may be associated with a normal mucosa. Moreover, Hindle and Creamer (1965) found that in 50 patients with a flat mucosa and steatorrhœa there was no method of distinguishing idiopathic steatorrhœa from that secondary to other causes except by the recognition of the under-lying disease process.

The list of conditions in which varying degrees of villous abnormality, and sometimes a flat mucosa, have been recognized is growing rapidly and includes: tropical sprue (Baker *et al.*, 1962), malignancy anywhere in the body (Creamer, 1964c), ulcerative colitis in active phase (Salem *et al.*, 1964) lymphoma of the bowel and/or the mesenteric lymph nodes (Sleisenger *et al.*, 1953), Crohn's disease (Shiner and Drury, 1962), hookworm disease (Sheehy *et al.*, 1962), various virus diseases (Sheehy *et al.*, 1964), following gastric operations, in the Zollinger-Ellison syndrome and in chronic pancreatitis (Creamer, 1964c), in diabetes mellitus (Ellenberg and Bookman, 1960) in sarcoidosis (Hindle and Creamer, 1965), in various skin diseases, e.g. dermatitis herpetiformis (Marks *et al.*, 1966), rosacea (Watson *et al.*, 1965b), eczema (Friedman and Hare, 1965), ichthyosis (Fry *et al.*, 1965). Minor abnormalities of the intestinal villi have been described in patients receiving neomycin (Jacobson *et al.*, 1960a, b). In this and in other instances where only minor abnormalities are seen it is probably well worth bearing in mind that there is also a racial variation in intestinal villous pattern (Rubin and Dobbins, 1965). Indians and Africans tend to show an increase in leaves and short ridges as compared to Europeans.

Other Abnormalities

1. **Whipple's Disease.** This is a rare disorder presenting with steatorrhœa, skin pigmentation and an arthropathy sometimes accompanied by a poly-serositis. The jejunal mucosa as seen under the dissecting microscope shows distinct, low, bulging or bloated villi. Sometimes the villi have white or

---

FIG. 11. Jejunal biopsy. Flat mucosa. (×14.)

FIG. 12. Jejunal biopsy. Mosaic pattern. (×14.)

FIG. 13. Histological appearance of mucosa seen in Fig. 11. (H. and E. ×90.)

FIG. 14. Histological appearance of mucosa seen in Fig. 12. (H. and E. ×90).

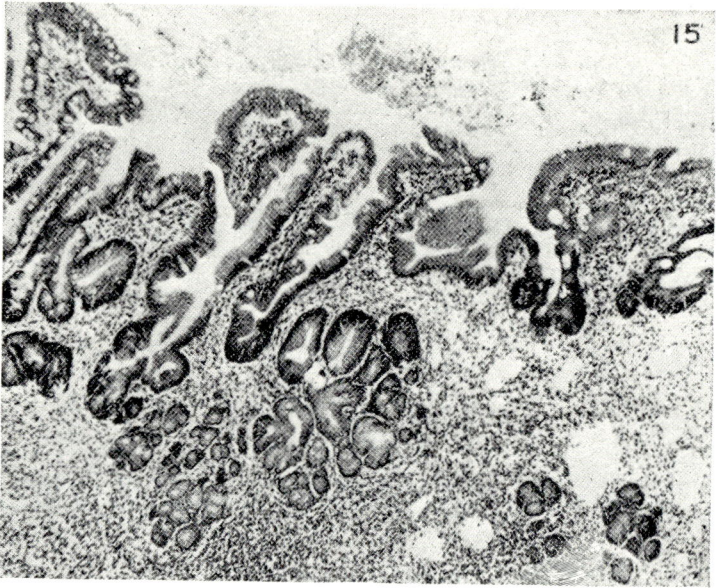

FIG. 15. Jejunal biopsy in Crohn's disease. There is pyloric gland metaplasia and overlying epithelium of gastric type detailed in Fig. 16. (H. and E. × 100.)

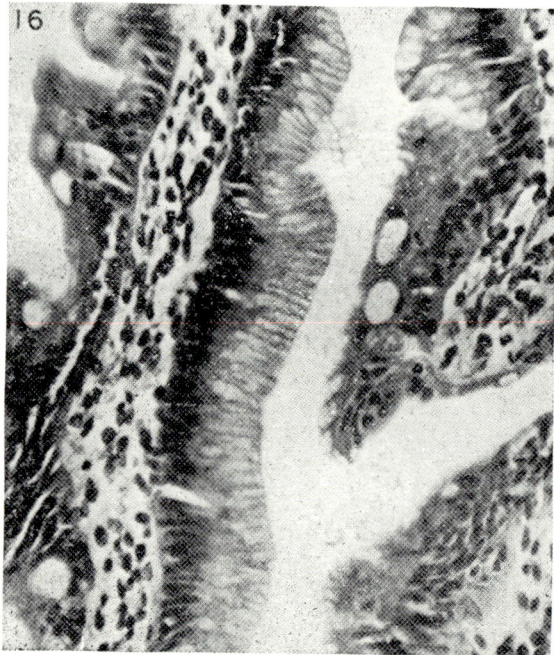

FIG. 16. Detail of Fig. 15. (H. and E. × 300.)

yellow tips (Gross *et al.*, 1959). Histologically the mucosa is stuffed with large macrophages (Fig. 17) whose cytoplasm contains PAS-positive diastase-resistant rods and granules. These macrophages accumulate especially at the villous tip but they are present also nearer the muscularis mucosa, where they may be slightly less PAS-positive. Sometimes the rod or sickle-shaped structures are seen in an extracellular situation. Hourihane (1963) has also demonstrated the presence of iron granules in these cells. Another characteristic feature is the presence of small spaces in the lamina propria which, in appropriately stained frozen sections, are seen to contain neutral fat. These spaces, although thought to be lacteals, have no endo-thelial lining and may be bordered by polymorphs. There is considerable doubt, therefore, as to their origin, especially in relation to lymphatics (Hourihane, 1963).

In addition to the intestinal changes, similar macrophages and spaces, often with marginal foreign body giant cells, are seen in mesenteric and other lymph nodes. Widespread involvement of the reticulo-endothelial system, the brain, liver and serosa can occur, and in several cases described by Enzinger and Helwig (1963) macrophages and associated thrombotic vegetations were present on the aortic and mitral valves. The nature of the condition is still in dispute; by some it is considered to be a bacterial infection not only because of the morphology of the macrophages but by the response to antibiotics which can partially reverse the intestinal lesions (Chears and Ashworth, 1961; Yardley and Hendrix, 1961; Ashworth *et al.*, 1964; Trier *et al.*, 1965). Others believe the condition to be a metabolic disturbance, the end-result of which is accumulation of polysaccharide substance within macrophages throughout the body (Taft *et al.*, 1959; Haubrich *et al.*, 1960). The earlier view that the condition was related to lymphatic obstruction has now been largely abandoned.

2. **Intestinal Lymphangiectasis.** Of the numerous causes of protein loss from the gut, the most recently recognized is the condition entitled intestinal lymphangiectasis (Waldmann *et al.*, 1961). This designation should probably be reserved for those cases showing an enlargement of villi which have œdematous tips, imparting to the mucosa a pebble-like appearance as seen in the dissecting microscope. Histologically there is œdema of the lamina propria and submucosa. The mucosal cells of the surface epithelium (Fig. 19) also show intracellular œdema, which pushes the nucleus away from its basal position towards the luminal surface (Mistilis *et. al.*, 1965). There is a dilata-tion of the mucosal lymphatics (Figs. 18 and 19) and outside these there are foamy macrophages which contain neutral fat. In relation to the dilated lymphatic there is an occasional multinucleate giant cell. Dilatation of submucosal and mesenteric lymphatics has been recorded, with collections of lipophages in regional nodes. In the cases associated with marked protein loss, lipofuscin pigmentation of the muscularis mucosa and other smooth muscle may occur. It now appears likely that the intestinal lymphatic dilatation is part of a more widespread abnormality. Pomerantz and Waldman (1963) and Mistilis *et al.* (1965) have shown ectasia of some and absence of other lymphatics in lower extremity lymphangiograms of patients with intestinal lymphangiectasis.

3. **Acanthocytosis** (*a β-lipoproteinæmia*). This is a syndrome comprising acanthocytosis of red cells, central nervous system manifestations, a

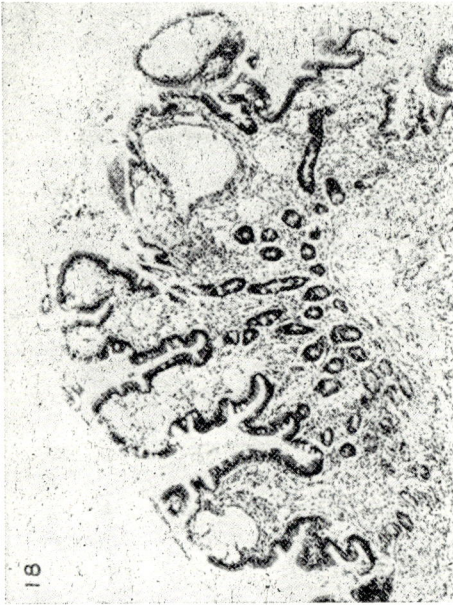

FIG. 17. Jejunal biopsy in Whipple's disease. Note simple spaces and dense accumulation of macrophages. (PAS. × 100.)

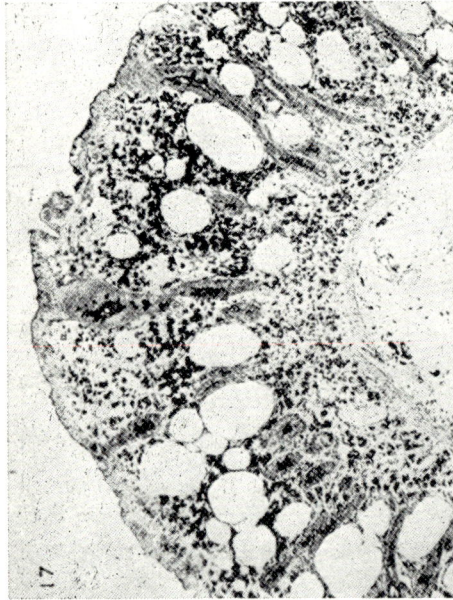

FIG. 18. Jejunal biopsy in intestinal lymphangiectasis. (H. and E. × 100.)

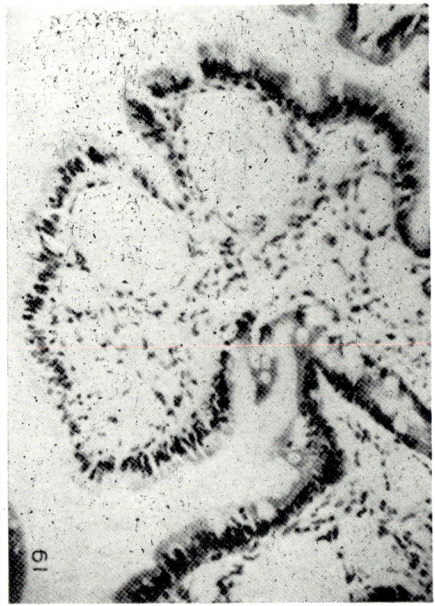

FIG. 19. Detail of surface epithelium and dilated lymphatics in intestinal lymphangiectasis. (H. and E. × 270.)

β-lipoproteinæmia and steatorrhœa. The jejunal mucosa, as described by Salt *et al.* (1960), exhibits abnormalities of the villi which are stunted and broad. Histologically there is a typical pallor of the surface epithelium. The cells retain their brush border, but they are distended by a clear substance which has been shown by Lamy *et al.* (1963) to be a lipid.

4. **Parasitic Infestations.** (a) *Hookworm Disease.* Until recently hookworm disease was a relative rarity in this country. This is no longer true, however, and infestation is being described with increasing frequency amongst many of the immigrant population (Miller and Bamforth, 1962; Salem and Truelove, 1964). In heavy infestation the small bowel often exhibits a picture of partial villous atrophy, but subtotal villous atrophy with a flat mucosa is also seen (Sheehey *et al.*, 1962). Frequently a dense eosinophil infiltration of the lamina propria is present and there are numerous small surface erosions. The latter are presumably the sites of attachment of the worms.

(b) *Strongyloidiasis.* This is an intestinal infestation which might increase in frequency in this country. It can give rise to variable villous changes and steatorrhœa (de Paola, 1961, 1962; Alcorn and Kotcher, 1961). The incidence in Jamaica, based on a small survey, was found to be 1 per cent (Bras *et al.*, 1964), and Wilson and Thompson (1964) describe a case in a West Indian female immigrant in London. Apart from abnormalities in villi, worms and ova can be seen in the crypts. The ova often bury themselves in the crypt epithelial cells and newly hatched rhabditiform larvæ may also be seen in the same location.

(c) *Lambliasis.* Infestation of the small bowel with *Giardia intestinalis* (*lamblia*), a flagellate protozoon, is a well-recognized cause of diarrhœa and steatorrhœa in childhood. Adult cases may also occur and the jejunal biopsy may reveal a partial villous atrophy with an increase in inflammatory cells in the lamina propria. Vegetative parasites, if searched for, can sometimes be seen overlying the surface epithelium (Fig. 20) or within the crypts (Cameron *et al.*, 1962). The vegetative form is pear-shaped, 10–18 μ in length, is bilaterally symmetrical and has two nuclei. A large sucking disc on one surface allows it to attach to the gut wall and it has four pairs of flagellæ. In ordinary (H. and E.) preparations it can be picked out as tiny grey structures similar to *Trichomonas vaginalis* as seen in Papanicolau preparations. In the PAS preparations of the intestinal biopsy the parasites are identified slightly more easily, since they are weakly positive.

5. **Miscellaneous.** Lipofuscin pigmentation of the muscularis mucosa in jejunal biopsies has already been mentioned in relation to idiopathic steatorrhœa and intestinal lymphangiectasis. It has also been described in Whipple's disease (Gresham *et al.*, 1958). It is probably only found in this site when pigmentation of other smooth muscle is heavy. The pigment is PAS-positive, autofluorescent in ultraviolet light, can be stained by Sudan Black, and is usually acid-fast with Zeil-Neilson's stain. The significance of the pigmentation is not fully understood but it is thought to be related to vitamin E deficiency (Toffler *et al.*, 1963; Ansanelli and Lane, 1957) or to hypoalbumenæmia (Ringsted, 1960). It is certainly seen in disorders commonly resulting in these two states. It has been described in a large number of the commoner malabsorptive syndromes in addition to cystic fibrosis of the pancreas, portal cirrhosis, biliary atresia and chronic pancreatitis. It is seen in idiopathic hypoproteinæmia and in other causes of protein loss from the gastro-intestinal tract, e.g. gastric rugal hypertrophy, neoplasms and peptic ulceration and its sequelæ, etc.

In systemic amyloidosis, deposits may be seen not only in submucosal vessels but also in the lamina propria. When present it can give rise to malabsorption (Golden, 1954). In systemic sclerosis, changes in the small bowel comparable to those seen in the œsophagus may occur, and can also result in malabsorption. Iron deposits may be seen in the lamina propria in hæmachromatosis, but they are sometimes present in the tips of villi in the absence of this disorder. The iron pigment which is presumed to be hæmosiderin has been seen in patients with chronic pancreatitis and in certain cases of human iron-deficiency anæmia treated by oral iron. Villous pigmentation can also be produced experimentally in animals by iron administration (Lillie and Geer, 1965), but clearly more work as to its significance is needed.

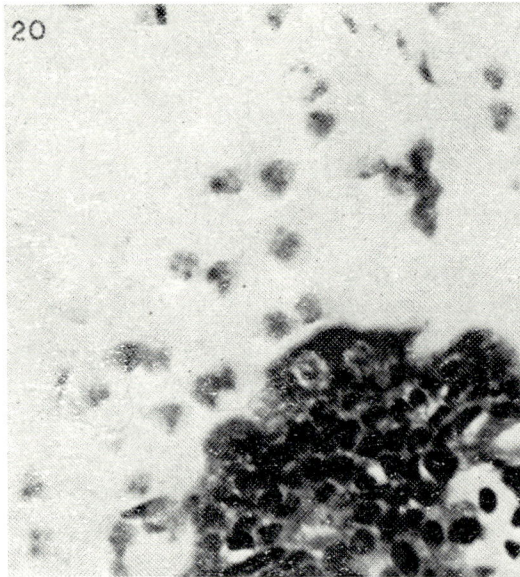

FIG. 20. Jejunal biopsy showing vegetative *Giardia lamblia*. (H. and E. × 500.)

COLONIC BIOPSY

Rectal and low colonic biopsies have long been employed in the diagnosis and management of local neoplasia. It is only more recently that their value in a wide range of other disorders is being appreciated.

Normal

The mucous membrane of the colon has a comparatively smooth surface for there are no villi (Fig. 21). Straight tubular glands extend from the surface down through the entire thickness of the lamina propria. The surface epithelium is of high columnar type with a thin striated border not visible on ordinary light microscopy. Interspersed amongst these cells are goblet cells. As the epithelium continues down into the glands the columnar cells become lower and the goblet cells exceedingly numerous, so that the wall of the gland may appear composed entirely of goblet cells. Occasional argentaffin cells can be seen, but Paneth cells are probably never present in the normal. The lamina propria contains a few plasma cells and eosino-phils and occasionally a solitary lymphoid follicle, which often extends into the submucosa.

Ulcerative Colitis and Crohn's Disease

Classically ulcerative colitis is a mucosal inflammatory process most commonly affecting the left side of the large bowel, but it may affect the whole colon and be associated with a terminal ileitis. In the past it was clearly distinguishable from the transmural inflammatory process of Crohn's disease, which arises mainly in the terminal ileum and which is associated with giant-cell granulomata. The distinction has, however, become blurred by the descriptions of local or patchy colonic lesions with a histological picture like that of Crohn's disease rather than ulcerative colitis. In some cases these colonic lesions have been associated with similar changes in the ileum and usually, in contrast to ulcerative colitis, the rectum has been spared. The condition has been called Crohn's disease of the colon (Wells, 1952; Brooke, 1959) or granulomatous colitis (Yarnis *et al.*, 1957). It does not seem to predispose to carcinoma of the colon as strongly as does ulcerative colitis (Janowitz and Present, 1966; Hawk and Turnbull, 1966) and auto-antibodies, though common in ulcerative colitis patients, are absent from patients with Crohn's colitis (Harrison, 1965). Ulcerative colitis affects women more commonly than men (Evans and Acheson, 1965), whereas in Crohn's colitis the sex incidence is equal. The clinical course and response to treatment of the two diseases is also different; Crohn's colitis is more often complicated by anal lesions (Lockhart Mummery and Morson, 1960) and internal fistulæ, and after surgical procedures recurrence is more frequent. This considerable evidence makes it probable that these two conditions are quite distinct and it is thus important to try to distinguish between the two in biopsy material.

In ulcerative colitis the bowel at different sites often shows phases of activity ranging from acute to quiescent and some areas may be normal. In the acute stage a biopsy may show ulceration or erosion and frequently a purulent surface exudate. The surface epithelium is flattened or cuboidal and frequently more basophilic than normal. Transmigration of polymorph leucocytes is a usual feature. The glands are often separated by œdema and some show dilation and are filled with polymorphs, constituting crypt abscesses (Fig. 22). The lamina propria is œdematous and shows capillary hyperæmia. There is an increase in plasma cells and eosinophils, and although neutrophils are plentiful in the surface exudate, in the capillaries and in the glands, they are less numerous in the lamina propria. Lymphoid aggregates, if included, show reactive hyperplasia. Clearly the reaction is chiefly a mucosal one, although in deeply ulcerated areas the inflammatory infiltrate may extend beyond the muscularis mucosæ into the submucosa. During the healing phase epithelial regenerative changes become obvious and mitotic activity is clearly visible in the surface and glandular epithelium. In the quiescent phase the inflammatory infiltrate in the lamina propria is less well marked and plasma cells predominate. The surface epithelium is often flattened and abnormal, but erosions and ulcers are absent. Crypt abscesses are small and inconspicuous and the gland pattern is often irregular, the glands being widely separated by infiltrate. In both active and quiescent phases one may observe metaplastic Paneth cells in the crypts (Watson and Roy, 1960), but their presence is not diagnostic since they occur in other ulcerative conditions. A point too frequently overlooked is that Paneth cell metaplasia is relatively much less common in the rectum than it is in the more proximal parts of the colon. When ulceration and subsequent regeneration and healing has been recurrent, another form of metaplasia can occur. This is a gastric pyloric gland metaplasia identical to that seen in some jejunal biopsies, but it is so rare as to be of no practical value in diagnosis. In the quiescent phase, differentiation from Crohn's disease is especially difficult.

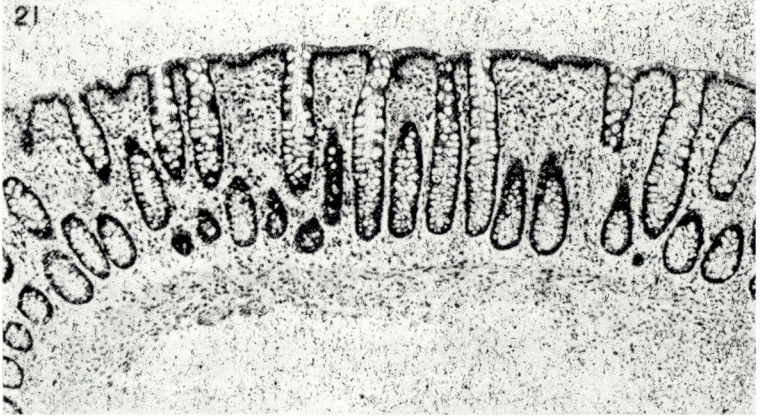

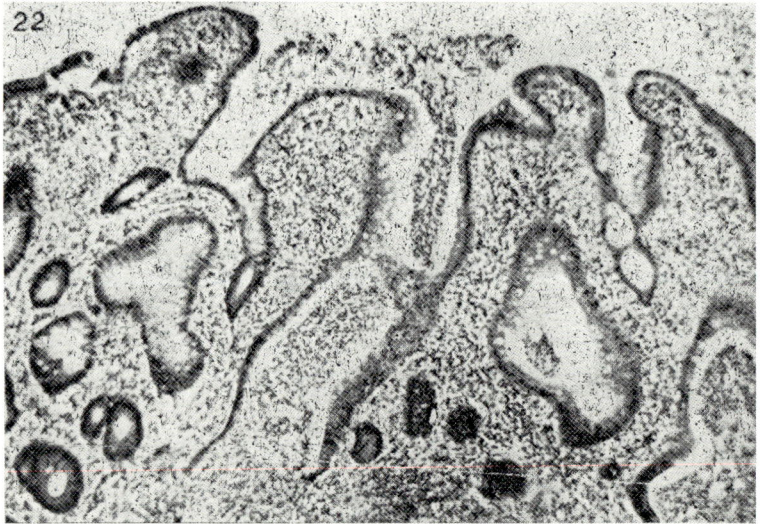

FIG. 21. Normal colonic mucosa. (H. and E. × 90.)
FIG. 22. Colonic mucosa in ulcerative colitis showing crypt abscesses. (H. and E. × 150.)

The infiltrate in Crohn's disease of the colon tends to be lymphocytic and is often distributed in focal collections. It is not limited to the lamina propria and is characterized by much œdema. The infiltrate and œdema are seen in the submucosa even in non-ulcerated areas. If ulcerated, however, a secondary polymorph infiltration appears and subsequently pyloric gland and Paneth cell metaplasia, in addition to crypt abscess formation, may be seen. Perhaps the only diagnostic feature of any real significance is the presence in Crohn's disease of epithelioid granulomata (Fig. 23) containing giant cells. In some cases of Crohn's disease they are few in number, but if a thorough search is made in several biopsies they can usually be found (Lockhart Mummery and Morson, 1964). Caution must be exercised in the interpretation of giant-cell granulomata, however. They have more significance in the absence of ulceration than in its presence, and if seen in the submucosa rather than the lamina propria. Such lesions can arise in relation to foreign material and morphologically it is not always possible to differ-

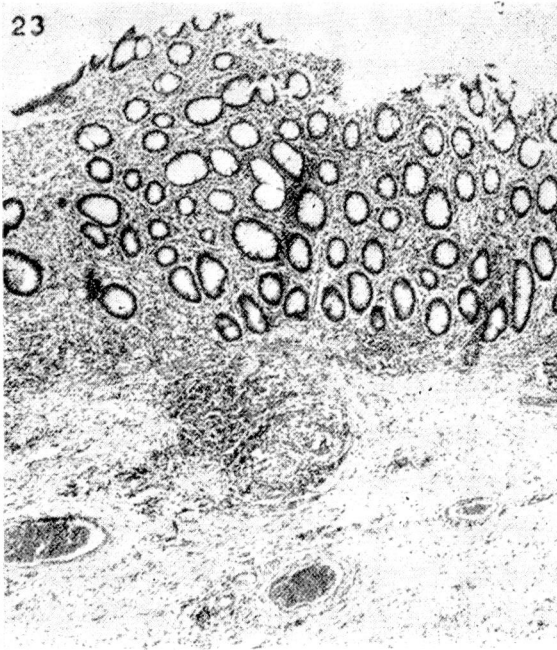

FIG. 23. Colonic mucosa in Crohn's disease. There is a granuloma in the submucosa together with marked oedema and lymphoid aggregates. (H. and E. × 40.)

entiate between these and true granulomata. Foreign body granulomata are seen in many ulcerative lesions of the colon and sometimes their true nature is disclosed when, by taking further sections through the blocks, foreign material is found in relation to them. Swollen ganglion cells and their schwannic satellite cells can mimic giant-cell granulomata (Figs. 24 and 25) especially if several occur in a group. Staining with a Nissl substance stain provides an easy means of recognizing these. In many biopsies, especially when the condition is of some standing, a differentiation between ulcerative colitis and Crohn's is not possible and indeed a diagnosis of neither may be made. Only too frequently is one able simply to report the presence of non-specific inflammatory changes.

Amœbic Colitis

In a country where amœbiasis is non-endemic, it is extremely important that this diagnosis be kept in mind. It is all too easy to miss the vegetative

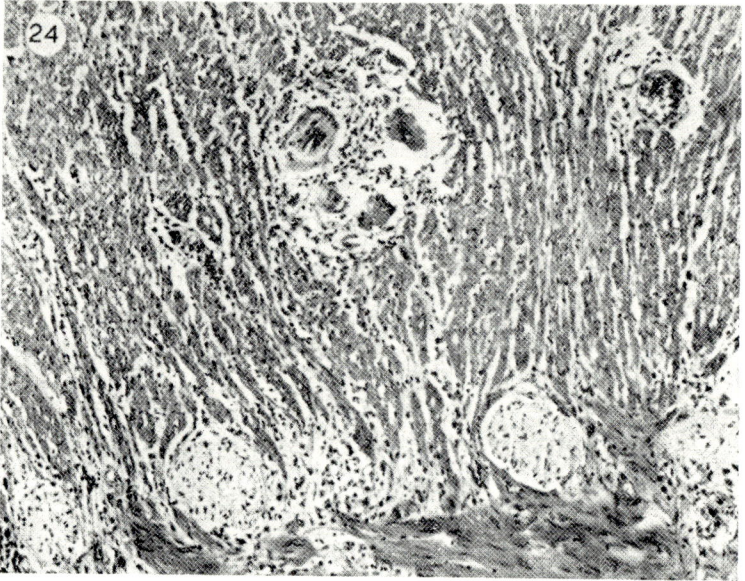

FIG. 24. Crohn's granuloma and swollen autonomic neural elements in muscularis of colon.   (H. and E. ×85.)

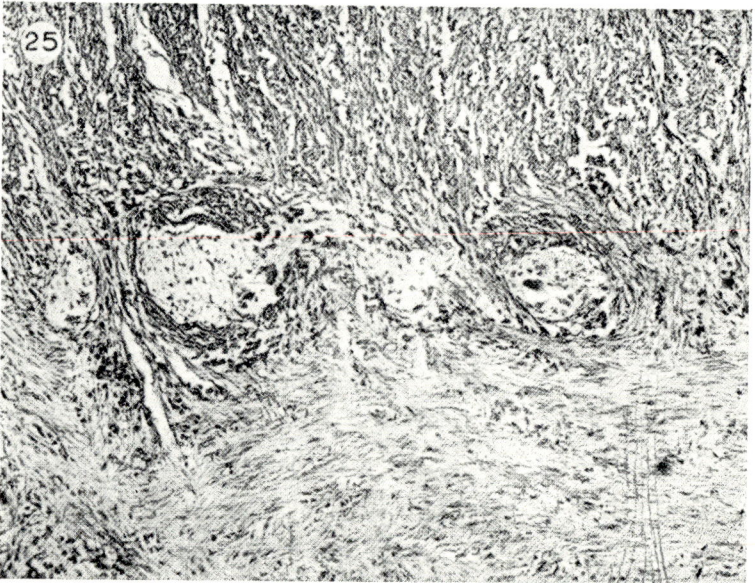

FIG. 25. Swollen autonomic neural elements closely mimicking Crohn's granulomata. Compare with Fig. 24. (H. and E. × 85.)

amœba in biopsy material even when the diagnosis is entertained.   Histologically the mucosal changes may be very similar to those seen in ulcerative colitis, and features such as crypt abscesses, pyloric gland and Paneth cell metaplasia may all be present, especially in the chronic case. As in ulcerative colitis, the inflammatory infiltrate is variable in type and in small biopsies one does not often see the characteristic flask-shaped ulceration, but the ulcer bases often have a marked surface zone of necrosis. Undermining of the ulcer edge may be present and it is in the region of the ulcers and in the surface mucus that a search for vegetative amœbæ should be made. These vary in size from 15 to 25 μ, have a single small spherical nucleus and a greyish-blue foamy cytoplasm. It is impossible in histological material to differentiate with certainty the vegetative forms of *entomœba histolytica* from non-pathogenic amœbæ. Furthermore, it is often difficult to differentiate amœbæ from macrophages (see later). The latter tend to be smaller and the nucleus more often oval or indented, but as with pathogenic amœba red cells may be seen within their cytoplasm. Whilst it is true also that the amœbæ are made more easily seen in iron hæmatoxylin, in PAS (Fig. 26) or in ultraviolet fluorescent preparations the same also applies to the macrophages which may have engulfed mucin or other carbohydrate material. An important histological feature in amœbic colitis is the presence of vegetative forms at the bases of the ulcers, in the actual tissues or within lymphatics or small vessel spaces. If amœbiasis is suspected on biopsy appearances, a thorough stool examination for both vegetative and cystic forms should follow and a definite diagnosis made in what is now a fairly easily treated condition.

Pneumatosis Cystoides Intestinalis

In this condition, air-filled gas cysts occur in the wall of the small or large intestine.

Koss (1952) noted a high incidence (58 per cent) in the reported cases of a coexistent organic lesion of the gut, e.g. ulceration, neoplasm, obstruction, etc., and it has also followed biopsy and sigmoidoscopy. In such cases a mechanical theory of origin was postulated whereby gas was forced into the wall via a breach in the mucosa. In many cases, however, no bowel lesion can be demonstrated and recently clinical (Doub and Shea, 1960) and experimental (Keyting et al., 1961) evidence has accumulated which strongly favours another origin. Rupture of lung alveoli producing mediastinal emphysema is followed by the movement of gas downwards around the aorta. The path upwards is blocked by the deep fascial attachments at the root of the neck. The gas moves along the branches of the aorta, into the mesentry, subsequently disrupting the bowel wall. It is easy to accept this ætiology in those cases arising in patients with chronic lung diseases, but it has also been suggested that all cases may have the same basis. Increased intrathoracic pressure and rupture of alveoli due to vomiting, straining, etc., may also occur in those cases associated with organic gastro-intestinal lesions.

At biopsy a hissing pop may be heard by the clinician and subsequent histological examination reveals characteristic features. The cysts will be seen in the lamina propria or submucosa (Fig. 27), which usually contains a mild chronic inflammatory cell infiltrate. They are usually lined by a single layer of flattened or plumper macrophages with multi-nucleate giant cells which may be numerous. Early cysts have no lining and the spaces can then be clearly seen not to be dilated lymphatics, as was once thought. The subsequent histiocytic and giant-cell reaction to the gas has its parallel in that which occurs in subcutaneous tissues after air or its individual component gases are injected (Wright, 1930).

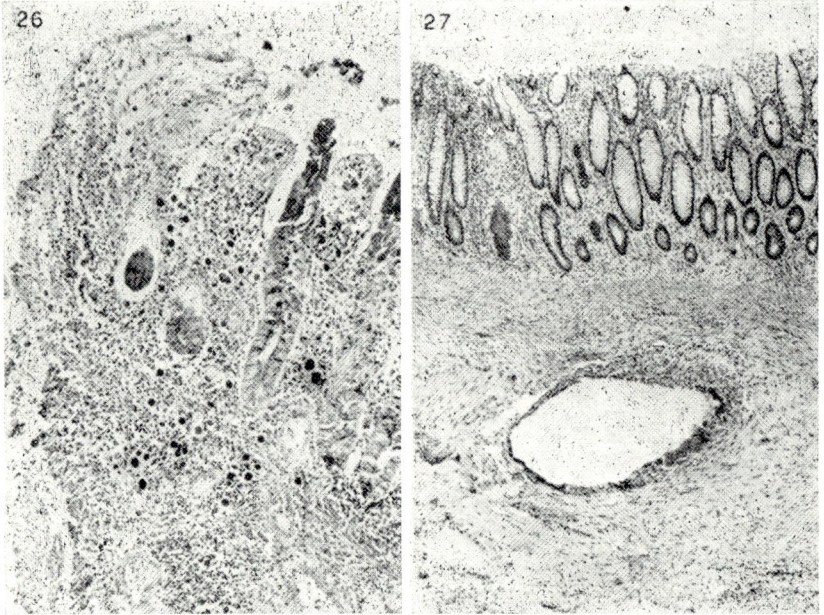

Fig. 26. Colonic biopsy in amoebic colitis. Obvious vegetative forms deep in the tissues·
(PAS. × 85.)
FIG. 27. Colonic biopsy in pneumatosis intestinalis. Gas cyst is lined by macrophages and giant cells. (H. and E. × 85.)

Amyloidosis

In primary amyloidosis there are no pathognomonic clinical manifestations and diagnosis by the Congo red test has proved valueless except in advanced cases.

The diagnosis of suspected cases by biopsy has therefore gradually developed. Aspiration biopsy of internal organs carries a small but nevertheless real risk, and gingival biopsy (Calkins and Cohen, 1960) or small intestinal biopsy (Green et al., 1961) gave too high a false negative rate. Rectal biopsy, however, furnished a diagnosis in 78 per cent of cases (Gafni and Sohar, 1960), results comparable to those obtained by renal biopsy and better than those from liver biopsy. The rectal biopsy must include the submucosa, for amyloid may be present there when absent in the lamina propria, a point stressed strongly by Kyle et al. (1966). Amyloid deposits may be seen in the small arterioles of the lamina propria and submucosa, also in the basement membrane of the epithelium and between the fibres of the muscularis mucosa.

In frozen sections amyloid can be demonstrated by its fluorescence in ultra-violet light after staining with thioflavine T (Vassar and Culling, 1959), and the metachromatic reaction with methyl violet is more consistently shown than in paraffin sections. Nevertheless, methyl violet and Congo red are the methods of choice for paraffin sections, although non-specific hyaline substances may be stained by the Congo red (Montgomery and Muirhead, 1954). Only true amyloid, however, gives dichroic birefringence with Congo red when examined under crossed polars (Missmahl and Hertwig, 1953), and by this method very small deposits of amyloid can be detected when other methods fail (Blum and Sohar, 1962).

Neurological Diseases

The histopathological diagnosis of Hirschsprung's disease in rectal biopsies has been dealt with fully in a previous edition (Series III) and needs no further consideration. Bodian and Lake (1963) and more recently Brett and Berry (1967) have published their experiences with rectal biopsy and the diagnosis of central nervous system disorders. In the neurolipidoses, metachromatic leukodystrophy and in Hurler's syndrome changes similar to these in the brain may be seen in the ganglion cells of the myenteric plexus. Jager and Bethlem (1960) have also reported the Lewy body inclusions of Parkinson's disease not only in the pigment containing neurones within the central nervous system but also in neurones of the autonomic ganglia, and in these cases rectal biopsy may be of diagnostic help. To be of value in the diagnosis of neurological disorders, however, all biopsies should include the muscularis proper and, although the technique is not without risk, it would seem preferable to the alternative of brain biopsy.

Cystic Fibrosis of the Pancreas (Mucoviscidosis)

The diagnostic specificity of the sweat test decreases with age (Anderson and Freeman, 1960; McKendrick, 1962) and it is sometimes negative in childhood (Schwachman and Antonowicz, 1962). In post-mortem material characteristic histological changes occur in most glandular epithelia and rectal biopsy suggests itself as a diagnostic procedure in cases not easily diagnosed by other methods. Parkins et al. (1963), in a preliminary evaluation, showed that characteristic changes are usually but not invariably present. Goblet cells were increased in number, the mouths of the colonic glands tended to gape and the crypts were widely dilated and filled with lamellated mucous. An inflammatory infiltrate in the lamina propria was noted in some cases. Similar changes can also occur normally in the region just above the mucocutaneous junction and, occasionally, in healed ulcerative colitis, regional enteritis, intestinal lymphoma and cœliac disease, but they tend to be focal or patchy in character. Differentiation from mucoviscidosis could well be attained if more than one high biopsy were examined.

Muciphages and Melanosis Coli

Macrophages containing mucin which are positively stained by mucicarmine, alcian blue and aldehyde fuchsin are commonly seen in the lamina propria of the colon (Arapakis and Tribe, 1963; Azzopardi and Evans, 1966), especially if there is a concomitant inflammatory reaction and ulceration. Azzopardi and Evans stressed the importance of their differentiation from the cells of Whipple's disease since both are PAS-positive and because rectal biopsy has been advocated in the diagnosis of Whipple's disease (Flemming et al., 1962). Whilst the above methods serve to differentiate muciphages from Whipple's cells, the latter being negative, muciphages are somewhat less easily differentiated from amœbæ. Some of the features which aid in this have been discussed already but further help is obtained by employing the PAS reaction after salivary diastase digestion. Whereas muciphages are diastase-resistant, amœba will show markedly decreased PAS-positivity, especially if the digestion is prolonged for a few hours (personal observation).

Not infrequently large macrophages containing dark-brown or black pigment are seen in the lamina propria of colonic biopsies. When they are present in large numbers the bowel mucosa appears brown or grey in the gross. The condition has been called melanosis coli although there is doubt as to the exact nature of the pigment. It gives a positive PAS reaction which is diastase-resistant and is autofluorescent. Lillie and Geer (1965) have shown that it has a protein component and a more or less closely bound glycolipid with free fatty acid residues. They claim that the pigment is homologous to the iron-containing macrophages seen in the villous tips of the small bowel, both in animals and man, and in some cases of melanosis, often subdivided as pseudomelanosis, the macrophages give a positive iron reaction. Clinically the condition appears to be related to chronic use of anthracene purgatives, but clearly there is need for further investigation into its true nature.

Acknowledgements

I would like to express my sincerest thanks to Dr. W. C. D. Richards, of the Ashford General Hospital, Middlesex, to whom I am deeply indebted. Much of the histological material upon which this paper is based was collected whilst he was in Oxford and many of the illustrations are the result of his work. He has made an invaluable criticism of the text and allowed me complete access to his collection of the relevant bibliography.

References

ALCORN, M. O., Jr. and KOTCHER, E. (1961). *Sth med. J.*, **54**, 193.
ANDERSON, C. M. and FREEMAN, M. (1960). *Arch. Dis. Childh.*, **35**, 581.
ANSANELLI, V. and LANE, N. (1957). *Ann. surg.*, **146**, 117.
ARAPAKIS, G. and TRIBE, C. R. (1963). *Ann. rheum. Dis.*, **22**, 256.
ARDEMAN, S. and CHANARIN, I. (1966). *Gut.*, **7**, 99.
ASHBY, B. S., APPLETON, P. J. and DAWSON, I. (1964). *Brit. med. J.*, **1**, 1141.
ASHWORTH, C. T., DOUGLAS, F. C., REYNOLDS, R. C. and THOMAS, P. T. (1964). *Amer. J. med.* **37**, 481.
AZZOPARDI, J. G. and EVANS, D. J. (1966). *J. Clin. Path.*, **19**, 368.
BADENOCH, J., EVANS, J. R. and RICHARDS, W. C. D. (1957). *Brit. J. Haemat.*, **3**, 175.
BAKER, S. J., IGNATIUS, M., MATHAN, V. I., VAISH, S. K. and CHACKO, C. C. (1962). In: *Ciba Foundation Study Group No. 14. "Intestinal Biopsy"*, p. 84. London: J. and A. Churchill Ltd.
BARDHAN, K. D. In: D. Phil. thesis to be submitted to Oxford University.
BARDHAN, K. D. and WHITEHEAD, R. To be published.
BLUM, A. and SOHAR, E. (1962). *Lancet*, **i**, 721.
BOCK, O. A., RICHARDS, W. C. D. and WITTS, L. J. (1963). *Gut*, **4**, 112.
BODIAN, M. and LAKE, B. D. (1963). *Brit. J. Surg.*, **50**, 702.
BRAS, G., RICHARDS, R. C., IRVINE, R. A., MILNER, P. F. A. and RAGBEER, M. M. S. (1964). *Lancet*, **ii**, 1257.
BRETT, E. M. and BERRY, C. L. (1967). *Brit. med. J.*, **iii**, 400.
BROOKE, B. N. (1959). *Lancet*, **ii**, 745.
BUTZ, W. C. (1960). *Gastroenterology*, **39**, 183.
CALKINS, E. and COHEN, A. S. (1960). *Bull. rheum. Dis.*, **10**, 215.
CAMERON, A. H., ASTLEY, R., HALLOWELL, M., RAWSON, A. B. MILLER, C. G., FRENCH, J. M. and HUBBLE, D. V. (1962). *Quart J. Med.*, **31**, 125.
CAPPER, W. M., LAIDLAW, C. D'A., BUCKLER, K., RICHARDS, D. (1962). *Lancet*, **ii**, 1200.
CHEARS, W. C., Jr. and ASHWORTH, C. T. (1961). *Gastroenterology*, **41**, 129.
GOGHILL, N. F. (1960). *Post-grad. med. J.*, **36**, 733.
GOGHILL, N. F. and WILLIAMS, A. W. (1958). *Proc. Roy. Soc. Med.*, **51**, 464.
COOKE, P. P., NASSIM, J. R. and COLLINS, J. (1959). *Quart, J. Med.*, **28**, 505.
CRANE, C. W. and EVANS, D. W. (1966). *Brit. med. J.*, **ii**, 1575.
CREAMER, B. (1964a). *Brit. med. J.*, **ii**, 1371.
CREAMER, B. (1964b). *Brit. med. J.*, **ii**, 1373.
CREAMER, B. (1964c.) *Brit. med. J.*, **ii**, 1435.

CREAMER, B. and PINK, I. J. (1967). *Lancet*, **i**, 304.
DE PAOLA, D. (1961). *Trop. dis. Bull.*, **59**, 281.
DE PAOLA, D. (1962). *Trop. dis. Bull.*, **60**, 348.
DONIACH, D., ROITT, I. M. and TAYLOR, K. B. (1963), *Brit. med. J*,, **i**, 1374.
DONIACH, D. and SHINER, M. (1957). *Gastroenterology*, **33**, 71.
DOUB, H. P. and SHEA, J. J. (1960). *J. Amer. med. Ass.*, **172**, 1238.
DU PLESSIS, D. J. (1965). *Lancet*, **i**, 974.
EDWARDS, F. C. and COGHILL, N. F. (1966). *Brit. med. J.*, **ii**, 1409.
ELLENBERG, M. and BOOKMAN, J. J. (1960). *Diabetes*, **9**, 14.
ENZINGER, F. M. and HELWIG, E. B. (1963). *Virchows. Arc. path. Anat.*, **336**, 238.
EVANS, J. G. and ACHESON, E. D. (1965). *Gut*, **6**, 311.
FILIPE, M. I. and CORREIA, J. P. (1963). *Gastroenterologia (Basel)*, **100**, 19.
FISHER, J. M. and TAYLOR, K. B. (1965). *New Eng. J. Med.*, **272**, 499.
FLEMMING, W. H., YARDLEY, J. H. and HENDRIX, T. R. (1962). *New Eng. J. Med.*, **267**, 33.
FONE, D. J., COOKE, W. T., MEYNELL, M. J., BREWER, D. B., HARRIS, E. L. and COX, E. V. (1960). *Lancet*, **i**, 933.
FRIEDMAN, M. and HARE, P. J. (1965). *Lancet*, **i**, 521.
FRY, L. T., SHUSTER, S. and McMINN, R. M. H. (1965). *Brit. med. J.*, **i**, 967.
GAFNI, J. and SOHAR, E. (1960). *Amer. J. med. Sci.*, **240**, 332.
GIRDWOOD, R. H., DELAMORE, I. W. and WYNN WILLIAMS, A. (1961). *Brit. med. J.*, **i**, 319.
GLASS, G. B. J., SPEER, F. D., NEIBURGS, H. E., ISHMORI, A., JONES, E. L., BAKER, H., SCHWARTZ,, S. A. and SMITH, R. (1960). *Gastroenterology*, **39**, 429.
GOLDEN, R. (1954). *Amer. J. Roentgenol.*, **72**, 401.
GREEN, P. A., HIGGINS, J. A., BROWN, A. L., Jr., HOFFMAN, H. N. and SOMMERVILLE, R. L. (1961). *Gastroenterology*, **41**, 452.
GRESHAM, G. A., CRUICKSHANK, J. G. and VALENTINE, J. C. (1958). *Nature*, **181**, 538.
GROSS, J. B., WOLLAEGER, E. E., HUIZENGA, K. A., DAHLIN, D. C. and POWER, M. H. (1959). *Gastroenterology*, **36**, 65.
HARRISON, W. J. (1965). *Lancet*, **i**, 1346.
HARRIS-JONES, J. N., SWAN, H. T. and TUDHOPE, G. R. (1957). *Blood*, **12**, 461.
HAUBRICH, W. S., WATSON, J. H. L. and SIERRACKI, J. C. (1960). *Gastroenterology*, **39**, 454.
HAWK, W. A. and TURNBULL, R. B. (1966). *Gastroenterology*, **51**, 802.
HINDLE, W. and CREAMER, B. (1965). *Brit. med. J.*, **ii**, 455.
HOURIHANE, D. O'B. (1963). *Proc. Roy Soc. Med.*, **56**, 1073.
IMERSLUND, O. (1960). *Acta Paediat. Suppl.*, **119**, 1.
IMERSLUND, O. and BJORNSTAD, P. (1963). *Acta Haemat. (Basel)* **30**, 1.
IRVINE, W. J., DAVIES, S. H., DELAMORE, I. W. and WILLIAMS, A. W. (1962). *Brit. med. J.*, **ii**, 454.
JACOBSON, E. D., CHODOS, R. B. and FALCON, W. W. (1960a). *Amer. J. Med.*, **28**, 524.
JACOBSON, E. D., PRIOR, J. T. and Falcon, W. W. (1960b). *J. Lab. clin. Med.* **56**, 245.
JAGER, W. A. DEN HARTOG and BETHLEM, J. (1960). *J. Neurol. Neurosurg. Psychiat.*, **23**, 283.
JAMES, A. H. (1964). *Gut*, **5**, 285.
JANOWITZ, H. D. and PRESENT, D. H. (1966). *Gastroenterology*, **51**, 778.
JOSKE, R. A., FINCKH, E. S. and WOOD, I. J. (1955). *Quart. J. Med.*, **24**, 269.
KEYTING, W. S., McCARVER, R. R., KOVARIK, J. L. and DAYWITT, A. L. (1961). *Radiology*, **76**, 733.
KOSS, L. G. (1952). *Arch. Path.*, **53**, 523.
KUIPERS, F. C., VANTHIEL, P. H. and ROSKAM, E. T. (1960a) *Ned. T. Geneesk*, **104**, 422.
KUIPERS, F. C., VANTHIEL, P. H., RODENBURG, W., WIELINGA, W. J. and ROSKAM, R. T. (1960b). *Lancet*, **ii**, 1171.
KYLE, R. A., SPENCER, R. J. and DAHLIN, D. C. (1966). *Amer. J. med. Sci.*, **251**, 501.
LAMY, M., NEZELOF, C., JOS, J. FREZAL, J. and REY, J. (1963). *Pr. med.*, **71**, 1267.
LAWSON, H. H. (1964). *Lancet*, **1**, 469.
LILLIBRIDGE, C. B., BRANDBORG, L. L. and RUBIN, C. E. (1967). *Gastroenterology*, **52**, 792.
LILLIE, R. D. and GEER, J. C. (1965). *Amer. J. Path.*, **47**, 965.
LOCKHART MUMMERY, H. E. and MORSON, B. C. (1960). *Gut*, **1**, 87.
LOCKHART MUMMERY, H. E. and MORSON, B. C. (1964). *Gut*, **5**, 493.
MACKAY, I. R. and HISLOP, I. G. (1966). *Gut*, 228.
McKENDRICK, T. (1962). *Lancet*, **i**, 183.
MAGNUS, H. A. (1958). *J. Clin. Path.*, **11**, 289.
MARKS, J., SHUSTER, S. and WATSON, A. J. (1966). *Lancet*, **ii**, 1280.
MILLER, G. A. H. and BAMFORTH, J. (1962). *Brit. med. J.*, **i**, 1661.
MISSMAHL, H. P. and HARTWIG, M. (1953). *Virchows. Arch. path. Anat.*, **324**, 489.
MISTILIS, S. P., SKYRING, A. P. and STEPHEN, D. D. (1965). *Lancet*, **i**, 77.
MONTGOMERY, P. O'B. and MUIRHEAD, E. E. (1954). *Amer. J. Path.*, **30**, 521.
MORSON, B. C. (1955). *Brit. J. Cancer*, **9**, 365.

PARKINS, R. A., EIDELMAN, S., RUBIN, C. E., DOBBINS, W. O. and PHELPS, P. C. (1963). *Lancet*, **ii,** 851.
POMERANTZ, M. and WALDMANN, T. A. (1963). *Gastroenterology*, **45,** 703.
RHODES, J. (1964). *Gut*, **5,** 454.
RINGSTED, J. (1960). *Med. Bull. Nat. Med. Cen.*, **i,** 103.
ROSS, J. R. (1965). *Amer. J. Gastroent.*, **43,** 285.
RUBIN, C. E. and DOBBINS, W. O. (1965). *Gastroenterology*, **49,** 676.
RUBIN, C. E., BRANDBORG, L. L., FLICK, A. L., PHELPS, P. C., PARMENTIER, C. and VAN NIEL, S. (1962). *Gastroenterology*, **43,** 621.
SALEM, S. N. and TRUELOVE, S. C. (1964). *Brit. med. J.*, **i,** 1074.
SALEM, S. N., TRUELOVE, S. C. and RICHARDS, W. C. D. (1964). *Brit. med. J.* **i,** 394.
SALT, H. B., WOLFF, O. H., LLOYD, J. K., FOSBROOKE, A. S., CAMERON, A. H. and HUBBLE, D. V. (1960). *Lancet*, **ii,** 325.
SCHEIN, J. (1947). *Gastroenterology*, **8,** 438.
SCHWACHMAN, H. and ANTONOWICZ, I. (1962). *Ann. N.Y. Acad. Sci.*, **93,** 600.
SHEEHY, T. W., ARTENSTEIN, M. S. and GREEN, R. W. (1964). *J .Amer. med. Ass.*, **190,** 1023
SHEEHY, T. W., MERONEY, W. H., COX, R. S., Jr. and SOLER, J. E. (1962). *Gastroenterology*, **42,** 148.
SHINER, M. (1965). In: *The Small Intestine. A Symposium of the 5th Congress of the Iner-national Academy of Pathology*, Oxford: Blackwell. p. 16.
SHINER, M. and DONIACH, I. (1957). *Gastroenterology*, **32,** 313.
SHINER, M. and DRURY, R. A. B. (1962). *Amer. J. dig. Dis.*, **7,** 744.
SLEISENGER, M. H., ALMY, T. P. and BARR, D. P. (1953). *Amer. J. Med.*, **15,** 666.
TAFT, L. I., LIDDELOW, A. G. and RALSON, M. (1959). *Aust. Ann., Med.*, **8,** 129.
TOFFLER, A. H., HUKILL, P. B. and SPIRO, H. M. (1963). *Ann. intern. Med.*, **58,** 872.
TOWNLEY, R. R. W., CASS, M. H. and ANDERSON, C. M. (1964). *Gut*, **5,** 51.
TRIER, J. S., PHELPS, P. C., EIDELMAN, S. and RUBIN, C. E. (1965). *Gastroenterology*, **48,** 684.
VASSAR, P. S. and CULLING, C. F. A. (1959). *Arch. Path.*, **68,** 487.
WALDMANN, T. A., STEINFELD,, J. L., DUTCHER, T. F., DAVIDSON, J. D. and GORDON, R. S. Jr. (1961). *Gastroenterology*, **41,** 197.
WATSON, A. J. and ROY, A. D. (1960). *J. Path. Bact.*, **80,** 309.
WATSON, A. J., WATSON, J. W. and WALKER, F. C. (1965a) *Amer. J. Path.*, **46,** 553.
WATSON, W. C., PATON, E. and MURRAY, D. (1965b). *Lancet*, **ii,** 47.
WELLS, C. (1952). *Ann. Coll. Surg.*, **11,** 105.
WILSON, S. and THOMPSON, A. E. (1964). *J. Path. Bact.*, **87,** 169.
WRIGHT, A. W. (1930). *Amer, J. Path.*, **6,** 87.
WRIGHT, R., WHITEHEAD, R., WANGEL, A. C., SALEM, S. N. and SCHULLER, K. F. R. (1966.) *Lancet*, **i,** 618.
YARDLEY, J. H. and HENDRIX, T. R. (1961). *Bull. Johns Hopkins Hosp.* **109,** 80.
YARNIS, H., MARSHAK, R. H. and CROHN, B. B. (1957). *J. Am. med. Ass.*, **164,** 7.

Chapter 22

QUANTITATIVE METHODS IN HISTOLOGY

M. S. DUNNILL

MORBID anatomy, although it claims to be the oldest branch of pathology, is the last of its disciplines to embrace measurement as one of its routine methods. Hæmatologists have been expressing their results in a quantitative manner for many years. Methods for measuring the amount of hæmoglobin and the numbers of erythrocytes and leucocytes in the blood were in use at the beginning of the century. Until recently, apart from measurement of certain linear dimensions with micrometer eye-pieces, little quantitative morphological data have been available. However, simple and accurate methods are available for the measurement of volumes of tissue components, estimation of the internal surface area of certain organs, e.g. the alveolar surface area in the lung, and the determination of the numbers of structures in an organ. Eranko (1954) gives an excellent account of earlier work in this field and Weibel (1963a) has written in a most comprehensive manner of the principles underlying many of the methods in use.

METHODS OF PREPARATION

The normal procedure at autopsy is to weigh the organs and then to slice them in order to obtain blocks of tissue to place in fixative for subsequent histological examination. This method is, in general, inappropriate for the purpose of quantitative histological analysis which requires that organs be fixed intact, their volume measured before and after fixation, and blocks selected by a suitable sampling method (*vide infra*). In certain cases special fixation procedures are needed. Thus, in the lung, inflation methods must be used and in this connection the formalin steam method of Weibel and Vidone (1961) is particularly useful. In other organs, for instance in the kidney, fixation by vascular perfusion may be indicated. These methods are simple, provided care is taken at the time of autopsy to remove the organ without damaging it in any way, and to leave a long vascular pedicle so that suitable cannulæ can be inserted.

VOLUME DETERMINATION

Measurement of the volume of the organ both before and after fixation is important in order that any shrinkage occurring during fixation can be estimated. It is necessary to make this measurement in every case as there is an individual variability, depending upon the disease process and the age of the patient. Simple water displacement methods are suitable for most organs. In those instances where the organ is too small for an accurate estimate to be made by water displacement, e.g. the pituitary, or where, as in the emphysematous lung, it is likely to undergo compression and deformation, volume determination can be accomplished using Simpson's rule. Adams, Daniel, Prichard and Venables (1963) used this method for measuring the volume of the pituitary gland and it has also been used for the measurement of fixed lung volume (Dunnill, 1964). To carry out this procedure, the organ is cut into slices of equal thickness. The area of one face of each slice is measured. In the lung the simplest way of accomplishing this is to lay each slice on a sheet of clean paper, trace its outline, and measure the area with a planimeter. With smaller organs, such as the pituitary, sections of the organ taken at given but equal intervals are projected, at suitable magnification, on to a screen, the outline is traced and the area measured as above. If n slices are taken and the area of each slice is A_0, A_1, A_2 . . ., then the volume of the organ, V, is given by

$$V = \tfrac{1}{3}h[(A_0 + A_n) + 4(A_1 + A_3 + \ldots A_{n-1}) + 2(A_2 + A_4 + \ldots A_{n-2})] \quad (1)$$

where h is the slice thickness. This gives an extremely good approximation of the actual volume and is at least as satisfactory as the method of water displacement.

Differential Volumetry

It is the difficulty encountered in measuring the volume of components making up an organ which has delayed much advance in quantitative pathology. Thus, at first sight, it appears a very difficult task to measure, for instance, the volume of the renal cortex or the volume of the blood vessels and bronchi in a lung. These difficulties are similar to the problems which have beset geologists for many years when making a quantitative analysis of the mineral content of rock: "If a field sample of rock is examined it can be seen to be made up of different kinds of particles. These are not mixtures; rather each is a distinct homogenous substance with definite chemical and physical characteristics. Some particles may be dull, earthy grains; others may be tiny brilliant flakes that reflect sunlight; and still others may be dense, transparent grains that resemble bits of glass" (Emmons et al., 1960). Each of these particles is a mineral and the geologist has the task of determining what are the relative volumes of each mineral in a given sample of rock. This problem was first approached successfully by the French geologist and mathematician Delesse in 1848. He annunciated a theorem which states that: "In a rock, composed of a number of minerals, the area occupied by any given mineral on a surface of a section of the rock is proportional to the volume of the mineral in the rock". This theorem is equally applicable to tissues and organs in biology and the task of differential volume determination thus resolves itself into the determination of areas, or ratios of areas, of various components on a cut surface.

Several methods are available for this type of area measurement. In the last century Delesse himself, Sorby and Charles Darwin traced the components seen on the cut surface of a rock on to paper. The paper over each component was then cut out and weighed, the weight for each component being proportional to its area. This method has been used recently by Restrepo and Heard (1963) to assess the mucous gland volume in normal bronchi and in cases of chronic bronchitis. Rosiwal (1898) introduced a system of linear sampling in which a series of lines are placed, preferably at random, across a section, or cut surface, and the length of line on each component measured. The total fractional length of line traversing the given component is proportional to the area of that component on the section whereas the total length of all the lines is proportional to the total area.

These methods are tedious, not always free from bias and difficult to use on gross anatomical and pathological specimens (Dunnill, 1962). A simpler procedure, which overcomes all these difficulties, is point sampling. This depends upon the fact that if a number of random points are placed on the section, or surface, of a composite substance, the number of points falling on each component is proportional to the area of the component on the surface and thus, from the Delesse theorem, to the volume of the component. In Figure 1, if N points are cast at random on the entire area of the square, A_t, and n points fall on the hatched area, A_s, it follows that

$$\frac{A_s}{A_t} = \frac{n}{N} \tag{2}$$

In practice, truly random points are not used; instead a grid, drawn on transparent plastic material, is employed. The grid is placed at random on the surface and thus sampling is systematic with a random start. Usually a grid with points placed at the angles of equilateral triangles is used. This method has the advantage that it is accurate, simple to use, independent of the shape of the components and applicable to organs of considerable complexity. It is important, in defining the components to be estimated, to make sure that together they make up the whole volume of the organ.Thus, in the kidney all points would have to be allocated, for instance, to the cortex, medulla or pelvis. Similarly, in the emphysematous lung the components would be defined as non-parenchyma, consisting of conducting blood vessels and airways down to $0 \cdot 1$ cm. in diameter, normal parenchyma and abnormal or emphysematous parenchyma.

In using this method it is desirable to know: (1) how many points it is necessary to count in order to achieve any given degree of accuracy and, (2) whether it is necessary to examine several slices of an organ or just one slice in order to obtain an accurate estimate of the volume proportions in the organ as a whole.

In answer to the first point it should be noted that the standard error, r, of a component on a surface is given by the equation

$$r = \sqrt{\frac{A(100-A)}{N}} \tag{3}$$

where A is the percentage of points lying on the component and N is the total number of points counted. From this equation two important conclusions can be drawn: (i) the smaller the proportion to be estimated, the larger the number of points that must be counted for a given standard error; (ii) since the error depends on the reciprocal of the square root of the number of observations, if it is desired to halve the standard error it is necessary to count four times the number of points. In order to assess the number of points that it is necessary to count, that is, the type of grid spacing to use,

N

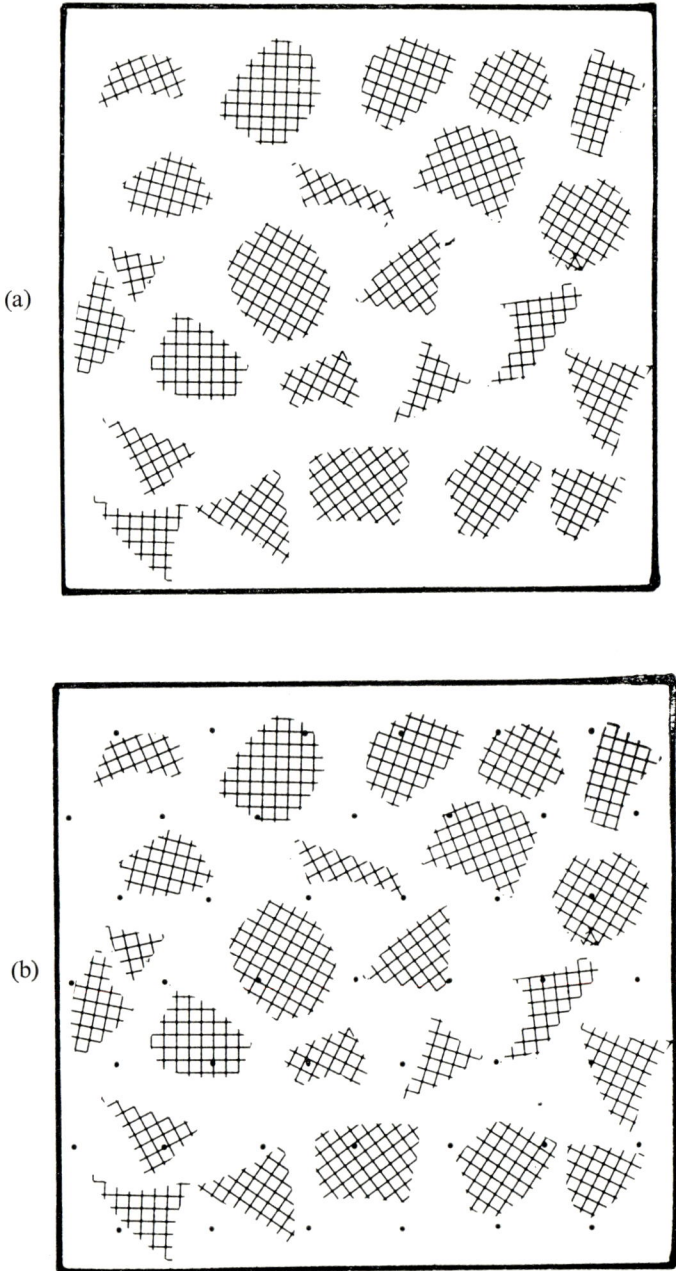

FIG. 1. The proportion of the square occupied by the hatched segments in (a) can be determined by placing a point-counting grid over the entire square as in (b). The points in this case are arranged at the angles of equilateral triangles. The number of points falling on the hatched segments is then proportional to their total area. In this example the hatched segments account for approximately one-third of the total area.

the graph shown in Figure 2, in which the percentage standard error is plotted against the proportion of the component to be assessed, is of value. Details of the errors involved in this method have been discussed by Anderson and Dunnill (1965).

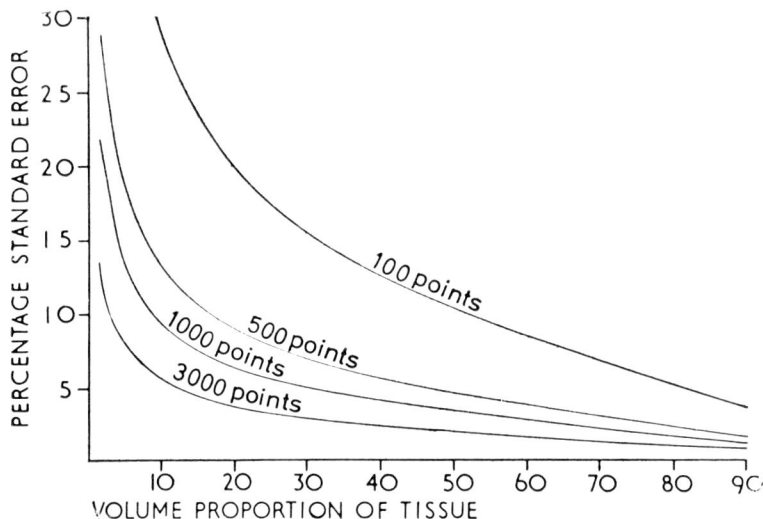

FIG. 2. A series of graphs showing the relationship between the total number of points sampled, the percentage volume of tissue estimated, and the percentage standard error of the estimate. (Reproduced by permission of the editors of *Thorax*.)

In answer to the second point, it can be shown that in the case of most organs there is a significant difference between slices indicating that the distribution of the components, of the organs, and indeed of disease processes, is by no means homogenous.

SAMPLING FOR HISTOLOGICAL ANALYSIS

In normal organs there may be few sampling problems as the parenchyma is fairly uniform, apart from a region near the hilum where the large conducting vessels and ducts predominate. In a diseased organ, such as the emphysematous lung, uniformity may be strikingly absent. It might be possible in this type of case to examine the entire organ histologically, but the labour, time and expense of this procedure render it expedient to select blocks of tissue of moderate dimensions and to submit these to detailed histological analysis. It is an important premise that the selection of these blocks must ensure that they give a representative picture of the whole organ, not just of the "interesting" areas.

Two methods are available. The first is a systematic sampling, and this involves taking blocks of tissue at given intervals throughout the lung. Its main disadvantage is that, if the diseased areas have a similar type of arrangement to the sampling pattern, the sample will be unrepresentative of the organ as a whole, and any results deduced from such samples will be wide of the true state of affairs. The second method is random sampling—that is, the selection of samples by means of a random number table. This method has the property of securing a small group of blocks of tissue possessing the same characteristics of the entire organ, i.e. the same proportion in which each special feature is present or absent. The method used, for instance in the lung, employs a transparent grid with squares of side 1 cm. The squares are numbered. The grid is placed over each slice of lung and blocks of tissue are selected by means of a random number table. In fact this is a method of stratified random sampling as slices are taken at regular intervals throughout the lung. The grid shown in Figure 3 has holes punched at the corners of the squares so that pins can be inserted into the organ at the appropriate points given by the random number table. In selecting blocks of tissue a convention is used that the pins are placed at the top left-hand corner of the block to be

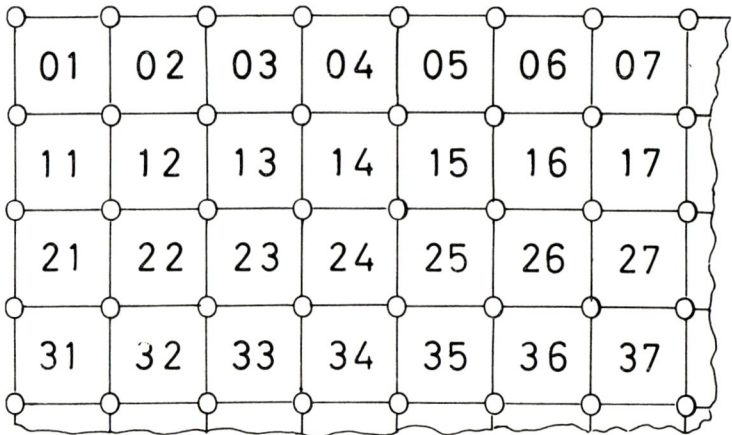

FIG. 3 A portion of a grid used for stratified random sampling. The length of the sides of the squares can be varied according to the size of the organ being investigated. The perforations at the corners of the squares should be large enough to admit a pin head.

selected. In sampling tissue it is important to avoid ragged or oblique angled blocks. The area of the face of each block which is to be cut is measured carefully. A block measuring approximately $2 \cdot 0 \times 1 \cdot 0 \times 0 \cdot 5$ cm. is convenient. The blocks of tissue are processed in the usual manner, embedded in paraffin wax and sections cut at 5 μ thickness. The area of each section is measured. The ratio of the area of the fixed block face to the area of the corresponding sections gives a measure, p^2, of the area shrinkage that occurs during processing. From this, values for linear shrinkage, p, and volume shrinkage, p^3, are easily calculated. The reciprocals of these values can be used to convert measurements made on processed tissues into values representative of fresh tissues.

Sampling of Histological Sections

In all the methods described below, which involve measurements on histological sections, similar problems of sampling arise. A comparable method of stratified random sampling can be employed in these cases.

Suitable microscopical fields can be selected by employing a six-digit random number table as a map reference for the micrometer gauges on the mechanical stage of the microscope. It is easier to select the first field in a random manner, and, by moving the mechanical stage a given distance, subsequent fields can be chosen systematically. It is usually sufficient to count ten fields for each slide (Dunnill, 1964).

In order to ascertain how many samples to take in any given case, the construction of a summation average graph is of great value. Figure 4 shows such a graph constructed for alveolar transections in a normal lung. The

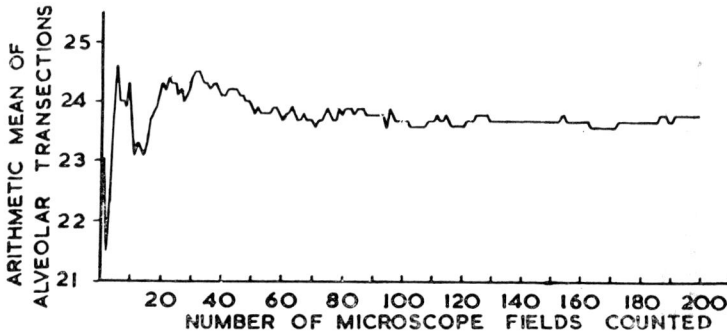

Fig. 4. A summation average graph plotted for alveolar transections of the normal lung. It can be seen that after 50 fields have been counted, i.e. five slides, the mean varies very little. (Reproduced by permission of the editors of *Thorax*.)

mean is calculated after each reading and at first it fluctuates a great deal, but after 50 or so readings, that is, after examination of five blocks with ten fields chosen from each section, the mean remains relatively steady and further readings will only alter it very slightly, if at all. At this point sufficient samples have been taken. A detailed evaluation of this method of sampling has been given elsewhere (Dunnill, 1964).

QUANTITATIVE ANALYSIS OF HISTOLOGICAL SECTIONS

Volume determination depends upon the Delesse principle which has already been discussed. There are two types of integrating eyepiece available for this work. The first uses the linear integration principle of Rosiwal (1898). This eyepiece is made by Leitz, and allows the procedure of linear integration —that is, measuring the sum of the portions of random lines lying on given components of tissue seen in histological sections—to be performed with comparative ease. The method is discussed very fully by Weibel (1963a) and there is no doubt that it gives very accurate results if only a small amount of tissue is available for analysis. Unfortunately it is very tedious if used for a large number of samples.

The second method depends on the point-counting principle already mentioned, and this was first employed in histology by Chalkley (1943). The original eyepiece designed by him had only four points, but Zeiss have produced one with 25 points (Hennig, 1958) placed at the angles of equilateral triangles (Fig. 5). This is a more precise procedure than that used on the gross specimen and different parameters are evaluated. Thus, in the renal cortex it is possible to determine the proportions of the volume occupied by the glomeruli, the tubules, the interstitial tissue and the blood vessels. The position of each point in the eyepiece is recorded according to which constituent it lies in on the histological section. A hand-operated counting device of the type used for differential blood counts has the advantage that results can be written down every 100 or 500 points instead of the laborious procedure of recording on paper the position of each point as it is observed. The entire section can be covered with about 500 points if the low-power objective is used. The objective chosen will depend upon what is required. Chalkley used this method for determining nuclear cytoplasmic ratios and for this purpsoe a high power P1 40 (Leitz) objective, or even an oil immersion

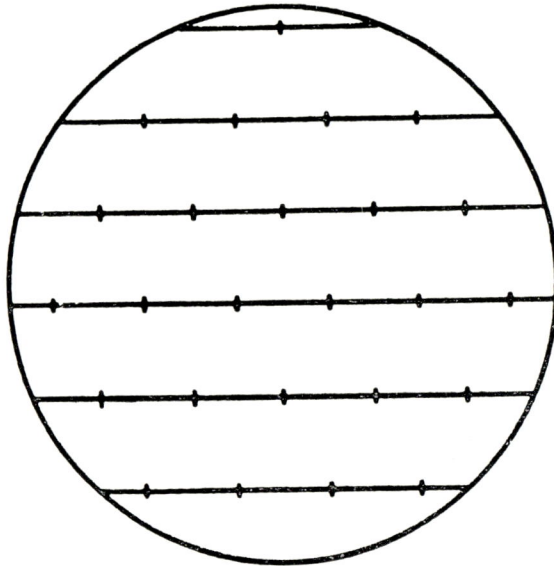

Fig. 5. The Zeiss I integrating eyepiece.

lens, is needed. At the higher powers of the microscope, plane objectives must be used as spherical aberration introduces significant errors. Corrections must be made for section thickness as described below.

The method of point-counting is of great value because it is simple, rapid, independent of the shapes of the various components, and its errors are easy to assess (Anderson and Dunnill, 1964).

Internal surface area estimation of complex randomly distributed structures, such as pulmonary alveoli, by the mean linear intercept method was first developed by Short (1950–51) but was also arrived at independently by Campbell and Tomkeieff (1952) and by Hennig (1956). The method depends upon the fact that if a line of known length is cast at random on a section of tissue it will be intersected a number of times by the component whose surface area is required; the mean distance between the intersections is termed the mean linear intercept, L_m. The surface area of the component can be shown to be inversely proportional to the mean linear intercept.

In practice, lines of known length are placed at random on histological sections. Crossed hair-lines can be used, but there is a special Zeiss integrating eyepiece available (Fig. 6). Any deformation which may occur in cutting and processing the sections can be compensated for by using the eyepiece in two positions at right angles to one another on any one microscope field. The

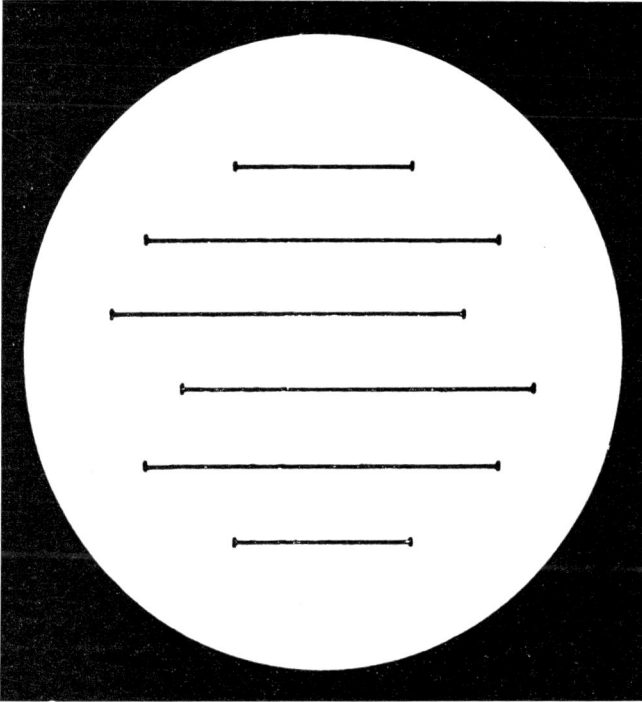

FIG. 6. The Zeiss II integrating eyepiece.

fields are selected on each histological section by the method of the sampling described above. The total number of intercepts, m, is counted. The mean linear intercept is then calculated from the total length of line in the eyepiece, L, and N the number of fields examined from

$$L_m = \frac{NL}{m}$$
(4)

The surface area, S, of the component is then given by

$$S = \frac{2V}{L_m}$$
(5)

where V is the volume of the processed parenchyma of the organ under examination. This value for the surface area has to be corrected for the shrinkage which occurs during processing and fixation.

Estimation of the number of particles in a given volume from counting the number of transections of the particles on a section has been one of the difficulties which has provided a great drawback to the quantitative approach to histology. Figure 7 illustrates the difficulty, showing that, in a histological section of finite thickness, portions of the particles, as well as whole particles, will be counted. The number of fragments of particles increases when the section thickness decreases, and when it is less than the diameter of the particles only portions of particles will be present. The actual number of particles per unit volume will thus always be smaller than the number

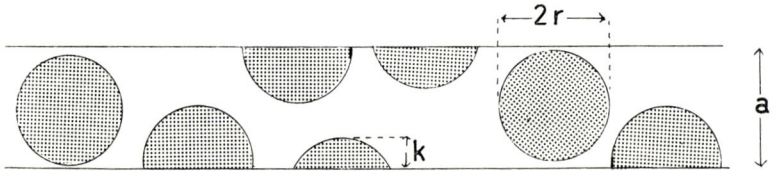

FIG. 7. A diagrammatic view of a histological section of finite thickness, a. It can be seen that in counting the number of structures in the section an overestimate will be made because portions of particles, as well as whole particles, will be counted. The notation refers to the Floderus formula for correcting this error (see text).

deduced from counting the sections. Floderus (1944) gives a formula for obtaining the number of particles, N, in a unit volume providing the particles are spherical and randomly distributed:

$$N = \frac{an}{a + 2r - k} \tag{6}$$

where a = the section thickness in μ, r = radius of the particles, k = the vertical height of the smallest particle in μ, and n = the number of particles counted per c.cm. of tissue.

Weibel and Gomez (1962), using the principle of Delesse, have recently provided a very elegant solution to this problem which has been expanded by Weibel (1963). They have shown that the number, N, of structures in a unit volume is given by

$$N = \frac{n^{3/2} K}{\beta \rho^{\frac{1}{2}}} \tag{7}$$

where n = the number of transections of the structures in a unit area, β = a dimensionless coefficient depending solely on the shape of the structures, ρ = the volume of proportion of the structures, and K = a distribution coefficient which is $\left(\dfrac{D_3}{D_1}\right)^{3/2}$, where D_1 and D_3 are the first and third moments of the distribution of the characteristic linear dimension, D, of the structure.

Weibel (1963a) gives a series of values of β for various commonly shaped bodies; for a sphere the value is 1·382. It is important that the structures be randomly distributed, that they have a well-defined shape, that their size distribution is such that the largest body is small compared to the total containing volume, and that the sections which are counted are very thin compared with the smallest dimension of the structure. The error involved in neglecting the distribution coefficient, K, is probably small where the distribution of the characteristic linear dimension of the structures is not very widespread. Thus, in the glomeruli in the kidney, Weibel found a value for K of 1·014 which gives an error of 1·4 per cent if K is neglected, and this is not significant.

Measurement of diameter of structures should be performed on sections which are the same thickness as, or thicker than, the structures being examined (Eranko, 1954). It is necessary for the central portion of the structure to be included in the section and this can be ascertained by focusing from the upper surface of the slide to the under surface of the cover-slip, and observing the diameter of the structure to increase and then decrease. The largest cross-sectional diameter is then estimated. Using this method a large number of structures can be measured and the frequency distribution of diameters constructed. If the structures are all spheres of the same size, then the true diameter, D, can be calculated from the mean diameter, D', of the transections of the spheres on thin histological sections, or on a surface, as

$$D = \frac{4D'}{\pi} \tag{8}$$

Measurement of individual cell volume may sometimes be of importance. In this connection the work of D. T. Chalkley (1953) is relevant. He used the fact that the shape of cells in compact tissues, such as the liver, approaches that of a regular 14-sided polygon or tetrakaidecahedron. In sections of such cells the only easily measured dimension is the mean chord length or mean linear intercept. He showed that in such an organ the mean volume of a cell, v, is given by

$$v = 2 \cdot 34 c^2 \tag{9}$$

where c is the mean chord length. The main criticism of this method lies in the fact that corrections must be made, the mean chord length being of the same order of magnitude as the section thickness, and thus considerable errors, due to spherical aberration, may occur.

Estimating Blood Vessel Surface Area and Length. A method for estimating blood vessel surface area and length in tissue has been given by Haynes (1964). The total volume of the vessels, V, is estimated by the point-counting method already described. The diameters of the vessels are then measured and arranged in classes in the following manner:

Diameters	$d_1 \ d_2 \ d_3 \ d_4 \ \ldots d_K$
Number of vessels	$n_1 \ n_2 \ n_3 \ n_4 \ \ldots n_K$

The proportion of vessels in the ith class is defined by

$$Pi = \frac{n_i}{\Sigma n_i} \tag{10}$$

then the estimate of the total length of blood vessels, L, in the tissue is given by

$$L = \frac{4V}{\pi \Sigma p_i d_i^2} \tag{11}$$

The total surface area of the vessels, A, is given by

$$A = 4V \left(\frac{\Sigma p_i d_i}{\Sigma p_i d_i^2} \right) \qquad (12)$$

This method has been used for estimating the total length of blood vessels and their surface area in tumour tissue.

Surface to volume ratios can be determined by using a combination of the point-counting and the linear intercept methods. This was originally described by Chalkley, Cornfield and Park (1949). They showed that if a line of known length, L, was cast at random on a composite structure and the number of times, h, the end-points of the line fell inside the structures, together with the number of times the line intercepted the perimeter of the structures, c, was recorded, then it followed that

$$\frac{rh}{c} = 4 \frac{\text{volume}}{\text{surface}} \qquad (13)$$

If a given space contained numerous structures of different volumes and surfaces then it followed that

$$\frac{rh}{c} = 4 \frac{\text{sum of the volumes}}{\text{sum of the surface areas}} \qquad (14)$$

Weibel, Kistler and Scherle (1966) have devised a multi-purpose graticule composed of short linear probes arranged in an equilateral triangular network so that this estimation can be performed with ease.

Measurement of section thickness is difficult to perform with accuracy, not only due to lack of a simple method but also because of lack of uniformity in the thickness of most histological sections. A rough approximation can be obtained from the microtome reading at the time of section cutting. Simple optical methods have been described of which the easiest, but least accurate, is to focus on the lower surface of the cover-slip and then on the upper surface of the slide, the distance travelled by the microscope stage being equal to the section thickness and being read on the micrometer attached to the fine adjustment. Methods have been described which are dependent on refractive index differences (Casperson, 1956) and interference methods (Richards, 1947).

APPLICATIONS

Lung

Until quite recently the emphasis in work on chronic non-specific lung disease has been on defining the terms chronic bronchitis and emphysema, and on classifying these diseases. The description of centrilobular emphysema (Leopold and Gough, 1956) was a notable landmark, as was the quantitative assessment of chronic bronchitis by Reid (1960). This work was well summarized by a Ciba Symposium on the classification of these diseases, published in *Thorax* (1960).

In pathophysiological circles there was increasing dissatisfaction with such phrases as "a considerable amount of emphysema" or "the emphysema was mainly of the centrilobular type", and there was a demand for a more quantitative approach. Pulmonary physiologists were among the first to take an interest in the morphometric techniques given by Weibel (1963b), who described for the first time many of the parameters in normal lung. In pathological material, the point-counting technique for gross specimens affords a simple, quick and accurate method whereby the volume of abnormal and normal lung parenchyma and the volume of conducting tissues can be determined (Dunnill, 1965). The more sophisticated techniques of counting the number of alveoli and measuring the alveolar surface area have also been used (Dunnill, 1965; Hicken, Heath and Brewer, 1966a, 1966b). It has been clearly shown that there is no simple direct relationship between either the volume of emphysema or between the internal surface area of the lung and the weight of the right ventricle, suggesting that obliteration of the pulmonary capillary bed is not a major factor in the ætiology of *cor pulmonale*. In this disease any attempt at clinicopathological correlation requires careful quantitative assessment of both the clinical and pathological processes.

Up to the present the lack of positive results has been a little disappointing but this is due to the fact that in emphysema, in addition to the volume and number of abnormal air spaces it is necessary to measure their distribution, and there is at the moment no satisfactory simple method of quantifying this parameter. However, it is well to bear in mind that, as Melville Arnott has stated: "The real function of structural and functional concepts occurs only on the basis of mathematics".

Bone

In the assessment of bone biopsy material, quantitative techniques are likely to prove of immediate value. Bone disease is often defined in quantitative terms; thus osteoporosis is a condition in which there is a deficiency of osteoid, but little histological information is available on the normal volume of osteoid tissue, or of bone, at the various sites which are selected for biopsy. Recently Dunnill, Anderson and Whitehead (1967), using a point-counting method, estimated the volume of bone, hæmopoietic marrow and fatty marrow in the body of the second lumbar vertebra in 95 normal subjects suffering a traumatic death and aged 10 to 90 years. The volume proportion of bone remained constant from childhood until the third decade, when there was a decrease with advancing age. These normal subjects were compared with a group of cases diagnosed clinically as suffering from osteoporosis and there was a considerable overlap between the two groups, although the mean value for the volume proportion of bone in the osteoporotic cases was lower. It was suggested that rather than making a hard and fast distinction between normal and diseased bone it would be more logical to give a numerical value for the volume proportion of bone in a given biopsy site. In addition it was shown that iliac crest samples did not give an acceptable quantitative indication of the percentage volume of bone, hæmopoietic or fatty marrow in the vertebra, which was somewhat disappointing in view of the popularity of this site for biopsy.

Garner and Ball (1966) have reported the results of quantitative observations on bone in chronic renal azotæmia and in the intestinal malabsorption syndrome, also using point-counting, on samples consisting of undecalcified sections of bone taken from the iliac crest. They found a normal range for total bone volume to be 12·3 to 24·7 per cent. They defined osteoporosis as a value less than 12·3 per cent, values greater than 24·7 per cent indicating osteosclerosis. The normal range for osteoid was 0·47 per cent and for the proportion of bone which was mineralized, 97·9 to 99·6 per cent. In cases diagnosed as osteomalacia, the amount of osteoid was greater than 1·0 per cent and the mineralized bone less than 90 per cent. The malabsorption syndromes were associated with a gross reduction in both the mineralized bone mass and the total bone mass; cases with simple osteoporosis were sometimes found. Azotæmic renal disease with osteomalacia was characterized by an increased total bone mass, the mineralized bone being within normal limits; osteoporosis was not encountered.

The Placenta

The placenta is an organ which lends itself admirably to a quantitative anatomical approach. The nutrition of the fœtus is dependent on the integrity of the placenta and any assessment of pathological change requires objective measurement of the degree of damage or deficiency. Thus, in instances where the fœtus is abnormally small for dates the placenta may appear qualitatively normal but show striking quantitative changes on histological examination, The same is often true of a fœtus born to a mother suffering from hypertension. though here there may be infarction of the placental parenchyma or excess intervillous fibrin disposition. Until recently rather tedious planimetric methods have been used to determine the chorionic villous surface area. Results in a normal placenta have varied from 6·5 sq. m. (Dodds, 1922–23) to 14·7 sq. m. (Dees-Mattingly, 1936). More recently the much quicker and more accurate methods of point counting and mean linear intercept determination have been applied to the problem of normal and abnormal placental anatomy by Aherne and Dunnill (1966a, 1966b). They showed that in normal placentas at term the mean value for the chorionic villous surface area was 11·0 sq. m. In infarcted placentas associated with maternal hypertension it was significantly lower at 8·4 sq. m., and in placentas associated with normotensive pregnancies, but abnormally small infants, it was 6·4 sq. m. In contrast to this, in cases of hæmolytic disease of the newborn, the villous surface area was considerably greater than normal and this was not due merely to œdema. In all cases, whether normal or abnormal, there was a highly significant correlation between chorionic villous surface area and the infant's birth weight. There was some evidence that stunting of fœtal growth was due to primary placental hypoplasia. The mean proportion by volume of the intervillous space and of the chorionic tissue, including fœtal capillaries, did not differ significantly from normal in any of the abnormal placentas, though the absolute volumes varied considerably. It was possible, using morphometric methods, to show that in normal placentas new villi were formed right up until term.

No pathological examination of the placenta is really complete without measurement of the placental volume, the chorionic villous surface area and the volume proportions of the intervillous space, villous tissue and villous capillaries.

The Kidney

In view of the frequency of percutaneous renal biopsy in clinical practice, it is somewhat surprising that quantitative methods have not been applied in this field to any great extent. In diseases of a focal nature, such as chronic pyelonephritis, there are considerable sampling difficulties which cannot be easily overcome without multiple biopsies which are obviously impractical. Quantitative methods might, however, have much to offer in studying the progress of renal disease in serial biopsies. Little quantitative information is available on the normal kidney, but recently Elias and Hennig (1967) have published a comprehensive article on the stereology of the normal renal glomerulus. This may well form the basis of work on abnormal glomeruli, and on the remainder of the renal parenchyma in both normal and abnormal kidneys.

In conclusion, it must be noted that if the work of the clinical histo-pathologist is to be related, in meaningful terms, to that of the clinical physiologist then his observations must be made in a truly quantitative manner. The words of Lord Kelvin, spoken in 1883, are of significance here: "I often say that when you can measure what you are speaking about and express it in numbers you know something about it; but when you cannot express it in numbers your knowledge is of a meagre and unsatisfactory kind; it may be the beginning of knowledge, but you have scarcely, in your thoughts, advanced to the stage of science".

ADDENDUM

After this chapter was written an excellent paper, by W. A. Aherne, on counting discrete structures in microscopical sections, was published in the *Journal of the Royal Microscopical Society* (1967), **87**, 493.

References

ADAMS, J. H. DANIEL, P. M., PRICHARD, M. M. L. and VENABLES, P. H. (1965). *J. Physiol.*, **166**, 37 P.
AHERNE, W. A. and DUNNILL, M. S. (1966a). *J. Path. Bact.*, **91**, 123.
AHERNE, W. A. and DUNNILL, M. S. (1966b). *Brit. med. Bull.*, **22**, 5.
ANDERSON, J. A. and DUNNILL, M. S. (1965). *Thorax*, **20**, 462.
CAMPBELL, H. and TOMKIEFF, S. I. (1952), *Nature (Lond).*, **170**, 117.
CASPERSON, T. O. (1950). *Cell Growth and Cell Function: A Cytochemical Study*. New York and London.
CHALKLEY, D. T. (1953). *Science*, **118**, 599.
CHALKLEY, H. W. (1943). *J. Nat. Cancer Inst.*, **4**, 47.
CHALKLEY, H. W., CORNFIELD, J. and PARK, H. (1949). *Science*, **110**, 295.
DEES-MATTINGLY, M. (1936). *Amer. J. Anat.*, **59**, 485.
DELESSE, A. (1848). *Annls. Mines*, **13**, 378.
DODDS, G. S. (1922-23). *Anat. Rec.*, **24**, 287.
DUNNILL, M. S. (1962.) *Thorax*, **17**, 320.
DUNNILL, M. S. (1964). *Thorax*, **19**, **443**.
DUNNILL, M. S. (1965). *Med. thorac.*, **22**, 261.
DUNNILL, M. S., ANDERSON, J. A. and WHITEHEAD, R. (1967). *J. Path. Bact.*, **93**, 275.
ELIAS, H. and HENNIG, A. (1967). In *Quantitative Methods in Morphology*, p. 130. Ed. E. R. Weibel and H. Elias. Berlin and New York.
EMMONS, W. H., ALLISON, I. S., STAUFFER, C. R. and THEIL, G. A. (1960). In *Geology: Principles and Progresses*. McGraw Hill, New York and London.
ERÄNKÖ, O. (1954). *Quantitative Methods in Histology and Microscopic Histochemistry*. Basel and New York.
FLODERUS, S. (1944). *Acta. Pathol. Microbiol. Scand., Suppl.* **53**, 93.
GARNER, A. and BALL, J. (1966). *J. Path. Bact.*, **91**, 545.
HAYNES, J. D. (1964). *Nature (Lond.)*, **201**, 425.
HENNIG, A. (1956). *Microskopie*, **11**, 1.
HENNIG, A. (1958). *Zeiss-Werkz.*, **6**, 78.
HICKEN, P., BREWER, D. and HEATH, D. (1966). *J. Path. Bact.*, **92**, 529.
HICKEN, P., HEATH, D. and BREWER, D. (1966). *J. Path. Bact.*, **92**, 519.

LEOPOLD, J. G. and GOUGH, J. (1957). *Thorax*, **12**, 219.
REID, L. McA. (1960). *Thorax*, **15**, 132.
RESTREPO, G. and HEARD, B. E. (1963). *J. Path. Bact.*, **85**, 305.
RICHARDS, O. W. (1947). In *Medical Physics*. Ed. O. Glasser. Chicago.
ROSIWAL, A. (1898). *Verh. Kongr. geol. ReichsAnst. Wien*, **6**, 143.
SHORT, R. H. D. (1950-51). *Phil. Trans.*, B, **235**, 35.
WEIBEL, E. R. (1963a). *Lab. Invest.*, **12**, 131.
WEIBEL, E. R. (1963b). *Morphometry of the Human Lung*. Berlin.
WEIBEL, E. R. and GOMEZ, D. (1962). *J. appl. Physiol.*, **17**, 343.
WEIBEL, E. R., KISTLER, G. S. and SCHERLE, W. F. (1966). *J. Cell Biol.*, **30**, 23.
WEIBEL, E. R. and VIDONE, R. A. (1961). *Amer. Rev. resp. Dis.*, **84**, 856.

Section V

IMMUNOLOGY

Section Editor

P. G. H. GELL,
M.B., B.Ch.

Professor of Experimental Pathology
University of Birmingham

Chapter 23

"FARMER'S LUNG" AND PULMONARY ASPERGILLOSIS

J. PEPYS

PULMONARY hypersensitivity diseases, caused by the inhalation of organic dusts and their micro-organismal flora, vary according to the immunological reactivity of the affected subject. The two main types of allergic disease produced affect predominantly the bronchi on the one hand, or the alveoli on the other. The production of asthma by organic dusts, based upon immediate, Type I, allergic reactions in the bronchi has long been known. These Type I reactions are mediated by non-precipitating skin-sensitizing antibody, known as *reagin*. Equally important, though less familiar, is the production of allergic alveolitis by the same dusts in other subjects. These reactions are associated with the presence of precipitating antibody and it is thought that the tissue-damaging Type III Arthus reaction is responsible.

ORGANIC DUST REACTIONS IN ATOPIC AND NON-ATOPIC SUBJECTS

The factors which determine what type of allergy, and therefore of disease, is produced by a particular inhaled organic dust, are now becoming understood. Atopic subjects, for example, are constitutionally predisposed to develop immediate, Type I allergy in response to everyday exposure to allergens. The rapidly developing reactions which may be elicited are mediated by non-precipitating, skin-sensitizing reagin. This antibody is best demonstrated *in vivo* by skin or inhalation tests.

In atopic subjects the reactions to inhaled dust take place in the eyes, nose and bronchi with the production of conjunctivitis, rhinitis and asthma. Œdema of the tissues, local eosinophil cell infiltration and blood eosinophilia are characteristic features. In non-atopic subjects, however, the same inhaled organic dust leads to the appearance of precipitating antibody, capable of mediating Type III Arthus reactions. These reactions take place chiefly in the alveoli. Consequently, the particle size of the inhaled organic antigen must be small enough for the antigen to penetrate to and be retained in the alveoli.

The response of the non-atopic subjects to inhaled organic dusts has many of the features of serum sickness following on the injection of heterologous serum. The larger the dose injected the more subjects develop serum sickness, in which Arthus, precipitin mediated reactions are important. It is common in serum sickness for Type I allergy to be present as well. The presence together of Types I and III allergy in non-atopic subjects is seen in patients with other allergic alveolar diseases, such as bird fancier's lung, in which the serum protein antigens present in the bird droppings play a leading part.

The distinction between the two types of allergic reaction and the different lung diseases they produce is important in practice. Diagnostic accuracy depends upon clear differentiation of the clinical features of disease affecting predominantly either the bronchi or the alveoli. This is aided by pulmonary function tests and by skin and serological tests and by inhalation tests where indicated. In general, the serological tests must be interpreted as evidence of exposure to particular environmental agents. The allergy tests show whether the antibodies demonstrated have a pathogenetic rôle. Correlation of these findings with the clinical findings is the next step in linking the immunological changes to the disease process.

EXTRINSIC ALLERGIC ALVEOLITIS

The term "hypersensitivity granulomatous interstitial pneumonitis" has been used to describe farmer's lung and related diseases. In view of the fact that granulomata are a feature of well-established disease and may be lacking earlier and that the alveolus, which is chiefly affected, has capillaries between its walls and no interstitial tissue, it is suggested that these diseases be called extrinsic allergic alveolitis. Farmer's lung is the classical example of this disease. The discovery that thermophilic actinomycetes of mouldy hay are the main source of the antigens responsible for farmer's lung and that precipitins are present against these antigens in the serum of affected subjects, has helped in the understanding of this and related diseases. The clinical and other features of extrinsic allergic alveolitis, whatever the cause, are identical with or closely similar to those of farmer's lung, which will be described.

Farmer's Lung

The production of lung disease in farmers by the inhalation of the dust of mouldy overheated hay was first described in the U.K. by Campbell (1932) and later, among others, by Studdert (1953), Fuller (1953) and in the U.S.A. by Dickie and Rankin (1958). Farmer's lung was registered in 1965 as a prescribed disease under the National Insurance (Industrial Injuries) Act of 1946. It is defined for this purpose as "pulmonary disease due to inhalation of the dust of mouldy hay or of other mouldy vegetable produce, and characterized by symptoms and signs attributable to a reaction in the peripheral part of the broncho-pulmonary system, and giving rise to a defect in gas exchange". It has been prescribed in relation to any occupation involving exposure to the dust of mouldy hay or other mouldy vegetable produce, such as sugar cane bagasse (H.M.S.O., 1964) (Watkins-Pitchford, 1966).

Clinical Features. The attacks of the disease may come on acutely, some six hours or so after exposure to the dust, or equally frequently the disease may develop insidiously without obvious acute attacks. Both pulmonary and systemic reactions are produced. The systemic manifestations usually precede the pulmonary changes and consist of fever, malaise and chills, which are followed by a characteristic loss of weight. The pulmonary symptoms and signs are, as indicated, attributable to reactions in the peripheral part of the respiratory tract, the alveoli; these manifest themselves by cough, often very severe dyspnœa, and the appearance of crepitant râles. Pulmonary function tests show that the CO gas transfer factor is decreased and that there is also a decrease in the elasticity of the lungs.

Asthma is not a feature of the disease; it was present prior to the farmer's lung in only four out of 205 affected subjects (Pepys and Jenkins, 1965). In asthma, provoked for example by mouldy hay, the bronchi are affected by a reaction developing rapidly within minutes and characterized by wheezing and expiratory difficulty and eosinophilia of the sputum and blood.

Acute attacks of farmer's lung may last for hours or days. Diffuse fibrosis of the lungs resulting in chronic disease may follow isolated or more commonly after repeated attacks. Radiographic examination during the acute attacks shows a ground glass, miliary micronodular infiltration of the lungs not unlike that of sarcoidosis, in which, however, the hilar nodes are usually enlarged.

In affected subjects the sensitivity to the inhaled dust may become very acute so that even minimal exposure is sufficient to induce severe attacks; in such the recurrent febrile episodes and pulmonary symptoms may well be regarded as infections.

Etiology of Farmer's Lung. The production of farmer's lung by mouldy hay and other mouldy vegetable produce and not by so-called "good" hay has been recognized from the outset. Many possible causes have been considered, such as irritation of the respiratory tract by the dust; infection by fungi, which caused confusion, especially with aspergillosis due to infection with *A. fumigatus*; and allergy to mouldy hay or its abundant microflora.

Skin tests with extracts of fungi and of good and mouldy hays have not been helpful. The discovery of precipitins against *A. fumigatus* in the serum of patients with pulmonary aspergillosis (Pepys *et al.*, 1959) led to similar studies in patients with farmer's lung, in whom precipitating antibodies were found against extracts of good and mouldy hay (Pepys *et al.*, 1961, 1962, 1965).

In the initial studies agar-gel precipitin tests by the double-diffusion method showed the presence, especially in affected farmers, of precipitins against extracts of mouldy hay in almost all cases, good hay in 50 per cent; *Mucor* sp. 52 per cent; *A. fumigatus* 25 per cent; *C. herbarum* 16 per cent; *P. notatum* 6 per cent; *Humicola* (*Monotospora*) *lanuginosa* 11 per cent and *Actinomycetes* and bacteria 18 per cent (Pepys *et al.*, 1962). These precipitins reflected only a part of the wide variety of antigens present in mouldy hay to which the farmers were exposed.

Absorption tests of the sera by the addition of the various extracts showed that precipitins were present in affected subjects against additional antigens not present in the fungi, though there was limited and, at the time, unappreciated evidence that the actinomycetes might contain them.

Inhalation tests by Williams (1963) confirmed these findings. Extracts of mouldy hay provoked typical attacks of farmer's lung coming on after six to seven hours, whereas extracts of good hay and of the fungal and other extracts described above had no effect. It was clear that the additional antigens which developed in hay in the course of moulding were responsible for the disease.

Development of Farmer's Lung Hay (FLH) Antigens in Mouldy Hay. The changes in hay in the course of moulding and their relationship to the appearance of the additional antigens of farmer's lung hay, termed FLH antigens, have been studied.

Examinations of hay dust blown through wind tunnels (Corbaz, Gregory and Lacey, 1963; Gregory and Lacey, 1963a, b; Gregory, Lacey, Festenstein and Skinner, 1963) showed good hays to contain about 3 million spores/g. dry weight consisting of *Aspergillus glaucus*, *Cladosporium herbarum* and *Hemitospora stellata*. Mouldy hay dust differed in composition, containing 5–250 million spores/g. weight, of *Aspergillus glaucus, fumigatus* and *nidulans Penicillium* spp., *Absidia* spp., *Mucor pusillus*, bacteria and over 10^9 actino-mycete spores/g. dry weight hay.

The thermophilic actinomycetes are of particular importance, growing well at temperatures of 40°–60°C; such temperatures are attributable in large part to the rapid growth in the hay of bacteria and fungi, which is influenced by the initial moisture content. Thus, hay with a moisture content of 16 per cent heated little and had a small but diverse microflora; hay baled at 25 per cent moisture heated to about 45° and moulded mainly with *A. glaucus*; wet bales containing 40 per cent moisture reached temperatures of 60°–65° and contained a large flora of thermo-philic fungi and of actinomycetes. Stacks of hay behave in a similar way. The vast numbers of spores in mouldy hay is shown by the calculation of Lacey and Lacey (1964) that the air in farm buildings in which mouldy hay was being used contained 1,600 million spores/m³, of which 98 per cent were *Actinomycete* spores, 0·8–1·3 μ in diam. They estimated that a man doing light work in these conditions would have $\frac{3}{4}$ million spores per minute deposited in the lung spaces.

Immunological investigation of the antigens in serial specimens of hay from experimental stacks and bales showed that the additional FLH antigens of mouldy hay appeared within four days, when the temperature of mouldy hay had risen and actinomycetes were present in large numbers (Pepys, Jenkins, Festenstein, Gregory, Lacey and Skinner, 1963). Further studies of small samples of hay sterilized with propylene oxide, inoculated with the fungal and actinomycete flora of mouldy, and incubated in Dewar flasks under conditions like those in moulding hay, showed that the thermophilic actinomycete *M. faeni* (*Thermopolyspora poly-spora*) was the tmain source of the FLH antigens and that *Thermoactinomyces* (*Micromonospora vulgaris*) also produced one of the FLH antigens, showing that the hay was acting as a substrate (Festenstein, Lacey, Skinner, Jenkins and Pepys, 1965).

M. faeni (*T. polyspora*) forms in culture yellow colonies; whitish aerial hyphæ, mostly simple, are present, bearing lateral chaines of 1 to 10 globose spores, 0·8–1·3 μ diam. *T. vulgaris* has abundant ærial mycelia, cottony white to light lavender in colour. The ærial hyphæ are mostly simple and the spores are globose and sharp cornered, single and sessile, and are 0·5–0·8 μ diameter. A number of species of *Streptomyces* are also present in mouldy hay (Corbaz, Gregory and Lacey, 1963). *M. faeni* and an unidentified actinomycete have been cultured from a lung biopsy of an affected subject (Wenzel *et al.*, 1964). It is uncertain whether sputum culture can be used for diagnosis because such vast numbers of the spores are inhaled by exposed subjects, whether or not they are suffering from farmer's lung.

Serological Tests

Carbol-saline extracts of acetone treated mouldy hay yield the FLH antigens which give reactions of identity in agar-gel precipitin tests with the antigens of *M. faeni* and absorption of sera with each of them inhibits the reactions to the other.

In tests on sera from urban dwellers and other subjects who have not been exposed to mouldy hay, no reactions are given to the FLH antigens (Pepys and Jenkins, 1965). Precipitation reactions are given by about 90 per cent of the sera of affected subjects and by 17–18 per cent of the sera of farmers who are exposed but are unaffected or are suffering from other lung diseases. The use of latex agglutination tests (Murray, Pepys and Brighton, 1967), together with the precipitin test, increases the proportion of positive reactions in affected subjects to about 93 per cent.

Double-diffusion tests are more sensitive but less discriminating than the immuno-electrophoresis test. Weak reactions in both tests are best seen by the drying of the agar-gel plates after one week and staining with protein stains which reveal arcs of precipitation that might otherwise be difficult to see. The immuno-electrophoresis test shows three main FLH antigens, labelled A and B which are negatively charged and faster moving, and antigen C which is positively charged and slow moving. The FLH antigen of *T. vulgaris* corresponds with antigen C of *M. faeni*.

The grading of reactions according to the presence in the serum of precipitins against 0 to all three of the main antigens shows that affected farmers have stronger reactions than unaffected but exposed farmers. In patients giving stronger reactions there was also a statistically significant correlation with the number and severity of attacks and with the degree of clinical sensitivity to the dust. Nevertheless, a heavy exposure may produce severe disease in subjects with weakly reacting sera and a small proportion of affected subjects may give no reaction.

Davies and Yull (1966) report that the FLH reaction was positive in all subjects with recent disease and in 19 out of 30 asymptomatic subjects, some of whom had been affected many years previously, suggesting that the test may become negative on avoidance of the mouldy hay. Rankin *et al.* (1965) also obtained positive reactions in all symptomatic subjects and in 59 per cent of subjects who were asymptomatic. Emanuel *et al.* (1964) found reactions to be negative if the sera were tested more than five years after the last attack.

In isolated cases reactions may be given to extracts of other actinomycetes. The possibility that other organisms may be responsible in some cases is suggested too by the fact that only one-half of the farmers affected by mouldy corn or oats gave reactions to the FLH antigens of *M. faeni* (Pepys and Jenkins, 1965). It should be noted that only a small number of the actinomycetes of mouldy hay have been cultured.

Cattle suffering from fog-fever caused by feeding on mouldy hay also have precipitins against the FLH antigens in 71 per cent of cases. Exposed but unaffected animals or animals suffering from other lung diseases have FLH precipitins in 21–26 per cent of cases, whereas animals not exposed to mouldy hay seldom have them. These findings are comparable with those in man. (Jenkins and Pepys, 1965).

Nature of the FLH Antigens

Kobayashi *et al.* (1963) using a trichloroacetic acid extract of mouldy hay, followed by precipitation with 90 per cent ethanol, obtained an antigen which corresponded with the C antigen of carbol saline extracts of *M. faeni* (Pepys and Jenkins, 1965). It was claimed that the trichloroacetic acid extract reacted more specifically and only with sera of affected subjects. C-reactions, however, were given by less than one half of the F.L.H. reactors in the U.K., and particularly with the sera giving the strongest reactions, which tended to come from the most severely affected subjects. Consequently reactions to the

C-antigen might appear to be highly specific. Davies and Yull (1966) have also reported that antibody against the C antigen was present in 14 out of 19 reactions to a *M. faeni* (*T. polyspora*) extract which contained the A, B and C antigens. Trichloroacetic acid precipitation of carbol saline extracts of *M. faeni* gave a precipitate containing the predominantly protein A and B antigens whilst the glycopeptide C antingen was in the supernatant (Jenkins, 1964; Pepys and Jenkins, 1965).

Laberge and Stahmann (1966) treated trichloroacetic acid extracts of mouldy hay, of the type used by Kobayashi *et al.* (1963), by fractionation with ethanol; the material precipitated by 50–60 and 60–70 per cent contained antigens which they label "A" and "B" and the material precipitated by 70–90 per cent ethanol contained antigen C. Identical antigens were present in similar extracts of *M. faeni* and of mouldy hay. It should be noted that these fractions of antigen C which they label "A" and "B" are different from the antigens A and B described in carbol-saline extracts by Pepys and Jenkins (1963). These latter are predominantly protein and are precipitated by trichloroacetic acid. They are faster moving than the fractions of antigen C, on which Laberge and Stahmann (1966) base their observations, and they produce more crescentic and well-defined arcs which lie nearer to the anode.

Inhalation Tests

The causal rôle of the FLH antigens of *Micropolyspora* in farmer's lung has been confirmed by inhalation tests which reproduce the features of attacks of farmer's lung of acute onset (Pepys and Jenkins, 1965; Rankin *et al.*, 1965; Barbee *et al.*, 1965) in the same way as extracts of mouldy hay (Williams, 1963). A systemic reaction, consisting of fever and chills, appears after five to six hours and is followed by pulmonary reactions, affecting chiefly the alveolar tissues. Reactions like this are produced by inhalation tests in patients with attacks of insidious onset as well as those with acute onset. The mode of onset of the attacks with which the patient presents reflects the frequency and intensity of exposure to the dust, rather than a difference in the nature of the disease.

Skin Tests

Reaction to extracts of mouldy hay and fungi were obtained to prick tests only in patients who had a previous history of asthma. Intracutaneous tests with carbol-saline extracts of *M. faeni* were not satisfactory because of non-specific and irritant reactions.

Pathology

The pathological changes affect the alveoli chiefly, although organizing endobronchial exudative bronchiolitis obliterans, commonly caused by inhalation of volatile chemicals such as nitrogen dioxide, was found in about one-quarter of the cases by Emanuel *et al.* (1964). Dickie and Rankin (1958) and Rankin *et al.* (1962) found acute granulomatous interstitial pneumonitis consisting chiefly of epithelioid cells and a few giant cells or fibrosis with patchy collections of lymphocytes. Emanuel *et al.* (1964) examined biopsies taken during the acute stage of the illness when the infiltration of the alveolar walls consisted predominantly of lymphocytes, large numbers of plasma cells in many cases and a variety of mononuclear and "histiocytic forms". Small numbers of neutrophils were present and scattered lymphoid nodules were common. Varying numbers of large histiocytes with abundant foamy to finely vacuolated lipid-filled cytoplasm were present in most cases and similar cells were also present in some cases within the alveolar spaces. Compact epithelioid cell granulomata with Langhans giant cells and peripheral lymphocytes were found. Complete obliteration of normal architecture of the lung was present in some cases. Multi-nucleated foreign body giant cells and foreign body material, some doubly refractile, was present. The doubly refractile basophilic elements varied in shape and ranged from 8 to 12 μ in diameter. Birefringent cores surrounded by homogenous basophilic or acidophilic material were present in some cells and empty cleft-like spaces surrounded by amorphous eosinophilic material were also seen. These biopsies were taken soon after exposure, which may account for the common finding of foreign material. Control specimens from farmers and others showed little evidence of foreign material and the larger and more bizarre forms of foreign body were not seen.

The amount of fibrosis was very variable and corresponded to the distribution of the cellular infiltration. Focal zones of alveolar wall thickening were present which progressed to more widespread distribution by irregular extension into the surrounding tissues. Fibrosis was present in the alveoli in the early stages and discrete nodular formations of loosely arranged fibroblasts were noted in the alveolar spaces or walls, at which time secondary collagen desposition became apparent. The bronchiolitis obliterans consisted of nodular fibroblastic masses with an admixture of chronic inflammatory cells projecting into and occluding the lumen. In about one-third of the cases granulomata were present.

Diagnostic Criteria of Farmer's Lung

A clinical history of exposure to mouldy hay, with attacks of acute onset occurring after some hours or equally frequently a more insidious onset, is usual. Pulmonary function tests show a decrease in the CO gas transfer factor and a decrease in lung compliance with, as a rule, little or no bronchial reaction or ventilatory impairment. There is no past history of infantile eczema, rhinitis, hay fever or asthma, nor is there the eosinophilia of the blood or sputum which is a feature of allergic asthma.

Serological tests for FLH precipitins are now made by the Public Health Laboratory Service, and by providing evidence of exposure to FLH antigens are strong supporting evidence of the diagnosis. In doubtful cases, an inhalation test with FLH antigens may be of help. On X-ray examination there is often, though not always, a fine miliary infiltration or changes suggestive of fibrosis.

Differential Diagnosis

The acute effects of the inhalation of nitrogen dioxide which is formed in silos within a few hours up to 10–14 days of filling may be indistinguishable clinically and radiographically from farmer's lung (Lowry and Schuman, 1956). Acute œdema is present in fulminating cases and subacute bronchopneumonia with bronchiolitis fibrosa obliterans in chronic cases. Sarcoidosis also has to be considered and scalene node biopsy and the Kveim test may be helpful. Tuberculin sensitivity is also said to be decreased in farmer's lung. Fibrosing alveolitis of the Hamman-Rich type can be excluded by the history, the occupation and the serological tests, though there may be instances where a farmer with lung disease other than farmer's lung, may have FLH precipitins because of exposure to mouldy hay.

EXTRINSIC ALLERGIC ALVEOLITIS DUE TO OTHER ORGANIC DUSTS

Bagassosis. In bagassosis caused by mouldy overheated sugar-cane bagasse, Salvaggio, Buechner, Leabury and Arquembourg (1966) found that extracts of certain old, mouldy bagasse specimens gave precipitin reactions with affected but not unaffected subjects, whereas extracts of others reacted with the sera of both affected and unaffected subjects. Precipitins have been found against *T. vulgaris* in the U.S.A. (Salvaggio, Seabury, Buechner and Kundur, 1967).

Bird Breeder's or Fancier's Lung. Systemic and pulmonary symptoms like those of farmer's lung occurring in persons plucking the feathers of geese and ducks was first reported by Plessner (1960). Barboriak, Sosman and Reed (1965) and Reed *et al.* (1965) reported the disease in pigeon fanciers, in whom precipitins were found in affected subjects against extracts of the droppings, feathers, serum and egg white, though they were also present in some unaffected pigeon fanciers. Hargreave, Pepys, Longbottom and Wraith (1966) showed that both budgerigar and pigeon fanciers could be affected and cases have now also been found in parrot fanciers. Precipitins are present against extracts of droppings, serum and egg of pigeons and budgerigars. Extracts of droppings may give weak reactions with some sera which do not react to the antigens in the avian test sera, and it seems that these reactions may not be specific for bird fancier's lung; care is therefore needed in the interpretation of these reactions to droppings. In subjects affected by pigeons more precipitins are present, probably because of the intermittent exposure to large amounts of dust. For the same reason attacks of acute onset tend to occur in these patients. The affected budgerigar fanciers have less precipitins and tend to have an insidious and probably therefore more dangerous development of the disease. The keeping of a single buderigar may be associated with severe pulmonary fibrosis in a patient with precipitins, in whom dual reactions to skin tests with sterile pigeon or budgerigar serum are elicited and inhalation tests reproduce the disease. There are cross-reactions between the pigeon and budgerigar antigens.

Extrinsic allergic alveolitis should not be confused with asthma, in which Type I skin test reactions are obtained to the test extracts but in which precipitins are not present, nor are there the same systemic and pulmonary manifestations. It should also not be confused with psittacosis, which differs clinically and does not recur with each exposure, and in which ornithosis antibodies are present. In rare cases a high titre of ornithosis antibodies are present together with avian precipitins. The gravity of the allergic alveolitis and the benefit obtained from complete avoidance of the birds makes it imperative that bird fanciers with pulmonary disease should be investigated to see if they are suffering from bird fancier's lung.

Maple Bark Disease. The production of a farmer's lung type disease originally thought to be asthma, by the spores of *Cryptostroma* (*Coniosporium*) *corticale*, was reported by Towey, Sweany and Huron (1932). Precipitins against extracts of the fungus have now been found in affected subjects by Emanuel, Wenzel and Lawton (1966), who have also described pathological changes like those of farmer's lung.

Pituitary Snuff Taker's Lung. Farmer's lung type disease in patients with diabetes insipidus, resulting from the nasal insufflation of bovine or porcine pituitary snuff, has been reported by Pepys, Jenkins, Lachmann and Mahon (1966) and by Mahon, Scott, Ansell, Manson and Fraser (1967). Some patients get asthma, others alveolar disease, and some both. Precipitins have been shown against bovine and porcine serum, against the pituitary antigens and also against human pituitary antigen. An iatrogenic auto-reactive antibody has been produced in response to heterologous cross-reacting pituitary antigens.

Wheat-weevil Disease. Frankland and Lunn (1965) and Lunn and Hughes (1966) have described asthma and alveolar disease in persons exposed to the wheat weevil, *Sitophilus granarius*. Dual reactions to skin test and precipitins were demonstrated against extracts of the weevil.

Mushroom-worker's Lung. Bringhurst, Byrne and Gershon-Cohen (1959) have reported a farmer's lung type of disease in mushroom workers. It is likely that this is caused by thermophilic actinomycete spores growing at the high temperatures in which mushrooms are grown. Precipitins have been found against *T. vulgaris* and *M. faeni* in cases in the U.K. (Sakula, 1967).

General Problems

Among other examples of allergic alveolitis are suberosis caused by cork dust and smallpox handler's lung in nurses (Morris-Evans and Foreman, 1963). Vegetable dusts in general, e.g. sisal and coffee, also stimulate precipitins in exposed workers (Pepys, Longbottom and Jenkins, 1964) though there is no proof of related disease as yet. Care is required with extracts of this type since vegetable dusts contain fungal and other antigens, as well as antigens specific for the particular plant, and they may contain glycopeptides which combine with C-reactive protein. Other precipitation reactions of unknown origin are also given. The report of precipitins against extracts of thatched-roof materials in hut dwellers in New Guinea suffering from chronic lung disease (Blackburn and Green, 1966) must be examined in this light, since it is not clear whether the precipitation reactions are due to fungal or other antigens and the evidence is not strong enough yet to justify the assumption that the precipitins and their corresponding antigens are causally related to the disease. Non-specific reactions to a fast-moving negatively charged antigen of vegetable dusts lying nearer the anode than the B line of the FLH antigens and labelled the D line is produced by extracts of many vegetable dusts, in tests against a wide range of sera from diverse sources. This too may be a source of error, since the responsible antigen has been observed in extracts made from bird droppings mixed with seed foodstuffs.

PULMONARY ASPERGILLOSIS

The Aspergillus genus is ubiquitous. The most important in respiratory disease in man is *A. fumigatus*, which is pathogenic for birds and other animals. It may participate in respiratory disease in a number of different ways, largely depending upon the immunological reactivity of the subject. The spores may provoke Type I reactions causing rhinitis and asthma. Skin tests give immediate whealing reactions in from 10 to 20 per cent of patients with extrinsic asthma. In an appreciable proportion of these patients the asthma later becomes complicated by the appearance of transitory pulmonary infiltrations around medium-sized bronchi or by collapse-consolidation of parts of lobes, lobes and even whole lungs. These pulmonary changes are often accompanied by febrile episodes and by the coughing up of characteristic tough brownish sputum plugs and of small hard brown particles. Because the episodes occur commonly in the winter months they may be mistaken for infection or aspiration pneumonia. Bronchograms show a characteristic cylindrical bronchiestasis at the sites of the infiltrations, with normal filling of the bronchi peripheral to the dilatation. Allergic broncho-pulmonary aspergillosis should be suspected in all cases of asthma with pulmonary infiltrations or with bronchiectasis.

In more than 90 per cent of patients in the U.K. with asthma and pulmonary eosinophilia, precipitins are present against extracts of *A. fumigatus*, though the serum had to be concentrated to show them in one-third of the cases (Pepys, 1966). In a previous report on tests on unconcentrated sera two-thirds had precipitins (Longbottom and Pepys, 1964). In patients with uncomplicated asthma, 9 per cent had precipitins. Skin tests gave immediate wealing reactions in almost all cases, and the simple prick test is of diagnostic importance, since if it is negative allergic bronchopulmonary aspergillosis is unlikely. Furthermore, intracutaneous tests especially with purified protein fractions of *A. fumigatus* give dual, Type I followed by Type III, reactions in almost all cases. It is exceptional for dual reactions to be elicited in a patient in whom precipitins cannot be demonstrated. Corticosteroid drugs inhibit the Type III component of the reaction and are also effective in resolving the pulmonary infiltrations, suggesting that the skin and lung reactions are analogous.

Sputum Examination. Culture of the sputum for *A. fumigatus* often yields negative cultures in these patients, followed by periods during which repeated positive cultures may be obtained. In view of the fact that the fungus can be grown from the sputum of unaffected as well as affected subjects, culture is not of high diagnostic value (Pepys, Riddell, Citron, Clayton and Short, 1959). The sputum of asthmatics gives positive cultures more often than that of non-asthmatics.

Examination of the sputum plugs is of value, since silver staining may show growing mycelium. The sputum may be purulent in appearance, suggesting a bacterial infection, yet on examination a high proportion of the cells may be shown to be eosinophils. It is common to find that such sputum, giving positive cultures, rapidly clears up in colour, diminishes in amount and becomes culture negative with corticosteroid treatment, suggesting that the allergic reaction is favouring the retention and growth of the fungus in the bronchi.

The fungus may grow in damaged lung such as the open-healed cavities of treated pulmonary tuberculosis giving rise to the aspergilloma or fungal-ball which shows on X-ray a characteristic halo of air around the mass. The aspergilloma tends to occur chiefly in non-atopic subjects, but it may also develop in atopic subjects in whom it may be accompanied by asthma and pulmonary eosinophilia. The large mass of antigen present is probably responsible for the very strong precipitation reactions observed in agar-gel in almost all patients in whom the diagnosis has been confirmed by surgery or autopsy. The positive precipitin reaction tends to decrease or become negative if the aspergilloma is removed or coughed up.

Nature of Antigens of A. Fumigatus

Test extracts may be prepared from the "cell-sap" of homogenized mycelium, which is a richer source of antigens than the culture filtrates; the latter are neverthe-less a good source (Longbottom and Pepys, 1964). Surface cultures at 37° in Sabouraud liquid medium for three to five weeks give optimal yields of antigen. Antigen production varies, even under constant conditions, from one culture to another, and a battery of extracts is of value.

The extracts contain predominantly protein antigens giving well-defined "R" type arcs in agar-gel double-diffusion tests and predominantly polysaccharide antigens giving infrequent, fuzzy "H" type reactions. The "R" type reactions are more species specific, whilst the "H" type reactions are given by those sera showing extensive cross-reactions with extracts of species of other fungal genera (Pepys, Riddell and Clayton, 1959; Longbottom, Augustin and Hayward, 1960; Feinberg and Temple, 1963). The glycopeptide antigen contains several fractions with increasing amounts of bound nitrogen linked to a glucogalactomannan (ratio 1 : 5 : 20) polysaccharide moiety. The N content consisted of a high proportion of the hydroxy-amino acids serine with threonine, together with alanine. Highly antigenic protein fractions are obtained by precipitation with ammonium sulphate followed by filtration through Sephadex G-25 (Longbottom, 1964).

It is worthy of a note that glycopeptides capable of combining with C-reactive protein are present in the dermatophytes (Longbottom and Pepys, 1964) in vegetable dusts (Pepys, Longbottom and Jenkins, 1964) and in nematode parasites (Capron, Biguet, Van Ky and Rose, 1964) and are probably present in many other materials.

Agar-gel double diffusion tests have been used with these antigens, the grading of intensity of reactions being measured by the number of precipitation arcs observed in immuno-electrophoresis tests. In patients with asthma and pulmonary eosinophilia, the majority of the sera gave weak double-diffusion reactions or reactions in immuno-electrophoresis of one to four arcs. In patients with asper-gilloma the majority gave stronger reactions of from five to eight arcs or more.

The majority of aspergillomata are caused by A. fumigatus. In certain cases giving negative reactions to A. fumigatus, specific reactions may be given by extract of the species of Aspergillus responsible for the mass, e.g. A. nidulans, A. flavus and A. niger (Longbottom, Pepys and Temple-Clive, 1964).

References

BARBEE, R. A., DICKIE, H. A. and RANKIN, J. (1965). Pathogenicity of specific glycopeptide antigen in farmer's lung. Proc. Soc. exp. Biol. Med., 118, 546.
BARBORIAK, J. J., SOSMAN, A. J. and REED, C. E. (1965). Serological studies in pigeon-breeder's disease. J. Lab. Clin. Med. 65, 600.
BLACKBURN, C. R. B. and GREEN, W. (1966). Precipitins against extracts of thatched roofs in the sera of New Guinea natives with chronic lung disease. Lancet, ii, 1396.
BRINGHURST, L. S., BYRNE, R. N. and GERSHON-COHEN, J. (1959). Respiratory disease of mushroom-workers. J. Amer. Med. Ass., 171, 15.
CAMPBELL, J. M. (1932). Acute symptoms following work with hay. Brit. Med. J., 3, 1143.

CAPRON, A., BIGUET, J., and VAN KY, P. T. and ROSE, G. (1964). Possibilities nouvelles dans le diagnostic immunologique de la distomatose humaine a *Fasciola hepatica*. *Presse. Med.*, **72**, 3103.

CORBAZ, R., GREGORY, P. H. and LACEY, M. E. (1963). Thermophilic and mesophilic actinomycetes in mouldy hay. *J. Gen. Microbiol.*, **32**, 449.

DAVIES, D. G. and YULL, A. J. (1966). A comparison of the precipitin test in asymptomatic and symptomatic cases of farmer's lung. *Mon. Bull. Minist. Health*, **25**, 75.

DICKIE, H. A. and RANKIN, J. (1958). Farmer's lung. An acute granulomatous interstitial pneumonitis occurring in agricultural workers. *J. Amer. Med. Ass.*, **167**, 1069.

EMANUEL, D. A., WENZEL, G. J., BOWERMAN, C. I. and LAWTON, B. R. (1964). Farmer's Lung. Clinical Pathologic and immunologic study of twenty-four patients, **37**, 392.

EMANUEL, D. A., WENZEL, F. J. and LAWTON, B. R. (1966). Pneumonitis due to *Cryptostroma corticale*. (Maple-bark disease). *New Engl. J. Med.*, **274**, 1413.

FEINBERG, J. G. and TEMPLE, A. (1963). An investigation on precipitins to moulds in asthamtic sera. *Int. Arch. Allergy, N.Y.*, **22**, 274.

FESTENSTEIN, G. N., LACEY, J., SKINNER, F. A., JENKINS, P. A. and PEPYS, J. (1965). Self-heating of hay and grain in Dewar flasks and the development of farmer's lung antigens. *J. Gen. Microbiol.*, **41**, 389.

FRANKLAND, A. W. and LUNN, J. A. (1965). Asthma caused by the grain weevil. *Brit. J. Med.*, **22**, 157.

FULLER, C. J. (1953). Farmer's lung. Review of present knowledge. *Thorax*, **8**, 59.

GREGORY, P. H. and LACEY, M. E. (1963a). Liberation of spores from mouldy hay. *Trans. Brit. Mycol. Soc.*, **46**, 73.

GREGORY, P. H. and LACEY, M. E. (1963b). Mycological examination of dust from mouldy hay associated with farmer's lung disease. *J. gen. Microbiol.*, **30**, 75.

GREGORY, P. H., LACEY, M. E., FESTENSTEIN, G. N. and SKINNER, F. A. (1963). Microbial and biochemical changes during the moulding of hay. *J. gen. Microbiol.*, **33**, 147.

HARGREAVE, F. E., PEPYS., J., LONGBOTTOM, J. L. and WRAITH, D. G. (1966). Bird breeder's (fancier's) lung. *Lancet*, **i**, 445.

H.M.S.O. CMND. 2403. Farmer's Lung (1964). Report by the Industrial Injuries Advisory Council.

JENKINS, P. A. (1964). Immunological studies in farmer's lung. Ph.D. Thesis. Univ. Lond.

JENKINS, P. A. and PEPYS, J. (1965). Fog-fever. Precipitin (F.L.H.) reactions to mouldy hay. *Vet. Rec.*, **77**, 464.

KOBAYASHI, M., STAHMANN, M. A., RANKIN, J. and DICKIE, H. A. (1963). Antigens in mouldy hay as the cause of farmer's lung. *Proc. Soc. exp. Biol. Med.*, **113**, 472.

LA BERGE, D. E. and STAHMANN, M.A. (1966a). Antigens from mouldy hay involved in farmer's lung. *Proc. Soc., exp., Biol. Med.*, **121**, 458.

LA BERGE, D. E. and STAHMANN, M.A. (1966b). Antigens from *Thermopolyspora polyspora* involved in farmer's lung. *Proc. Soc. exp., Biol., Med.*, **121**, 463.

LACEY, J. and LACEY, M. E. (1964). Spore concentrations in the air of farm buildings. *Trans. Brit. Mycol. Soc.*, **47**, 547.

LONGBOTTOM, J. L., AUGUSTIN, R. and HAYWARD, B. J. (1960). Antigenic relationships in moulds. *Acta Allerg. (Kbh.)* **15**, (Suppl. VII) 94.

LONGBOTTOM, J. L. (1964). Immunological investigation of *Aspergillus fumigatus* in relation to disease in man. Ph.D. Thesis. Univ. London.

LONGBOTTOM, J. L. and PEPYS, J. (1964). Pulmonary aspregillosis. Diagnostic and immunological significance of antigens and C-substance in *Aspergillus fumigatus*. *J. Path. Bact.*, **88**, 141.

LONGBOTTOM, J. L., PEPYS, J. and TEMPLE-CLIVE, F. (1964). Diagnostic precipitin test in *Aspergillus* pulmonary mycetoma. *Lancet*, **i**, 588.

LOWRY, T. and SCHUMAN, L. M. (1956). Silo-filler's disease—Syndrome caused by nitrogen dioxide. *J. Amer. Med. Ass.*, **162**, 153.

LUNN, J. A. and HUGHES, D. T. D. (1966). Pulmonary hypersentitivity to the Grain weevil. *Brit. J. Indust. Med.*, **24**, 158.

MAHON, W. E., SCOTT, D. J., ANSELL, G., MANSON, G. L. and FRASER, R. (1967). Hypersensitivity to pituitary snuff with miliary shadowing in the lungs. *Thorax*, **22**, 13.

MORRIS-EVANS, W. H. and FOREMAN, W. H. (1963). Smallpox-handlers lung. *Proc. Roy. Soc. Med.*, **56**, 274.

MURRAY, I. A., PEPYS, J. and BRIGHTON, W. D. (1967). Latex agglutination test in farmer's lung. *Mon. Bull. Minist. Health*, **26**, 96.

PEPYS, J., RIDDELL, R. W. and CLAYTON, Y. M. (1959). Human precipitins against common pathogenic and non-pathogenic fungi. *Nature, Lond.*, **184**, 1328.

PEPYS, J., RIDDELL, R. W., CITRON, K. M., CLAYTON, Y. M., SHORT, E. I. (1959). Clinical and immunologic significance of *Aspergillus fumigatus* in the sputum. *Amer. rev. Respy. Dis.*, **80**, 167.

PEPYS, J., RIDDELL, R. W., CITRON, K. M. and CLAYTON, Y. M. (1961). Precipitins against extracts of hay and fungi in the serum of patients with farmer's lung. *Acta. allerg. (Kbh)*, **16**, 76.

PEPYS, J., RIDDELL, R. W., CITRON, K. M. and CLAYTON, Y. M. (1962). Precipitins against extracts of hay and moulds in the serum of patients with farmer's lung, aspergillosis, asthma and sarcoidosis. *Thorax*, **17**, 366.

PEPYS, J., JENKINS, P. A., FESTENSTEIN, G. N., GREGORY, P. H., LACEY, M. E. and SKINNER, F. A. (1963). Farmer's Lung. Thermophilic actinomycetes as a source of "Farmer's Lung Hay" antigen. *Lancet*, **ii**, 607.

PEPYS, J., LONGBOTTOM, J. L. and JENKINS, P. A. (1964). Vegetable dust pneumoconioses. *Amer. rev. Respy. Dis.*, **89**, 842.

PEPYS, J. and JENKINS, P. A. (1965). Precipitin (FLH) test in farmer's lung. *Thorax*, **20**, 21.

PEPYS, J. (1966). Pulmonary hypersensitivity disease due to inhaled organic antigens. *Postgrad. Med. J.*, **42**, 698.

PEPYS, J., JENKINS, P. A., LACHMANN, P. J. and MAHON, W. E. (1966). An iatrogenic auto-antibody immunological responses to "pituitary snuff" in patients with diabetes insipidus. *Clin. exp. Immunol.*, **1**, 377.

PLESSNER, M. M. (1960). Une maladie des trieurs de plumes, la fievre de canard. *Arch. mal. Profess.*, **21**, 67.

RANKIN, J., JAESCHKE, W. H., CALLIES, Q. C. and DICKIE, H. A., (1962). Farmer's Lung. Physiopathologie features of the acute interstitial granulomatous pneumonitis of agricultural workers. *Ann. Int. Med.*, **57**, 606.

RANKIN, J., KOBAYASHI, M., BARBEE, R. A. and DICKIE, H. A. (1965). Agricultural dusts and diffuse pulmonary fibrosis. *Arch. Environ. Health*, **10**, 278.

REED, C. E., SOSMAN, A. and BARBEE, R. A. (1965). Pigeon-breeder's lung. *J. Amer. Med. Ass.*, **193**, 261.

SAKULA, A. (1967). Mushroom workers lung. *Brit. med. J.*, **ii**, 708.

SALVAGGIO, J. E., BUECHNER, H. A., SEABURY, J. H. and ARQUEMBOURG, P. C. (1966). Bagassosis I. Precipitins against extracts of crude bagasse in the serum of *Ann. int. Med.*, **64**, 748.

SALVAGGIO, J. E., SEABURY, J. H., BEUCHNER, H. A. and KUNDUR, V. G. (1967). Bagassosis: demonstration of precipitins against extracts of thermophilic actinomycetes in the sera of affected individuals. *J. Allergy*, **39**, 106.

STUDDERT, T. C. (1953). Farmer's Lung. *Brit. Med. J.*, **i**, 1305.

TOWNEY, J. W., SWEANY, H. C. and HURON, W. H. (1932). Severe bronchial asthma apparently due to fungus spores found in maple-bark. *J. Amer. Med. Ass.*, **99**, 453.

WATKINS-PITCHFORD, J. (1966). Farmer's Lung. A review. *Brit. J. Indust. Med.*, **23**, 16.

WENZEL, F. J., EMANUEL, D. A., LAWTON, B. R. and MAGNIN, G. E. (1964). Isolation of the causative agency of farmer's lung. *Ann. Allergy.*, **22**, 533.

WILLIAMS, J. V. (1963). Inhalation and skin tests with extracts of hay and fungi in patients with farmer's lung. *Thorax*, **18**, 182.

Chapter 24

THE KVEIM TEST

D. N. MITCHELL

Introduction

IN 1935, Williams and Nickerson, working from a hypothesis based on the Frei test in lymphogranuloma inguinale, reported their findings following the intradermal injection of a sterile particulate saline suspension prepared from a *sarcoid* skin lesion. When graded doses of this suspension were injected at intervals of three days in four patients with histologically proven sarcoidosis, a firm red papule developed at each injection site within 24 hours and slowly increased in size until the end of 36 hours after injection. Thereafter, the papules slowly decreased in size and redness but were still present as small papules one week after injection. No such reactions were observed in four control subjects. Appel (1941), reporting his findings with a test suspension prepared by Nickerson's technique, mentions that the latter had excised the papule at the site of a strongly positive reaction, the histology being identical to that of sarcoid tissue.

Harrell (1940) attempted to confirm the findings of Williams and Nickerson using three test suspensions prepared according to their technique. One suspension gave questionably positive reactions in three sarcoidosis patients; the other two suspensions gave negative reactions in four.

Kveim (1941) gave the first comprehensive description of the test which bears his name. Using a suspension prepared from sarcoid lymph nodes he showed that in 12 of 13 patients with sarcoidosis papules developed at the test site between nine days and four weeks after injection; that these papules may persist for a period of several months and that on excision their histology was indistinguishable from sarcoid tissue. No papules developed in control subjects including those with tuberculosis, lupus vulgaris and syphilis.

Sources of Test Material

Test suspensions may be prepared from sarcoid spleen, lymph nodes, skin, or other affected tissues. Since at the present time it is hazardous to pool material such as lymph glands taken from different patients with sarcoidosis (Chase, 1961), sarcoid spleens removed at operation for reasons of hypersplenism offer the ideal source of continued supplies of potentially satisfactory test material. Spleens should only be used from sarcoidosis patients with no history of transmissable or other relevant illness and who have not had a recent blood transfusion. The spleen should be cut into narrow slices (e.g. $1.5 \times 1.5 \times 7.0$ cm.) under sterile conditions and rinsed free of blood with sterile normal saline. After setting aside a representative sample for preservation in formal saline, the remaining tissue should be stored in one or more containers, preferably not glass to avoid breakage on change of temperature, and transferred as soon as possible to a deep freeze at $-20°C$ or lower. The tissue should be free from detectable bacteria or fungi when stained and cultured by appropriate methods. It is impossible to postulate prior to validation in man which sarcoid spleen will yield a potent test suspension, but tissue showing histological evidence of relatively fresh sarcoid granulomas with only a minor degree of hyalinization is usually most suitable (Siltzbach, 1964). It is noteworthy that the donor of a sarcoid spleen yielding a highly potent and specific test suspension may show only a weak positive or even a negative Kveim reaction. Putkonen (1943, 1964) stresses that the most active test suspensions were obtained from patients whose Kveim test showed only a weak positive reaction.

Test Suspensions

Preparation. Samples of the tissue from which a suspension is to be pre-pared should be examined by acid-fast stains, by culture, and by guinea-pig inoculation to exclude *M. tuberculosis* and by culture for fungi.

Earlier, so-called "crude" or "conventional" suspensions were prepared (Nelson, 1948; Danbolt, 1951). The sarcoid tissue was weighed and cut up with scissors as finely as possible, after which it was ground to a paste without the addition of abrasive materials in a sterile mortar or mechanical blender. Sterile normal saline was then added in sufficient quantities to give a final dilution of about 1 : 10 by wet weight of tissue. Phenol was used as a preservative.

More recently Chase (1961), working in collaboration with Siltzbach, described the preparation of a "Type 1" test suspension. After thawing, the tissue is teased and cut up as finely as possible with scissors; using a sterile technique in the cold, the tissue is then disintegrated in cold buffered saline. It is then washed twice by centrifugation (5,500 g. for 20 minutes on each occasion) following which it is suspended, dispersed and strained through 40-mesh, 80-mesh and 100-mesh sieves. The suspension is heated to $58°C$ for 75 minutes on two successive days at pH 7·2 to 7·4. Sterility checks are made and the alcohol precipitable dry weight ascertained. The bulk suspension is then phenolized (0·25 per cent) and after checking the pH the suspension is dispensed.

This "Type 1" suspension may be prepared in several concentrations, their use in Kveim testing being determined by subsequent biological assay among sarcoidosis patients alongside tests with a suspension of known potency and specificity. The concentration of the Chase-Siltzbach suspension used in the International Kveim Test Study, referred to later, was 3 mg./ml., the amount deposited in the skin at the test site in a test dose of 0·15 ml. being 450 gamma. Chase (1961) points out that the activity of such a test dose would be approximately that of a 5 per cent crude suspension of the same spleen containing about 1,000 gamma of alcohol-precipitable material.

A "crude" or "conventional" suspension is heavily particulate and may not pass easily through a 26-gauge or wider needle suitable for intracutaneous injection; it is also more likely to produce a greater degree of inflammatory reaction at the test site. Hence, the use of such suspensions is now usually limited to the preliminary tests required to ascertain the potency of a test suspension derived from a new source.

Douglas (1964) reported the preparation of a freeze-dried Kveim test material from a 10 per cent "conventional" saline suspension of a sarcoid cervical lymph node, using phosphorous pentoxide as a desiccant. When required, the ampoules were opened and the test material reconstituted by mixing with distilled water. Kennedy (1967) reported an evaluation of simultaneous tests made with this freeze-dried test material and with a fluid suspension from the same source. He concluded that following storage for a period of up to 10 months, the freeze-dried Kveim material showed no loss of potency or specificity.

It should be emphasized that individual workers with a special interest in this field remain responsible for the preparation, validation and dispensing of reliable Kveim test suspensions.

Dispensing. Ideally, the test suspension should be dispensed in sterile rubber-capped 2-ml. glass vials each containing about 1·2 ml. in preference to larger vials. Such vials will suffice for six separate tests each of 0·15 ml.; limited re-entry guards against the possible danger of contamination and wastage of test material which is in very short supply is minimal. Further, the surface area of the vial over which the particulate material is spread when the suspension is shaken is limited, thus avoiding marked disparity in the amount of particulate material contained in each succeeding test dose. Finally, limited re-entry to the vial guards against possible damage to the rubber cap, whereby bits of rubber might become admixed with the test suspension and be introduced at the test site giving rise to a foreign body reaction. Single-dose glass vials each containing about 0·2 ml. of suspension necessitate repeated wastage.

Injection of Test Suspensions

Syringes and Needles. All glass 1-ml. syringes of tuberculin type, with short shank needles of adequate gauge to allow free passage of the particulate suspension (e.g. 26 gauge), should be used. Syringes set aside for Kveim testing should be cleaned thoroughly after use and rinsed with sterile pyrogen free water before autoclaving preferably in glass containers to avoid contamination with fibre such as cotton or dust particles. Chase (1961) advocates the use of 26-gauge needles with Huber point and closed bevel. Sterile ½-ml. or 1-ml. disposable syringes are readily available and have the advantage of inherent safety and ease of use. Our experience of their use in Kveim testing has been limited, but a preliminary assessment and that of Siltzbach (personal communication) suggests that their use is unlikely to be followed by an increase in the incidence of refractile material or of foreign body granulomas at the test site.

Skin Cleaning. The skin in the area of the test site should be cleaned with 70 per cent alcohol. The use of cotton-wool or gauze must be avoided. Alcohol dabs as manufactured by leading pharmaceutical houses or skin-cleaning tissues provide convenient substitutes.

Test Sites. Tests may be made at any site from which a biopsy can conveniently be taken. The skin overlying the deltoid and suprapatellar areas has been used, but the most convenient sites are provided by the skin over the middle third of the ulnar aspect of the anterior forearm. This area will normally suffice for four or more equally spaced test sites. It should be emphasized that any minimal residual scar following biopsy of test sites is less easily visible when tests are confined to the ulnar aspect of the forearm.

The Injection. After cleaning the rubber cap the vial is thoroughly shaken to ensure uniform dispersion of the particulate material within the suspension. The test dose (usually 0·15 ml.) is then drawn into the syringe. The Kveim suspension must be injected intracutaneously and as superficially as possible so as to raise a bleb at the test site with "peau d'orange" of the overlying skin. If the suspension is injected more deeply into the skin a positive test might only be felt as a palpable induration, without the appearance of a papule at the test site.

For ease of location at the time of reading and biopsy the method advocated by Siltzbach (personal communication) is simple, allows of precise identification and does not interfere with interpretation of the histological findings following biopsy of the Kveim test site. The test site is marked by a single tattoo speck using a sterile needle dipped into autoclaved Gunter-Wagner Pelican Ink at a point within the periphery of the injection site (Fig. 1). The tattoo speck serves as a marker

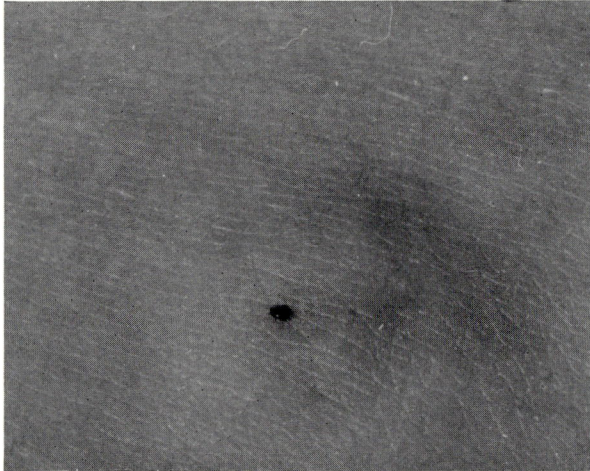

FIG. 1. Marking of test site. The epidermis is just broken by a single "tattoo speck" of autoclaved Gunter-Wagner "Pelican "ink at a point well within the periphery of the bleb raised by the intracutaneous injection of Kveim suspension.

and is subsequently included in the area of skin punch biopsy. Such a technique is essential if tiny areas of induration at test sites are not to be missed or if the test site is to be biopsied routinely, as is now standard practice.

The Kveim Reaction

Evolution of the Macroscopic Reaction. An area of induration of some 3–4 mm. in diameter with an overlying erythema develops at the test site within 24–48 hours following injection. This reaction is attributed to trauma and to inflammatory response following the injection of a tissue suspension and is seen in nearly all subjects tested, whether Kveim-positive or Kveim-negative. During the first week after injection this inflammatory reaction slowly recedes and in Kveim-negative subjects disappears completely within 7–14 days. In Kveim-positive subjects the initial inflammatory reaction is slowly replaced, usually during the second week, by an area of palpable induration or by a visible violaceous papule at the test site which slowly increases in size, attaining a diameter of 3–5 mm. or more by about 14 days

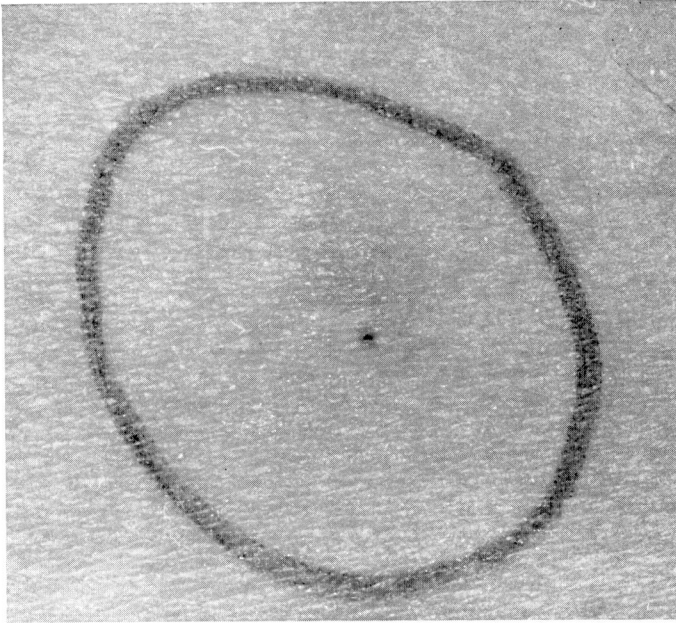

FIG. 2a. To show the value of "marker" in defining the Kveim test site prior to biopsy. (Only a little diffuse erythema and a tiny deep-seated nodule 2-3 mm. in diameter were present. Microscopically the test was positive.)

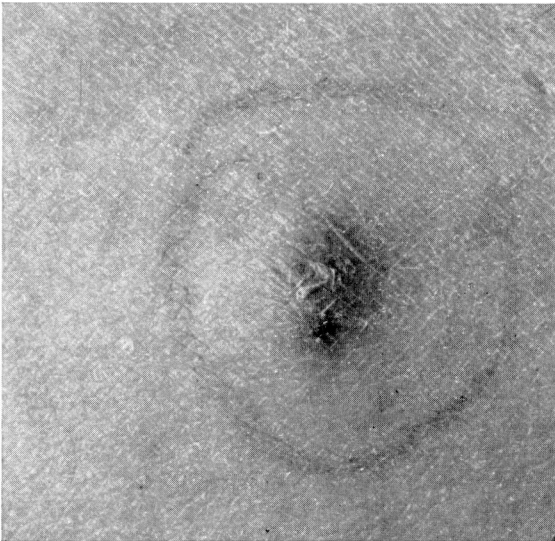

FIG. 2b. Positive Kveim reaction. Note "marker" at edge of raised, indurated violacious nodule, 6 mm. in diameter.

O

after injection. Thereafter, the reaction at the test site persists, perhaps even increasing in diameter during the ensuing two to four weeks. The important point is that this late reaction is not evanescent and may persist unchanged throughout the active phase of the disease, thereafter fading slowly and eventually leaving only a little residual pigmentation at the test site. Møller (1952) described a patient with generalized sarcoidosis including skin lesions in whom positive Kveim reactions on the left thigh persisted through a period of nine years. Siltzbach (1964) reported that racial factors may influence the size of developing Kveim papules, some 30 per cent of white males and some 17 per cent of white females developing a papule of 5 mm. or more in diameter at the test site six weeks after injection, whereas amongst Negro subjects some 70 per cent of males and 60 per cent of females attained Kveim papules of this diameter after a similar interval. Very infrequently a papule representing a positive Kveim reaction may appear at the test site after an unduly long interval following injection (Putkonen, 1952). Rarely a very large Kveim papule may result in a highly reactive subject and this may ulcerate, healing only with remission of the illness or following treatment with steroids which suppress the disease, and likewise the reaction.

Reading and Recording of Macroscopic Reaction. Ideally, examination of the test site should be made at two weeks, and is obligatory not later than four weeks after injection. Biopsy of the test site is made not less than four weeks and more usually after an interval of six weeks following injection (see below). If biopsy is deferred to this later date, a further reading is of course made at six weeks after injection and immediately prior to biopsy of the test site. Great care must be taken not to overlook a tiny papule or more deeply situated area of induration.

Biopsy of the Test Site. The test site is defined and any visible or palpable reaction recorded. A circle approximately 1·5 cm. in diameter and extending just beyond the periphery of any reaction is then drawn around this (Figs. 2 and 2A). With the patient seated and the arm extended in a comfortable position, the skin of the forearm is cleaned thoroughly with a detergent followed by 70 per cent alcohol. About 0·5–1·0 ml. of 1 per cent procaine without adrenaline is then injected into and just beneath the skin at the test site. Using a no-touch technique, a skin biopsy punch of Hays-Martin type with a circular knife 4 mm. in diameter is then placed so as to encircle the centre of any reaction or the test site, and is gently rotated so as to cut through the full thickness of skin. The pedicle of the biopsy is then raised gently with fine non-toothed forceps and after dissecting clear with scissors (Fig. 3) is transferred to neutral 10 per cent formalin. Hæmostasis is secured by the use of a simple "band-aid" and overlying elastoplast gauze dressing which can be removed by the patient some five days later.

The 4-mm. "core" of tissue, consisting of the full thickness of skin and including the injection site is fixed in neutral 10 per cent formalin. After embedding in paraffin wax, sections, 5–7 μ in thickness are cut at right angles to the epithelium. The sections mounted must include the midline through the biopsy. Ideally all or a sequence of sections should be mounted in ribbon formation and stained by H. and E. Dornetzhuber (1966) recommended that serial sections be performed, since moulds in granulomas may be detected only in some layers.

Evolution of the Microscopic Reaction. Rogers and Haserick (1954) observed the early development of the Kveim reaction in serial biopsies of two Kveim-positive and two Kveim-negative subjects. In the two with negative reactions the test sites showed only minimal perivascular infiltration with lymphocytes during the early period. After 13 days the test site in one of these subjects showed a small collection of lymphocytes with a few small giant cells, but by 42 days the test sites in both showed virtually normal skin.

In one of the two Kveim-positive subjects who developed an intense positive reaction with a small central area of necrosis, the changes after three days were not significantly different from those seen at a Kveim-negative

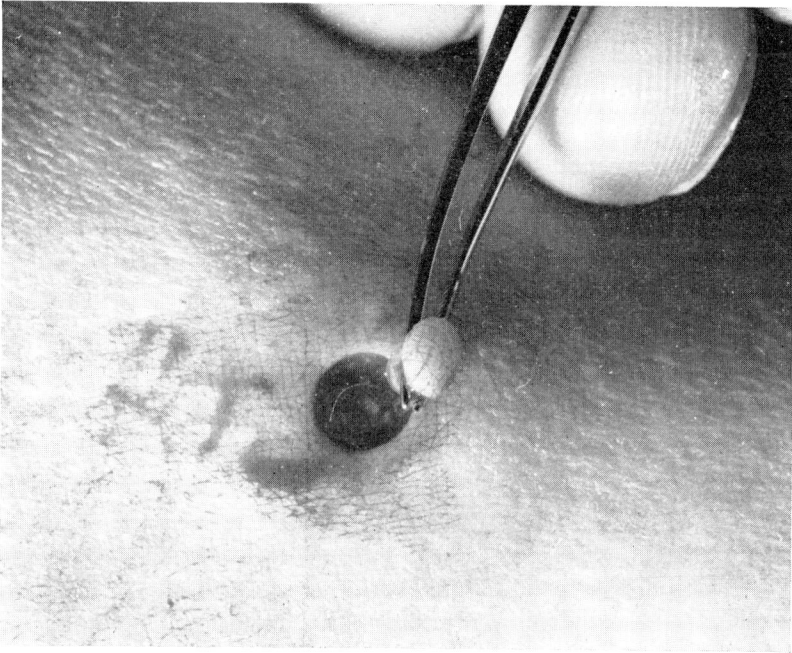

FIG. 3. To show pedicle of biopsy raised from wound before dissecting clear at base.

test site after the same interval. After six days a dense perivascular infiltration containing large pale-staining histiocytes, small deeply staining mononuclear leucocytes and some pleomorphic atypical cells were seen. After 10 days there was some degeneration of collagen in the central area with a few foci of complete necrosis; this area was diffusely infiltrated with polymorphonuclear leucocytes. Surrounding this were mononuclear leucocytes with histiocytes and many pleomorphic and atypical cells. A few giant cells containing from two to six nuclei were present. After 13 days fewer atypical cells were seen and there was a dense perivascular infiltration with lymphocytes. Near the vessels small collections of epithelioid cells were recognizable and were surrounded by deeper-staining mononuclear cells. Occasional well-formed giant cells of the Langhans type were seen in the areas of greatest activity. After 16 days the epithelioid characteristics of the reaction were more evident. Epithelioid cell tubercles were loosely packed with an eosinophilic strauma and there was a tendency to whorl formation. Within the larger collections of epithelioid cells lymphocytes were present but in smaller numbers. No further significant changes were observed after 20 days, but after 25 days large aggregations of epithelioid cells were present with a minimal peripheral zone of lymphocytes. The microscopic appearance at 42 days showed almost confluent epithelioid tubercles surrounded by a few lymphocytes. The central necrotic area seen earlier was now a well-defined area of complete necrosis in which no cells were seen.

Siltzbach (1964) studied the microscopic changes of the positive Kveim reaction in serial sections by means of injections given at intervals of one to four weeks. During the first week the reaction at the test site was predominantly a mononuclear cell response with small numbers of neutrophils, eosinophils and plasma cells. It was not clear whether the mononuclear cells with dark-staining nuclei which appeared early in the reaction gave rise to the epithelioid cells with vesicular nuclei or whether the epithelioid cells evolved from cells which replaced the mononuclear cells. The neutrophils, eosinophils and plasma cells present during the early part of the reaction diminished during subsequent weeks as the characteristic epithelioid cell follicles appeared at about three weeks after injection and continued to mature. Subsequently, as in the healing of spontaneous sarcoid lesions, the epithelioid cell follicles became surrounded and eventually replaced by hyalinized connective tissue. This process takes some six months to one year and proceeds more quickly in a patient receiving corticosteroid therapy.

Siltzbach and Ehrlich (1954) reported that they had not encountered Shaumann bodies in epithelioid cell granulomas of the Kveim test. Asteroids were rarely seen within the multinucleated cells in positive reactions and were occasionally found also in negative reactions. The cytoplasm of the epithelioid cells frequently appeared vacuolated. Biopsy of the scar several months after excision of the test sometimes showed a residual granulomatous reaction. Progressive cutaneous lesions after removal of the test area were not encountered.

Dornetzhuber *et al.* (1966) described their microscopic findings following biopsy of Kveim test sites at increasing intervals after injection. The only microscopic differences between the appearances seen in the positive Kveim reaction and those of florid sarcoid lymph node, were the absence of Shaumann's inclusion bodies and of fibrinoid necrosis in the Kveim reactions seen in their patients. They concluded that the most suitable interval at which to read the result of the test microscopically was five to six weeks after injection, by which time fully developed epithelioid cell follicles have appeared.

Assessing the Result of the Test. In earlier studies the test was regarded as positive or negative according to the evolution of the macroscopic reaction at the test site. Putkonen (1943) placed no time-limit on the interval after which the test should be read but considered the reaction negative unless the papule at the injection site attained a diameter of 5 mm. or more. Nelson (1948) regarded the test as positive if a papule or an area of induration of any size occurred at the injection site and remained palpable for at least 60 days from the date of its appearance. Danbolt (1951) considered no reaction positive which did not show a marked and distinct papule one month after injection and which did not persist distinctly for at least one month thereafter. Siltzbach and Ehrlich (1954) performed biopsy of all test sites whether or not a reaction at the test site could be seen or felt. They concluded that biopsy of all test sites was imperative; they were convinced that if they had relied on the macroscopic reading of the test site there would have been a substantial error in their findings.

Microscopic Reading of Test

Careful microscopic examination of all sections representative of each Kveim test site, including examination under the polarized light, is essential for an accurate assessment of the result.

Positive Reactions. Microscopically, the essential feature for diagnosis of a positive test is the presence of one or more granulomas composed principally of epithelioid cells and resembling those of sarcoidosis. Within the granuloma there may be a central area of fibrinoid necrosis of collagen devoid of cells and staining pink in sections stained by H. and E. Surrounding the granuloma there may be a peripheral infiltrate in which lymphocytes predominate, but in which histiocytes, neutrophils and occasional eosinophils or plasma cells are sometimes seen. Several granulomas may be present. Siltzbach and Ehrlich (1954) pointed out that but for the admixture of the cells of inflammation the microscopic appearances of the positive Kveim reaction and those of the naturally occurring sarcoid lesion would be hard to differentiate.

The brown granules or brown fibres, or the doubly refractile particles which are present in some Kveim test suspensions are never seen in sections from spontaneous sarcoid lesions. The presence of doubly refractile material in sections from Kveim test sites should call attention to microscopic changes which may be attributable to a foreign body reaction; their presence in itself does not necessarily exclude the diagnosis of a positive Kveim test.

The microscopic findings in "positive", "equivocal" or "negative" Kveim reactions may be conveniently summarized in tabular form:

(*a*) **Positive** (Figs. 4, 5 and 6)

Discrete epithelioid cell granulomas.

Compact or confluent epithelioid cell granulomas.

Diffuse epithelioid cells infiltrating between collagen bundles, but with satellite epithelioid granuloma present.

(*b*) **Equivocal**

Epithelioid cells diffusely infiltrating between collagen bundles, but with no satellite epithelioid cell granuloma.

Predominantly histiocytes (with less abundant cytoplasm and smaller round nuclei) in focal collections, with few or no epithelioid cells.

(*c*) **Negative** (Figs. 7 and 8)

Non-specific inflammatory cells, mononuclear cells, lymphocytes, neutrophils, plasma cells, eosinophils.

Foreign body reaction.

Scar with fibroblasts or fibrocytes.

Normal skin.

Specificity of the Kveim Reaction

Kveim Tests in Sarcoidosis and Controls. The initial studies of Williams and Nickerson (1935) and of Kveim (1941) are described in the introductory section, and the results of tests made by these and subsequent authors in sarcoidosis and controls, are summarized in Table I.

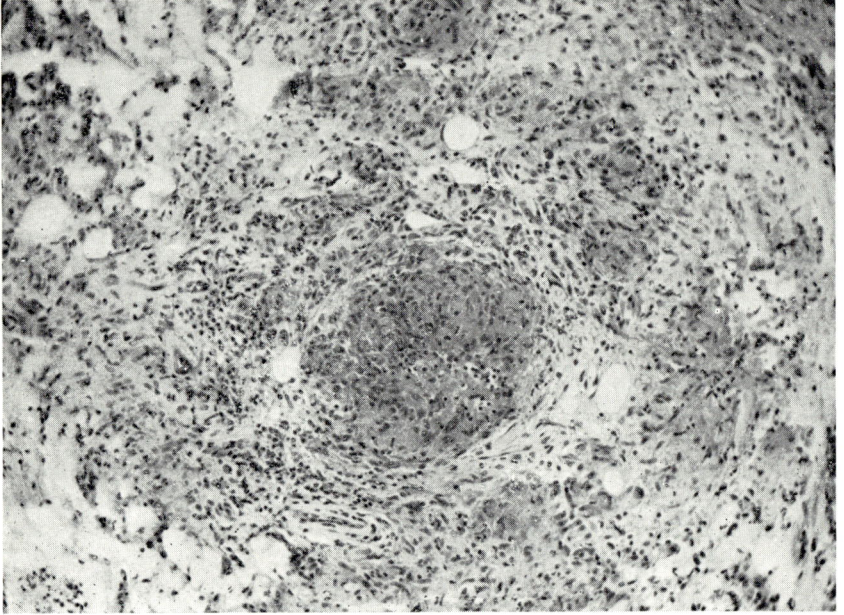

FIG. 4. Positive Kveim reaction. Confluent epithelioid cell granulomata. (Stained H. and E. × 160.)

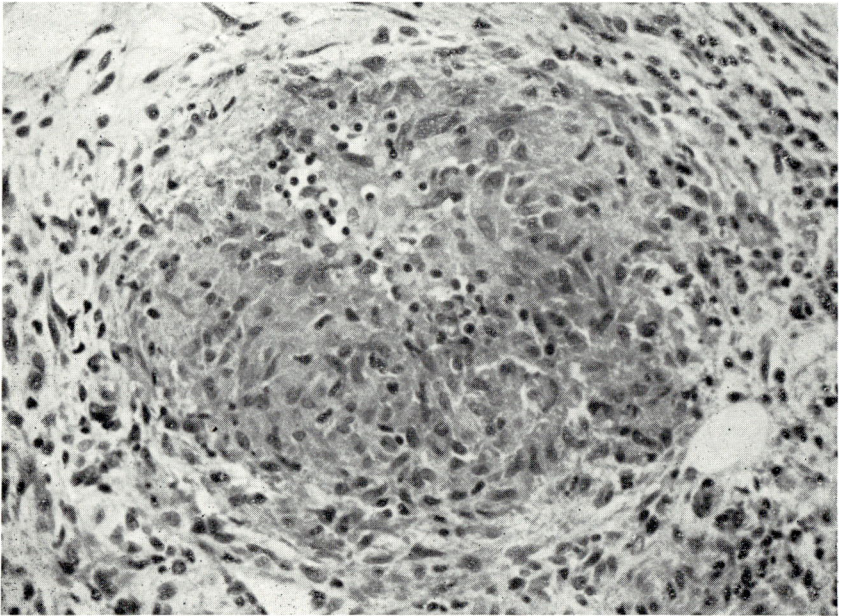

FIG. 5. Positive Kveim reaction. Showing characteristic epithelioid cells and then "whorled" arrangement within the granuloma. (Stained H. and E. × 400.)

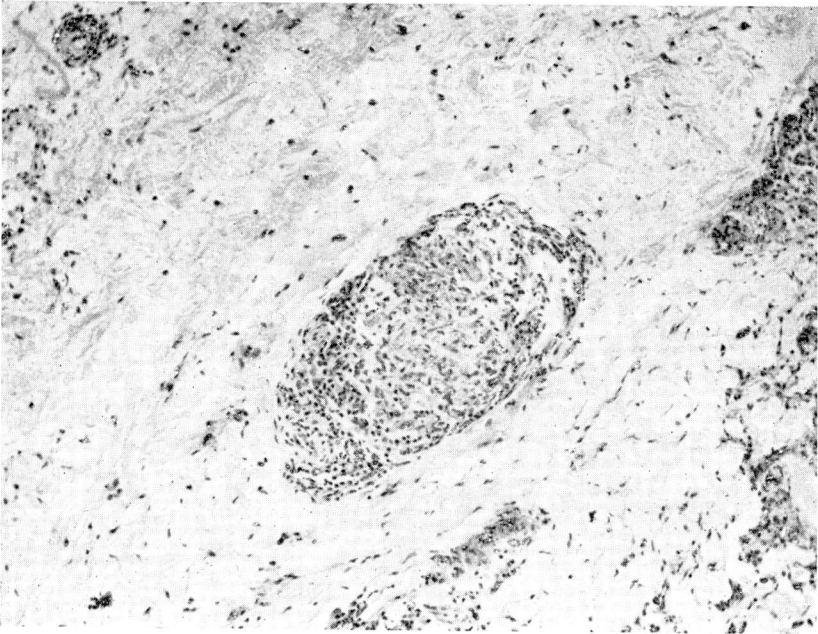

FIG. 6. Positive Kveim reaction. Showing solitary epithelioid cell granuloma. (Stained H. and E. × 160.)

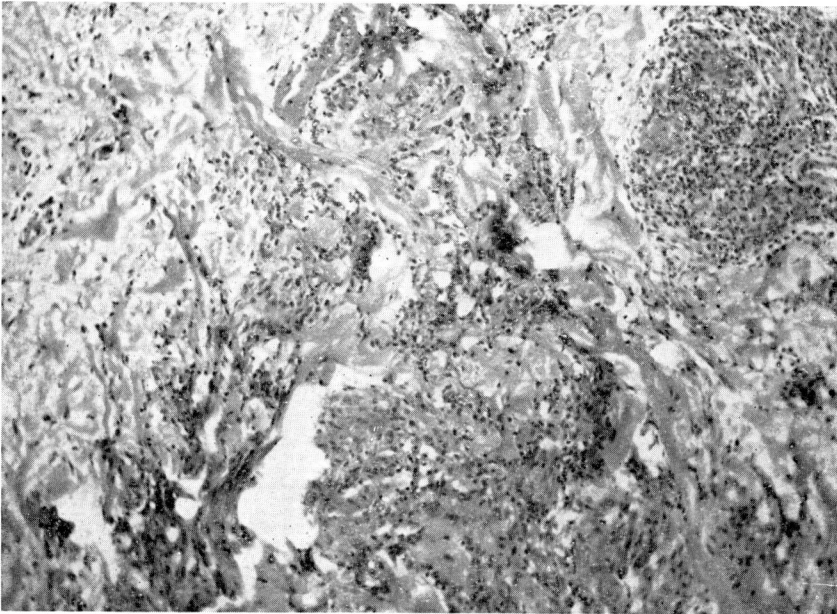

FIG. 7. Negative Kveim reaction. Showing non-specific inflammatory reaction. (Stained H. and E. × 160.)

TABLE I

Kveim Tests in Sarcoidosis and Controls

Reference	Origin of test suspensions	Macroscopic or microscopic reading	Series	Subjects	Total tested	Negative	Equivocal	Positive No.	Positive %
Williams and Nickerson, 1935	Sarcoid skin lesion	Macroscopic	Sarcoidosis	Clinical, with histological proof	4	0	0	4	100
			Controls	Healthy adults	4	4	0	0	0
Kveim, 1941	Sarcoid lymph nodes	Both	Sarcoidosis	Clinical, with histological proof	13	1	0	12	92
			Controls	Non-sarcoid patients	?	All	0	0	0
Putkonen, 1943	Sarcoid lymph nodes; suspensions also from skin and tonsil lesions	Macroscopic	Sarcoidosis	Clinical, with histological proof	42	9	0	33	78
				Doubtful clinical sarcoidosis	10	?	?	0	0
			Controls	Non-sarcoid patients	65	65	0	0	0
Danbolt and Nilssen, 1945	? Sarcoid lymph nodes	Macroscopic	Sarcoidosis	Definite clinical	36	2	0	34	94
			Controls	Non-sarcoid patients and a few healthy persons	68	68	0	0	0
Nelson, 1948	Sarcoid lymph nodes; suspensions also from skin lesions	Macroscopic	Sarcoidosis	Clinical, with histological proof: Active	11	0	0	7	64
				Healed or inactive	6	0	0	0	0
			Controls	Non-sarcoid patients	8	0	0	0	0
				Apparently healthy subjects	12	0	0	0	0
Nelson, 1949	Sarcoid lymph nodes and skin lesions	Macroscopic	Sarcoidosis	Clinical, with histological proof: Active	15	0	0	11	73
				Healed or inactive	9	0	0	0	0
Danbolt, 1951	Sarcoid lymph nodes; suspensions also from skin and distal finger joint lesions	Macroscopic	Sarcoidosis	Definite clinical	46	5	0	41	89
				Doubtful clinical	65	41	0	24	37
			Controls	Non-sarcoid patients	51	46	0	5 (or 4)	Up to 6·5
				Apparently healthy subjects	25	25	0	0	0
Sondergaard, 1951	? Sarcoid lymph nodes	Macroscopic	Sarcoidosis	Definite clinical, pulmonary	29	?	?	14	48
Nitter, 1953	Sarcoid lymph nodes	Both	Sarcoidosis	Clinical, with histological proof	50	7	5*	38	76
				Clinical, biopsy negative	18	3	4*	11	60
				Clinical, no biopsy	22	8	2*	12	54

Study	Antigen	Route	Group	Clinical	N				%
Rogers and Haserick, 1954	Sarcoid spleen and lymph nodes	Both	Sarcoidosis	Definite clinical: Active	51	2	0	49	96
				Regressed	6	6	0	0	0
			Controls	Non-sarcoid patients	46	42	4	0	0
Siltzbach and Ehrlich, 1954	Sarcoid spleen and lymph nodes	Both	Sarcoidosis	Clinical, with histological proof	58	?	?	50	86
				Clinical suspects: Strong	33	?	?	28	85
				Intermediate	24	?	?	12	50
				Weak	33	?	?	1	4
			Controls	Non-sarcoid patients	54	?	?	2	4
James and Thomson, 1955	Sarcoid spleen	Both	Sarcoidosis	Definite clinical	16	?	?	12	75
			Controls	Non-sarcoid patients	47	44	3	0	0
Israel and Sones, 1955	Sarcoid lymph nodes	Both	Sarcoidosis	Definite clinical	28**	?	?	12†	21·1††
			Controls	Active pulmonary tuberculosis	33	?	?	14†	42·1††
				Non-sarcoid patients and 9 apparently healthy adults	20+	?	?	2†	8·3††
Nelson and Schwimmer, 1957	Sarcoid spleen	Both	Sarcoidosis	Clinical, with histological proof: Including 16 inactive cases	72	?	?	53	74
				Excluding 16 inactive cases	56	?	?	53	94
			Controls	Non-sarcoid patients	234	232	0	2	0·8
Israel and Sones, 1958	Sarcoid lymph nodes	Both	Sarcoidosis	Definite clinical	46	?	?	13†	28·3++
			Controls	Active pulmonary tuberculosis	29	26	3†x	0†	0++,‡
Siltzbach, 1961	Sarcoid spleen	Both	Sarcoidosis	Clinical, with histological proof: <2 years duration	115	?	?	?	87
				>2 years duration	50	?	?	?	78
				Clinical suspects	282	?	?	?	52
			Controls	Tuberculosis	63	?	?	1	<1
				Other non-sarcoid patients	240	?	?	1	<1
Siltzbach (International Kveim test study), 1964	Sarcoid spleen	Both	Sarcoidosis	Clinical, with histological proof: Clinical suspects: Subacute	307	?	?	?	52
				Chronic					30
			Controls	Non-sarcoid patients	173	?	?	2	1·2

* Doubtful and inconclusive categories combined.
** 57 tests on 28 subjects.
† Only those with nodules were biopsied.
†† Percentage of tests performed.

+ 24 tests on 20 subjects.
++ Percentage of those completing test.
x Non-specific granulomas.

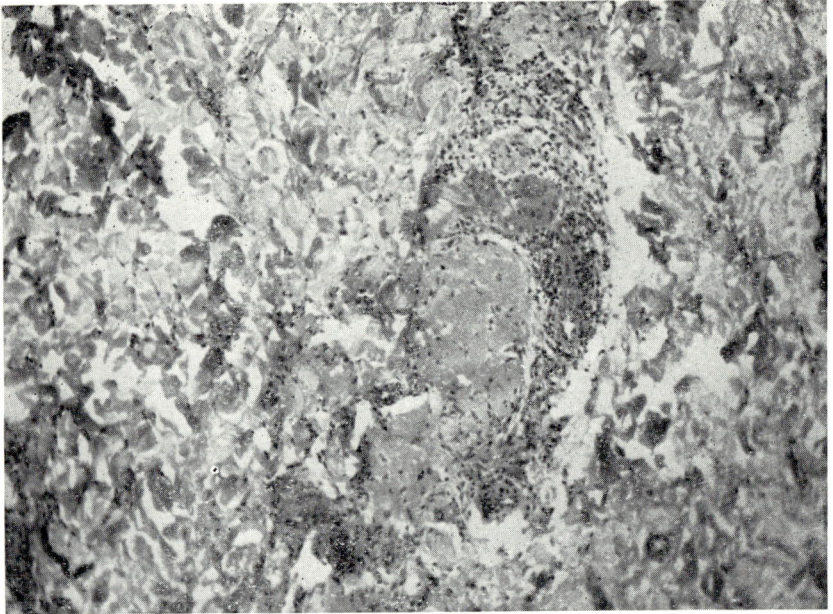

FIG. 8. Negative Kveim reaction. Showing foreign body giant cell reaction. (Stained H. and E. × 160.)

Tests with Normal Spleen Suspensions

Nelson (1948; 1949), reported his findings following the use of two test suspensions, prepared in the same manner as the sarcoid test suspension used in these studies, from normal spleens obtained at autopsy from two subjects who died from cardiovascular disease and who showed no evidence of sarcoidosis. Following simultaneous intracutaneous tests with normal spleen and with sarcoid test suspensions, the sarcoidosis patients who showed a positive test in response to the sarcoid test suspensions (Table I), also developed a typical Kveim response at the site of injection of the normal spleen suspension. Biopsy of these normal spleen suspension test sites between 6 and 10 months after injection, showed a microscopic picture comparable to that of spontaneous sarcoid. The characteristic skin reactions which followed the injection of either normal spleen or sarcoid test suspensions were found with one exception only, in each of these two studies, in patients with active cutaneous sarcoid lesions at the time of testing. Moreover as with the sarcoid test suspensions (Table I), these normal spleen suspensions did not produce a characteristic Kveim response when injected intracutaneously in 12 apparently healthy subjects and in eight patients with various illnesses including leprosy, granuloma annulare, lymphogranuloma venereum, tuberculosis and metastatic carcinoma. When cutaneous reactions did occur in these subjects they were always evanescent, and disappeared completely within two or three weeks following injection. However, in a later report, Nelson (1957) states that his finding that patients who show a positive cutaneous reaction following the injection of a sarcoid test suspension may also give a Kveim-like response following the intracutaneous injection of suspensions prepared from certain normal spleens, has been confirmed in only one instance (Lovelock, personal communication) and that other investigators, notably Danbolt (1951), Siltzbach and Ehrlich (1954) and Rogers and Haserick (1954), have been unable to corroborate this.

Tests on Patients with Leprosy. Wade (1951) made simultaneous Kveim tests with two sarcoid spleen suspensions among 10 bacteriologically positive lepromatous leprosy patients and seven healthy "control" subjects. Marked erythema and induration was present at all test sites 24 and 48 hours after injection. After 72 hours the erythema had subsided and the induration which persisted in all subjects during the first seven-day period after injection thereafter showed a slow subsidence. Wade concluded that following rather marked non-specific 24–48 hour reactions, the two Kveim suspensions had failed to give any positive reaction among the 10 lepromatous leprosy patients and the seven healthy subjects tested. Kooij and Gerritsen (1958) reported Kveim papules about 5 mm. in diameter among patients with tuberculoid leprosy following simultaneous tests with two different Kveim suspensions among these patients. Grotepass et al. (1962) confirmed the finding of Kooij and Gerritsen following tests among leprosy patients with preparations from normal liver, but found that the responses obtained were considerably weaker in evoking the lepromin reaction pattern. Leiker (1961) found that normal skin suspensions may produce "positive" reactions in leprosy patients. It should be noted, however, that Wade (1951) found no correlation between the results of lepromin and Kveim tests with sarcoid spleen suspensions amongst lepromatous leprosy patients and healthy "control" subjects. Kooij (1964) emphasizes that the 10 patients studied by Wade (1951) were all suffering from lepromatous leprosy and describes his findings using three Kveim test suspensions simultaneously injected among 14 patients with tuberculoid leprosy and 12 patients with lepromatous leprosy. After four weeks the average diameter of induration at the Kveim test site was greater for each test suspension amongst the patients with tuberculoid than for those with the lepromatous form of leprosy. As assessed by the evolution of the reaction at the Kveim test site about one-third of the patients with tuberculoid leprosy were considered to show a positive Kveim test.

Trend of Sarcoidosis and the Results of the Kveim Test after varying Intervals. Siltzbach (1961) reported that of 97 Kveim-positive patients who were retested, about one in ten became negative after two to six months, and one in four after one year. After three to five years one in two patients remained positive, and after 15 years one in three. The test sometimes became negative without detectable change in the course of the illness; one such patient who showed positive tests repeatedly for 13 years became negative in the fourteenth year, another remained positive for 11 years and became negative in the thirteenth year. Occasionally, recrudescence of sarcoidosis was preceded by a sudden resurgence of activity at unbiopsied test sites months and sometimes years after injection of the test suspension. A similar resurgence of activity was noted at test sites in the postpartum period, and after termination of corticosteroid therapy. Recrudescence of sarcoidosis however did not always restore Kveim positivity to patients who had previously lost their capacity to respond.

Effect of Corticosteroid Drugs

In general, corticosteroid therapy suppresses the Kveim reaction, although this effect is not constant. Rogers and Haserick (1954) noted that patients who showed little response to corticosteroid drugs continued to develop positive Kveim tests. Rogers and Haserick (1954) investigating the effect of the injection of hydrocortisone (5 mg.) with the Kveim test suspension in patients with active sarcoidosis found that the histology of these test sites six weeks later failed to show the cellular response seen in control tests made with Kveim suspension alone. They concluded that the injection of hydrocortisone at Kveim test sites effectively suppressed the stimulus responsible for granuloma formation and dispersed partially and fully developed Kveim test granulomas. Similarly, Siltzbach (1961, 1964) reported that in general the systemic administration of coricosteroids or local injection along with Kveim test suspensions may abolish it completely.

Diagnostic Value of the Kveim Test

Given an extensively validated test suspension of known potency, the test provides a reliable and specific diagnostic aid among patients in whom the diagnosis of sarcoidosis is suspected or in doubt. Fortunately, one of the common forms of sarcoidosis, bilateral hilar adenopathy, with or without erythema nodosum, is often so characteristic in presentation, and its subsesequent course in European patients so benign, that the clinician experienced in this field oftens feels justified in retaining the patient under surveillance without recourse to histological proof of the diagnosis. However, among patients with this form of sarcoidosis the test can be expected to yield a high incidence (60–85 per cent) of positive results, and since the tissues of involved organs are not readily accessible for biopsy, the test provides valuable confirmatory evidence where an atypical presentation leaves the clinical diagnosis open to doubt. In such cases the delay of a minimum of four weeks in obtaining a result following biopsy of a relatively simple Kveim test must be weighed against the increased risk to the patient in attempting to obtain more immediate histological proof of the diagnosis by liver aspiration or biopsy.

Where pulmonary mottling is associated with bilateral hilar adenopathy the Kveim test can again be expected to give a similar high level of positive results provided that the onset of the disease is relatively recent. The results of the test compare favourably with those of other diagnostic procedures such as bronchial biopsy (Schiessle *et al.*, 1961; Friedman *et al.*, 1963; Turiaf, 1964) or open-fringe lung biopsy (Levinsky *et al.*, 1964).

Although direct recourse to affected tissue may yield sections showing epithelioid cell granulomas, these are often regarded as compatible with rather than as confirmatory diagnostic proof of sarcoidosis (Refvem, 1954). Hirsch *et al.* (1961) and Siltzbach (1964) reported that the Kveim test gave negative results in a wide variety of other conditions in which similar granulomas may be found histologically. The Kveim test is therefore useful in deciding upon the cause of erythema nodosum and in differentiating sarcoidosis from such conditions as tuberculosis, brucellosis, Hodgkin's disease, pneumoconiosis, carcinomatosis, beryllium poisoning, chronic allergic inflammatory reactions and connective tissue disorders.

Likewise the test can be used to differentiate from generalised sarcoidosis the local sarcoid tissue reactions sometimes seen histologically following a granulomatous response to neoplasm, reticulosis, infection, chemicals or trauma.

Where sarcoidosis is the cause of uveitis, cranial nerve palsies, subacute meningitis, hypercalcæmia, hypercalciurea or of isolated hepatic or cardiac lesions, a positive Kveim test is not only of diagnostic value but may be a deciding factor in the treatment of these conditions with corticosteroid therapy.

Conclusion

Given a properly validated test suspension of known potency, the Kveim test is a relatively simple and highly specific diagnostic test for sarcoidosis which can be conveniently carried out on an out-patient basis. Moreover, since loss of Kveim reactivity is generally associated with regression of sarcoidosis, the test also has some prognostic significance. Sarcoid spleens suitable for the preparation of a regular supply of test suspensions are only rarely available and only a small proportion will yield suspensions having the potency and specificity needed for Kveim testing. Although essentially simple, the technique of the test requires careful attention to detail at all stages. A delay of four to six weeks prior to biopsy of the test site is obligatory and unavoidable. Finally, although a high degree of correlation can be expected between the microscopic readings of the test by different observers (Siltzbach, 1964), non-specific reactions of a foreign body type may occasionally interfere with the microscopic assessment of the test and differences may be encountered in the evaluation of the weak positive or equivocal Kveim reaction.

References

CHASE, M. W. (1961). The preparation and standardisation of Kveim testing antigen. *Amer. Rev. Resp. Dis.*, **84**, (5 pt 2), 86-8.

DANBOLT, N. and NILSSEN, R. W. (1945). Investigations on the course of Kveim's reaction and its clinical value. *Acta Dermativneer* (Stockholm), **25**, 489-502.

DANBOLT, N. (1951). On the skin test with sarcoid-tissue-suspension (Kveim's reaction). *Acta Dermatovener* (Stockholm), **31**, 184-93.

DANIEL, T. M. and SCHNEIDER, G. W. (1962). Positive Kveim tests in patients without sarcoidosis. *Amer. Rev. Resp. Dis.* **86**, 98-9.

DORNETZHUBER, V. (1966). Routine investigation of the Kveim reaction in sarcoidosis. *Amer. Rev. Resp. Dis.* **93**, 459.

DOUGLAS, A. C. (1964). Discussion following section on "Results of Kveim testing". Proceedings of the Third International Conference on Sarcoidosis, Stockholm 1963. *Acta. Med. Scand. Supplement*, **425**, 189.

FRIEDMAN, O. H., BLAUGRUND, S. M. and SILTZBACH, L. E. (1963). Biopsy of the bronchial wall as an aid in diagnosis of sarcoidosis. *J.A.M.A.*, **183**, 646-50.

GROTEPASS, F. W. K., DE KOCK, D. H. and KOOIJ, R. (1962). Some biochemical aspects of the lepromin reaction pattern evoked by normal liver preparations. *Leprosy Review*, **33**, 129.

HARRELL, G. T. (1940). Generalised sarcoidosis of Boeck: Clinical review of eleven cases, with studies of blood and etiological factors. *Arch. Intern. Med.*, **65**, 1003.

HIRSCH, J. G., COHN, Z. A. MORSE, S. I., SCHAEDLER, R. W., SILTZBACH, L. E., ELLIS, J. T. and CHASE, M. W. (1961). Evaluation of the Kveim reaction as a diagnostic test for sarcoidosis. *New Engl. J. Med*, **265**, 827-30.

ISRAEL, H. L. and SONES, M. (1955). The diagnosis of sarcoidosis with special reference to the Kveim reaction. *Ann. Intern. Med*, **43**, 1269-82.

ISRAEL, H. L., SONES, M., BEERMAN, H. and PASTRAS, T. (1958). A further study of the Kveim reaction in sarcoidosis and tuberculosis. *New Engl. J. Med.*, **259**, 365-9.

JAMES, D. G. and THOMSON, A. D. (1955). The Kveim test in sarcoidosis. *Quart. J. Med.*, **24**, 49-60.

JAMES, D. G. (1961). Clinical concept of sarcoidosis. *Amer. Rev. Resp. Dis.*, **84**, 14.

KENNEDY, W. P. U. (1967). An evaluation of freeze-dried Kveim reagent. *Brit. J. Dis. Chest*, **61**, 4.

KOOIJ, R. and GERRITSEN, T. (1958). On the nature of the Mitsuda and the Kveim reaction. *Dermatologica*, **116**, 1.

KOOIJ, R. (1964). The nature of the Kveim reaction. Proceedings of the Third International Conference on Sarcoidosis, Stockholm 1963. *Acta Med. Scand. Supplement*, **425**, 79.

KVEIM, A. (1941). En ny og specifikk kutan-reaksjon ved Boecks sarcoid, en forelobig meddelelse. (On a new and specific cutaneous reaction in Boeck's sarcoid; a preliminary report.) *Nord. Med.* **9**, 169-72.

LEIKER, D. L. (1961). Studies on the lepromin test. 1. The influence of the bacillary and tissue components in dilution of lepromin. *Int. J. Leprosy*, **29**, 157.

LEVINSKY, L, REHÁK, F. and ZÁKOVÁ, N. (1964). The value of lung biopsy in diagnosis of pulmonary sarcoidosis. Proceedings of the Third International Conference on Sarcoidosis, Stockholm 1963. *Acta. Med. Scand. Supplement*, **425**, 241.

MACKAY, J. B., LAING, M. C. and REID, J. D. (1964). Sarcoidosis: Some observations on present status, prevalence and treatment. *New Zeal. Med. J.*, **63**, 264.

MØLLER, P. (1952). Case of Boeck's sarcoid with Kveim reactions persisting through nine years. *Acta. Dermatovener* (Stockholm) **32**, 435-6.

NELSON, C. T. (1948). Observations on the Kveim reaction in sarcoidosis of the American negro. *J. Invest. Derm*, **10**, 15-26.

NELSON, C. T. (1949). Kveim reaction in sarcoidosis. *Arch. Derm. Syph.* (Chicago), **60**, 377-89.

NELSON, C. T. and SCHWIMMER, B. (1957). The specificity of the Kveim reaction *J. Invest. Derm*, **28**, 55-61.

NELSON, C. T. (1957). The Kveim reaction in sarcoidosis. *J. Chronic. Dis.* **6**, 158-77.

NICKERSON, D. A., quoted by APPEL, B. (1941). Sarcoid. *Arch. Derm. Syph.* (*Society Trans.*) **43**, 172.

NITTER, L. (1953). Changes in the chest roentgenogram in Boeck's sarcoid of the lungs; a study of the course of the disease in 90 cases. *Acta Radiol.* (Stockholm), Supplement, **105**, 1-202.

PUTKONEN, T. (1943). Uber die intrakutarekation von Kveim (KvR) bei lymphogranulomatosis benigna und uber das bild dieser krnakheit in lichte der reaktionsergebnisse. (On intracutaneous reaction of Kveim in benign lymphogranulomatosis and the clinical manifestations of the illness in the light of results of the reaction.) *Acta Dermatovener* (Stockholm), **23** (Supplement 10), 1-194.

PUTKONEN, T. (1952). A case of skin tuberculosis with a positive Kveim reaction as late as five years after injection of antigen. *Acta Dermatovener* (Stockholm), **32**, 294-6.

PUTKONEN, T. (1964). Source of potent Kveim antigen. Proceedings of the Third International Conference on Sarcoidosis, Stockholm 1963. *Acta Med. Scand. Supplement*, **425**, 83.

REFVEM, O. (1964). The pathogenesis of Boeck's disease (sarcoidosis); investigations on the significance of foreign bodies, phospholipides and hypersensitivity in the formation of sarcoid tissue. *Acta Med. Scand*, **149** (Supplement 294), 1-146.

ROGERS, F. J. and HASERICK, J. R. (1954). Sarcoidosis and the Kveim reaction. *J. Invest. Derm*, **23**, 389-406.

SCHIESSLE, W., WURN, K. and REINDELL, H. (1961). Engebnisse und bedeutung bronchologischer untersuchungen bei der lungen sarkoidose (morbus Boeck). (Results and significance of bronchologic investigation in lung sarcoidosis—Boeck's disease.) *Munchen Med. Wschr*, **103**, 726-30.

SILTZBACH, L. E. and EHRLICH, J. C. (1954). The Nickerson-Kveim reaction in sarcoidosis. *Amer. J. Med.*, **16**, 790-803.

SILTZBACH, L. E. (1961). The Kveim test in sarcoidosis; a study of 750 patients. *J.A.M.A.*, **178**, 476-82.

SILTZBACH, L. E. (1964). Significance and specificity of the Kveim reaction. Proceedings of the Third International Conference on Sarcoidosis, Stockholm, 1963. *Med. Scand. Supplement*, 425, 79.

SILTZBACH, L. E. (1964). The Kveim test in tuberculosis, beryllium disease, leprosy and sarcoidosis. *Amer. Rev. Resp. Dis,*. **90**, 308.

SILTZBACH, L. E. (1964). An international Kveim test study. Proceedings of the Third International Conference on Sarcoidosis, Stockholm 1963. *Acta Med. Scand. Supplement*, **425**, 178.

SILTZBACH, L. E. (1966). An international Kveim test trial. Progress report (1960-1966). Proceedings of Fourth International Conference on Sarcoidosis, Paris. (In press.)

SØNDERGAARD, G. (1951). Kveims reaktion anvendt ved diagnosen af den pulmonale form af lymfogranulomatosis benign, Schaumann. (Kveim reaction of pulmonary form of Schaumann's benign lymphogranulomatosis.) *Ugeskr. laeg.*, **113**, 1412-5.

TURIAF, J. (1964). Bronchial biopsy. Proceedings of the Third International Conference on Sarcoidosis, Stockholm 1963. *Acta Med. Scand. Supplement*, **425**, 228.

WADE, H. W. (1951). Leprosy and sarcoid; the Kveim test in leprosy patient and contacts. *J. Invest. Derm.*, **17**, 337.

WILLIAMS, R. H., NICKERSON, D. A. (1935). Skin reactions in sarcoid. *Proc. Soc. Exp. Biol. Med.*, **33**, 403-5.

Chapter 25

THE THYMUS IN THE DEVELOPMENT
OF IMMUNOLOGICAL RESPONSIVENESS

Delphine M. V. Parrott

THE unique importance of the thymus has been realized only in recent years mainly as a consequence of experimental observations on the effect of removing the thymus from certain laboratory animals shortly after birth. Such animals fail to achieve complete immunological responsiveness, and show a profound deficiency of lymphocytes throughout the whole of the lymphoid tissue; they may develop a severe wasting disease culminating in death. These dramatic effects of thymectomy are only revealed when the thymus is removed prior to or very early in the development of the whole immunological system. In most species this development commences in fœtal life (see reviews by Good and Papermaster, 1964; Good, Gabrielsen, Peterson, Finstad and Cooper, 1966) and removal of the thymus at or after birth has little effect. The advantage of using mice and rats stems from their tardy development in this respect and thus most experimental studies in mammals have been carried out in these species.

Structure of the Thymus. The thymus is a lobed structure, located in most species in the upper anterior part of the chest; in the guinea-pig and the chicken it is in the neck. The lobules, which are incompletely divided, are composed of a medulla of mixed epithelial-reticular cells and lymphoid cells surrounded by a cortex of tightly packed lymphoid cells in a network of epithelial-reticular cells. The presence of this network is an important difference between the thymus and other lymphoid organs in the mammal. Other differences are the presence of Hassall's corpuscles only in the thymus, and the irregular presence in the normal thymus of lymphoid follicles and germinal centres and paucity of plasma cells, structures which in other lymphoid organs are associated with response to antigenic stimulus.

Immunological Deficiencies of Neonatally Thymectomized Animals

In many of the first observations it was implied that all of the immunological capabilities of animals thymectomized within 24 hours of birth, especially mice, were equally and uniformly impaired, but it is now realized that this is not so (Table I). Serum immunoglobulin levels are usually normal, and although there may be irregular increases of $\gamma_1 A$ in mice (Humphrey, Parrott and East, 1964; Fahey, Barth and Law, 1965), this globulin is reduced in neonatally thymectomized rats (Arnason, de Vaux, St.-Cyr and Relyveld, 1964). One so far unexplained aspect of immunoglobulin production in neonatally thymectomized mice is that although synthesis of $7S\gamma_2$- and $7S\gamma_1$-globulin is normal or increased, catabolism is often accelerated, especially in wasting animals (Humphrey *et al.*, 1964; Fahey *et al.*, 1965).

Effects of

Age at thymec-tomy	Wasting syndrome		Immunological parameters			
	Incidence	Age at onset	Immuno-globulins	Antibody production		Cellular sensitivity reactions reduced
				Reduced	Normal	
< 24 hours after birth	Mice: up to 100 per cent depending upon strain Very variable in rats and hamsters	Mice: 2–4 months variable between strains (normal life span 1½–3 years)	Normal. γ_1A slightly increased in mice	SRBC Salmonella typhii H and O BSA BGG	Hæmocyanin Ferritin SSSIII Polyoma virus	Allogeneic skin and tumour grafts Allogeneic leukæmic cells Skin reaction to tuberculin and BSA Resistance to G-V-H reduced Resistance to tumour induction reduced
3–7 days	Very slight incidence	Late onset 5–9 months	Normal	Normal		Allogeneic skin grafts (closely related) Allogeneic leukæmic cells Resistance to G-V-H slightly reduced Resistance to tumour induction reduced
30 days	None	—	Normal	Normal		Normal
Adult	None	—	Normal	Normal (except after 6–9 months' interval)		Normal

Immunological Deficiency

Disease	Type (authors who first described it)	Main clinical features	Immunological parameters		
			Immuno-globulins	Antibody production	Cellular sensitivity reactions
Thymic alymphoplasia	"Swiss type" agamma-globulinæmia (Glanzman and Riniker, 1950)	Familial Early onset (2–6 months) Poor growth; pulmonary infection; diarrhœa; monilial infections	—	—	—
	"French type" normal globulinæmia (Nezelof et al., 1964)	Spleen and lymph nodes not palpable No thymus shadow on chest X-ray (regular or oblique)	+	±	—
Congenital agamma-globulinæmia	"Bruton type" (Bruton, 1952)	Familial Sex-linked-boys Later onset (6 months to 3 years) Usual childhood infections (pneumonia, meningitis, otitis media, etc.) unusually frequent and severe Small tonsils No adenoid shadow on lateral X-ray of the nasopharynx	—	—	+

I

Thymectomy

		Lymphoid system	
		Spleen and lymph nodes	
Blood lymphocyte	Thoracic duct lymphocytes	Thymus-dependent areas	Follicles, plasma cells and germinal centres
Very low (< 1,000 cu./mm. in some strains of mice)	Very low	Severely depleted of lymphocytes No response to immunological stimuli	Normal development in most animals Follicular necrosis in wasting mice Normal response to immunological stimuli
Low	Low	Depleted Slight response to immunological stimuli	Normal
Reduced	Reduced	Slight depletion	Normal
Slightly reduced	Reduced	Very slight depletion	Normal

II

Diseases of Infancy

Lymphomyeloid system			Thymus	
Blood	Bone marrow aspiration	Lymph node biopsy	Macroscopic	Microscopic
Lymphopenia	No lymphocytes No plasma cells	Few lymphocytes No plasma cells	Hypoplastic	Rare lymphocytes No demarcation between cortex and medulla Epithelial foci No Hassall's corpuscles
Lymphopenia	No lymphocytes Plasma cells present	Few lymphocytes Plasma cells present		
Normal	—	Lymphocytes No germinal centre or plasma cell development after local antigenic stimulation	Normal	Lymphocytes Clear demarcation between cortex and medulla Hassall's corpuscles present

Neonatally thymectomized animals show extremely random and variable responses to administered antigen. Thus, for example, the response to sheep red blood cells, whether measured by serum hæmolysin and agglutinin production (Miller, 1962; Humphrey et al., 1964; Law, Trainin, Levey and Barth, 1964) or by the Jerne plaque technique (Friedman, 1965) is usually reduced, the response to other antigens such as pneumococcus polysaccharide-type 3 (SSSIII), hæmocyanin and ferritin can be completely normal (Humphrey et al., 1964; Fahey et al., 1965). By contrast, almost all cellular sensitivity (delayed hypersensitivity) reactions are drastically impaired. Thus, skin reactions in rats to tuberculin and bovine serum albumin (BSA) (Janković, Waksman and Arnason, 1962) are reduced, and skin grafts, except from other species, are retained for long periods (Miller, 1961; Miller, 1962; Janković et al., 1962; Miller, 1965). Mice remain extremely susceptible to graft-versus-host reaction (Runt disease) caused by the injection of unrelated lymphoid cells well beyond the neonatal period (Parrott, 1962; Parrott and East, 1962) and the induction of tumours by the tumour viruses, such as polyoma (Malmgren, Rabson and Carney, 1964). It is interesting to note that whilst these animals apparently cannot detect new tumour antigens induced by polyoma virus they are perfectly capable of making hæmagglutinating antibody to the virus itself (Miller, Ting and Law, 1964), thus providing a very clear example of the partial immunological impairment resulting from neonatal thymectomy (Law, 1966). When mice are thymectomized between three days and seven days the resulting immunological deficiencies are much less severe (Law and Ting, 1965) and their measurement is dependent upon methods which call into play maximum immunological capacity as, for example, in resisting large doses of allogeneic leukæmic cells (Parrott and East, 1965) or in detecting the subtle antigenic differences between closely related skin donors (Miller, 1965). Thymectomy in the adult animal has none of the drastic effects on immunological responsiveness which follow neonatal thymectomy, although there is ample evidence that the thymus continues to function throughout adult life. For if sufficient time, 9–18 months, is allowed to lapse between thymectomy and administration of an antigen, deficiencies in responsiveness can be detected (Metcalf, 1965; Taylor, 1965); and if adult thymectomy is followed by lethal whole-body irradiation plus bone marrow therapy, then such animals show immediately all the immunological deficiencies of neonatally thymectomized animals (Miller, Doak and Cross, 1963) including failure to reject skin grafts.

Effect of Thymectomy on the Lymphoid System

Neonatal thymectomy prevents the normal rise in the numbers of lymphocytes in the circulating blood and thoracic duct lymph which normally follows birth, so that when the animals are 2–3 months of age the number of lymphocytes may be less than 30 per cent of that in intact litter mates (Miller, 1962; Parrott and East, 1962). Thymectomy at later ages also causes depression of circulating lymphocytes though not so profound as that resulting from neonatal thymectomy (Metcalf, 1960; Schooley and Kelly, 1964).

The development of organized structures as follicles and germinal centres within the lymphoid organs is not delayed or prevented by neonatal thymectomy. However, it becomes apparent during the first three weeks after birth that certain specific areas, termed thymus-dependent, in both lymph nodes and spleen remain permanently depleted of lymphocytes (Parrott, de Sousa and East, 1966). These areas are in the mid and deep cortex of the lymph nodes and immediately around the central arteriole of the spleen (Figs. 1–4). The rest of the white pulp of the spleen, the follicles and medullary cords of the lymph nodes, remain primarily unaffected by thymectomy although secondary destruction caused by mouse hepatitis virus (MHV) is sometimes seen in mice with severe wasting symptoms. From all these findings it is assumed that the primary lymphoid deficiency in thymectomized mice is in the mobile or recirculating pool of lymphocytes and not in the fixed structures. Recent work has demonstrated (Parrott and de Sousa, 1966; Parrott, 1967) a direct correlation between the failure of neonatally thymectomized mice to mount a cellular sensitivity reaction whilst maintaining some antibody production with the specific deficiencies in the lymphoid organs. Application of skin sensitizing agents such as oxazolone or the application of a skin graft (Oort and Turk, 1965; Scothorne and McGregor, 1955) characteristically provokes a proliferation of pyroninophilic blast cells in the mid and deep cortex of the draining lymph nodes of non-thymectomized animals. This proliferation does not occur in neonatally thymectomized mice (Parrott, 1967) and it seems reasonable to relate the failure of these animals to respond by cellular means to this failure of blast cell proliferation and the absence of small lymphocytes. On the other hand, the response to antigens such as pneumococcus polysaccharide is by plasma cell proliferation and germinal centre development; the response does occur in the thymectomized mouse and thus accords well with their ability to respond to this antigen (Humphrey et al., 1964; de Sousa and Parrott, 1967).

Wasting Disease in Neonatally Thymectomized Animals

Many animals, including mice, rats and hamsters, thymectomized within 24 hours of birth ultimately die from a curious syndrome known as wasting disease (Parrott and East, 1964). They grow normally until they are about 6–8 weeks old; they then deteriorate in general appearance and progressively lose weight. Coat condition is poor, mice in particular become haunched, walk with a curious high-stepping gait and often have diarrhœa. The most obvious post-mortem features are the thinness of skin and bone, lack of subcutaneous fat and necrotic lesions in the liver of many mice. There is a considerable variability in the susceptibility of different species and different strains to wasting disease (Parrott, 1962; Parrott and East, 1962; Janković et al., 1962) and a delay of thymectomy of only one or two days will cause both a considerable reduction in the incidence of wasting and a delay in the onset and severity of symptoms (Parrott and East, 1962; Law, 1966). It appears certain that infection is involved in the pathogenesis of wasting disease because neonatally thymectomized mice raised under germ-free conditions do not show any symptoms of the disease (McIntire, Sell and Miller, 1964; Wilson, Sjodin and Bealmear, 1964); however, microscopic lesions characteristic of wasting may still be present in these mice (de Vries, unpublished data, 1966) and only one virus has been regularly isolated from wasting mice, mouse hepatitis virus (East, Parrott, Chesterman and Pomerance, 1963).

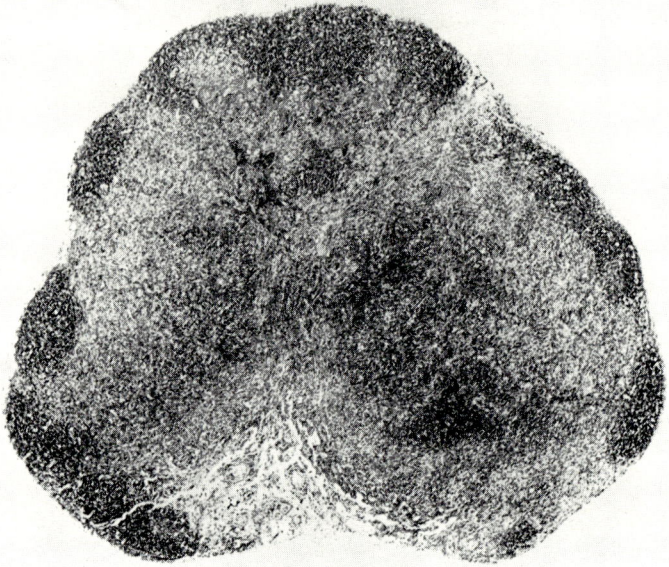

FIG. 1. Lymph node form a control non-thymectomized mouse. Note primary and secondary follicles in the outer cortex and even distribution of lymphocytes through the mid and deep cortex. (Methyl green pyronin × 50.)

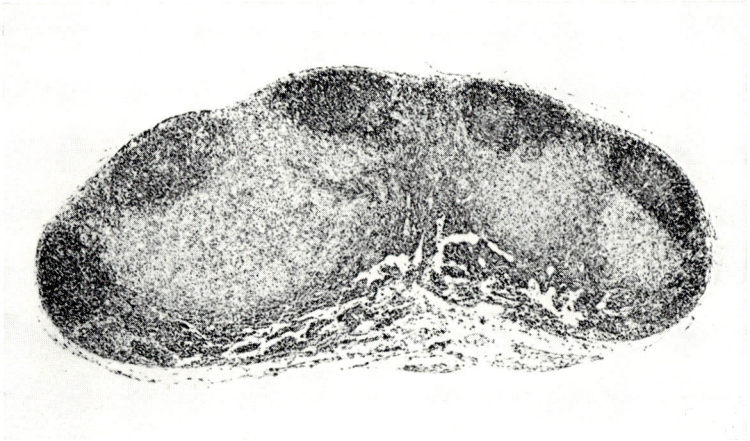

FIG. 2. Lymph node from a neonatally thymectomized mouse. Note primary and secondary follicles in the outer cortex but depletion of lymphocytes from the mid and deep cortex (the thymus-dependent area). (Methyl green pyronin × 50.)

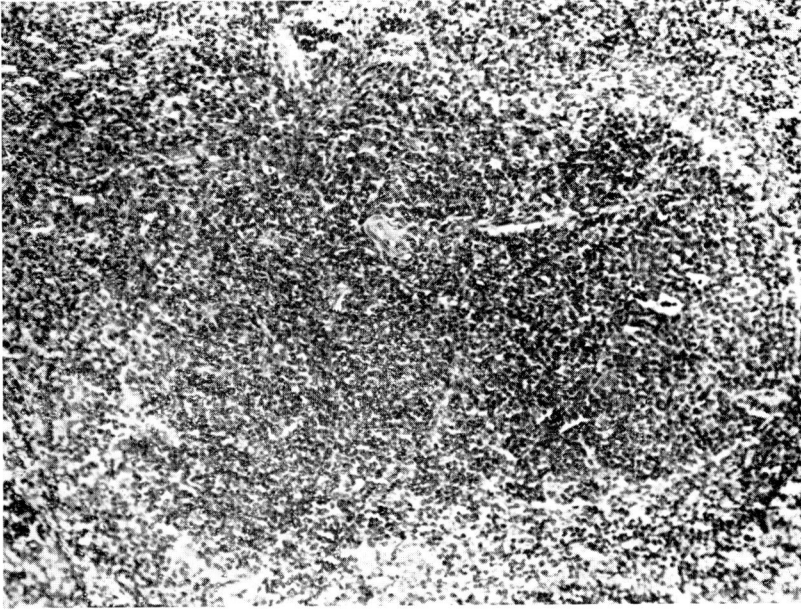

FIG. 3. Spleen follicle from a control non-thymectomized mouse. Note closely packed lymphocytes around the central arteriole. (Hæmatoxylin and eosin × 225.)

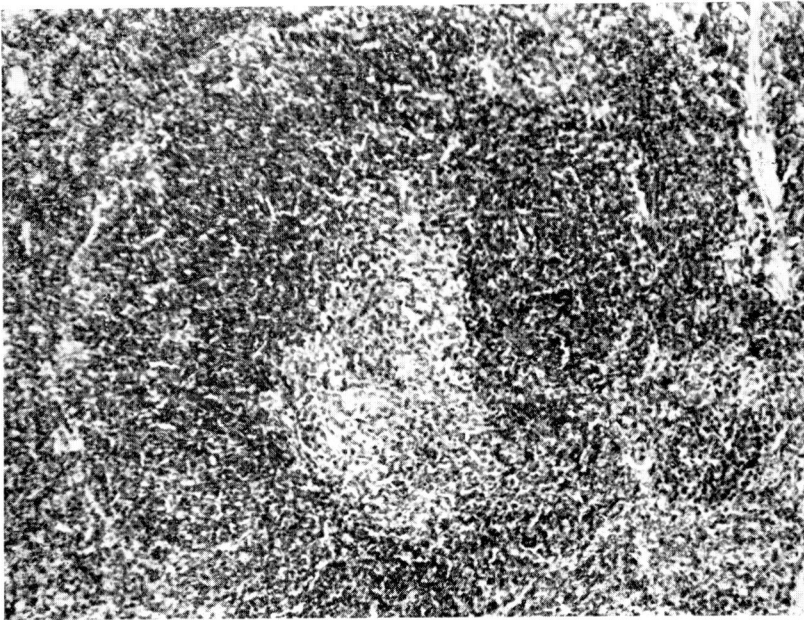

FIG. 4. Spleen follicle from a neonatally thymectomized mouse. Note pale area around the central arteriole depleted of lymphocytes (the thymus-dependent area). (Hæmatoxylin and eosin × 225.)

Restoration of the Deficiencies of Neonatally Thymectomized Animals

The most rapid way of "curing" a neonatally thymectomized mouse already on the brink of wasting and restoring its immune responses is by the intravenous injection of spleen cells from an intact adult donor of the same strain (syngeneic) (East and Parrott, 1964). Also partially successful are cells from bone marrow, multiple thymus cell injections from syngeneic donors and spleen from allogeneic but closely related donors (East and Parrott, 1964; Yunis, Hilgard, Sjodin, Martinez and Good, 1964; Law, Dunn, Trainin and Levey, 1964). The presence of lymphoid cells is essential, repeated injections of serum from intact adult donors, presumably containing normal quantities of immunoglobulins, is completely ineffective (Humphrey *et al.*, 1964); single suspensions of lymphoid cells do not always restore the lymphocyte population and may "run out", resulting in a form of late wasting disease (East and Parrott, 1964; Law *et al.*, 1964). The only permanent and complete method of restoration, preventing wasting and restoring both the total lymphocyte population and immune responses, is by a thymus graft. The tissue is only effective when from a neonatal donor and when grafted well before any wasting symptoms appear (East and Parrott, 1964). The best site of implantation is under the kidney capsule (Parrott and East, 1964).

Mode of Action of the Thymus

The thymus does not play any immediate part in immunological reactions itself. All functions of the thymus whether as a graft or in its orthotopic site, are fulfilled by its effect on the other lymphoid organs and the total population of circulating lymphocytes. It has been shown by several groups of workers (Miller, 1962; Harris and Ford, 1963; Miller, de Burgh, Dukor, Grant, Allman and House, 1966) using special strains of mice carrying an easily identifiable chromosome marker that cells migrate from a thymus graft to the lymph nodes and spleens of recipient mice. Such cells advertise their presence by dividing, and thus enabling their chromosomes to be identified, on appropriate immunological stimulation as the application of a skin graft (Miller *et al.*, 1966; Davies, Leuchars, Wallis and Koller, 1966). Other experiments using autoradiographic techniques have shown that cells from $[3]$H-thymidine labelled thymus tissue either as a graft (Parrott and de Sousa, 1967) or *in situ* (Weissman, 1967) or intravenously injected $[3]$H-adenosine labelled thymus cells (Parrott *et al.*, 1966) localize specifically in the thymus-dependent areas of the lymph nodes and spleens. However, although the lymphoid cells which migrate from the thymus may be vital for maintaining the mobile lymphocyte population, the structure within the thymus which endows it with its uniqe characteristics is the epithelial reticular network. These cells survive transplantation (Dukor, Miller, House and Allman, 1965) and persist (Parrott and de Sousa, 1967) when all other cells in a thymus graft have been replaced (Metcalf and Wakonig-Vaartaja, 1964; Dukor *et al.*, 1965) by cells apparently derived from the bone marrow (Micklem, Ford, Evans and Gray, 1966); all that is necessary is the epithelial-reticular framework, which in some way converts bone marrow derived cells into thymic lymphocytes (Micklem *et al.*, 1966).

The epithelial-reticular network can even survive and continue to function when enclosed in a diffusion chamber consisting of a millipore membrane which is impermeable to cells, although allowing liquids and substances of low molecular weight to pass through. The fact that thymus tissue enclosed in such a chamber can restore some of the immune responses in neonatally thymectomized animals (Osoba and Miller, 1963; Levey, Trainin and Law, 1963; Osoba, 1965) has given rise to the theory that the thymus produces a hormone which is responsible for the maturation of immunologically competent cells (Osoba and Miller, 1963). This hormone has not yet been isolated, nor is it certain that the thymus produces a hormone in the normally accepted sense of the word. However, it seems likely that the epithelial-reticular network does have an inductive effect on other cells and that this effect can be mediated through a millipore membrane. Nevertheless, the question remains open as to whether the thymus acts by "seeding" new lymphocytes to other organs, by "processing" or "instructing" lymphocytes from other sources, e.g. the bone marrow or by a hormonal action on peripheral lymphocytes; possibly a combination of all these mechanisms is essential.

The exact role of the thymus-derived cell once it has entered the recirculatory pool of lymphocytes remains to be defined. These cells respond first in time to immunological stimuli (Davies et al., 1966; de Sousa and Parrott, 1967) and are especially concerned in reactions of the cell mediated type (Parrott and de Sousa, 1966; Parrott, 1967). However, we do not yet know the exact relationship of the thymus-derived cell to the immunologically competent small lymphocyte as defined by Gowans (Gowans and McGregor, 1965) or yet if it has any effector role in the actual cell-mediated processes such as rejection of a skin graft. Recently, however, additional information has been gained from the response of this cell to the widely used antigen SRBC. The thymus-derived cell in the spleen responds to an intravenous injection of SRBC in a very similar way to the same cell type in the lymph node draining a skin graft, that is by prompt and rapid cell division (Davies et al., 1966), thus it may be termed antigen reactive (Miller, Mitchell and Weiss, 1967). But it has been clearly demonstrated by several workers that despite being antigen-reactive the thymus-derived cell is not the effector antibody producing cell (Davies et al., 1967; Taylor, Wortis and Dresser, 1967; Mitchell and Miller, 1968), which is known to be derived from the bone marrow. However, both thymus derived and bone marrow derived cell types are necessary to ensure full response to the antigen, for neither is effective independently (Claman, Chaperon and Triplett, 1966; Davies et al., 1967; Mitchell and Miller, 1968).

IMMUNOLOGICAL DEFICIENCY DISEASES OF CHILDHOOD

The human diseases which throw the greatest light on the functions of the thymus are the immunological deficiency diseases of infancy and childhood (Table II). *Thymic alymphoplasia* (Glanzman and Riniker, 1950; Hitzig and Willi, 1961; Gitlin and Craig, 1963) is a familial disease exhibiting the most serious forms of immunological deficiency. As stated by Janeway (1966), the "characteristic clinical manifestations are depressingly uniform— onset of cough with pulmonary infiltration, thrush, and failure to thrive, with poor appetite, poor growth, abdominal distension, and loose stools at a few months of age". Response to therapy including injections of γ-globulin is usually very poor and the child dies before 2 years of age. These children are totally incompetent immunologically, they have no immunoglobulins, no capacity to form antibodies or develop cellular sensitivity reactions: blood lymphocyte counts are extremely low. At post-mortem examination the thymus is often difficult to find; it may still be in the neck, having failed to descend into the chest, and consisting of a few epithelial elements only, with no thymic lymphocytes and no differentiation into cortex and medulla.

Lymph nodes and tonsils are minute structures and there is a complete absence of follicular structures, germinal centres and plasma cells. Recently, however, reports of cases of thymic alymphoplasia have been appearing in the literature (Nezelof, Jammet, Lortholary, Labrune and Lamy, 1964; Fulginiti, Hathaway, Pearlman, Blackburn, Reiquam, Githens, Claman and Kempe, 1966) which vary from the original description of this syndrome but which are more analogous to the effects of experimental neonatal thymectomy in mice. These children have the same persistent illnesses, recurrent pseudomonas and monilia infections, depression of small lymphocytes and impaired cellular sensitivity responses. However, although response to specific antigenic stimuli may be defective, serum immunoglobulin levels are often normal. Pathological findings include thymic alymphoplasia, though occasionally some thymic lymphocytes may be present (Fig. 5), lymphoid depletion though some follicular structures are found (Fig. 6), but normal plasma cells particularly in the bone marrow. The primary defect in children with thymic alymphoplasia especially in the cases described by Nezelof et al., 1964, and Fulginiti et al., 1966, may be within the thymus itself with a subsequent failure in the development of other lymphoid tissues. However, in the more severe cases (Glanzman and Riniker, 1950; Hitzig and Willi, 1961; Gitlin and Craig, 1963) when there is total impairment of all immune responses and often some associated haematological disorder then it seems more likely that there are defects in the bone marrow as well as in the thymus. An interesting alternative explanation, that is, that the children are the victims of a type of auto-immune reaction has also been suggested (de Vries, Dooren and Cleton, 1967).

Treatment with mature lymphoid cells has had the same dire fatal consequences as injections of unrelated cells into neonatally thymectomized mice, namely acute graft-versus-host reaction (runt disease) (Fulginiti et al., 1966). Several attempts, so far unsuccessful (Rosen, Gitlin and Janeway, 1962; Hitzig, Kay and Cottier, 1965; Fulginiti et al., 1966), have been made to reconstitute the lymphoid system with thymic grafts usually from fœtal donors. It may be, again as with animals, that the graft must be placed in a well-vascularized site long before any adverse symptoms are apparent in order to be effective. Such therapy could, therefore, only be of value in an asymptomatic sibling of an affected child.

The finding in children with thymic alymphoplasia contrast strongly with cases of *congenital hypogamma-globulinæmia* (Bruton, 1952; Janeway, 1966) who also have recurrent infections but of a different type. In this syndrome severe bacterial infections predominate which respond to antimicrobial therapy and the administration of γ-globulin. Immunoglobulins and antibody production are defective, but the circulating small lymphocyte population and cellular sensitivity reactions are normal. At post-mortem examination the lymph nodes are very small, and contain no follicles, germinal centres or plasma cells. The thymus, however, is apparently normal.

Thymic Involvement in Immunological Diseases

In addition to thymic alymphoplasia, various other abnormalities of the thymus have been found in association with many clinical disorders. For example, hyperplasia of the medulla with the formation of germinal centres and plasma cells has

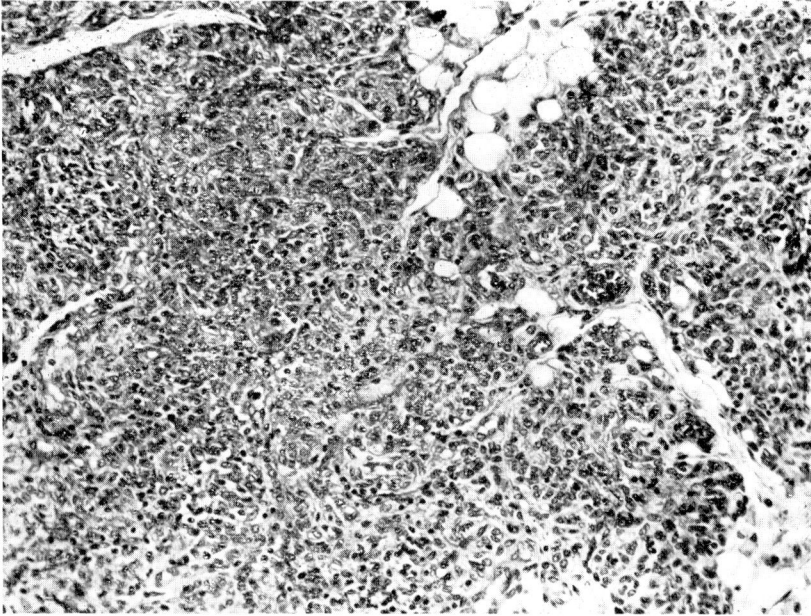

FIG. 5. Thymus from an infant with "Swiss-type" thymic alymphoplasia. Note undifferentiated spindle-shaped epithelial cells and a severe deficiency of lymphocytes. (Hæmatoxylin-phloxin-saffron × 225.)

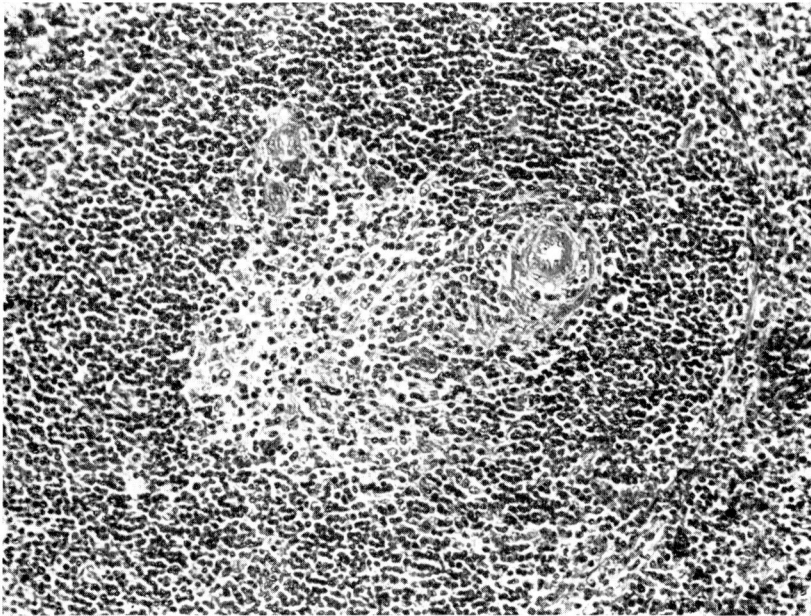

FIG. 6. Spleen from the same infant as Fig. 5. Note the similarity in appearance with the spleen from the neonatally thymectomized mouse (Fig. 4). Normal sized follicle and lymphocytes present at the periphery but absent from a pale stained area inside the follicles. (Hæmatoxylin-phloxin-saffron × 225.)

(Figs. 5 and 6 are reproduced by kind permission of Prof. M. J. de Vries. This case has been described in detail by M. J. de Vries et al., 1967).

long been associated with the muscular disease myasthenia gravis (reviewed by Castleman, 1955; Miller, Marshall and White, 1962); more recently such changes have been seen in patients with systemic lupus erythematosus (Mackay and de Gail, 1963) and rheumatoid arthritis (Burnet and Mackay, 1962). Thymomas with several different morphological characteristics have been observed in association with myasthenia gravis (Castleman, 1955) agammaglobulinæmia (Good and Varco, 1955), hypergammaglobulinæmia, autoimmune hæmolytic anæmia, systemic lupus erythematosus (see review, Strauss and van der Geld, 1966). Thymic abnormalities, germinal centre proliferation, plasma cells and mast cells have also been seen in the thymus of the mice of special inbred strains, NZB (Burnet and Holmes, 1962). These mice spontaneously develop autoimmune hæmolytic anæmia from 5–6 months of age (Bielschowsky, Helyer and Howie, 1959; Holmes and Burnet, 1963) and their hybrid progeny NZB × NZW mice develop lupus nephritis from 6 months of age and have positive LE tests (Helyer and Howie, 1963a). However, the precise functional relationships between all these syndromes in mice and in man and the associated pathological changes in the thymus have still to be defined. While it is reasonable to suppose that the thymus, which plays such an important part in the development of the lympho-myeloid complex, should often be involved in disease processes which concern other members of the complex, the idea that abnormality of the thymus was the primary cause of a whole variety of immunological diseases is no longer tenable. Thus, in human cases the onset of a thymoma and the associated diseases are often quite unrelated in time (Mackay, 1966), and the recent observation by Middleton (1967) that germinal centres are present in 72 per cent of apparently normal thymuses removed at post mortem has considerably reduced the significance of the finding of such structures in the thymuses of patients with myasthenia gravis or other auto-immune diseases. Similarly, there is no direct relationship between the appearance of germinal centres in the NZB mice and the onset of auto-immune symptoms (Parrott and East, 1965; East, de Sousa and Parrott, 1965) and germinal centres have been seen in other strains of mice without auto-immune symptoms (Seigler, 1966).

Excision of the thymus in patients often fails to cure the associated disease and may indeed precipitate the appearance of other abnormal symptoms (Alarçon-Segovia, Galbraith, Maldonado and Howard, 1963; Birch, Cooke, Drew, London, Mackenzie and Milne, 1964; Fisher, 1964; Mackay and Smalley, 1966).

Experiments with the NZB and NZB × NZW mice have also failed to inculpate the thymus as the primary cause of the spontaneous auto-immune disease in these animals, for thymectomy in the neonatal period, i.e. well before the usual time of onset of auto-immune symptoms, fails to prevent the disease (Helyer and Howie, 1963b; East, de Sousa, Parrott and Jaquet, 1967). Indeed, in some neonatally thymectomized NZB mice Coombs tests were positive earlier than usual in the hybrid NZB × NZW and the symptoms of lupus nephritis were of greater severity (Howie and Helyer, 1966). Nevertheless, mice of these strains show the same wasting disease and depletion of small lymphocytes from the blood and lymphoid organs as follows neonatal thymectomy in other strains (East et al., 1967). However, although thymectomy does not cure the spontaneous mouse auto-immune diseases in which the primary symptoms are the production of abnormal antibodies, there are certain experimental auto-allergic diseases (e.g. encephalomyelitis, thyroiditis) in which cellular sensitivity reactions play a major part (Roitt and Doniach, 1966) and it is, therefore, not surprising to find that these are prevented by neonatal thymectomy (Arnason, Janković, Waksman and Wennersten, 1962; Janković, Isvaneski, Popeskovic and Mitrovic, 1965).

SUMMARY AND CONCLUSIONS

During the initial discoveries on the immunological importance of the thymus it was concluded by many investigators that the thymus in the mammal was directly responsible for the development of all forms of immunological responsiveness both normal and abnormal, and although such generalizations are no longer valid, there is little doubt that the thymus does play a very important rôle.

The effects of neonatal thymectomy on experimental animals and examination of the defects of infants with immunological deficiency diseases show that the thymus exerts its major and primary effects upon cellular sensitivity reactions and the migratory population of small lymphocytes. The absence of the thymus and its thymic-dependent lymphocytes from birth results in a predictable pattern of infection in both human infants and experimental animals against which there is, as yet, no adequate therapy; although demonstrating that cellular sensitivity reactions do fulfil a useful defensive function, a fact which is often debated.

The problem of the mode of action of thymic control remains unsolved. In neither normal nor abnormal reactions does the thymus itself play any immediate part, thus its excision cannot be expected to influence any existing immune reaction. There is evidence that both the epithelial-reticular framework and the thymic lymphocyte population are involved in mediating control of and contributing cells to the other lymphoid organs.

Immunoglobulin production is to a considerable extent independent of the thymus and although specific antibody responses to some antigens may be impaired in neonatally thymectomized animals, especially those which are particularly dependent on circulating lymphocytes, others are completely normal. Conversely, there are many immunological diseases in which production of immunoglobulins and specific antibodies is impaired but which do not show either thymic involvement or impairment of the thymic responses. Does this mean that an alternative system primarily responsible for immunoglobulin and antibody production exist in mammals? (Peterson, Cooper and Good, 1965). It is well established that such an alternative system, the bursa of Fabricius, exists in chickens. Birds from which the bursa is removed immediately after hatching are unable to produce antibody responses and lack plasma cells although there is little or no interference with their capacity to express cellular sensitivity reactions (Szenberg and Warner, 1962; Cooper, Peterson, South and Good, 1966); this is only affected if the thymus is removed. Recent experimental work on rabbits (Cooper, Percy, McKneally, Gabrielson, Sutherland and Good, 1966) has suggested that the lymphoid tissues of the appendix, sacculus rotundus and Peyer's patches may be analogous to the bursa of Fabricius. Removal of these organs, plus sub-lethal doses of irradiation, has no effect on the response to skin grafts or the development of cellular sensitivity reactions to tuberculin, but antibody production to antigens is defective. The presence of such an alternative system to the thymus could explain not only the independence of some antibody production but it would also offer an explanation of some thymic abnormalities (hyperplasia, tumours), for these could be interpreted as a result of abnormal immunological reaction initiated elsewhere rather than as a primary cause of the abnormality. Such experiments in mammals are still in a preliminary stage but the fact that the thymus does not reign supreme must now be remembered when interpreting the effects of neonatal thymectomy in animals or when contemplating thymectomy as a therapeutic measure in patients.

ACKNOWLEDGMENT

I should like to thank Mr. J. Pringle for the photography.

References

ALARÇON-SEGOVIA, D., GALBRAITH, R. F., MALDONADO, J. E. and HOWARD, F. M. (1963). *Lancet*, **ii**, 662.

ARNASON, B. G., DE VAUX, ST.-CYR, C. and RELYVELD, E. H. (1964). Int. Arch. Allergy, **25**, 206.

ARNASON, B. G., JANKOVIĆ, B. D., WAKSMAN, B. H. and WENNERSTEN, C. (1962). *J. exp. Med.*, **116**, 117.

BIELSCHOWSKY, M., HELYER, B. J. and HOWIE, J. B. (1959). *Proc. Univ. Otago med Sch.*, **37**, 9.

BIRCH, C. A., COOKE, K. B., DREW, C. E., LONDON, D. R., MACKENZIE, D. H. and MILNE, M. D. (1964). *Lancet*, **i**, 693.

BRUTON. O. C. (1952). *Pediatrics*, **9**, 722.

BURNET, F. M. and HOLMES, H. (1962). *Nature, Lond*, **194**, 146.

BURNET, F. M. and MACKAY, I. R. (1962). *Lancet*, **ii**, 1030.

CASTLEMAN, B. (1955). In *Atlas of Tumor Pathology*, Section 5, fascicle 19. Washington D.C. Armed Forces Institute of Pathology.

COOPER, M. D., PETERSON, R. D. A., SOUTH, M. A. and GOOD, R. A. (1966). *J. exp. Med.*, **123**, 75.

CLAMAN, H. N., CHAPERON, E. A. and FASER TRIPLETT, R. (1966). *J. Immunol.* **97**, 828.

DAVIES, A. J. S., LEUCHARS, E., WALLIS, V. and KOLLER, P. C. (1966). *Transplantation*, **4**, 438.

DAVIES, A. J. S., LEUCHARS, E., WALLIS, V., MARCHANT, R. and ELLIOT, E. V. (1967). *Transplantation*, **3**, 639.

DE VRIES, M. J., DOOREN, L. J. and CLETON, F. J. (1967). *Proc. Third Immunology Workshop in the Immunological Deficiency Diseases in Men.* (In press).

DUKOR, P., MILLER, J. F. A. P., HOUSE, W. and ALLMAN, V. (1965). *Transplantation*, **5**, 639.

EAST, J., DE SOUSA, M. A. B. and PARROTT, D. M. V. (1965). *Transplantation*, **3**, 711.

EAST, J., DE SOUSA, M. A. B., PARROTT, D. M. V. and JAQUET, H. (1967). *Clin. exp. Immunol.*, **2**, 203.

EAST, J. and PARROTT, D. M. V. (1964). *J. natn. Cancer Inst.*, **33**, 673.

EAST, J., PARROTT, D. M. V., CHESTERMAN, F. C. and POMERANCE, A. (1963). *J. exp. Med.*, **118**, 1069.

FAHEY, J. L., BARTH, W. F. and LAW, L. W. (1965). *J. natn. Cancer Inst.*, **35**, 663.

FISHER, E. R. (1964). *The Thymus in Immunobiology*, p. 676. Hoever-Harper, New York.

FRIEDMAN, H. (1965). *Proc. Soc. exp. Biol., N.Y.*, **118**, 1176.

FULGINITI, V. A., HATHAWAY, W. E., PEARLMAN, D. S., BLACKBURN, W. K., REIQUAM, C. W., GITHENS, J. H. CLAMAN, H. N. and KEMPE, C. A. (1966). *Lancet*, **ii**, 5.

GITLIN, D. and CRAIG, J. M. (1963). *Pediatrics*, **32**, 517.

GLANZMAN, E., RINIKER, P. (1950). *Ann. paediat., Basel*, **175**, 1.

GOOD, R. A., GABRIELSEN, A. E., PETERSON, R. D. A., FINSTAD, J. and COOPER, M. D. (1966). p. 181 in *The Thymus: Experimental and Clinical Studies.* Ciba Foundation Symposium. J. and A. Churchill, Ltd., London.

GOOD, R. A. and PAPERMASTER, B. W. (1964). *Adv. Immunology*, **4**, 1.

GOOD, R. A. and VARCO, R. L. (1955). *Lancet*, **75**, 245.

GOWANS, J. L. and MCGREGOR, D. D. (1965). *Progr. Allergy*, **9**, 1.

HARRIS, J. E. and FORD, C. E. (1963). *Lancet*, **i**, 389.

HELYER, B. J. and HOWIE, J. B. (1963a). *Nature, Lond.*, **197**, 197.

HELYER, B. J. and HOWIE, J. B. (1963b). *Lancet*, **ii**, 1026.

HITZIG, W. H., KAY, H. E. M. and COTTIER, H. (1965). *Lancet*, **ii**, 151.

HITZIG, W. H. and WILLI, H. (1961). *Schweiz. med. Wschr.*, **52**, 1625.

HOLMES, M. C. and BURNET, F. M. (1963). *Ann. intern., Med.*, **59**, 265.

HOWIE, J. B. and HELYER, B. J. (1966). in *The Thymus: Experimental and Clinical Studies.* Ciba Foundation Symposium. p. 360. J. and A. Churchill, Ltd., London.

HUMPHREY, J. H., PARROTT, D. M. V. and EAST, J. (1964). *Immunol.*, **7**, 419.

JANKOVIĆ, B. D., ISVANESKIE, M., POPESKOVIC, L. and MITROVIC, K. (1965). *Int. Arch. All.*, **26**, 18.

JANKOVIĆ, B. D., WAKSMAN, B. H. and ARNASON, B. G. (1962). *J. exp. Med.*, **116**, 159.

JANEWAY, C. A. (1966). *Arch. Dis. Childh.*, **41**-, 358.

LAW, L. W. (1966). *Cancer Res.*, **26**, 551.

LAW, L. W., DUNN, T. B., TRAININ, N., and LEVEY, R. H. (1964). In *The Thymus*, p. 105. The Wistar Institute Press.

LAW, L. W. and TING, R. C. (1965). *Proc. Soc. Exp. Biol.* and *Med.*, **119**, 823.
LAW, L. W., TRAININ, N., LEVEY, R. H. and BARTH, W. F. (1964). *Science*, **143**, 1049.
LEVEY, R. H., TRAININ, N. and LAW, L. W. (1963). *J. natn. Cancer Inst.*, **31**, 199.
MACKAY, I. R. (1966). in *The Thymus: Experimental and Clinical Studies.* Ciba Foundation
    Symposium p. 449. J. and A. Churchill, Ltd., London.
MACKAY, I. R. and DE GAIL, P. (1963). *Lancet*, **ii**, 667.
MACKAY, I. R. and SMALLEY, M. (1966). *Clin. exp. Immunol.*, **1**, 129.
MALMGREN, R. A., RABSON, A. S. and CARNEY, P. G. (1964). *J. natn. Cancer Inst.*, **33**, 101.
McINTIRE, K. R., SELL, S. and MILLER, J. F. A. P. (1964). *Nature, Lond.*, **204**, 151.
METCALF, D. (1960). *Brit. J. Haemat.* **6**, 324.
METCALF, D. (1965). *Nature, Lond.*, **208**, 1336.
METCALF, D. and WAKONIG-VAARTAJA, R. (1964). *Proc. Soc. Exp. Biol. Med.*, **115**, 731.
MICKLEM, H. S., FORD, C. E., EVANS, E. P. and GRAY, J. (1966). *Proc. roy. Soc. B.*, **165**, 78.
MIDDLETON, G. (1967). *Austr. J. exp. Biol. Med. Sci.*, **45**, 189.
MILLER, J. F. A. P. (1961). *Lancet*, **ii**, 748.
MILLER, J. F. A. P. (1962). *Proc. roy. Soc. B.*, **156**, 415.
MILLER, J. F. A. P. (1965). *Brit. med. Bull.*, **21**, No. 2, p. 111.
MILLER, J. F. A. P., DE BURGH, P. M., DUKOR, P., GRANT, G., ALLMAN, V. and HOUSE, W.
    (1966). *Clin. exp. Immunol.*, **1**, 61.
MILLER, J. F. A. P., DOAK, S. M. A. and CROSS, A. M. (1963). *Proc. Soc. exp. Biol. Med.*,
    112, 785.
MILLER, J. F. A. P., MARSHALL, A. H. E.and WHITE, R. G. (1962). In *Advances in Immunology*
    2, p. 111. Academic Press, London.
MILLER, J. F. A. P., TING, R. C. and LAW, L. W. (1964). *Proc. Soc. exp. Biol. Med.*, **116**,
    334.
MILLER, J. F. A. P., MITCHELL, G. F. and WEISS, N. S. (1967). *Nature*, **214**, 992.
MITCHELL, G. F. and MILLER, J. F. A. P. (1968). *Proc. nat. Acad. Sci.*, **59**, 296.
NEZELOF, C., JAMMET, M. L., LORTHOLARY, P., LABRUNE, B. and LAMY, M. (1964). *Arch.
    franc. pediat.*, **21**, 897.
OORT, J. and TURK, L. J. (1965). *Brit. J. exp. Path.*, **46**, 117.
OSOBA, D. (1965). *J. exp. Med.*, **122**, 663.
OSOBA, D. and MILLER, J. F. A. P. (1963). *Nature, Lond.*, **199**, 653.
PARROTT, D. M. V. (1962). *Transplant. Bull.*, **29**, 102.
PARROTT, D. M. V. (1967). *Suppl. J. Clin. Path.*, **20**, 456.
PARROTT, D. M. V. and DE SOUSA, M. A. B. (1966). *Nature. Lond.*, **212**, 1316.
PARROTT, D. M. V. and DE SOUSA, M. A. B. (1967). *Immunology*, **13**, 193.
PARROTT, D. M. V., DE SOUSA, M. A. B. and EAST, J. (1966). *J. exp. Med.*, **123**, 191.
PARROTT, D. M. V. and EAST, J. (1962). *Nature, Lond.*, **207**, 487.
PARROTT, D. M. V. and EAST, J. (1964). p. 523. In *The Thymus in Immunobiology.* Hoever-
    Harper, New York.
PARROTT, D. M. V. and EAST, J. (1965). In *Autoimmunity*, p. 95. Blackwell, Oxford.
PARROTT, D. M. V. and EAST, J. (1965). *Nature, Lond.*, **207**, 487.
PETERSON, R. D. A., COOPER, M. D. and GOOD, R. A. (1965). *Am. J. Med.*, **38**, 579.
ROSEN, F. S., GITLIN, D. and JANEWAY, C. A. (1962). *Lancet*, **ii**, 380.
ROITT, I. M. and DONIACH, D. (1967). *Brit. med. Bull.*, 23, p. 66.
SCHOOLEY, J. C. and KELLY, L. S. (1964). In *The Thymus in Immunobiology*, p. 236. Hoever-
    Harper, New York.
SCOTHORNE, R. J. and McGREGOR, I. A. (1955). *J. Anat.*, **89**, 283.
SIEGLER, R. (1966). *J. exp. Med.*, **122**, 929.
DE SOUSA, M. A. B. and PARROTT, D. M. V. (1967). *In Germinal Centres in Immune Res-
    ponses.* Springen-verlag, Berlin, p. 361.
STRAUSS, A. J. L. and VAN DER GELD, H. (1966). In *The Thymus: Experimental and Clinical
    Studies.* Ciba Foundation Symposium p. 416. J. and A. Churchill, Ltd., London.
SZENBERG, A. and WARNER, N. L. (1962). *Nature, Lond*, **194**, 146.
TAYLOR, R. B. (1965). *Nature, Lond.*, **208**, 1334.
TAYLOR, R. B., WORTH, H. H. and DRESSER, D. W. (1967). In *The Lymphocyte in Immuno-
    logy and Haemopiesis.* Edward Arnold, London, p. 242.
WEISSMAN, I. L. (1967). *J. exp. Med.*, **126**, 291.
WILSON, R., SJODIN, K. and BEALMEAR, M. (1964). *Proc. Soc. exp. Biol. Med.*, **117**, 237.
YUNIS, E. J., HILGARD, H., SJODIN, K., MARTINEZ, C. and GOOD, R. A. (1964). *Nature,
    Lond.* **201**, 784.

Chapter 26

BYSSINOSIS

Geoffrey Taylor and A. A. E. Massoud

Byssinosis is a chronic respiratory disease affecting a proportion of workers involved in the early stages of the manufacture of cotton, flax, jute and hemp fibres. The dusty stages of the manufacturing process in which the relatively crude natural product is cleaned provide the majority of cases.

TABLE I

Country	Raw material	Industry	Incidence	Reference
			%	
England (Lancashire)	Cotton (coarse)	Carding and blowing	60	Schilling et al., 1955
		Waste	30	Dingwall-Fordyce et al., 1966
		Winding	17	Mekky et al., 1967
		Ring spinning	1·5	Lammers et al., 1964
Scotland	Flax	All workers	30	} Mair et al., 1960
	Jute		Nil	
N. Ireland	Flax	Pre-preparers	43	} Elwood et al., 1965
		Other workers	35	
Egypt	Cotton	Pressing	53	
		Ginning	38	} Batawi, 1962
		Carding	27	
	Flax	All workers	48	Batawi et al., 1964
Italy	Cotton	Card-room	62	Vigliani, 1962
France	Cotton	Card-room	47	Marchand and Weiner, 1962
Netherlands	Cotton	Card-room	17	} Lammers et al., 1964
		Ring spinning	1·6	
	Flax	Card-room	67	Bouhuys et al., 1961
Belgium	Flax	Card-room	12	Tupens, 1961
Sweden	Flax	Card-room	68	Belin et al., 1965
Greece	Flax	Ginning	Nil	Kendakis et al., 1965
Yugoslavia	Soft hemp	All workers	39	Zuskin et al., 1966
Spain	Hemp	All workers	77	Bouhuys et al., 1967
W. Germany	Cotton	Cleaning room	11·4	Antweiler et al., 1967

The disease is characterized by a sensation of chest tightness after returning to work following a weekend or holiday and hence is known as "Monday tightness" or "return to work tightness". A further characteristic is the delay of several years between first employment in the industry and the occurrence of symptoms. The disease appears to have a world-wide distribution (Table I).

CLINICAL FEATURES

A typical history as given by a worker who has worked in a dusty room for several years (3 to 40) is that, between one and six hours after commencing work on Mondays he notices "tightness across his chest" which makes physical effort difficult. This discomfort commonly increases until he leaves the mill at the end of the day. On his way home he may find it difficult to walk quickly, particularly up hill, and at home he may find it necessary to rest for the remainder of the day. On the other days of the week he is free of symptoms. Should he continue to work in the dusty situation, these symptoms may extend to other days of the week, but Monday will still be his worst day. This does not mean that progression of the disease is the rule; the symptoms may remain slight and static in some individuals and progress in others. In the latter cases the rates of progression may vary considerably.

PATHOLOGY AND PATHOGENESIS

No specific pathological lesions have been described in the lungs of byssinotic individuals. Several workers have described the changes of chronic bronchitis and emphysema (Greenhow, 1869; Landis, 1925; Ruszczewski et al., 1954), but these changes are so common in the population at risk as to cast doubt on their relationship to byssinosis. A further problem is that the material investigated has invariably been from post-mortems carried out on individuals who have usually ceased to work in the hazardous section of the textile industry several years before death. It is hardly surprising that there is no record of the histology of the lung at the time the individual is suffering from chest tightness. Such information would be of utmost value in elucidating the pathogenesis of the disease.

The mechanism by which the characteristic chest tightness of byssinosis occurs is still obscure. Theories have been postulated on possible mechanisms, but supporting evidence is either slender or completely lacking. One theory suggests that the sensation of tightness is due to increased airways resistance consequent upon inhalation of dust (McKerrow et al., 1962; Bouhuys, 1967). This is to some extent supported by a fall in the forced expiratory volume in $1 \cdot 0$ second ($FEV_{1 \cdot 0}$) found in byssinotics. The explanation does, however, ignore the fact that some byssinotics do not show such a fall in $FEV_{1 \cdot 0}$ whilst other symptom-free textile workers do show falls which in some cases are greater than those found in byssinotics (Gandevia and Milne, 1965). It would seem therefore that increase in airways resistance is unlikely to be the mechanism producing the sensation of tightness in affected workers.

The observation of severe disability due to dyspnœa in cases of byssinosis quoted by Schilling (1956), who at post-mortem had only minor degrees of emphysema, suggests that perhaps the interference with pulmonary physiology in byssinosis is in the pulmonary vascular bed rather than in the airways. This has not been postulated formally as a theory, and requires further investigation.

DIAGNOSIS

As byssinosis does not show any specific physical sign, pathological lesion or radiological change, and is without a specific diagnostic laboratory test, the diagnosis depends entirely on the characteristic history of "return to work tightness". This means that the diagnosis depends completely on the worker's own account of his symptoms. The disease has a very insidious onset, and it is almost impossible for the worker to remember when his Monday symptoms started. Careful history-taking by an experienced physician is at the moment the only method of diagnosis. There has been a tendency to consider the increase in airways resistance as measured by a $FEV_{1.0}$ determination to be an objective method of diagnosis. This is not justifiable for the reasons discussed under pathogenesis. Studies on airways resistance may be a help in epidemiological studies, but are valueless in the individual case.

Legally byssinosis is a prescribed disease only in Britain and in Egypt, and to qualify for compensation the worker must fulfil the following criteria:

(a) have worked in a card-room or blowing-room for at least 10 years using raw cotton, waste cotton or flax;
(b) have typical symptoms of byssinosis on each "return to work";
(c) be disabled by breathlessness unexplained by any other disease.

This does not cover all cases of the disease. Some individuals develop disease before the 10-year period required by law, and also occasional cases, who do not work in the card- or blowing-rooms, are found from time to time.

There has, on occasion, been confusion between byssinosis and other specific chest diseases which occur in textile workers. The main confusing condition is "mill fever" (Arlidge, 1892; Oliver, 1902). This occurs amongst new employees or visitors to the mill. Symptoms usually develop within 12 hours of exposure when the patient complains of a dry cough, headache, sneezing and general malaise. The temperature is usually raised. The symptoms usually clear quickly, but may occur again on next exposure. The worker soon fails to respond to exposure and does not suffer in this manner again. Complications have not been described and the ætiology is not known. Exposure to foreign proteins and bacterial endotoxins have been suggested as possible causes (Doig, 1949). Another condition which could be confused with byssinosis is "weaver's cough" (Collis, 1915; Bridge, 1924; Middleton, 1926). This occurs as outbreaks of an acute febrile illness in cotton weaving sheds and in velvet-cutting factories. The disease is characterized by an irritating productive cough, breathlessness, wheezing and pyrexia. It appears to be related to applying size to the warp and was originally attributed to fungal growth on the sized threads, but an outbreak reported by Murray *et al.* (1957) was investigated by Tuffnell and Dingwall-Fordyce (1957), who attributed symptoms to hypersensitivity to the tamarind seeds used in the size.

There are as yet insufficient data available to explore the relationship between byssinosis and chronic bronchitis. As in any dusty occupation the incidence of chronic bronchitis is high in the textile industry. In addition symptoms of byssinosis often occur in individuals clearly suffering from

P

chronic bronchitis. Individuals rarely consider themselves severely disabled when suffering from "Monday tightness" alone; it is those individuals with symptoms of both byssinosis and chronic bronchitis who are disabled. Physiological studies by Massoud (1964) and by Massoud *et al.* (1967) distinguish between bronchitic byssinotics and non-bronchitic byssinotics. This difference they attribute to the bronchial irritability found in chronic bronchitis.

ÆTIOLOGY

The ætiology of byssinosis is still obscure, and as in all diseases of obscure causation many theories have been proposed. Most theories fail by not taking into account the natural history of the disease. The facts which must be fitted into any theory are summarized below:

1. The disease has a world-wide distribution.
2. The incidence of the disease is related to the concentration of ambient dust.
3. The disease occurs amongst workers exposed to different dusts of vegetable origin.
4. Only a proportion of the workers are affected.
5. There is a long latent period (greater than three years) between the first exposure and first occurrence of symptoms.
6. In an established byssinotic symptoms occur with a delay of between one and six hours after exposure to dust.
7. In an established byssinotic recovery from chest tightness is delayed for a period often of several hours after exposure to dust has ceased.
8. In the more mildly affected subjects symptoms only occur on return to work after a period away from dust—usually on Monday after the weekend break.
9. In more severely affected byssinotics symptoms occur on days other than Monday, but these are less severe than the Monday symptoms.
10. Symptoms are most severe following a long period away from work.
11. Symptoms tend not to occur when working seven days per week.
12. Symptoms of byssinosis cease when the worker leaves the industry.

The dust present in the cotton card-room contains many things. It is made up largely of fine cotton fibres but also contains bacteria and fungi and plant material from the cotton plant, mainly from the fruiting body of the plant. Analysis of the dust has shown 96–98 per cent cellulose, 1·5 per cent protein and traces of inorganic materials, organic acids, vitamins, and pigments of unidentified nature (Ward, 1955). Much effort has been employed in attempts to identify the byssinogen present in the dust, and to demonstrate its mode of action. The theories arising from this work are discussed below.

Mechanical Irritation Theory. Mechanical irritation of the epithelial surfaces of the air passages in the lungs by the short cotton fibres has been suggested as a possible mechanism of causation (Leach, 1863; Arlidge, 1892; Middleton, 1926; Prausnitz, 1936). Two facts contradict this suggestion. The rare occurrence of byssinosis in workers carding fine cotton as opposed to those carding coarse cotton, although the cotton fibre content of the dust is similar, would exclude the cotton fibre itself as the byssinogen. This is further confirmed by the absence of byssinosis in workers carding medical cotton-wool in which much if not all of the non-cellulose material has been removed before carding although the dust concentration is higher than in a normal card-room (Batawi and Shash, 1962).

Micro-organism Theories. A wide range of both bacteria and fungi have been isolated from cotton dust and have been held by various investigators to be the causal agents of byssinosis (Castellani, 1932; Furness and Maitland, 1952; Drummond and Hamlin, 1952; Tuffnell, 1960). For several reasons it is unlikely that this interpretation is correct. None of the organisms isolated are known to be respiratory pathogens, nor can they be isolated from the sputum of individuals suffering from the disease (Prausnitz, 1936). Again, there is no correlation between the incidence of byssinosis and the presence of any particular micro-organism, and also the type of organism isolated from dust is variable both from place to place and from time to time in the same factory.

The endotoxins of Gram-negative bacteria are present in cotton, flax and hemp dusts, and this has led several investigators to incriminate them in the causation of byssinosis (Pernis et al., 1961; Cavagna et al., 1966). Endotoxins characteristically produce pyrexia, and byssinosis is a disease in which pyrexia does not normally occur. The hypothesis also fails to explain the long lag-period between first employment in the mill and first occurrence of symptoms and also the occurrence of symptoms on Mondays, but not on other days of the week. Endotoxins may well be involved in the causation of "mill fever" and this has led to considerable confusion in the past. There is, however, no similarity between "mill fever" and byssinosis.

Pharmacological Agent Theories. A number of agents with either direct or indirect activity on smooth muscle have been described as being present in extracts of cotton dust. These are histamine, histamine liberators, 5-hydroxytryptamine and smooth muscle contracting agents of unknown nature. All these agents have been implicated by various workers in theories on the causation of byssinosis.

Histamine. The presence of histamine was first detected by Maitland, Heap and Macdonald in 1932. The concentration in dust is low—0·001 mg./ml. (Bouhuys et al., 1960). It has been suggested by Bouhuys that this is far too low a concentration to produce any pulmonary effect. This has been confirmed by Massoud et al. (1967), who showed that inhalation of aerosols of histamine did not produce the typical symptoms or influence lung function tests in uncomplicated byssinotic subjects. Further, although hemp workers suffer from byssinosis, Jimenez Diaz and Lahoz (1944) failed to find histamine in hemp dust.

Histamine Liberator Substances. Substances which cause the liberation of histamine from its bound form in tissues were found in cotton dust by Bouhuys et al. (1960) and by Antweiler (1961). Similar criticisms to those above apply to any suggestion that these agents are involved in the causation of byssinosis. In addition, even though cotton dust extracts may be capable of releasing histamine in pharmacological quantity from tissues, there is no suggestion that byssinotics suffer from symptoms attributable to systemic dissemination of histamine, as would be expected were large amounts in fact released.

Other Smooth Muscle Contractor Substances. The fall in $FEV_{1\cdot0}$ observed to occur in many byssinotics at the end of the day following return to work (McKerrow et al., 1958) has resulted in a search for other agents which, by causing smooth muscle spasm, might account for increased airways resistance. Workers have suggested that 5-hydroxytryptamine or other smooth muscle contractors which have yet to be characterized might cause the symptoms of byssinosis (Davenport and Paton, 1962; Nichols, 1962). These suggestions fail in common with the other pharmacological theories in neither explaining the long latent period between first exposure and first occurrence of symptoms nor the occurrence of symptoms on return to work but not on other days.

Theories involving Hypersensitivity. The possibility that allergy to some component of cotton dust might be involved in the ætiology of byssinosis was suggested and investigated many years ago (Bramwell and Ellis, 1932; Van Leeuwen, 1932; Prausnitz, 1936). Skin tests using crude extracts of the dust were carried out then and by subsequent workers. The results have varied from highly significant correlation of positive skin test with Monday tightness (Prausnitz, 1936) to lack of such correlation (Cayton et al., 1952). The results using skin testing are shown in Table II. With such a vague entity as card-room dust it is hardly surprising that results should vary from investigator to investigator particularly when it is realized that the dust itself contains traces of pharmacologically active agents which themselves could cause skin capillary changes.

The major advantage of a theory involving allergy to a component of card-room dust is that it can explain the delay between first exposure and onset of symptoms by considering this as the period required for sensitization. Such a theory can also explain the great individual variation in response to chronic exposure to card-room dust in that some workers develop the disease early and progress to disability quickly whilst others, no less exposed, do not develop the disease during their working lifetime. A difficulty with allergic theories has been the great difference between byssinosis and the usual pulmonary allergic disease—asthma. The two are different in so many respects both objectively and subjectively that it is not likely that they have a common ætiological mechanism. More recently, with the discovery of pulmonary disease associated with the presence of circulating precipitating antibody in Farmer's Lung (Pepys et al., 1962; Bishop et al., 1963) and in pulmonary aspergillosis (Pepys et al., 1959) and bird-fancier's lung (Hargreaves et al., 1966), these difficulties may be resolved. In these diseases, already discussed in Chapter 23, the site of damage appears to be the capillaries in the smaller air passages, the symptoms are not typically asthmatic in nature and the increased airways resistance typical of asthma is not necessarily present. The work of Massoud and Taylor (1964) has demonstrated the occurrence of precipitating antibody to parts of the cotton plant which invariably contaminates raw cotton and hence is present in card-room dust. They have suggested that this antibody is involved in the production of the symptoms of byssinosis.

Massoud and Taylor demonstrated the presence in all sera tested of antibody to an antigen present in the receptacle and epicalyx of the cotton plant. They carried out semi-quantitative titrations using a diffusion in gel technique on normal individuals, on cotton workers not working in hazardous sections of the factory, and on both byssinotic and non-byssinotic card-room workers. Comparing "normals" with cotton workers a highly significant difference in the distribution of titres was found with the textile workers having the higher range of titres. Again comparing those workers operating the carding machines (the most hazardous occupation) with other cotton workers a highly significant difference was found; the carding machine operatives having the higher range of titres. Finally, a significantly higher range of titres were found in byssinotic subjects as compared with cotton workers not suffering from this disease. Thus an association has been shown between antibody to the "cotton antigen" and working in the cotton industry and also between the antibody and byssinosis. The occurrence of antibody in individuals who had never been exposed to card-room dust may be explained by assuming that the antigen is a fairly common one, perhaps widely distributed in the plant kingdom. The observations suggest the following hypothesis. During the early years of work in those parts of the cotton mill in which cotton-antigen-containing dust is found, the worker builds up his level of antibody from that found in the "normal" group to that found in the group of card-room workers. The

TABLE II

Skin Test Results

Investigators	Group	Diagnosis	No.	Skin test with cotton dust	
				+	−
Bramwall and Ellis (1932)	Card-room workers	Byssinotic	48	37 (77%)	11
	Card-room workers	Free of symptoms	10	1 (10%)	9
	General population	Free of symptoms	11	4 (35%)	7
Van Leeuwien (1932)	General population	Asthmatics	?	100%	...
		Normals	?	...	100%
Prausnitz (1936)	Card-room workers	Byssinotic	30	28 (93%)	2
	Card-room workers	Free of symptoms	14	4 (28%)	10
	General population	Asthmatics	11	4 (36%)	7
	General population	Free of symptoms	7	2 (28%)	5
Cayton et al. (1952)	Card- and blowing-room workers	Advanced byssinosis	31	For details of results consult original publication. Ten different types of cotton extract were used in different dilutions. The results of early and late reactions failed to distinguish between the groups tested.	
	Card- and blowing-room workers	Early byssinosis	16		
	Card- and blowing-room workers	Free of symptoms	21		
	Other mill workers	Free of symptoms	16		
	General population	Allergic	61		
	General population	Free of symptoms	146		
Gernez-Rieux et al. (1962)	Card-room workers	Byssinotics	25	10 (40%) (react only to cotton dust)	15
	Card-room workers	Asthmatics	15	10 (66%) (react vigorously to other dusts)	5
	General population	Free of symptoms	68	3 (5%)	65

amount of antibody produced will depend on the worker's own inherent ability to produce antibody. The better antibody producers will have the highest antibody levels, as found in byssinotic card-room workers. Following exposure to dust on Monday morning, an antigen-antibody reaction takes place in the lungs. The magnitude of the reaction will be largely determined by the amount of available antibody. The symptoms of byssinosis are produced directly by the action of antigen-antibody complex on the capillaries in the peripheral part of the lung. In normal subjects or in card-room workers with low-antibody titres, the amount of antigen-antibody complex produced is small, and the resulting lung changes are insignificant and unnoticed. In the byssinotic subjects exposure to cotton antigen results in a large amount of antigen-antibody complex, and symptoms appear. As a result of the reaction, the amount of circulating antibody decreases, and on further exposure to dust on Tuesday there is not sufficient complex formed to produce symptoms. In advanced cases of byssinosis with symptoms on Tuesdays and sometimes on other days of the week, it may be postulated that absorption of antibody on Monday leaves sufficient still available to produce a reaction on exposure to cotton dust later in the week. Over the weekend, during which the card-room worker is not exposed to the cotton antigen, the antibody is no longer removed daily from the circulation and the antibody titre rises. The amount of antibody is again high enough on Monday to produce further symptoms. The most severe attacks of byssinotic symptoms are after the annual holidays, when a longer period away from the antigen may have resulted in much higher antibody levels than are found after the two-day weekend absence from work.

Since this publication, attempts have been made to confirm or deny this theory. The cotton antigen has been found to occur in other parts of the cotton plant as well as those already described (Taylor, 1965). It has been extracted from dust obtained from around the carding machines and has been demonstrated in respirable dust taken by an air sampler from the card-room. The antigen has been obtained in a relatively pure state which has enabled further serology to be carried out. The antigen appears to be a complex flavanoid polyphenol of molecular weight in the range of 10,000–15,000 and is probably in the group of substances known as condensed tannins (Lucas and Taylor, 1966). Antibody is present in considerable amount in byssinotic subjects being in the range 150–200 μg. Ab N/ml. in several byssinotics tested by quantitative precipitation. Normal subjects had less and were in the range 50–100 μg. Ab N/ml.

Further serology using more sensitive techniques is currently being used in a large survey of cotton workers. Preliminary analysis of the results bear out those obtained using the gel diffusion technique (Massoud and Taylor, 1964). Bronchial challenge tests, using the purified antigen, have been carried out on 25 normal volunteers and on 20 byssinotic card room workers. Varying doses have been administered, and although no symptoms or abnormal signs of any description have been produced in the normal group, 4 of 8 byssinotics given the higher dosages suffered from typical symptoms of byssinosis 3-8 hours after challenge. Challenges were carried out on Monday morning after the usual weekend away from the card room. It is of considerable interest that following the 'laboratory induced' byssinosis on Monday the symptoms of 'card room induced' byssinosis on Tuesday were either much milder or did not occur at all. This supports the view that exposure to the antigen results in a period of desensitisation, possibly by an antibody-absorption effect.

The work so far carried out suggests that it may be possible to develop a laboratory test for byssinosis, alternatively the bronchial challenge test with suitable controls could be used for diagnostic purposes. The ætiology of byssinosis still requires further investigation, particularly in respect of its patho-physiology. Laboratory induced byssinosis provides a very promising approach to this problem.

BYSSINOSIS 473

References

ANTWEILER, H. (1961). *Brit. J. industr. Med.*, **18**, 130.
ANTWEILER, H., KLOSTERDOTTER, W. and SIEBOFF, F. (1967). *Arbmed, Sozmed. Arbhyg.* **2**, 154.
ARLIDGE, J. T. (1892). *The Hygiene Diseases and Mortality of Occupations.* Percival, London.
BATAWI, M. A. (1962). *Brit. J. industr. Med.*, **19**, 126.
BATAWI, M. A. and HUSSIEN, M. (1964). *Brit. J. industr. Med.*, **21**, 231.
BATAWI, M. A. and SHASH, S. E. (1962). *Int. Arch. Gewerbepath und Gewerbehyg.*, **19**, 393.
BELIN, L., BOUHUYS, A., HOCKSTRA, W., JOHNSSON, M. B., LINDELL, S. E. and POOL, J. (1965). *Brit. J. industr. Med.*, **22**, 101.
BISHOP, J. M., MENICK, S. C. and RAINE, J. (1963). *Quart. J. Med.*, **32**, 257.
BOUHUYS, A. (1967). *Amer. Rev. Resp. Dis.*, **95**, 89.
BOUHUYS, A., BARBERO, A., LINDELL, S. E., ROACH, S. A. and SCHILLING, R. S. F. (1967). *Arch. Environ. Hlth.*, **14**, 533.
BOUHUYS, A., LINDELL, S. E. and LUNDIN, G. (1960). *Lancet*, **1**, 423.
BOUHUYS, A., VAN DUYN, J. and VAN LENNEP, H. J. (1961). *Arch. Environ. Hlth.*, **3**, 499.
BRAMWELL, J. C. and ELLIS, R. (1932). Home Office. Report of the Departmental Committee on Dust in Cardrooms in the Cotton Industry. pp. 43. H.M.S.O., London.
BRIDGE, J. C. (1924). Ann. Rep. Chief Inspector of Factories, p. 80.
CASTELLANI, A. (1923). Home Office. Report on the Department Committee on Dust in Cardrooms in the Cotton Industry. p. 31, H.M.S.O., London.
CAVAGNA, G., FOA, V., NICHELATTI, T., CALGARO, N. and LOCATI, G. (1966). *Proc. 15th Int. Cong. Occup. Hlth.*, **3**, 299. Verlag der Weiner Mid. Akademie, Vienna.
CAYTON, H. R., FURNESS, G. and MAITLAND, H. B. (1952). *Brit. J. industr. Med.*, **9**, 186.
COLLIS, E. L. (1951). Milroy Lecture. Publ., London. **28**, 260.
DAVENPORT, A. and PATON, W. O. M. (1962). *Brit. J. industr. Med.*, **19**, 19.
DINGWALL-FORDYCE, I. and O'SULLIVAN, J. G. (1966). *Brit. J. industr. Med.*, **23**, 53.
DOIG, A. T. (1949). *Post Grad. Med. J.*, **25**, 639.
DRUMMOND, D. G. and HAMLIN, M. (1952). *Brit. J. industr. Med.*, **9**, 309.
ELWOOD, P. C., PEMBERTON, J., MERRETT, J. O., CAREY, G. C. R. and MCAULAY, I. R. (1965). *Brit. J. industr. Med.*, **22**, 27.
FURNESS, G. and MAITLAND, H. B. (1952). *Brit. J. industr. Med.*, **9**, 138.
GANDEVIA, B. and MILEN, J. (1965). *Brit. J. industr. Med.*, **22**, 295.
GERNEZ-RIEUX, G., VOISIN, G., JACOB, M., CORSIN, L. and LEFERBORE, J. (1962). *Poumon et le Cœur*, **18**, 651.
GREENHOW, E. H. (1869). *Trans. path. Soc. Lond.*, **20**, 48.
HARGREAVE, F. E., PEPYS, J., LONGBOTTOM, J. L. and WRAITH, D. G. (1966). *Lancet*, **i**, 445.
JIMENEZ DIAZ, C. and LAHOZ, C. (1944). *Rev. Clin. Esp.*, **14**, 366.
KONDAKIS, X. G. and POURNARAS, N. (1965). *Brit. J. industr. Med.*, **22**, 291.
LAMMERS, B., SCHILLING, R. S. F. and WALFORD, J. (1964). *Brit. J. industr. Med.*, **21**, 124.
LANDIS, H. R. M. (1952). *J. industr. Hyg.*, **7**, 1.
LEACH, J. (1863). *Lancet*, **2**, 648.
LUCUS, F. and TAYLOR, G. (1966). *Unpublished observations.*
MCKERROW, C. G., MCDORMETT, M., GILSON, J. C. and SCHILLING, R. S. F. (1958). *Brit. J. industr. Med.*, **15**, 75.
MCKERROW, C. B., ROACH, S. A., GILSON, J. C. and SCHILLING, R. S. F. (1962). *Brit. J. industr. Med.*, **19**, 1.
MAIR, A., SMITH, D. H., WILSON, W. A. and LOCKHART, W. (1960). *Brit. J. industr. Med.*, **17**, 272.
MAITLAND, H. B., HEAP, H. and MACDONALD, A. D. (1932). Home Office. Report of the Departmental Committee on Dust in Cardrooms in the Cotton Industry. p. 87., H.M.S.O., London.
MARCHAND, M. and WERNER, G. C. H. (1962). Symposium on Byssinosis, Manchester. Reported by R. S. F. Schilling *et al.*, *Proc. 14th Int. Cong. Occup. Hlth.*, Madrid, 1963. Excerpta media, Amsterdam.
MASSOUD, A. A. E. (1964). *Ph.D. Thesis*, Manchester University.
MASSOUD, A. A. E., ALTOUNYAN, R. E. C., HOWELL, J. B. L. and LANE, R. E. (1967). *Brit. J. Industr. Med.*, **24**, 38.
MASSOUD, A. A. E. and TAYLOR, J. (1964). *Lancet*, **2**, 607.
MEEKY, S., ROACH, S. A. and SCHILLING, R. S. F. (1967). *Brit. J. industr. Med.*, **24**, 123.
MIDDLETON, E. L. (1926). *J. industr. Hyg.*, **8**, 432.
MURRAY, R. DINGWALL-FORDYCE, I. and LANE, R. E. (1957). *Brit. J. industr. Med.*, **14**, 105.
NICHOLLS, P. J. (1962). *Brit. J. industr. Med.*, **19**, 33.
OLIVER, T. C. (1902). *Dangerous Trades, p.* 273, Murrey, London.
PEPYS, J., RIDDELL, R. W., CITRON, K. M. and CLAYTON, Y. M. (1962). *Thorax*, **17**, 366.

PEPYS, J., RIDDELL, R. W., CITRON, K. M., CLAYTON, Y. M. and SHORT, E. I. (1959). *Amer. Rev. Resp. Dis.*, **80**, 167.
PERNIS, B., VIGLIANI, E. C., CAVAGNA, C. and FINULLI, M. (1961). *Brit. J. industr. Med.* **18**, 120.
PRAUSNITZ, C. (1936). *Spec. Rep. Ser. Med. Rec. Coun. Lond.*, No. 212.
ROSZEZEWSKI, Z., ZAWADZKI, R., GRYNSZTAZN, A., KAPSUCINSKA, W., RIEWINSKI, B. WIECZ-OREK, M. and SZOZDA, M. (1954). *Pol. Med. Wkly.*, **8**, 1602.
SCHILLING, R. S. F. (1956). *Lancet*, **2**, 261, 319.
SCHILLING, R. S. F., HUGHES, J. P. W., DINGWALL-FORDYCE, I. and GILSON, J. C. (1955). *Brit. J. industr. Med.*, **12**, 217.
TAYLOR, G. (1965). *Acta. Aller.*, **20**, 505.
TUFFNELL, P. (1960). *Brit. J. industr. Med.*, **17**, 307.
TUFFNELL, P. and DINGWALL-FORDYCE, I. (1957). *Brit. J. industr. Med.*, **14**, 250.
TUPENS, E. (1961). *Brit. J. industr. Med.*, **17**, 307.
VAN LEEUWEN, W. S. (1932). Home Office. Report of the Departmental Committee on Dust in Cardrooms in Cotton Industry, p. 90, H.M.S.O., London.
VIGLIANI, E. C. (1962. Symposium on Byssinosis, Manchester. Reported by R. S. F. Schilling, *Proc. 14th Int. Cong. Occup. Hlth.*, Madrid, 1963. Excerpta media. Amsterdam.
WARD, K. J. (1955). Chemistry and Chemical Technology of Cotton, Interscience Publishers, New York.
ZUSKIN, E. and VALICE, F. (1966). *Proc. 15th Int. Cong. Occup. Hlth.*, **3**, 291, Verlag der Weiner Med. Akademie, Vienna.

Chapter 27

TISSUE COMPATIBILITY TESTS

J. R. BATCHELOR

INTRODUCTION

THE transplantation of tissues from one animal into a genetically dissimilar recipient normally excites an immune response which leads to graft rejection. The antigens which are responsible for provoking the destructive immune reaction are known as histocompatibility or H antigens. Although there is no reason for excluding interspecies differences, traditionally the term is used for antigenic disparities between different members of the same species, i.e. iso-antigens.

In man the investigation of H antigens has only just begun. With the development of effective immuno-suppressive agents, it has become evident that prolonged survival of kidney transplants is possible even if graft donor and recipient are unrelated. The feasibility of transplanting other organs is also being actively investigated. Since it is reasonable to expect that improved clinical results will be obtained if histocompatibility differences between a graft donor and recipient are reduced to a minimum, the practical importance of studying human H systems is considerable.

Studies upon H systems of experimental animals have been going on for many years, and therefore there is a good deal of comparative evidence on which to base human studies. The mouse, which has been studied in great detail, is known to have at least 14–15 independently segregating H-antigen systems (Barnes and Krohn, 1957; Prehn and Main, 1958). Many of them have been individually identified and "fixed" in the genome of a series of specially bred mouse strains (see Graff, Hildemann and Snell, 1966, for references). Less is known about other species, but multiple systems appear to be the general rule (see Batchelor, 1965a, for references). Man like other species probably also possesses a number of independent H systems.

One might expect that tissue matching would be an impossible achievement because of the large number of independent loci. However, the outlook is not quite so bleak because the different loci vary greatly in their influence upon the survival of foreign grafts. For example, one system of the mouse, the H-2 system, consists of a series of strongly immunogenic antigens. If a skin graft contains several H-2 antigens lacked by the recipient, it provokes a very brisk immune response and rejection is usually complete in less than two weeks. In contrast antigenic differences determined by the H-1 locus will allow skin grafts to survive 20–124 days (Snell and Stevens, 1961). Another factor has also to be taken into account, namely the susceptibility of the grafted tissue to the immune reaction of the host. Skin grafts are extremely sensitive as indicators of incompatibility, whereas other organs or tissues are much less vulnerable to immunological attack. For example, kidney grafts and ovarian tissue grafts will survive in the face of an incompatibility strong enough to produce rejection of a skin graft from the same donor (Moseley, Shiel, Mitchell and Murray, 1966; Linder, 1962). Therefore, for certain purposes in clinical transplantation, matching graft and recipient only with respect to the strongly immunogenic antigens may be satisfactory. The first priority in man is clearly to identify the strongest H antigens, and then to find out whether they belong to the same or different systems.

In order to carry out any analysis of human H antigen systems it is necessary to know on what cells the antigens are to be found. Judging from experience in mice (Gorer and Mikulska, 1954; Amos, Gorer and Mikulska, 1955), rats (Bogden and Aptekman, 1960), chickens (Schiermann and Nordskog, 1961), and possibly rabbits (Zotikov, 1958) and dogs (Puza, Rubinstein, Kasakura, Vlahovic and Ferrebee, 1964), one might expect that strong human H antigens would be present on red cells. At present the only erythrocyte antigens known to influence the survival of allogeneic tissue, other than red cells, are those of the ABO and P systems (Dausset and Rapaport, 1966; Ceppellini, Curtoni, Mattiuz, Leigheb, Visetti and Colombi, 1966; Gleason and Murray, 1967). ABO system antigens affect the survival of foreign skin grafts in accordance with the principles established for red cells. The studies of Ceppellini *et al.* (1966) show that it is legitimate to use group O donors for all recipients.

Although the ABO and P systems influence tissue compatibility, it is clear that other and more potent H antigens exist because matching donor and host with respect to ABO and P systems is not sufficient to procure extended survival of kidney grafts (Woodruff, Robson, Nolan, Lambie, Wilson and Clark, 1963). A number of lines of evidence show that some, possibly all, human H antigens are present on leucocytes. Whole leucocytes (Friedman, Retan, Marshall, Henry and Merrill, 1961) or their extracts (Rapaport, Dausset, Converse and Lawrence, 1965) are capable of sensitizing an individual against allogeneic skin grafts. Immunization with skin grafts elicits antileucocyte antibodies (Colombani, Colombani and Dausset, 1964; Walford, Gallagher and Sjaarda, 1964; Batchelor, 1965b). At least four leucocyte iso-antigens or blocks of antigens have been already identified as H antigens (Dausset, Rapaport, Ivanyi and Colombani, 1965; van Rood, van Leeuwen, Schippers, Vooys, Frederiks, Balner and Eernisse, 1965). The results of clinical renal transplantation are significantly improved if donor and recipient show good correspondence of white cell iso-antigens, as determined by the cytotoxic test (Terasaki, Vredevoe, Mickey, Porter, Marchioro, Faris and Starzl, 1966). Finally, comparative evidence from other species points to the conclusion that potent H antigens are carried by leucocytes.

Interest has therefore been concentrated heavily on the iso-antigens of leucocytes. In the ensuing sections, some of the more commonly used methods of detecting leucocyte iso-antigens will be discussed.

SEROLOGICAL METHODS

These methods have certain advantages. They are relatively quick and simple. If for some reason direct testing is inapplicable, it is possible to detect the presence of any particular antigen by performing absorption tests. There is also the advantage that antisera are easy to transport and this will help ultimately towards the use of standardized reagents and nomenclature.

Leucocyte Agglutination. There are several variations of this test. At the 1st Histocompatibility Testing Workshop held in 1964, the participants gave detailed descriptions of their own methods (*Histocompatibility Testing*, Publication 1229, National Acad. of Sciences-National Research Council, Washington, D.C.). This publication is a useful guide for anyone wishing to carry out the tests.

In brief freshly drawn blood is either defibrinated or treated with sequestrene anticoagulant. The former method makes the test more sensitive but also more liable to give false positive results. A red cell sedimenting agent is then added— gelatin, polyvinylpirrolidone, or dextran—and after sedimentation the white cell rich supernate is removed and the cell concentration adjusted. Different workers favour slightly different concentrations for testing, but 3,000–6,000 cells per mm^3 is a usual level. For testing, a convenient volume of white cell suspension is mixed with 1–3 volumes of inactivated antiserum. The test is read microscopically after incubation for 90 minutes at 37°C. Some workers prefer to lyze the remaining red cells by adding dilute acetic acid to each tube just before reading is begun.

Although essentially simple, agglutination tests require careful execution if reliable results are to be obtained. In practised hands, using selected antisera, the results are consistent. It is important to note that polymorpho-nuclear leucocytes are the target cells in this test and that pure lymphocyte suspensions are inagglutinable. There is one pitfall associated with leuco-agglutination tests which merits special mention. In some cases direct testing of a cell suspension may show no agglutination, but positive absorption tests indicate that the leucocytes do possess the particular antigen under study. Van Rood has termed this the agglutination negative, absorption positive or ANAP phenomenon (van Rood, 1962). Some sera are more liable to produce ANAP reactions than others and it is advisable not to use these sera in critical genetic or transplantation studies. The reasons for occurrence of the ANAP reactions are not properly understood.

A second problem which may be of clinical importance should also be mentioned. Zmijewski (1965) has demonstrated that if suspensions of leucocytes which do not react with a particular antiserum are contaminated with small numbers of positively reacting cells, the mixed cell suspensions will then give positive reactions with the test antiserum. The contamination necessary to produce a positive result may be as little as 1–8 per cent depending on the agglutination test used. Such contamination is possible as a result of transfusion and Zmijewski warns against testing the cells of a patient too soon after transfusion.

Cytotoxic Test. In this test, target cells are incubated with antiserum and complement. If sufficient complement-fixing antibody combines with the test cells to allow activation of the complement system, lysis occurs. Viability of the test suspension is then quantitatively assessed.

In the original test (Gorer and O'Gorman, 1956) cell viability was determined by adding a solution of trypan blue or eosin and examining a sample of the suspension microscopically. Dead cells permit the entry of dye and become stained whereas live cells remain colourless. The percentage of dead cells can therefore be counted directly. Under the conditions of the test, the number of cells which disintegrate completely and therefore are not counted is too small to affect the test significantly. Technical details of the test can be found in Gorer and O'Gorman (1956) and Batchelor (1967).

When testing for human H antigens it is convenient to use lymphocytes from peripheral blood as target cells. Granulocytes have been used to a small extent (Engelfriet, 1965) but they are extremely susceptible to damage by factors other than iso-antibody and therefore are less suitable than lymphocytes. Fibroblasts, neoplastic cells, and probably many other cell types, if obtainable as monodiscrete cell suspensions can be used.

Lymphocytes may be prepared from peripheral blood by several methods. The one favoured by the author is a slight modification of that described by Walford, Gallagher and Troup (1965). Heparin-treated blood is mixed with a sedimenting agent and left to stand for 30–60 minutes. The white cell rich supernate is then removed and incubated with two successive changes of brushed nylon wool. After each incubation, the nylon wool is gently squeezed against the side of a small funnel to express the cell suspension. Granulocytes adhere to the nylon wool and are removed from the suspension, whereas lymphocytes do not attach to the nylon fibres and are squeezed out with the fluid. Two treatments for 30 minutes at 37°C with nylon wool usually produces a suspension in which 95–100 per cent of the white cells are lymphocytes. The cells are then centrifuged and resuspended in veronal buffered saline for the purpose of testing. Preparation of good lymphocyte suspensions from severely ill patients is sometimes difficult. For unknown reasons, polymorphs from these patients may not adhere to nylon wool. It is advisable, therefore, to type prospective kidney graft recipients after they have been adequately dialyzed. If a significant percentage of the test cell suspension consists of polymorphs, the background cell mortality level is usually raised and this will obscure the difference between negative and weak positive reactions. In difficult cases, many of the residual polymorphs may be removed by incubating the cell suspension with fresh normal rabbit serum which contains a natural cytotoxic antibody for polymorphs. Lymphocytes are not noticeably affected by the rabbit serum. The polymorph contaminated cell suspension is incubated for 20 minutes at 37°C with rabbit serum and then gently centrifuged. A large proportion of the polymorphs either disintegrate entirely or become so swollen that they are not deposited in the cell button. The lymphocyte containing cell button is resuspended after removal of the supernatant and used for testing.

More recently the technique of preparing lymphocytes as for the ^{51}Cr assay has been increasingly used. Further details are given in the section on this assay.

If heparin-treated blood is sent to another laboratory for typing, satisfactory lymphocyte suspensions can usually be obtained provided transportation time is limited to six hours and the blood sample is maintained at approximately 4°C. If transportation time exceeds this, it becomes increasingly difficult to obtain polymorph-free suspensions. Probably this is because the polymorphs die and therefore subsequent attempts to make them adhere to nylon wool fail. If transportation time is expected to be more than six hours, either nylon wool should be added to the sample before dispatch so that the granulocytes may adhere to it during transit, or a lymphocyte suspension should first be prepared. Polymorph-free suspensions of lymphocytes keep well at 4°C for 24–48 hours, and sometimes longer. In liquid nitrogen, they may be preserved indefinitely (Terasaki, Vredevoe and McClelland, 1965).

The performance of cytotoxicity tests varies slightly between different laboratories. In the author's laboratory, lymphocyte suspensions are made up in veronal buffered saline and adjusted to 1–3 million cells/ml. though less concentrated suspensions are occasionally used. One volume (20 μl.) of antiserum dilution, one volume of cell suspension and one volume of normal rabbit serum (complement source) are mixed and incubated for 30 minutes at 37°C. After incubation, titration racks are kept at 4°C. Before reading, the supernate is removed from each tube, leaving the sedimented lymphocytes behind, and two volumes of trypan blue solution are added. Samples from each tube are then examined microscopically for the percentage of dead cells. In the test described above, the lymphocyte suspension is contaminated with small numbers of red cells which are not removed during the original sedimentation. If preferred, these red cells can be removed before setting up the test by lysis with distilled water since white cells are considerably more resistant to osmotic shock than are red cells (Walford, Gallagher and Troup, 1965). However, the few contaminating red cells are easy to recognize and do not usually interfere with the reading of a test. Furthermore, they are considerably reduced in number after the addition of normal rabbit serum, which contains a natural hæmolytic antibody active against certain human red cells.

Terasaki and his colleagues (Terasaki and McClelland, 1964; Vredevoe, Terasaki, Mickey, Glassock, Merrill and Murray, 1965) have developed a microdroplet cytotoxic test which is both sensitive and remarkably economical in its use of reagents. Other variations in the test include different methods of assessing cell viability—such as the use of phase contrast microscopy instead of dye exclusion.

In the author's laboratory microdroplet cytotoxic tests are carried out with some modifications of the Terasaki method. Lymphocyte suspensions are prepared as described in the section on the ^{51}Cr assay. The plastic trays designed by Terasaki (available from Falcon Plastics, Los Angeles, California) which have numbered wells in them are employed. These trays are filled with paraffin oil containing 0·5 per cent wax and individual antisera are inoculated in 2 μl amounts into the wells. (Micro-dispensing syringes obtainable from the Hamilton Company, P.O. Box 307, Whittier, California 90608.) The trays, each of which contains a complete set of antisera available, are stored at $-25°C$ until required. They are thawed just before use and 4 μl of a lymphocyte suspension in complement is added to each serum-containing well. Two wells which contain normal serum or buffered saline provide controls. The lymphocyte/complement mixture is made up by adding non-toxic rabbit complement to an equal volume of lymphocytes at a concentration of 1×10^6 cells per ml. After incubating the test for either 30 or 60 minutes, all fluid is removed from each well by gentle suction. The removal of fluid must be complete, but care should be taken not to suck too vigorously or the target lymphocytes may be swept out of the well. 1-2 μl of a 0·15 per cent trypan blue is then injected into each well. The test is read by placing the tray on an inverting microscope stage and examining each well for the presence of trypan blue stained cells.

Chromium-51 Assay. The principle of this test is that when lymphoid cells labelled with ^{51}Cr react with specific iso-antibody and complement, isotope is quantitatively released. The test was developed using mouse lymphoid tissues and iso-antisera (Sanderson, 1964, 1965). It has proved to be a precise and sensitive way of measuring mouse H-2 antibodies. The major difficulty in its application to human systems has been that it requires the use of highly purified lymphocyte preparations, free not only of other leucocytes but also of red cells. Until recently all methods for obtaining pure lymphocyte preparations also caused enough damage to the lymphocytes to interfere with uptake or release of the label. This difficulty has now been overcome (Sanderson, 1967).

After the usual preliminary sedimentation of most of the red cells with dextran or gelatin, the supernatant plasma containing white cells and the remaining unsedimented red cells, is treated with chicken anti-human red cell antibody. This antibody agglutinates the red cells but leaves the white cells unaffected. After allowing chicken antibody to react with the mixed cell suspension for 5 minutes at 37°C, the polymorphs and larger red cell clumps are removed by passing the suspension through a 10 cc. column of 40-60 mesh styrene divinylbenzene copolymer (Dow Chemical Co., P.O. Box 512, Midland, Michigan). A convenient column can be made of a 10 ml. disposable syringe with the barrel removed and held vertically, the needle joint downwards. The barrel of the syringe is packed with a small pledgelet of cotton wool and then nearly filled with a slurry of copolymer in saline. Excess saline is allowed to drip out, and the crude white cell rich suspension is applied to the column with a pasteur pipette. It is advisable to concentrate the white cell rich suspension into a volume of approximately 0·5 ml. by a preliminary centrifugation before applying it to the column. This procedure makes the chicken antibody coated red cells adhere to each other, and also ensures that the column is not overloaded with too much fluid. After the cell suspension has been run on to the column, it is incubated at 37°C for 20 minutes. Lymphocytes and a few remaining red cells are eluted from the column by applying approximately 10 ml. of buffered saline to the top of the column. The remaining red cells in the column eluate are firmly clumped by gentle centrifugation and the white cells lying on top of the agglutinated red cell button can be resuspended by tapping the tube lightly. With care, suspensions containing less than 1 per cent red cells may be prepared in this way. The use of a column of styrene divinylbenzene copolymer is of course not essential, and if preferred one can obtain equally good suspensions by incubating the original mixed-cell suspensions with chicken antiserum in the presence of nylon wool. The polymorphs adhere to the wool, and the suspension obtained by squeezing the wool contains lymphocytes and red cells. The latter are then firmly clumped by gentle centrifugation and the white cells are resuspended as described previously by tapping the centrifuge tube lightly. The highly purified lymphocyte cell suspension is then labelled with ^{51}Cr, washed and used. Details of the test performance are given in Sanderson (1967).

In order to determine whether the ^{51}Cr assay and the trypan blue cytotoxic test detected the same antigenic specificities in man, a comparison has been carried out using several human iso-antisera and lymphocyte preparations (Sanderson and Batchelor, 1967). The two techniques gave virtually identical reactions and it is clear that not only do they detect the same antigenic specificities but that they are of equal sensitivity. For cheap and rapid typing, the dye-exclusion method is preferable. For automated mass testing, the isotope method appears to be more suitable.

Other Serological Methods. Complement fixation may be employed for detecting leucocyte iso-antigens (Shulman, Marder, Hiller and Collier, 1964). The technique has the advantages that viable target cells are not required, and it can permit precise quantitative measurements. Nevertheless, it is more cumbersome and less sensitive than the agglutination or cytotoxic tests.

Mixed agglutination tests with cell cultures may also be used (Metzgar and Flanagan, 1965; Milgrom and Kano, 1965). Human cell cultures are incubated with iso-antiserum, washed and then re-incubated with an indicator system. The indicator systems consist of red cells coated with human γ-globulin and agglutinated with anti-human globulin antibody. If human iso-antibody has combined with the cultured cells, red cells of the indicator system adhere to the culture, linked by the divalent anti-human globulin antibody. Mixed agglutination is probably the most sensitive method available today for the detection of human iso-antigens. Milgrom and Kano (1965) record titres of over 1/2,000 with some of their antisera. The main disadvantage of the test is that it is necessary to maintain a range of cell cultures which possess the particular iso-antigens one wishes to detect.

Antiglobulin consumption (Colombani, Colombani and Dausset, 1966) has now been superseded by other tests of greater convenience and precision.

Source of Antisera

Iso-antisera may be obtained from patients receiving multiple blood transfusions, from multiparous women or by the artificial immunization of volunteers. Sera from patients who have received multiple transfusions are usually unsatisfactory as typing reagents because they show poor specificity due to the repeated immunizations with antigenically varied material. Antisera from multiparous women are readily obtainable and show considerable specificity. Artificial immunization has been invaluable for several reasons. Immunizations involving specific antigenic differences may be carried out. If immunization is performed by successive skin grafts, the survival time of the primary skin graft is a measure of the incompatibility that exists between the donor and recipient. When antigenic stimulation is kept to a minimum, the number of different antibodies elicited is correspondingly reduced and therefore large quantities of highly specific reagents can be obtained. Finally, cells from the immunizing donor which contain all antigens detectable with the particular antiserum are readily obtainable for use in absorption analysis of the serum. The chief problem posed by artificial immunization is the possibility of transmitting viral jaundice. Immunization itself if kept to a minimum does not entail serious risk; this is apparent when one considers the large number of mothers who have been naturally immunized during successive pregnancies. To avoid the risk of transmitting jaundice, volunteers should be blood donors of good standing and known not to transmit disease.

LEUCOCYTE ISO-ANTIGENS

In the preceding sections, the more commonly used serological methods for detecting leucocyte iso-antigens have been described. We must now consider what information has been obtained from these tests and how it may be interpreted. It was recognized at an early stage that most antisera reacting with leucocytes contained a mixture of antibodies against a number of different iso-antigens. Such multispecific reagents obviously were not suitable for making precise antigenic classifications. A way out of the difficulty was found by van Rood, who argued that if antisera which contained only a few antibodies were tested on a large number of different white cells, those sera which contained the same antibody should show patterns of reactivity that were significantly alike (van Rood, 1962; van Rood and van Leeuwen, 1963). The patterns of activity of the different sera might be compared in χ^2 tests, a technique used with success in the investigation of red cell antibodies (see Race and Sanger, 1962). This approach has been extremely valuable and is worth considering in greater detail. The first step is to test the battery of antisera on the cells of a large number of individuals. The reactions of each serum are then compared with those of each other serum in a series of χ^2 tests, preferably with the help of computers to handle the large amount of data. The χ^2 tests indicate which antisera show significant positive or negative associations. Initially it was assumed that those antisera which showed significant positive associations must contain a common antibody, and that the discrepant reactions of the two antisera were due to the presence in them of other antibodies. Significant negative associations, which are also observed, were believed to indicate that the pertinent antisera were defining allelic antigens. Absorption analysis and family studies are then used to confirm the integrity of the provisionally defined antigen.

As a result of this approach van Rood and co-workers defined six white cell groups containing a total of 12 antigens (see van Rood, van Leeuven, Schippers, Vooys, Frederiks, Balner and Ernisse, 1965, for references). The groups and their component antigens were as follows: 4a, 4b; 5a, 5b; 6a, 6b; 7a, 7b, 7c(6c), 7d; 8a; 9a. 6c is placed in brackets next to 7c because the

TABLE I

Some Common Antigens which are either Identical or Closely Associated, defined by Different Workers*

Amos	...	...	2	...	1
Batchelor	3	4	...	1 & 2	5
Ceppellini	Buf	...	...	...	...
Dausset	3	7	9	8	1 (Mac)
Payne	...	...	...	LA1	LA2
Shulman	...	...	...	...	B1
Terasaki**	3	7	5	1	2
van Rood	4a	4b	6b	7d	8a

* Compiled from van Rood et al., 1966; Vredevoe et al., 1966; and unpublished data.
** Terasaki has described a series of antigenic groups, each of which are probably compound.

antigen was originally thought to be part of group 6, but was later placed in group 7 and designated 7c.

Other laboratories have also employed this technique for the analysis of their serological results, and have obtained similar though not identical results (Dausset, Ivanyi, and Ivanyi, 1965; Payne, Tripp, Weigle, Bodmer and Bodmer, 1964; Bodmer, Bodmer, Adler, Payne and Bialek, 1966; Amos, 1965; Vredevoe, Mickey, Goyette, Magnuson and Terasaki, 1966). Because of the lack of standard antigens, each laboratory has been forced to use its own private nomenclature. Collaborative studies (Bruning, van Leeuven and van Rood, 1965) and exchange of reagents have done something to minimize the proliferation of different terminologies, but it is difficult, and probably premature, at this stage to obtain general agreement on terminology. Despite the lack of a general terminology many specificities defined by different laboratories are known to be either the same or very closely associated—see Table I.

The fact that two antisera show significantly similar patterns of reactivity when tested on a random sample of the general population does not necessarily mean that they are detecting the same antigenic specificity.

Association between different antigens is a characteristic feature of compound histocompatibility systems, and the two sera may well be detecting two different specificities which are significantly associated.

Another approach to the problem of defining white cell iso-antigens is by orthodox *absorption analysis*. Here, one absorbs antiserum with a selection of positively reacting cells, and tests the absorbed serum for evidence of residual antibody. If residual serological activity is found after absorption, provided quantitative factors can be excluded as an explanation, one can assume that the serum contains at least two antibodies. By a series of absorption tests it is possible to work out how many antibodies each serum contains, and the pattern of reactivity of each separate antibody. In this way, using the cytotoxic test, Batchelor and Chapman (1966, 1967) have been able to identify a minimum of 26 different antigenic specificities. Some of these antigens are known to be either the same or closely associated with those defined by van Rood—see Table I. From some recent data it appears possible that certain of the antigens originally defined by van Rood are compound, being made up of frequently associated but separable antigenic specificities (Batchelor and Sanderson, 1967). If this possibility proves correct, it would explain the difference in the number of antigens recognized by the different laboratories.

Antigen Relationships

What relationship do the different antigens bear to each other? There are several reasons for suspecting that they might belong to the same genetic system. The first is the analogy of data obtained from experimental animals— particularly the compound H-2 system of mice. Secondly, as mentioned earlier, population studies showed that many of the antigens are distributed in association, not independently of one another as would be expected if they belonged to independent genetic systems. Lastly, clinical renal homo-transplantation results fit the concept of a single genetic system reasonably well (Simonsen, 1965). The family studies which have been carried out to investigate this question support the idea of a large and complex system. Most of the antigens recognized by Batchelor and Chapman (1967) were found to be inherited in association. The evidence of van Rood *et al.* (1966) indicates that leucocyte groups 6 and 7, and also groups 4 and 7 are closely linked. Probably groups 7 and 8 are also linked. The data did not support close linkage between groups 4 and 6. It seems likely that this unexpected observation is due to unsuspected polyspecificity of the antisera used in the studies or to technical problems of the test system. Group 5 antigens did not show linkage with group 6 antigens. Neither 5a nor 5b have been detected on lymphocytes and it appears that they belong to another system.

In contrast to the concept of a single large system embracing most of the currently recognized leucocyte iso-antigens (except 5a and 5b), Bodmer *et al.* (1966) postulate the existence of two independent systems on the basis of a single family which they maintain demonstrates the absence of close linkage between the two systems. The most recent family studies (Histo-compatibility Testing 1967) carried out by twelve collaborating teams of investigators have shown conclusively that most of the white cell iso-antigens identified so far, belong to a single genetic system. It has been agreed that this system will be called HL-A. Subsequently discovered human H systems will be termed HL-B, HL-C etc.

Before leaving the subject of leucocyte iso-antigens it should perhaps be emphasized that although there is good evidence to show that at least some of them function as tissue-compatibility antigens, we do not yet know enough about their relative antigenic potency. Naturally transplantation units must aim for the ideal of minimum incompatibility that is possible, but the definition of a clinically acceptable "minimum" has yet to be made. It is known that kidney homografts can survive despite some degree of incompatibility (Terasaki, Vredevoe, Porter, Mickey, Marchioro, Faris, Herrmann and Starzl, 1966). We have yet to learn whether certain antigenic differences are of particular importance or whether they are all equally dangerous, and it is merely the number of differences that is the critical factor.

NON-SEROLOGICAL TESTS FOR MATCHING

Normal Lymphocyte Transfer (NLT) Test. This test was originally devised by Brent and Medawar (1963) to help in selecting for a particular recipient the least incompatible subject from amongst a panel of genetically heterogeneous, living, potential tissue donors. Aliquots of a lymphocyte suspension prepared from the recipient are injected intradermally into members of the potential donor panel. An inflammatory lesion later develops at the injection site, and this is believed to be a local graft-versus-host immune reaction. Brent and Medawar argued that the violence with which the injected lymphocytes would react against the foreign antigens of the potential tissue donor would depend upon the amount of incompatibility. The greater the incompatibility, the more extensive would be the inflammatory lesion. This idea was supported by experiments on guinea-pigs in which the rate at which allogeneic skin grafts were rejected correlated well with the size of the NLT reaction.

As a result, similar tests have been performed on man (Gray and Russell, 1963; Bridges, Nelson and McGeown, 1964; Moorhead and Patel, 1964) and these papers should be consulted for details of lymphocyte preparation, injection and measurement of lesions. While there has been some dispute as to whether host-versus-graft reactions significantly influence the early lesion observed during the first two days after injection (Amos, Nicks, Peacocke and Sieker, 1965), Brent and Medawar's latest experiments on guinea-pigs are firmly in favour of their original concept (Brent and Medawar, 1966). However, there are several drawbacks to the test in man. Satisfactory lymphocyte preparations free of polymorphs may not be obtained very easily from uræmic patients (Russell, Nelson and Johnson, 1966). The results of the test depend greatly on the accuracy of the intradermal injection (Amos et al., 1965; Harris, 1965). The test does not give any information as to the particular antigens by which any two individuals differ, although there seems to be a correlation between the outcome of the test and leucocyte antigen incompatibility (van Rood et al., 1965). Finally the test exposes potential donors to the risks of immunization and serum transmitted jaundice. Recent outbreaks of serum transmitted jaundice epidemics in chronic dialysis units emphasize the seriousness of the risks. In the author's view, most of the serological tests are more satisfactory than the NLT, but if serological typing is not available, use of the NLT test may be preferable to having no guide at all.

Mixed Lymphocyte Cultures (MLC). When lymphocytes from genetically dissimilar individuals are cultured together, a proportion of cells transform into large blast forms (Bainvas and Lowenstein, 1964; Bach and Hirschorn, 1964). Since the same changes are induced in lymphocytes of sensitized individuals by antigen, it seemed possible that the transformation occurring in mixed lymphocyte cultures was a response to foreign histocompatibility antigens. Experiments on cells derived from twins (Bain, Vas and Lowenstein, 1964), other blood relatives (Ceppellini *et al.*, 1965) and the effect of immunization against transplantation antigens (Oppenheim, Whang and Frei, 1965) support this interpretation. There are numerous technical variations possible in setting up cultures which cannot be discussed here. So far the test has been of little practical help in donor selection because it requires considerable experience before reproducible results can be obtained, and furthermore each test requires several days for performance. But in circumstances where kidney or other tissues are being taken from live donors and therefore "cold" operations performed, the MLC test may be useful in selecting the best possible donor.

There are a number of other non-serological tests which may ultimately prove to be of some value in tissue typing, but at their present stage of development, it would be premature to consider their use in detail here.

References

Amos, D. B. (1965). *Histocompatibility Testing* 1965. Munksgaard, Copenhagen.
Amos, D. B., Gorer, P. A. and Mikulska, Z. B. (1955). *Proc. roy. Soc. B.*, **144**, 369.
Amos, D. B., Nicks, P. J., Peacocke, N. and Sieker, H. O. (1965). *J. Clin. Invest.*, **44**, 219.
Bach, F. and Hirschhorn, K. (1964). *Science*, **143**, 813.
Bain, B., Vas, M. R. and Lowenstein, L. (1964). *Blood*, **23**, 108.
Barnes, A. D. and Krohn, P. L. (1957). *Proc. roy. Soc. B.*, **146**, 505.
Batchelor, J. R. (1965). *Brit. med. bull.*, **21**, 100.
Batchelor, J. R. (1967). *Handbook of Experimental Immunology*, Blackwell, Oxford.
Batchelor, J. R. and Chapman, B. A. (1966). *Ann. N.Y. Acad. Sci.*, **129**, 529.
Batchelor, J. R. and Chapman, B. A. (1967), *J. clin. Path.*, Supp. **20**, 415.
Batchelor, J. R. and Sanderson, A. S. (1967). *Histocompatibility Testing* 1967, Munksgaard, Copenhagen.
Bodmer, W., Bodmer, J., Adler, S., Payne, R. and Bialek, J. (1966). *Ann. N.Y. Acad. Sci.*, **129**, 473.
Bogden, A. E. and Aptekman, P. M. (1960). *Cancer Res.*, **20**, 1372.
Brent, L. and Medawar, P. B. (1963). *Brit. med. J.*, **2**, 269.
Brent, L. and Medawar, P. B. (1966). *Proc. roy. Soc. B.*, **165**, 281.
Bridges, J. M., Nelson, S. D. and McGeown, M. (1964). *Lancet*, **i**, 581.
Bruning, J. W., van Leeuwen, A. and van Rood, J. J. (1965). *Histocompatibility Testing* 1965, Munksgaard, Copenhagen.
Ceppellini, R., Curtoni, E. S., Leigheb, G., Mattiuz, P. L., Miggiano, V. C. and Visetti, M. (1965). *Histocompatibility Testing* 1965, Munksgaard, Copenhagen.
Ceppellini, R., Curtoni, E. S., Mattiuz, P. L., Leigheb, G., Visetti, M. and Colombi, A. (1966). *Ann. N.Y. Acad. Sci.*, **129**, 421.
Colombani, J., Colombani, M. and Dausset (1964). *Ann. N.Y. Acad. Sci.*, **120**, 307.
Dausset, J., Ivanyi, P. and Ivanyi, D. (1965). *Histocompatibility Testing* 1965, Munksgaard, Copenhagen.
Dausset, J., Rapaport, F. T., Ivanyi, P. and Colombani, J. (1965). *Histocompatibility Testing* 1965, Munksgaard, Copenhagen.
Dausset, J. and Rapaport, F. T. (1966). *Ann. N.Y. Acad. Sci.*, **129**, 408.
Engelfriet, C. P. (1965). *Histocompatibility Testing* 1965, Munksgaard, Copenhagen.

FRIEDMAN, E. A., RETAN, J. W., MARSHALL, D. C., HENRY, L. and MERRILL, J. P. (1961). *J. clin. Invest.*, **40**, 2162.

GLEASON, R. E. and MURRAY, J. E. (1967). *Transplantation*, **5**, 343.

GORER, P. A. and MIKULSKA, Z. B. (1954). *Cancer Res.*, **14**, 651.

GORER, P. A. and O'GORMAN, P. (1956). *Transplant Bull.*, **3**, 142.

GRAFF, R. J., HILDEMANN, W. H. and SNELL, G. D. (1966). *Transplantation*, **4**, 425.

GRAY, J. G. and RUSSELL, P. S. (1963). *Lancet*, **2**, 863.

HARRIS, R. (1965). *Histocompatibility Testing* 1965, Munksgaard, Copenhagen.

LINDER, O. (1962). *Immunology*, **5**, 195.

METZGAR, R. S. and FLANAGAN, J. F. (1965), *Histocompatibility Testing*, publication 1229, *Nat. Acad. Sci.*, National Research Council, Washington, D.C.

MILGROM, F., ABEYOUNIS, J. and KANO, K. (1965). *Histocompatibility Testing*, publication 1229, *Nat. Acad. Sci.*, National Research Council, Washington, D.C.

MOORHEAD, J. F. and PATEL, A. R. (1964). *Brit. med. J.*, **2**, 1111.

MOSELEY, R. V., SH'EL, A. G. R., MITCHELL, R. M. and MURRAY, J. E. (1966). *Transplantation*, **4**, 678.

OPPENHEIM, J. J., WHANG I. and FREI, E. (1965). *J. exper. Med.*, **122**, 651.

PAYNE, R., TRIPP, M., WEIGLE, J., BODMER, W. and BODMER, J. (1964). *Symposia on Quant. Biol.*, **29**, 285.

PREHN, R. T. and MAIN, I M. (1958). *J. nat. Cancer Inst.*, **20**, 207.

PUZA, A., RUBINSTEIN, P., KASAKURA, S., VLAHOVIĆ, S. and FERREBEE, J. W. (1964). *Transplantation*, **2**, 722.

RACE, R. R. and SANGER, R. (1962). *Blood Groups in Man*, Blackwell, Oxford.

RAPAPORT, F. T., DAUSSET, J., CONVERSE, J. M. and LAWRENCE, H. S. (1965). *Transplantation*, **3**, 490.

VAN ROOD, J. J. (1962). *Leucocyte Grouping*, Ph.D. thesis, Univ. Leiden, Leiden.

VAN ROOD, J. J. and VAN LEEUWEN, A. (1963). *J. clin. Invest*, **42**, 1382.

VAN ROOD, J. J., VAN LEEUWEN, A., BRUNING, J. W., EERNISSE, J. G. (1966). *Ann. N.Y. Acad. Sci.*, **129**, 446.

VAN ROOD, J. J., VAN LEEUWEN, A., SCHIPPERS, A. M. J., VOOYS, W. H., FREDERIKS, E., BALNER, H. and EERNISSE, J. G. (1965). *Histocompatibility Testing* 1965, Munksgaard, Copenhagen.

RUSSELL, P. S., NELSON, S. D. and JOHNSON, G. J. (1966). *Ann. N.Y. Acad. Sci.*, **129**, 368.

SANDERSON, A. R. (1964). *Brit. j. exp. Path.*, **45**, 34.

SANDERSON, A. R. (1965). *Immunology*, **9**, 287.

SANDERSON, A. R. (1967). *Nature*, **216**, 23.

SANDERSON, A. R. and BATCHELOR, J. R. (1967). *Histocompatibility Testing* 1967, Munksgaard, Copenhagen.

SCHIERMAN, L. W. and NORDSKOG, A. W. (1961). *Science*, **134**, 1008.

SHULMAN, N. R., MARDER, U. J., HILLER, M. C. and COLLIER, E. M. (1964). *Progress in Hematology*, vol. 4, Grune & Stratton, New York.

SIMONSEN, M. (1965). *Lancet*, **i**, 415.

SNELL, G. D. and STEVENS, L. C. (1961). *Immunology*, **4**, 366.

TERASAKI, P. I., McCLELLAND, J. D. (1964). *Nature*, **204**, 998.

TERASAKI, P. I., VREDEVOE, D. L., PORTER, K. A., MICKEY, M. R., MARCHIORO, T. L., FARIS, T. D., HERRMANN, T. J. and STARZL, T. E. (1966). *Transplantation*, **4**, 688.

TERASAKI, P. I., VREDEVOE, D. L., McLELLAND, J. D. (1965). *Histocompatibility Testing* 1965, Munksgaard, Copenhagen.

VREDEVOE, D. L., MICKEY, M. R., GOYETTE, D. R., MAGNUSON, N. S. and TERASAKI, P. I. (1966). *Ann. N.Y. Acad. Sci.*, **129**, 521.

VREDEVOE, D. L., TERASAKI, P. I., MICKEY, M. R., GLASSOCK, R., MERRILL, J. P. and MURRAY J. E. (1965). *Histocompatibility Testing* 1965, Munksgaard, Copenhagen.

WALFORD, R. L., GALLAGHER, R. and SJAARDA, J. R. (1964). *Science*, **144**, 868.

WALFORD, R. L., GALLACHER, R. and TROUP, G. M. (1965). *Transplantation* **3**, 387.

WOODRUFF, M. F. A., ROBSON, J. S., NOLAN, B., LAMBIE, A. T., WILSON, T. I. and CLARK, J. G. (1963). *Lancet*, **2**, 675.

ZOTIKOV, E. A. (1958). *Transplant Bull.* **5**, 67.

ZMIJEWSKI, C. M. (1965). *Histocompatibility Testing* 1965, Munksgaard, Copenhagen.

Chapter 28

IMMUNOLOGICAL ADJUVANTS

Robert G. White

INTRODUCTION

IMMUNOLOGICAL adjuvants are usually regarded as agents which when mixed with immunogens increase the production subsequently of antibody by the injected animal. Ever since it was realized by Pasteur that the ravages of microbes in the human host could be counteracted by immunization, much effort has been directed to inducing immunogens to produce a better response. Two current developments in theoretical immunology have spurred this effort. First, the resounding defeat of the unitarian hypothesis of antibody means that specific adjuvant activities may apply to each of a wide range of processes for the biosynthesis of different immunoglobulins of different molecular form and distinct biological functions. Secondly, extension of knowledge of cell-mediated immunological responses, such as delayed hypersensitivity, cellular immunity, homograft and tumour rejection, means that we must seek out the adjuvants which may operate specifically in such processes. If development of a neoplasm can only occur after a failure of immunological surveillance (Burnet, 1963), then we might hope to find adjuvants to reinforce such defects. We also have to think of adjuvants in relation to the production of certain experimental disease states such as thyroiditis (McMaster, Lerner and Exum, 1961), allergic encephalitis (Kabat, Wolf and Bezer, 1947), adrenalitis (Colover and Glynn, 1954), or arthritis and iridocyclitis (so-called adjuvant disease of Pearson, 1956a, b).

Such is the importance in practice of adjuvants that it is seldom nowadays that antigens intended for immunization are injected alone, either in man or experimental animals. Their activity can be regarded as an essential second dimension of the response, and the analysis of the mode of action of such non-specific factors becomes basic to an understanding of the cellular and molecular workings of antibody production.

Influence of the Chemical and Physical State of the Antigen

Built-in Adjuvanticity. Following the work of Carl Landsteiner in the early years of this century an immunogen came to be envisaged as a carrier macromolecule provided with a surface which is divided like a mosaic into *determinants* of small size. In the case of a native protein these would be configurations of 4 or 5 amino acids. The specificity of the resultant antibody came to be interpreted as wholly dependent on the chemical configuration of these determinant areas. The rest of the molecule was interpreted as an inert carrier for such determinants. However, it is now clear that both the quality and quantity of antibody produced are affected by non-specific factors appertaining to the whole of the immunogenic moiety.

Artificial determinants can be constructed by attaching small chemically defined molecules to protein macromolecules. Antibody which is formed against such hapten-protein conjugates can be shown to react with the hapten alone (Landsteiner, 1945). However, a stronger antibody response to the hapten determinant will, in general, develop if the protein carrier comes from an animal species other than that injected. Also, if the number of haptens attached to the carrier is 3–5, antibodies to the hapten are more likely to be formed than if less haptens are attached to the same protein.

It is also well known that the molecular weight of the carrier molecule determines whether a substance is a good immunogen. There is no obvious explanation why this should be so, but it may relate to the fact that larger molecules contain more of the same antigenic determinant. Thus the immunogenicity of many small organic substances, e.g. the penicillin derivatives such as penicillenic acid or penicillinoyl, appears to depend on their ability to form a stable covalent bond with a carrier protein. This concept of increase in antigenicity with particle size has been extended as the "schlepper" concept to account for the observed increase in antigenicity of haptenic substances when adsorbed to particles like collodion, polyvinyl-pyrrolidone (Amies, 1962), silica particles (Vigliani and Pernis, 1959), or silicates such as bentonite (Torrigiani and Roitt, 1965).

Built-in adjuvant may exist in solutions of simple proteins such as bovine gammaglobulin in the form of aggregates of the protein molecules. A solution of this protein can thus be rendered non-immunogenic in the mouse by centrifuging away the higher polymers (Dresser, 1960). Heat aggregation of certain simple proteins can increase their immunogenicity. In an analogous manner the satisfactory immunogenicity of certain crude diphtheria toxoid preparations can be explained by their content of toxin (Glenny, Hopkins and Pope, 1924). Sela and Arnon (1960) observed that the configuration of the determinant groups at the surface of the molecule must be rigidly maintained. If they are not, as with gelatin, immunogenicity can be improved by adding a few tyrosine groups to stiffen up the surface stereo-chemical arrangement.

Adjuvant Effect of Antibody. It is well known that immunogenicity may depend on the levels of homologous antibody circulating at the time of the injection and that the presence of maternally derived IgG antibody in the circulation of infants may prevent injections of diphtheria toxoid or inactivated poliomyelitis vaccine from exerting their normal immunogenicity (Barr, Glenny and Randall, 1950). Alum-precipitated antigens are known to be more effective than the equivalent amount of fluid toxoid in breaking through a given level of diphtheria antitoxin. The same facts have been made use of recently to prevent immunization against Rhesus factor released from the foetus into the maternal circulation at the end of pregnancy.

Under other circumstances antibody can play an opposite or adjuvant role. Thus Glenny and Pope (1925) obtained increased antibody production from diphtheria toxoid by mixing it with antitoxin as an *underneutralized* mixture. A similar enhancing effect of small amounts of antibody in the mouse has been described by Terres and Wolins (1961). Stoner and Terres (1963) have shown that the antibody portion of the complex may consist of homologous antibody and that the greatest degree of enhancement occurs when the complexes are prepared in the region of antigen excess or equivalence.

Concepts of Adjuvant Activity

In the present state of understanding of the cellular mechanisms concerned in antibody production and the induction of delayed hypersensitivity it is not possible to state precisely how most of the adjuvants work. In general terms, adjuvants may act either (i) by preserving the activity of antigen by preventing rapid catabolism or by regulating its release from a depot, or

(ii) by preventing the antigen from inducing specific immunological tolerance, or (iii) by causing proliferation of the precursors of the cells with specific ability to make antibody (or mediate hypersensitivity), or (iv) by prolonging the effective life of plasma cells (or the effector cells in delayed hyper-sensitivity), or (v) by eliminating feed-back inhibition of the immunological response.

Possibly the simplest adjuvants are those which delay the release of antigen from a depot. Simple water-in-oil antigen mixtures (incomplete Freund-type) would appear to act almost entirely in this manner. Herbert (1967-8) has shown that the adjuvant effect of a single subcutaneous dose of a protein antigen in water-in-oil emulsion can be closely simulated by a series of very small and frequent injections of a saline solution of the antigen. Similar prolongation of antigen effect occurs with the mineral salt adjuvants such as aluminium hydroxide or phosphate and calcium phosphate.

White, Coons and Connolly (1955) compared the cellular responses in the popliteal node of a rabbit injected in the footpad with 10 Lf. of alum-precipitated diphtheria toxoid and 150 Lf. of soluble toxoid. Antibody-containing cells had almost completely disappeared from the regional node at three weeks after injection of soluble toxoid, whereas with the precipitated toxoid the cellular response in the node was still very evident at three and four weeks, implying longer antigenic stimulus in this case. The effect of the depot of antigen is further shown by a local production of antibody by the granuloma which develops at the site of injection of alum-precipitated (Oakley, Batty and Warrack, 1951) or a water-in-oil suspension of antigen (White, Coons and Connolly, 1955). A local alum granuloma consists of a mass of macrophages laden with antigen adsorbed to the mineral salt or hydroxide forming a circumferential zone around the central amorphous mineral mass. Beyond the macrophages are perivascular collections of lymphocytes and antibody-containing plasma cells. These antibody-containing cells persist for at least seven weeks and presumably make an important contribution to the later and persisting antibody production.

An example of an adjuvant which acts by the postulated mechanism (ii) above, i.e. by preventing the antigen from inducing tolerance, is provided by the protein adsorbent bentonite (aluminium silicate). Claman (1963) showed that bovine gamma-globulin injected intravenously produces tolerance in the mouse, whereas the same amount of antigen adsorbed to bentonite and given by the same route produces a vigorous antibody response.

Adjuvants which act directly on the immunologically competent cells rather than via the antigen might be expected to be able to exert their effects without local granuloma formation. It might also be expected that such adjuvants might work best if given later than the antigen injection. Bacterial endotoxin may be an example of this kind. Thus endotoxin does not give rise to granuloma formation, and becomes ineffective as an adjuvant on antibody production when given days or even as short a time as several hours before the antigen (Johnson, 1967). It is suggested that the adjuvant effect of endotoxin could depend on a rapid cytotoxic effect on the cells, mainly the small lymphocytes of lymphoid tissue. Nucleic acid breakdown products could be released and act as a stimulus for antibody-producing cells. Colchicine gives an adjuvant effect which is very similar in many respects to that of endotoxin. This surprising effect of a drug which is widely known for its antimitotic effects may depend on early cell damage and release of nucleic acid breakdown products. The paradoxical finding that an antimitotic agency can exert an adjuvant effect is further illustrated by X-radiation. Thus total-body irradiation at two hours before the injection of antigen leads to an adjuvant effect on antibody production. Such irradiation needs to be critically timed in relation to the injection of antigen, and irradiation at 24 hours before the injection of antigen results in a maximal depression of the immunological response (Taliaferro and Taliaferro, 1954). Braun (1965) has suggested that the effective nucleic acid derivatives are oligoribonucleotides.

In seeking for common factors having a role in the mechanism of adjuvant action, it has often been pointed out that many of the substances with known activity as adjuvants consist of surface-active materials. Recently Gall (1966) investigated a large number of aliphatic nitrogenous bases as adjuvants in the guinea-pig, and found high activity among a number of quaternary ammonium compounds, guanidines and benzamidines. Activity appeared to depend on a combination of basicity and a long aliphatic chain of 12 or more carbon atoms. Such adjuvants tended to be hæmolytic and to cause cytopathic effects in culture cells and it is suggested that their activity was connected with their ability to alter cell membranes.

Mineral Salt Adjuvants. Until recently aluminium salts have proved the most popular adjuvants in man and have been used very extensively for diphtheria prophylaxis. The initial search for an adjuvant able to facilitate the production of diphtheria antitoxin in horses took place in 1925. Research began with the idea of rendering the antigen less soluble and led to precipitation with alum by Glenny, Pope, Waddington and Wallace (1925).

The early history of immunization with this preparation was characterized by some severe reactions and by variations in potency of different samples of alum precipitated toxoid (APT). Later Holt (1950) adsorbed purified toxoid on to hydrated aluminium phosphate (PTAP) and Schmidt and Hensen (1933) used purified toxoid adsorbed to a preformed aluminium-hydroxide gel. Recently Relyvaud and Raynaud (1967) have made use of antigens adsorbed to calcium phosphate gel (brushite). The main value of such mineral absorbents appears to be in relation to the primary response. Thus, aluminium phosphate precipitated toxoid could not be shown to have any advantage over soluble toxoid as judged by the serum antibody levels attained in a secondary response (Barr and Cunliffe, 1954).

In immunization programmes, aluminium or calcium salts are probably more acceptable than mineral-oil adjuvants since they are less likely to result in a local granuloma of excessive size or which undergoes necrotic liquefaction, ulceration and chronic sinus formation. However, aluminium salts are usually found to be inferior to water-in-oil emulsions in respect of maintenance of high antibody levels. Based on data from the guinea-pig, Holt (1950) stated that the residual nodule from APT exercised no immunological activity from about 14 days after inoculation. Tiny injections of antigen made into the same limb as the injection granuloma produce secondary responses. The antigen is presumably unable to penetrate the zone of fibrous tissue which limits the granuloma, especially in the presence of antibody. Antigen-antibody precipitates among the fibres of the peripheral zone of the granuloma may act like the precipitin band in an agar plate of the Ouchterlony type, and prevent the penetration of antigen out and of antibody inwards (Germuth et al., 1959).

Bacterial Endotoxin. The ability of Gram-negative bacteria to enhance antibody levels has proved of great practical importance in mixed vaccines such as typhoid vaccine and tetanus toxoid (TABT). The phenomenon was established on a broad basis by the work of Johnson, Gaines and Landy (1956), who obtained the same enhancement of antibody to proteins, with purified lipopolysaccharide preparations from *Salmonella typhi* and several other Gram-negative bacterial species. Their data indicated that the ability of the host to respond with the stress symptomatology which characterizes endotoxin was essential if the lipopolysaccharide was to exert its adjuvant effect. Rabbits rendered tolerant to endotoxin by repeated dosage failed to show an adjuvant effect. Also, endotoxin was found to be relatively ineffective in those animal species (guinea-pig, chicken and mouse) which are insusceptible to endotoxic activity, although others (Farthing, 1961; Luecke and Sibal, 1962) found that small doses, which caused no untoward reactions, acted as adjuvants in guinea-pigs and chickens respectively.

The action of endotoxin has usually been studied after intravenous injection, and although the highest antibody levels have been achieved when this lipopolysaccharide was administered simultaneously with the antigen, it is apparent that endotoxins do not require to be injected in close association with the antigen, as do mycobacterial peptidoglycolipoids. In mice, endotoxin was effective when given seven days before or six days after the antigen (Merritt and Johnson, 1962).

Recently, much use has been made of *Bordetella pertussis* as an adjuvant in combined vaccines in man and in animal experiments. Some authors (*see* discussion in Munoz, 1963) have questioned whether all the adjuvant activity of *Bordetella pertussis* can be attributed to its contained endotoxin (Pittman, 1957). However, Farthing (1961) described a good correlation between extracted lipopolysaccharide and the equivalent number of whole organisms. Nevertheless, there is much evidence that *Bordetella* occupies a rather unique position as an adjuvant. *B. pertussis* also seems unique in increasing the formation of "mast cell sensitizing antibody" in the rat (Mota, 1964a, b). Other adjuvants (Austen and Humphrey, 1961) did not produce the same effects although antibody levels increased. This effect of *B. pertusiss* can possibly be regarded in terms of ability to change the antibody response qualitatively. Endotoxin effects upon delayed hypersensitivity are seldom recorded but Levine and Wenk (1964) successfully used *Bordetella pertussis*, and Shaw, Alvord, Fahlberg and Kies (1964) have used endotoxin from *Escherichia coli* for the induction of allergic encephalomyelitis with homologous brain in water-oil emulsion in guinea-pigs.

Water-in-oil Emulsions with added Mycobacteria (Complete Freund-type Adjuvant). Dienes (1928) showed that when a protein antigen is injected into a guinea-pig's tuberculous focus the immunogenicity is enhanced and production of delayed-type sensitivity greatly facilitated. Later, Freund (1956) and his associates found that antibody production could be greatly increased by incorporating the antigen as a water-in-oil emulsion either with (Freund's complete) or without (Freund's incomplete) added killed *Mycobacteria*. It has been maintained that tubercle bacilli are essential in such emulsions for pronounced sensitization of the delayed type to occur and also for the production of allergic encephalomyelitis. These statements are based on the guinea-pig, and do not necessarily apply to other animal species. Thus encephalitis was originally produced in the monkey with suspension of brain in saline, although repeated injections over several months were required.

Several different species of *Mycobacteria* or *Nocardia* or *Corynebacteria* have been successful in oily adjuvant mixture with homologous brain for the induction of encephalitis or for the production of an adjuvant effect on serum antibody levels or delayed hypersensitivity. Shaw, Alvord and Kies (1964) found several mycobacteria about equally effective, while *Nocardia asteroides* was somewhat less so. Gram-positive organisms other than mycobacteria and nocardia are relatively ineffective as adjuvants. An apparent exception is *Corynebacterium rubrum*. The uniqueness of the role of mycobacteria and corynebacteria for induction of delayed-type hypersensitivity has been recently challenged. In the guinea-pig Gram-negative bacilli could be used effectively for the production of allergic encephalitis (Shaw *et al.*, 1964), but required to be used in at least tenfold greater doses.

It has been argued that the action of mycobacteria in increasing delayed hypersensitivity is independent of the effect in increasing serum levels of antibody, but most recent work seems to be consistent with the view that the two effects are related. Indeed, an explanation of the adjuvant effect on antibody production could depend on the fact that an antigen which is introduced into an animal having delayed hypersensitivity to it yields an increased antibody response (Humphrey and Turk, 1963). Also, the extensive use of purified peptidoglycolipids extracted from *M. tuberculosis* shows that in the guinea-pig they affect both hypersensitivity and antibody production (White and Marshall, 1958).

The antibody which is increased by the mycobacterial component of adjuvant mixtures is of a different immunoglobulin form (White, Jenkins and Wilkinson, 1963). Thus, in the guinea-pig, a protein antigen injected alone or in water-in-oil emulsion leads to an antibody response at three weeks which is almost entirely confined to the fast or γ_1-immunoglobulin. But when mycobacteria are added to the water-in-oil emulsion a new peak of slow or γ_1-immunoglobulin appears. This antibody of γ_1 mobility can be readily separated from γ_1-antibody by chromatography on DEAE cellulose: both are split by reduction, alkylation and dialysis against 0·5 M proprionic acid into heavy and light peptide chains, of which the heavy chain is distinct from that of γ_1-globulin (Askonas, White and Wilkinson, 1965), although identical antigenic determinants are present in the Fd portion of the heavy chain (Nussenzweig and Benacerraf, 1964). On current evidence it would seem that the stimulation of delayed-type hypersensitivity in the guinea-pig is linked with the enhancement of γ_2-immunoglobulin. Both of these effects of mycobacterial adjuvant can be blocked simultaneously by prior injection of the antigen as a water-in-oil emulsion or as an aluminium phosphate precipitate. The subsequent injection of antigen in complete Freund's adjuvant then fails to induce delayed hypersensitivity or enhance γ_2-immunoglobulin.

The chemical and physical nature of the active principle of the mycobacteria and related micro-organisms has been the subject of much investigation. A chloroform-soluble waxy material (wax D) can reproduce the adjuvant effect of human type *M. tuberculosis* in enhancing delayed hypersensitivity and serum

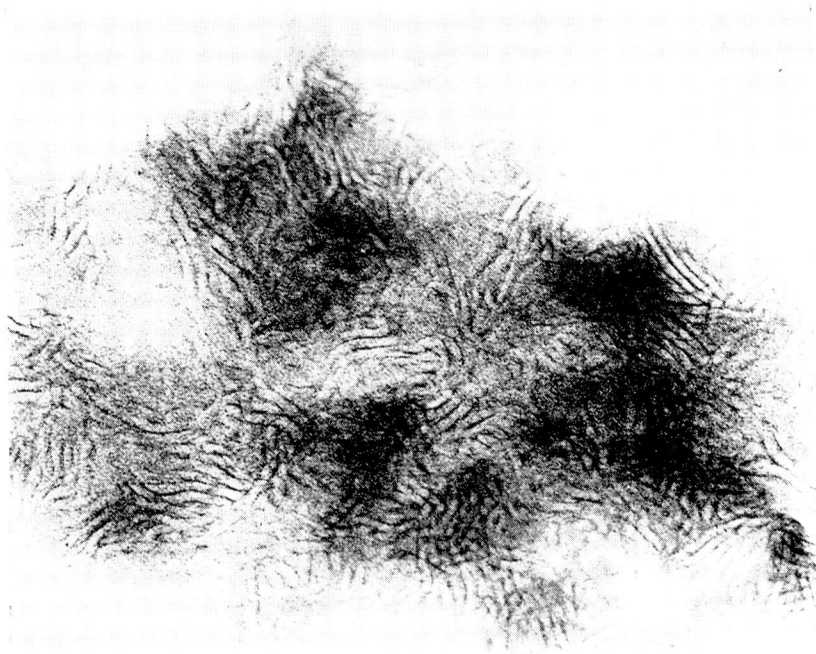

FIG. 1. Electron-micrograph of a centrifugal fraction of wax D from the human strain of *Mycobacterium tuberculosis* Brevannes. Negative staining technique with phosphotungstic acid. Magnification before reproduction 174,000. *Note* that the thin layer of wax is made up of unit filaments of uniform width (133 ± 15 Å).

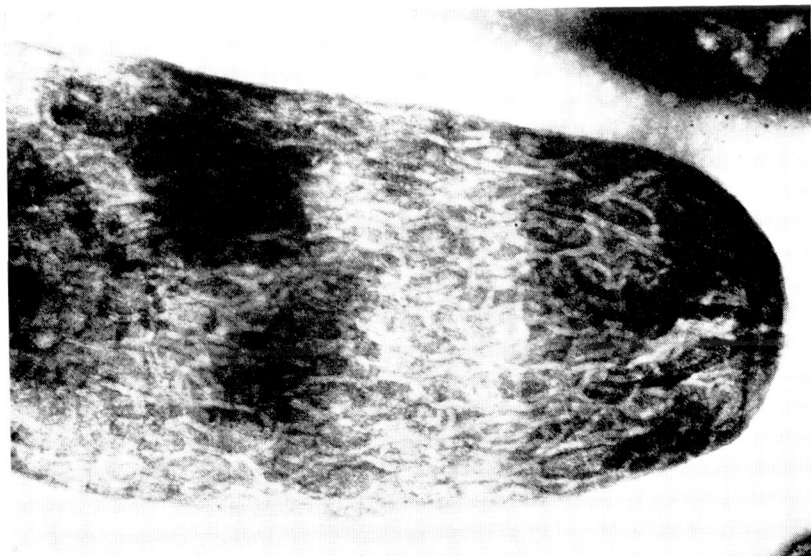

FIG. 2. Electron-micrograph of the rounded end of one bacillary cell of *Mycobacterium phlei*, Negative staining technique with phosphotungstic acid. Note the dense surface multilayered network of filaments (diameter 133 Å). Magnification before reproduction 30,000.

antibody levels in the guinea-pig (White, Bernstock, Johns and Lederer, 1958). The wax D fractions derived from bovine strains of *M. tuberculosis*, or *M. avium* and the saprophytic strains of mycobacteria, were all inactive although the whole bacillary cells of these same bacteria were fully active.

The main chemical components of the chloroform soluble wax D fractions are glycolipids and peptidoglycolipids. The variability in composition of wax D from different mycobacteria depends mainly on variation in the relative proportions of glycolipid and peptidoglycolipid. In the case of the bovine types of *M. tuberculosis* *M. avium* and saprophytic mycobacteria, the major part of the wax D is composed of biologically inactive glycolipids. This stresses the essential rôle of peptide in the adjuvant. Amino acids which compose this peptide moiety are alanine (D and L), glutamic acid (D) and α,ϵ di-aminopimelic acid; i.e. the same aminoacids which make up the mucopeptide of the cell wall of mycobacteria and related Gram-positive bacteria. By making use of its rapid sedimentation in ether, purified peptido-glycolipid fractions can be obtained which produce allergic encephalomyelitis in 50 per cent of injected guinea-pigs in a single dose of 50 μg. Four or five times as much whole dried bacteria were required to produce the same result (White, 1965).

Gordon and White (reported in White, 1965) have shown that adjuvant-active peptidoglycolipids can be visualized by the phosphotungstic acid negative stain technique in the electron microscope as homogeneous filaments of uniform width (133 ± 10A) (Fig. 1). Preparations from different adjuvant active mycobacteria showed identical filaments. The same negative staining technique applied to whole mycobacterial cells reveals similar filamentous structure ramifying in a multi-layered network over the outer surface of a variety of mycobacteria (Fig. 2).

Complete Freund adjuvant is unique in its ability to stimulate the prolifera-tion of antibody-producing plasma cells over a wide area of lymphoid tissues, including the spleen, bone marrow and remote lymph nodes of the guinea-pig after a footpad injection (White, Coons and Connolly, 1955b). In most species, the adjuvant effect is accompanied by the development of a large macrophage (epithelioid cell) granuloma at the site of injection, which often undergoes massive necrosis. In the rabbit and the horse (but not the guinea-pig) the local granuloma makes a major contribution to the antibody produced. When the rabbit is injected with complete Freund adjuvant, including mycobacteria but no other added antigen, a very large increase in the serum level of gamma-globulin results. If an antigen is present in the adjuvant, about half or more of the increased gamma-globulin becomes specific antibody (Humphrey, 1963) and it is suggested that globulin made by cells which are stimulated non-specifically by the adjuvant can acquire specific antibody character when antigen is present.

Adjuvants in the Treatment of Malignant Neoplasia

The possibility that immunological capacity can be increased by the use of adjuvants so as to inhibit the growth of tumours has been investigated in several laboratories. Since surveillance mechanisms *contra* malignant cells are possibly of the nature of cell-mediated delayed-type hypersensitivity responses, it is natural that mycobacterial adjuvants should have been used for such trials. However, the action of Freund's complete adjuvant in inducing a large granuloma at the site of injection and the tendency for this subsequently to undergo massive necrosis provides a strong deterrent for its use in man. Graham and Graham (1959) prepared a vaccine from the patient's own tumour and injected it together with Freund's adjuvant. The authors concluded that this procedure could have exerted a beneficial effect in potentiating the radiotherapy given subsequently.

Chorioncarcinoma presents a particularly favourable immunological situation for such a trial, since this tumour would be expected to possess paternally-derived homotransplantation antigens. Cinader, Hayley, Rider and Warwick (1961) used Freund's complete adjuvant to immunize a rabbit with a husband's seminal fluid. Serum from the rabbit was used in the patient, together with active immunization with the husband's leucocytes in order to secure a successful regression of chorioncarcinoma.

In experiments in rats and mice, BCG vaccine, *Corynebacterium parvum*, and zymosan have been used successfully to increase the frequency of rejection of allogeneic tumours (Woodruff and Boak, 1966). Mice treated in these ways showed an increased immunological response to various antigens and also a hyper-reaction and proliferation of the reticulo-endothelial system.

References

AMIES, C. R. (1962). *J. Hyg.*, **60**, 483.
ASKONAS, B. A., WHITE, R. G. and WILKINSON, P. C. (1965). *Immunochemistry*, **2**, 329.
AUSTEN, K. F. and HUMPHREY, J. H. (1961). *J. Physiol.* (London), **158**, 36.
BARR, M. and CUNLIFFE, A. C. (1954). *Mon. Bull. Minist. Hlth. Lab. Serv.*, **13**, 98.
BARR, M., GLENNY, A. T. and RANDALL, K. J. (1950). *Lancet*, **i**, 6.
BRAUN, W. (1965). In *Molecular and Cellular Basis of Antibody Formation*, Proc. Symposium, Ed. Šterzl, J. Prague (1964), p. 525. Czechoslovak Acad. Sci, Prague.
CINADER, B., HAYLEY, M. A., RIDER, N. D. and WARWICK, O. M. (1961). *Can. med. Ass. J.*, **84**, 306.
COLOVER, J. and GLYNN, L. E. (1958). *Immunology*, **1**, 172.
CLAMAN, H. N. (1963). *J. Immunol.*, **91**, 833.
DIENES (1928). *J. Immunol.*, **15**, 153.
DRESSER (1960). *Immunology*, **3**, 289.
FARTHING (1961). *Brit. J. exp. Path.*, **42**, 614.
FREUND (1956). *Advanc. Tuberc. Res.* **7**, 130.
GALL (1966). *Immunology*, **11**, 369.
GERMUTH, F. G., Jr., MAUMENEE, A. E., PRATT-JOHNSON, J. A., SENTERFIT, L. B., VAN ARNAM, C. E. and POLLOCK, A. D. (1959). In Schaffer, J. H., Lo Grippo, G. A. and CHASE, M. W. eds. *Mechanisms of hypersensitivity*, p. 155, Churchill, London.
GLENNY, A. T. and POPE, C. G. (1925). *J. Path. Bact.*, **28**, 273.
GLENNY, A. T., HOPKINS, B. E. and POPE, C. G. (1924). *J. Path. Bact.*, **27**, 261.
GLENNY, A. T., POPE, C. G., WADDINGTON, H. and WALLACE, U. (1926). *J. Path. Bact.*, **29**, 31.
GRAHAM, J. B. and GRAHAM, R. M. (1959). *Surgery Gynec. Obstet.*, **109**, 131.
HERBERT, W. J. (1967). In *Round Table Conference on Adjuvants*, ed. Cohen, H. Springer, Berlin.
HERBERT, W. J. (1968). *Immunology*, **14**, 301.
HOLT, L. B. (1950). *Developments in Diphtheria Prophylaxis*, pp. 86-94, Heinemann, London.
HUMPHREY, J. H. (1963). Intl. Colloqium C.N.R.S. (Paris) No. **116**, p. 401.
HUMPHREY, J. H. and TURK, J. L. (1963). *Immunology*, **6**, 119.
JOHNSON, A. G. (1967). In *International Symposium on Adjustments of Immunity*, No. 6 (Symposiar Series). Ed. Regamey, R. H., Hennessen, W., Ikič, D. and Ungar, J., p. 221. Karger, Basel.
JOHNSON, A. G., GAINES, S. and LANDY, M. (1956). *J. exp. Med.*, **103**, 225.
KABAT, E. A., WOY, A. and BEZER, A. E. (1947). *J. exp. Med.*, **85**, 117.
LANDSTEINER, K. (1946). The specificity of Serological Reactions, 2nd ed., p. 158, Harvard, Boston.
LEVINE, S. and WENK, E. J. (1964). *Science, N.Y.*, **146**, 1681.
LUECKE, D. H. and SIBAL, L. R. (1962). *J. Immunol.*, **89**, 539.

McMaster, P. R. B., Lerner, E. M. and Exum., E. D. (1961). *J. exp. Med.*, **113**, 611.
Merritt, K. and Johnson, A. G. (1962). *Bacteriol. Proc.*, p. 75 (abstract).
Mota (1964a). *Immunology*, **7**, 681.
Mota (1964b). *Immunology*, **7**, 700.
Munoz, J. J. (1963). *Bact. Rev.*, **27**, 325.
Nussenzweig, V. and Benacerraf, B. (1964). *J. Immunol.*, **93**, 1008.
Oakley, C. L., Batty, I. and Warrack, G. H. (1951). *J. Path. Bact.*, **63**, 33.
Pearson, C. M. (1956a). *Ann. rheum. Dis.*, **15**, 379.
Pearson, C. M. (1956b). *Proc. Soc. exp. Biol. Med.*, **91**, 95.
Pittman, M. (1957). *Fed. Proc.*, **16**, 867.
Relyvaud, E. H. and Raynaud, M. (1967). In *International Symposium on Adjuvants of Immunity*. Ed. Regamey, R. H., Hennessen, W., Ikič, D. and Ungar, J., p. 77, Karger, Basel.
Schmidt and Hensen (1933). *Acta path. microbiol. scand.*, **16**, 407.
Sela, M. and Arnon, R. (1960). *Biochem. J.*, **75**, 91.
Shaw, C. M., Alvord, E. C., Jr. and Kies, M. W. (1964). *J. Immunol.*, **92**, 24.
Shaw, C. M., Alvord, E. C., Jr., Fahlberg, W. J. and Kies, M. W. (1964). *J. Immunol.*, **92**, 28.
Stoner, R. D. and Terres, G. (1963). *J. Immunol.*, **91**, 761.
Taliaferro, W. H. and Taliaferro, L. G. (1954). *J. infect. Dis.*, **95**, 134.
Terres, G. and Wolins, W. (1961). *J. Immunol.*, **86**, 361.
Torrigiani, G. and Roitt, I. M. (1965). *J. exp. Med.*, **122**, 181.
Vigliani, E. C. and Pernis, B. (1959). *J. occup. Med.*, **1**, 219.
White, R. G. (1965). In *Molecular and cellular basis of antibody formation*. Ed. Šterzl, J., p. 71. Czechoslovak Acad. Sci., Prague.
White, R. G., Bernstock, L., Johns, R. G. S. and Lederer, E. (1958). *Immunology*, **1**, 54.
White, R. G., Coons, A. H. and Connolly, J. M. (1955a). *J. exp. Med.*, **102**, 73.
White, R. G., Coons, A. H. and Connolly, J. M. (1955b). *J. exp. Med.*, **102**, 83.
White, R. G., Jenkins, G. C. and Wilkinson, P. C. (1963). *Int. Arch. Allergy*, **22**, 156.
White, R. G. and Marshall, A. H. E. (1958). *Immunology*, **1**, 111.
Woodruff, M. F. A. and Boak, J. L. (1966). *Brit. J. Canc.* **20**, 345.

Chapter 29

AUTO-IMMUNE AND HYPERSENSITIVITY PHENOMENA IN ALIMENTARY DISEASES

W. J. IRVINE

Introduction

DURING the past decade immunological phenomena, with special reference to auto-immunity and hypersensitivity, have been the subject of much study in relation to diseases of the alimentary system. My object has been to review the present state of knowledge in this area, indicating where the existence of immunological phenomena has been clearly established and where its existence is less certain. In so doing, reference is made to the various immunological techniques that have been applied to the study of alimentary diseases. The diagnostic value of certain auto-antibody tests is stated and the possible role of immunological mechanisms in the pathogenesis of various diseases of the alimentary system is discussed.

Aphthous Ulceration

Recurrent aphthous ulceration of the mouth is a chronic disorder of unknown ætiology which occurs more frequently in females. The histology is characterized by lymphocytic and plasma cell infiltration and the condition is said to be associated with idiopathic steatorrhœa, Crohn's disease and ulcerative colitis, although the evidence for this is far from satisfactory. Aphthous ulceration also occurs as part of Behçet's syndrome (recurrent oral and genital ulceration with associated eye lesions, especially iritis). Using tanned cell hæmagglutination, complement fixation and precipitin techniques with a saline extract of fœtal oral mucosa, Lehner (1964, 1967) has described a higher incidence of positive results and titres with the sera of patients suffering from aphthous ulceration in its major form and also with the sera of patients with Behçet's syndrome than with the sera of control subjects. The antigen is said to reside in the prickle cells. Preliminary studies indicate that the active constituent in the serum is in the IgG and IgM globulin fractions.

A second immunological approach has been the demonstration of an increased incidence and titres of antibodies to milk proteins in the sera of patients with aphthous ulceration (Taylor, Truelove and Wright, 1964). As will be discussed later, this has also been described in patients with ulcerative colitis.

Sjögren's Syndrome

Sjögren's syndrome is a chronic benign disorder which occurs in middle-aged females and which is characterized by the triad of keratoconjunctivitis sicca, xerostomia and in one-half to two-thirds of patients, some form of connective tissue disease, usually rheumatoid arthritis and less commonly systemic lupus erythematosus, progressive systemic sclerosis, polymyositis or periarteritis nodosa. The term "sicca" syndrome is used to describe the association of keratoconjunctivitis sicca and xerostomia in the absence of connective tissue diseases. The lacrimal and salivary glands show extensive chronic inflammatory cell infiltration and acinar atrophy with failure of secretion. Similar pathological changes may be seen in other secreting glands and lead to dryness of the nose, pharynx, larynx, trachea, bronchi and vagina. In the salivary glands the intercalated ducts frequently show epithelial and myo-epithelial proliferation (Morgan and Castleman, 1953; Bloch et al., 1965).

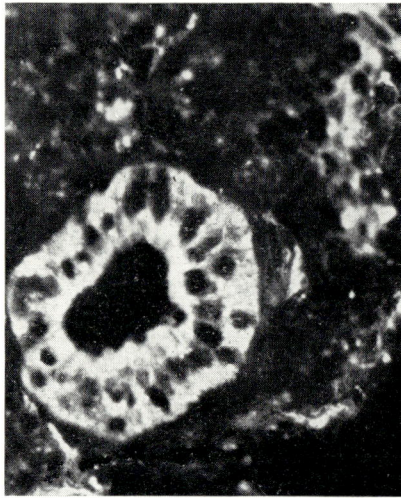

FIG. 1. Staining of direct epithelial cytoplasm in the indirect immunofluorescence test using an unfixed section of human parotid tissue, serum of a patient with Sjögren's syndrome and anti IgG conjugated with fluorescein (UV × 225).
(From Feltkamp and van Rossum (1968), Clin. exp. Immunol).

Bertram and Halberg (1964) using the indirect fluorescent antibody technique with unfixed sections of normal parotid, submaxillary and sublingual glands, have demonstrated antibodies to the salivary duct cell cytoplasm in 11 out of 19 patients. Feltkamp and van Rossum (1968) have confirmed these findings, obtaining an incidence of 16 sera positive for antibody to salivary duct cells out of a series of 30 patients (Fig. 1). The antibodies were always present in the IgG serum fraction, but some also occurred in the IgM fractions and a few in the IgA serum fractions. These observations are of importance since previous serological studies using complement fixation or precipitin test had revealed only non-organ-specific antibodies (Anderson et al., 1961; Bloch and Bunim, 1963). Some sera react in the immunofluorescent tests with epithelium of sweat glands, breast, prostate and bronchus. Feltkamp and van Rossum (1968) found no salivary duct antibodies in normal controls matched for age and sex. Bertram and Halberg (1965) describe a frequency of 27 per cent in controls above the age of 65 years.

Rheumatoid factor has been described in 48–100 per cent of sera from patients with Sjögren's disease. The prevalence and titre of rheumatoid factor is just as high in those patients with the sicca syndrome alone as in those with Sjögren's syndrome associated with a connective tissue disease, including rheumatoid arthritis.

Antinuclear antibodies (ANF) have been found in a high proportion of patients with Sjögren's syndrome. Positive L.E. cell tests appear to be related to associated connective tissue disease rather than to the sicca syndrome. By contrast, antinuclear antibodies have been detected by immunofluorescence techniques in approximately two-thirds of patients with Sjögren's syndrome. The increased prevalence of ANF in patients with the sicca syndrome is due to an increased incidence of "speckled" and "nucleolar" antibodies (Beck et al., 1965).

In Feltkamp and van Rossum's series, the incidence of antibodies to skeletal muscle, gastric parietal cell, thyroid antigens, adrenal cortex, and mitochondria did not differ significantly from those in matched controls. Anderson et al. (1965) found an increased incidence of gastric parietal cell antibody in British subjects with Sjögren's but not in patients with this disease who were studied at the National Institute of Health, U.S.A. He maintains that antibody to thyroglobulin is more common in Sjögren's than in controls but the titres were generally low. There is no convincing evidence for an increased prevalence of clinical chronic thyroiditis or atrophic gastritis in Sjögren's syndrome.

In a preliminary report it has been stated that family studies in Sjögren's syndrome suggest an increased prevalence of rheumatoid arthritis, decreased tear formation (as detected by the Shirmer test), thyroglobulin antibodies, auto-immune complement fixation tests and elevated IgG levels in relatives of patients with the disease (Burch, Bunim and Bloch, 1963).

Although attempts have been made to produce Sjögren's syndrome by immunological means in experimental animals, the results do not closely resemble the lesions in man. There was no epithelial or myo-epithelial hyperplasia, but these features might be regarded as a form of repair and not specific for any particular injury (Chan, 1964).

In conclusion, the immunological features of Sjögren's syndrome resemble the non-organ-specific group of auto-immune diseases (e.g. systemic lupus erythematosus, rheumatoid arthritis) more strongly than they do the organ-specific group (thyroiditis, pernicious anæmia and idiopathic Addison's disease). The role of the antibodies in the pathogenesis of the disease remains undetermined.

Atrophic Gastritis

A number of facts suggested that immunological phenomena may be important in the study of the atrophic gastritis of Addisonian pernicious anæmia. The histology of the gastric mucosa in pernicious anæmia is characterized by atrophy of the specialized cells of the body of the stomach accompanied by a variable but often marked degree of lymphocytic infiltration. Pernicious anæmia occurs predominantly in middle-aged females and has an increased

Q

incidence in auto-immune thyroid disease (thyrotoxicosis, Hashimoto goitre and primary atrophic hypothyroidism). It is known that corticosteroids can induce a reticulocyte response (Doig *et al.*, 1957) and improve absorption of radioactive vitamin B_{12} (Frost and Goldwein, 1958; Gordin, 1959, Kristensen and Friis, 1960) in Addisonian pernicious anæmia patients. During the past ten years auto-immune phenomena in relation to the gastritis of pernicious anæmia and in some cases of atrophic gastritis without pernicious anæmia have been clearly established.

Antibody to Gastric Parietal Cells. In a careful study of the relationship between pernicious anæmia and thyroid disease, Tudhope and Wilson (1962)

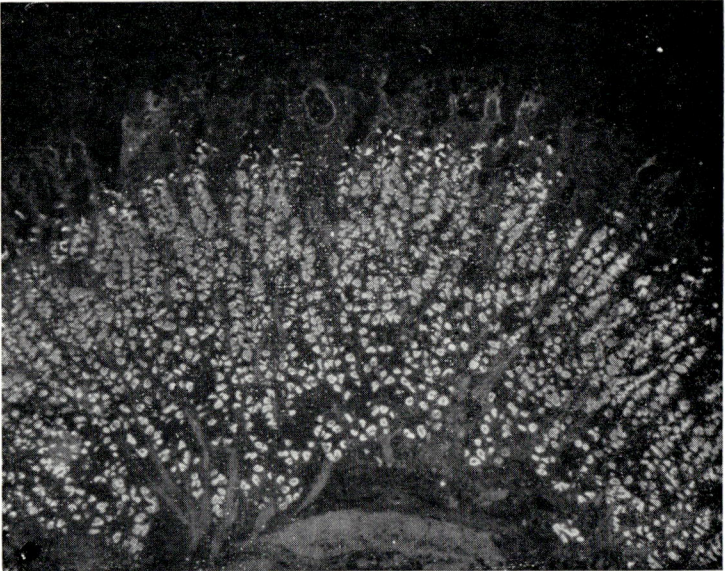

Fig. 2. Positive indirect immunofluorescence test for gastric parietal cell antibody using an unfixed section of body of human stomach, serum from a patient with Addisonian pernicious anæmia and human polyvarant gammaglobulin conjugated with fluorescein (UV × 50).

(From Irvine *et al.* (1965a), *Annals, N.Y. Acad. Sci.*).

found that 24 out of 52 patients with primary hypothyroidism had a histamine fast achlorhydria and that 12 per cent of 72 hypothyroid patients had Addisonian pernicious anæmia; immunological methods that had proved so rewarding in the investigation of thyroid disease were therefore applied to the study of pernicious anæmia. It was found that 75 per cent of the sera of patients with Addisonian pernicious anæmia gave a positive complement fixation test specific for a saline extract of gastric body mucosa and that the serum component responsible for this reaction was a gammaglobulin (Irvine *et al.*, 1962). Using the immunofluorescence technique Taylor *et al.* (1962) and Irvine (1963) demonstrated that the complement fixing gastric antibody was specific for parietal cell cytoplasm (Fig. 2), and it was shown that the gastric antibody would react equally well with the patient's own gastric mucosa provided it still contained an adequate concentration of parietal cells (Irvine, 1963). An overlap was shown to occur in the incidence of gastric and thyroid antibodies in pernicious anæmia and thyroid disease (Irvine, 1965a; Roitt, Doniach and Shapland, 1965). Approximately 30 per cent of patients with auto-immune thyroid disease (thyrotoxicosis, Hashimoto thyroiditis and primary atrophic hypothyroidism) have gastric parietal cell antibody and between 30–55 per cent of patients with pernicious anæmia have thyroid complement fixing antibody in the serum.

The parietal cytoplasmic antigen is associated with an insoluble lipo-protein microsomal element (Baur, Roitt and Doniach, 1965). Electron microscopic and ultraviolet absorption evidence suggests that the antigen component(s) of the microsomal fraction is associated with smooth membranes and not with the ribosomes (Ward and Nairn, 1967). The gastric parietal cell antigen is not species-specific; rat gastric mucosa (de Boer, Nairn and Maxwell, 1965) and pig gastric mucosa (Irvine, 1966a) reacting equally well. It is necessary to distinguish the gastric specific cytoplasmic fluorescence from that obtained with the mitochondrial antibodies in primary biliary cirrhosis (Doniach *et al.*, 1966; Goudie, MacSween and Goldberg, 1966) and from lysosomal (Wiedermann and Miescher, 1965) and ribosomal (Sturgill and Carpenter, 1965) antibodies described in connective tissue disorders. To exclude this possibility human kidney sections are included as a control in the fluorescent tests and fresh rat kidney homogenate is used for a control in the complement fixation reaction. The gastric complement fixation reaction, although usually carried out by the Takasi microtitre method, can be automated (Irvine, 1966a).

Jeffries and Sleisenger (1965) and Fisher, Rees and Taylor (1965) have shown the presence of antibodies to gastric parietal cells in gastric juice of subjects who have circulating parietal cell antibodies. Whether these have any special function has not yet been elucidated.

Antibodies to Intrinsic Factor. The first direct demonstration that immune phenomena may occur in association with pernicious anæmia is to be found in the work of Schwartz (1958, 1960). In patients given oral intrinsic factor, he looked for inhibitors to intrinsic factor using an *in vivo* assay and found them in the serum of the majority of pernicious anæmia patients so treated but also in some who had not. Likewise, Taylor (1959) observed intrinsic-factor-inhibiting substance in nine out of 19 patients either treated by parenteral administration of vitamin B_{12} or untreated.

In vitro methods for the detection of antibodies to intrinsic factor have been developed. The basis of the method of Jeffries, Hoskins and Sleisenger (1962) is to observe the alteration of the electrophoretic mobility of radio-active vitamin B_{12} intrinsic factor complex in the presence of test as opposed to normal serum. In the presence of antibody to intrinsic factor a larger complex is formed and is retained at the origin on starch gel electrophoresis. Other methods depend upon the property of intrinsic factor to bind vitamin B_{12} and that this can be inhibited by antibody to intrinsic factor (Abels *et al.*, 1963). The method of Ardeman and Chanarin (1963) has been modified by Gottlieb *et al.* (1965) and by Irvine (1966b), and is dependent upon the separation of bound from unbound radio-active vitamin B_{12} by protein coated charcoal. Abels *et al.* (1963) used dialysis to separate the unbound vitamin B_{12}.

Schade et al. (1967) have shown that there are two separate antibodies to intrinsic factor. Antibody I blocks the binding of B_{12} by intrinsic factor and antibody II unites with intrinsic factor-B_{12} or with intrinsic factor alone. Antibody I exchanges readily with the B_{12} of intrinsic factor-B_{12} complex. The complex of intrinsic factor and antibody I will absorb antibody II. Intrinsic factor would therefore appear to have at least two antigenic sites. The intrinsic factor antibodies are IgG immunoglobulins.

In man there is evidence that the gastric parietal cell is the site of secretion of intrinsic factor (Hoedemaeker et al, 1964).

Fisher, Rees and Taylor (1966) have produced circumstantial evidence that antibody to intrinsic factor may be present in the gastric juice of some patients with pernicious anæmia. Schade et al. (1966) studied one patient who did not absorb normal amounts of vitamin B_{12} from a standard dose of normal human gastric juice and vitamin B_{12} given by mouth. The patient's gastric juice was shown by in vitro and in vivo techniques to contain antibody to a complex of human intrinsic factor and vitamin B_{12}. The inhibition of vitamin B_{12} absorption by the presence of antibody to intrinsic factor in gastric juice would provide an interesting demonstration that an antibody can inhibit the physiological function of an endogenous antigen. Further studies are required to establish this point.

Incidence of Gastric Antibodies in Pernicious Anæmia and Related Disorders. Seventy-three to eighty-nine per cent of patients with Addisonian pernicious anæmia have gastric parietal cell antibody detectable in the serum irrespective of the duration of treatment that the patient may have had with vitamin B_{12} (Taylor et al., 1962; Irvine, 1965a; Jeffries and Sleisenger, 1965). There is a rising incidence with age, particularly in females, in control populations (Irvine et al., 1965a). As already mentioned, the incidence of parietal cell antibodies in the thyroid auto-immune diseases is 25-33 per cent. There is an increased incidence in patients with chronic iron deficiency anæmia (Dagg et al., 1964; Irvine et al., 1965a), in patients with idiopathic adrenal insufficiency (Irvine, Stewart and Scarth, 1967) and in the young diabetic subjects (Moore and Neilson, 1963; Irvine and Davies, 1963; Irvine, 1968). In all these groups the presence of parietal cell antibody in the serum correlates with some degree of atrophic gastritis. The incidence and titre of gastric parietal cell antibody shows a general correlation with the severity of the atrophic gastritis as indicated by a reduction in gastric acid secretion following stimulation by histamine and a reduction in the number of parietal cells and also chief cells in the gastric biopsy (Adams et al., 1964; Dagg et al., 1964; Irvine et al., 1965a; Irvine, 1965a). The incidence of parietal cell antibodies is increased in patients with simple atrophic gastritis without associated disease (Mackay, 1964; Coghill et al., 1965) but the incidence in gastric carcinoma, gastric ulcer, and in post-gastrectomy and post-gastro-enterostomy cases is low.

Intrinsic factor antibody I occurs in about 50–60 per cent of patients with Addisonian pernicious anæmia (Ardeman and Chanarin, 1963; Roitt, Doniach and Shapland, 1965; Irvine, 1965a) and intrinsic factor antibody II occurs in approximately 30 per cent (Jeffries, Hoskins and Sleisenger, 1962). Antibody to intrinsic factor shows a very high degree of correlation with malabsorption of vitamin B_{12} due to deficiency in secretion of intrinsic factor (Irvine, 1966b). A small number of patients have been described in whom intrinsic factor antibodies are present in the serum although no abnormality could be detected in the patient's vitamin B_{12} metabolism. These patients have occurred among those with thyroid auto-immune diseases (Ardeman and Chanarin, 1966), idiopathic adrenal insufficiency (Irvine, Stewart and Scarth, 1967) and in relatives of pernicious anæmia patients (te Velde *et al.*, 1964). The majority of these subjects had a histamine fast achlorhydria, although one patient described by Ardeman and Chanarin had a normal secretion of both acid and intrinsic factor; in this patient it was shown that the antibody to intrinsic factor was a true auto-antibody. In general, patients with simple atrophic gastritis, although they may have the same gastric histology as patients with pernicious anæmia, do not have intrinsic factor antibody in the serum (Coghill *et al.*, 1965; Fisher, Rees and Taylor, 1965). Very few control subjects have yet been found with antibody to intrinsic factor in the serum.

When pernicious anæmia of the Addisonian type occurs in children with gastric atrophy and loss of both acid and intrinsic factor secretion, there is a high incidence of both parietal cell and intrinsic factor antibodies in the serum (Doniach and Roitt, 1964). However, in infantile pernicious anæmia (in which there is normal gastric histology and acid secretion but an impairment of intrinsic factor synthesis) no gastric antibodies have been detected (Doniach, Roitt and Taylor, 1965). It would appear that infantile pernicious anæmia is a distinct and separate condition from Addisonian pernicious anæmia of the adult. The adult type of pernicious anæmia occasionally affects juveniles. Infantile pernicious anæmia is due to a highly selective deficiency in intrinsic factor synthesis and is genetically unrelated to adult pernicious anæmia and is not associated with auto-immunity (McIntyre *et al.*, 1965).

Immunoassay of Intrinsic Factor. Possibly the most direct application of the study of gastric auto-immunity has been the development of a sensitive and accurately quantitative immunoassay for gastric intrinsic factor using intrinsic factor antibody I. The most satisfactory methods (Gottlieb *et al.*, 1965; Irvine, 1966b) are modifications of the method of Ardeman and Chanarin (1963). The secretion of intrinsic factor in the post-histamine hour is less than 100–200 nanogram units in patients with pernicious anæmia (Ardeman and Chanarin, 1965a; Irvine *et al.*, 1965b; Irvine *et al.* 1968), and, as shown in Fig. 3, there is a good correlation between the direct immunoassay of intrinsic factor in gastric juice following histamine or pentagastrin in patients with achlorhydria and the absorption of vitamin B_{12} in the Schilling test correctable with exogenous intrinsic factor.

The immunoassay of intrinsic factor has also enabled the description of the pattern of intrinsic factor secretion following gastric stimulation with histamine or gastrin or pentagastrin. Immediately following stimulation intrinsic factor would appear to be washed out of the gastric secretory cells or from the gastric crypts. This is followed by a much lower but sustained intrinsic factor secretion at approximately twice the basal level, if stimulation is continued (Irvine, 1965b; Wangel and Callender, 1965; Irvine, 1966b; Lawrie and Anderson, 1967).

According to Ardeman and Chanarin (1965a) 500 ng. units of human intrinsic factor in a single dose usually restores the absorption of vitamin B_{12} in pernicious anæmia. Since intrinsic factor antibody is not strictly species-specific, it can also be used for the immunoassay of preparations of hog intrinsic factor and thereby provide a ready means of standardization. Three hundred to six hundred nanogram hog intrinsic factor is sufficient to correct vitamin B_{12} absorption in patients with pernicious anæmia (Irvine, 1966b).

Relation of Gastric Antibodies to Pathogenesis of Atrophic Gastritis. Achlorhydria and indeed frank Addisonian pernicious anæmia can occur without gastric parietal cell or intrinsic factor antibody being detectable in the serum. Electron microscopic studies (Irvine *et al.*, 1965a) have shown that lymphocytes may lie within the gastric tubules, invaginating the specialized cells of the gastric mucosa. Crabbé, Carbonara and Heremans (1965) have demonstrated the production of IgA, IgM and IgG immuno-globulins in the lamina propria of the small gut in man but the antigenic

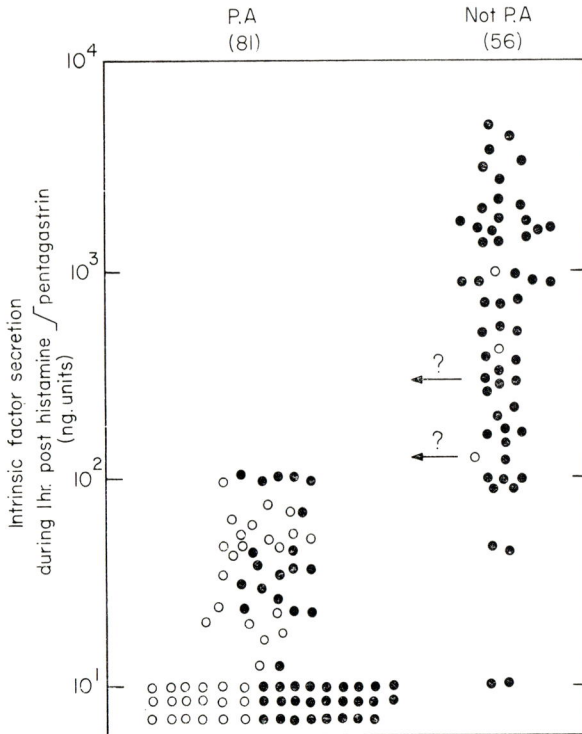

Fig. 3. Intrinsic-factor secretion in post-stimulation hour in 137 achlorhydric patients, 81 of whom had pernicious anæmia.
o = serum positive for intrinsic-factor antibody I.
(From Irvine *et al.* 1968, *Lancet.*)

specificities of these immunoglobulins is not known. A comparable study of the stomach in atrophic gastritis would be of interest. As already mentioned, parietal cell and intrinsic factor antibodies have been described in the gastric juice. The presence of intrinsic factor antibody in gastric juice may be inde-pendent of the level of the antibody in the serum. This suggests that gastric antibodies may be synthesised within the gastric mucosa.

Antibody to intrinsic factor may be effective at the site of vitamin B_{12} absorption in the distal ileum. The fact that vitamin B_{12} absorption can be corrected in Addisonian pernicious anæmia by the administration of oral intrinsic factor can be explained by assuming that the dose of intrinsic factor given is in excess of what can be inhibited *in vivo* by intrinsic factor antibody.

It has been argued that the presence of gastric parietal cell antibody in the serum of patients with chronic hypochromic anæmia may be a consequence of atrophy of the gastric mucosa as a result of the iron deficiency (McFadyen *et al.*, 1967). To others (Irvine, 1967) it would appear more probable that the chronic hypochromic anæmia may be due to atrophic gastritis as it has been shown that such subjects have some impairment of iron absorption (Goldberg, Lochhead and Dagg, 1963). The latter view is supported by the observations of Wright *et al.* (1965) that patients with certain diseases (e.g. auto-immune thyroid disease) are much more liable to produce gastric parietal cell antibodies than patients with other diseases (e.g. ulcerative colitis, idiopathic steatorrhœa), although the histological appearance of gastric atrophy is identical. Patients with achlorhydria may continue to form small amounts of intrinsic factor sufficient to maintain an adequate absorption of vitamin B_{12}. In only a relatively small proportion of patients with gastric atrophy is the impairment of vitamin B_{12} absorption of such a degree as to lead to pernicious anæmia. The transition from a state of achlorhydria with adequate absorption of vitamin B_{12} to that of pernicious anæmia with malabsorption of the vitamin has only infrequently been observed.

Although the histological appearance of the atrophic gastric mucosa of pernicious anæmia would suggest a static end stage of an antecedent destructive process, Croft, Pollock and Coghill (1966) have shown, from the measurement of DNA in gastric perfusates, that in pernicious anæmia the rate of cell loss (and therefore presumably the rate of cell turnover) in the gastric mucosa was not reduced below normal. The capacity of the gastric mucosa to regenerate is shown by the response of some patients with pernicious anæmia to prolonged treatment with therapeutic doses of corticosteroids (15–40 mg. prednisolone/day). In some there is an increase in the secretion of intrinsic factor to levels sufficient to restore the Schilling test to normal and small amounts of acid may be secreted. In serial biopsies histological evidence for some regeneration of parietal cells and chief cells has been observed. The improvement in the histology and function is not maintained after the steroids are withdrawn (Jeffries, 1965; Ardeman and Chanarin, 1965b; Jeffries, Todd and Sleisenger, 1966; Rødbro *et al.*, 1967; Wall *et al.*, 1968). In two patients with megaloblastic anæmia following partial gastrectomy there was no improvement in the absorption of vitamin B_{12} with steroid therapy; it is possible that ischæmic factors are important in producing atrophy of the gastric remnant (Ardeman and Chanarin, 1965b). It would therefore appear that corticosteroids may counteract an immuno-destructive process in patients with pernicious anæmia permitting mucosal regeneration to occur.

Convincing experiments have yet to be done to show that a state of chronic atrophic gastritis can be produced in rats, guinea-pigs or dogs by immunological techniques, but in monkeys atrophic gastritis can be produced; for example, by the repeated intradermal injection of gastric antigen emulsified with Freund's adjuvant. (Andrada and Rose, 1969). It has also not yet been possible to demonstrate a cytotoxic effect of humoral antibody or of lymphocytes on parietal cells in tissue culture, the difficulty being to get parietal cells to grow in tissue culture.

Familial Tendency to Pernicious Anæmia and Gastric Auto-immunity. The relatives of patients with pernicious anæmia show an increased incidence of

overt pernicious anæmia, latent pernicious anæmia and of histamine fast achlorhydria (Callendar and Denborough, 1957; McIntyre *et al.*, 1959). te Velde *et al.*
(1964) found gastric parietal cell antibodies in 20 per cent of 220 relatives of 21
patients with pernicious anæmia. They concluded from an analysis of the pedigrees
that the development of this antibody is controlled by a autosomal gene with
incomplete penetrance showing a sex controlled bias. Roitt and Doniach (1967)
in a careful re-assessment of the aggregation of auto-immunity in families of
thyroiditis patients showed that the increased incidence of gastric antibodies
which had been previously reported in the relatives was no longer evident.

It is often stated that the geographic distribution of pernicious anæmia shows
considerable variation. It is said to be rare in the coloured races. The incidence
of gastric parietal cell antibodies and intrinsic factor antibodies in a population
of Hong Kong Chinese thyrotoxic patients was the same as in a British population
of similar patients (Irvine, McFadzean, Todd, Tso and Young; in preparation). A
less complete reduction in intrinsic factor together with a high dietary intake of
vitamin B_{12} probably explains the lower incidence of PA in the Hong Kong Chinese.

Clinical Value of Gastric Antibodies. It is suggested that patients at risk
of developing pernicious anæmia (those with thyroid auto-immune disease,
idiopathic Addison's disease, early onset diabetes, chronic hypochromic
anæmia and relatives of patients with pernicious anæmia) should be screened
routinely for antibody to gastric parietal cells and for antibody to intrinsic
factor. While such a procedure may indicate considerable subclinical disease
it will also indicate a proportion of patients with latent or overt pernicious
anæmia that had previously escaped diagnosis. The immunoassay of gastric
intrinsic factor is recommended as a simple and direct diagnostic aid and
can be done on the samples obtained during routine gastric analysis for
acid secretion.

Subclinical Atrophic Gastritis. The study of gastric auto-immunity has
revealed that advanced atrophic gastritis without symptoms and without
vitamin B_{12} deficiency is a common occurrence. This observation, together
with the development of an accurate and quantitative technique for the
assay of intrinsic factor, should allow a better understanding of the natural
history of atrophic gastritis and its mode of inheritance.

Liver Disease

There is evidence that auto-immunity is concerned with three types of
chronic liver disease—active chronic hepatitis, cryptogenic cirrhosis and
primary biliary cirrhosis.

Active Chronic Hepatitis ("Juvenile" Cirrhosis; "Lupoid" Hepatitis).
Active chronic hepatitis is associated with the markers indicative of an auto-
immune disease—hypergammaglobulinæmia, circulating auto-antibodies in
a proportion of cases to antigens derived from cell nuclei and cytoplasm,
lymphoid and plasma cell infiltration and "piecemeal" necrosis in the liver,
response to cortisone and an occasional association with other auto-immune
diseases (Mackay, Weiden and Hasker, 1965). Lupoid hepatitis may be
regarded as those cases of active chronic hepatitis that have a positive LE
cell test and who may occasionally have manifestations, usually of a
minor nature, of systemic lupus erythematosus. Some cases of active
chronic hepatitis have an initial illness resembling infective hepatitis, but in

many the disease has an insidious onset. Some cases of active chronic hepatitis become quiescent, but others progress to post-necrotic cirrhosis.

Cryptogenic Cirrhosis. In this group of patients there is no history of alcohol abuse and the histology shows a post-necrotic cirrhosis.

Primary biliary cirrhosis describes a clinical picture of prolonged obstructive jaundice or cholestasis, but with demonstrable patency of the extrahepatic ducts. The disease begins in mid to late adult life and is relentlessly progressive; the majority of cases occur in females. The onset is insidious and the course prolonged. The early histological appearances on liver biopsy show destruction of bile ducts with lymphocytic infiltration, initially with minimal fibrosis and a well-preserved hepatic architecture. Subsequently, the development of fibrous tissue in the portal areas and regeneration of liver tissue produces a finely or coarsely nodular cirrhosis.

Immunological Features of Liver Disease

ANF. According to Doniach *et al.* (1966) by far the highest incidence of ANF is found in active chronic hepatitis (77 per cent compared to 2 per cent in matched controls for this young age group). Fifty-six per cent had moderate or high titres although only five of the total of 43 subjects gave a positive LE cell test. Seventy-nine per cent of patients' sera gave a diffuse nuclear staining pattern and 21 per cent were of the speckled variety.

In primary biliary cirrhosis 46 per cent of 41 cases were positive for ANF, the titres being moderate or high in 31 per cent. Speckled and diffuse staining reactions were found in equal proportions and LE cell tests were consistently negative. Thirty-eight per cent of patients with cryptogenic cirrhosis were positive for ANF.

Mitochondrial Antibodies. Antibodies to mitochondria ("M" antibodies) have been described by Doniach *et al.* (1966) in the sera of virtually all patients with primary biliary cirrhosis (98 per cent). They were also found in 31 per cent of patients with cryptogenic cirrhosis (particularly those with obstructive features) and 28 per cent of cases of active chronic hepatitis. In contrast only two patients out of 28 with extrahepatic biliary obstruction and one patient out of 25 with infective hepatitis gave reactions and these in very low titre. Uniformly negative results for "M" antibodies were obtained in alcoholic cirrhosis, cholestatic drug jaundice and cholestasis associated with ulcerative colitis.

These antibodies are clearly of value to the clinician in the differential diagnosis of surgical from non-surgical jaundice, although care must be taken in interpretation of the results in cases with associated connective tissue disorders where a significant incidence of positive reactions has been observed. In confirmation of the findings of Walker *et al.* (1965), Goudie, MacSween and Goldberg (1966) noted that out of 30 cases diagnosed as primary biliary cirrhosis 26 had anti-mitochondrial antibody whereas none of 77 cases with jaundice due to extrahepatic bile obstruction showed this serological abnormality. The incidence of the "M" antibodies in the different types of liver disease suggest that they do not arise merely in response to liver damage.

As implied by the name, antibodies to mitochondria are not specific to any tissue. In the indirect immunofluorescence procedure "M" antibodies give a bright uniform cytoplasmic fluorescence with renal distal tubules, gastric parietal cell, and thyroid Askanazy cells, and a characteristically coarse granular duller staining of renal proximal tubule, thyroid epithelial and gastric chief cells (Fig. 4). Human renal distal tubule is probably the best tissue to use for the detection of "M" antibodies so as to avoid confusion with other tissue specific antibodies that may also be present in the patient's serum.

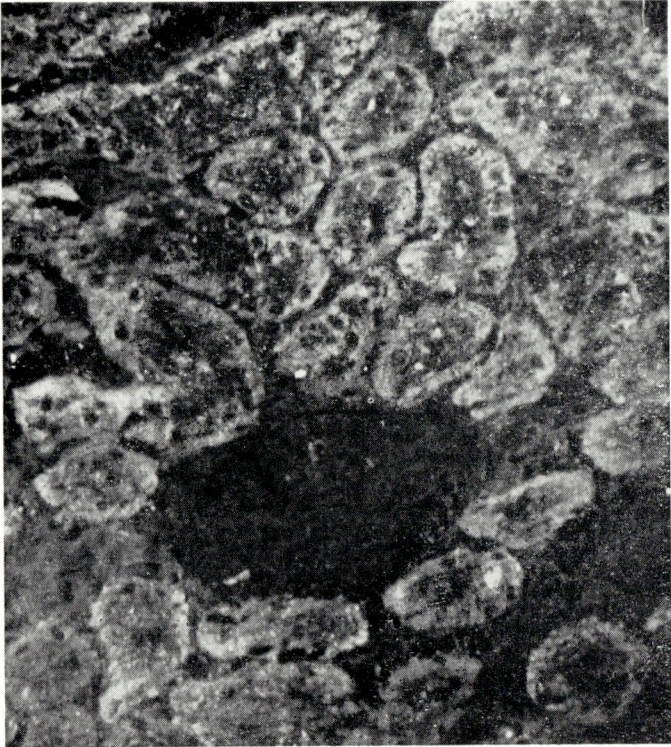

FIG. 4. Positive test for mitrochondrial ("M") antibodies using unfixed section of rat kidney, serum from a patient with primary biliary cirrhosis and anti-β, C conjugated with fluorescein. Note the bright uniform cytoplasmic fluorescence in the renal tubules. A glomerulus is seen to be unstained (UV $\times$ 350).

Complement Fixation Tests. Many authors have applied the complement fixation reaction to the study of antibodies in liver diseases, but in no instance was evidence for organ-specificity obtained. Doubt has been cast on the truly immunological nature of the so-called "auto-immune complement fixation test" of Gajdusek (Beall, 1963). Complement fixation tests with liver sera will detect antibodies to mitochondria and also to other cell constituents. They have been described in acute infective hepatitis (Holborow, *et al.*, 1963).

Pinckard and Weir (1966) have demonstrated a transient appearance of complement fixing antibodies which react mainly with mitochondrial fractions in rats developing liver cell necrosis after injections of carbon tetrachloride and other poisons. These reach a maximum 3–4 days after injury and disappear on recovery. Similar antibodies were obtained in rats by injections of homologous liver extracts, clearly showing that the rat responds immunologically to the products of liver cell breakdown. The finding of Doniach et al. (1966) of "M" antibodies in three out of five patients with drug related hepatic necrosis may be relevant in this context. These observations are difficult to reconcile, however, with the definite predilection of "M" antibodies for certain liver diseases and not for others as described above.

Smooth Muscle Antibodies. Smooth muscle antibodies as detected by the immunofluorescence test occur in about two-thirds of patients with active chronic hepatitis, about half of the patients with primary biliary cirrhosis and about a quarter of patients with cryptogenic cirrhosis (Johnson, Holborow and Glynn, 1965; Whittingham, 1966; Doniach et al., 1966). These antibodies were not found, or only in low incidence, in other forms of liver disease or in control subjects.

Rheumatoid Factor. The Latex fixation reaction is positive in 17–53 per cent of patients with viral hepatitis, primary biliary cirrhosis, and alcoholic, juvenile and cryptogenic cirrhosis. The incidence of a positive Rose-Waaler reaction is about half this figure except in primary biliary cirrhosis, when the incidence is comparable to that of the Latex fixation reaction (Bouchier, Rhodes and Sherlock, 1964).

Antibody to "Bile Canaliculi". Antibody staining bile canaliculi of the liver parenchymal cells has been claimed to occur using the immunofluorescence test by Johnson et al. (1966) in a proportion of patients with active chronic hepatitis. However, the staining pattern is not convincing with regard to bile canaliculi but may represent liver cell membranes. This would appear to be the first observation in liver disease of an antibody reacting with a component specific to the liver parenchyma. Antibody to bile ductual cells has been described in the immunofluorescence test by Paronetto, Schaffner and Popper (1964). Its existence requires further confirmation.

The demonstration that serum from some patients with putative auto-immune disease of the liver gives rise to staining of various tissue components by immunofluorescence raises the question whether some at least of these reactions are attributable to common elements in the tissues studied. The pattern of incidence of positive reactions with the different tissues and the observation that absorption of primary biliary cirrhosis serum with liver mitochondria leaves the smooth muscle staining intact without removing all the "M" fluorescence indicates that these are separate antigen antibody reactions (Johnson et al., 1966). On the other hand, Ironside, de Boer and Nairn (1966) have reported that the reaction with smooth muscle can be inhibited by absorption with homogenates of liver, kidney or stomach.

Thyroid and Gastric Antibodies. Thyroid and gastric antibodies have been observed more commonly in active chronic hepatitis and in primary biliary cirrhosis than in normal controls while this difference was not observed in alcoholic cirrhosis, extrahepatic obstruction or infective hepatitis (Doniach et al., 1966).

Immunosuppressive Therapy. A positive role of immune processes is suggested by the clinical improvement following steroids (Mackay and Wood, 1961) or other immunosuppressive drugs such as 6-mercaptopurine and azothioprine (Mackay, Weiden and Unger, 1964) in patients with active chronic hepatitis. However, Page, Condie and Good (1964) reported similar clinical and biochemical improvement in four patients with plasma cell hepatitis treated with 6-mercaptopurine in dosage insufficient to inhibit antibody production and expressed the opinion that the agent's beneficial effect could be related to suppression of a chronic virus infection.

Conclusion. In active chronic hepatitis, cryptogenic cirrhosis and primary biliary cirrhosis, there is evidence of a widespread immunological hyper-reactivity. The possibility of a co-existence of organ and non-organ specific antibodies in the sera of these patients requires further investigation, particularly in view of the demonstration of several liver-specific antigens (Milgrom, Tuggac and Witebsky, 1965). However, with the possible exception of antibody to"bile canaliculi" or to liver cell membranes there is no established evidence for the existence of antibodies that are specific for liver. Any causal relationship between the immune processes described so far and the pathogenesis of the disease remains unknown.

CHRONIC PANCREATITIS

Positive precipitin reactions with saline extracts of human pancreas have been reported in cases of chronic relapsing pancreatitis and pancreatic carcinoma (Thal, Murray and Enger, 1959; Fonkalsrud and Longmire, 1961). The serum from 14 of 16 patients with cystic fibrosis demonstrated clear and distinct precipitin lines to an extract of cystic fibrosis lung but only ill-defined precipitin lines were observed when the same sera were tested against an extract of cystic fibrosis pancreas (Stein *et al.*, 1964). Rhesus monkeys immunised with pooled Rhesus monkey pancreas extract and Freund's complete adjuvant developed pancreas-specific iso-antibodies, but auto-immunisation of rabbits with their now pancreas incorporated in Freund's complete adjuvant failed to elicit auto or iso-antibodies and the pancreas of the immunised animals were normal grossly and histologically. Further studies are required before the phenomenon of auto-immunity can be defined in relation to chronic pancreatitis in man.

MALABSORPTIVE DISEASE

In cœliac disease in children and its counterpart in adults, malabsorption is due to an idiosyncrasy to gluten, a complex heterogeneous protein in wheat and certain other cereals. The harmful factor resides in gliadin, the alcohol soluble portion of gluten. In gluten-induced enteropathy there is atrophy of the villi of the small intestine and heavy infiltration of the lamina propria with lymphocytes and plasma cells. (*See also* chap. 21.) Direct instillation of flour or gluten on to the histologically normal distal small intestine of patients with adult cœliac disease produces similar acute mucosal inflammation, whereas the intestinal mucosa of a normal subject remains unchanged (Rubin *et al.*, 1962). The malabsorption is usually correctable by a strict gluten-free diet, and corticosteroids are also effective.

In gluten-induced enteropathy of children and adults a significantly higher incidence and titre of antibodies to various fractions of wheat gliadin compared to controls has been shown (Heiner *et al.*, 1962; Taylor, Truelove and Wright, 1964). A high incidence of antibodies to other dietary proteins, particularly to milk proteins, has also been described in cœliac disease, but not all published results are in agreement. Sewell *et al.* (1963), for example, have confirmed the finding of high antibodies to milk proteins in cœliac disease but have failed to find antibodies to a gluten in the same sera. There is no apparent correlation between the clinical severity of the disease and the presence of the antibodies. The factors involved in determining such antibody responses could include proteolytic activities at all stages in the pathway of absorption, the activity of immunocytes in the gut wall, the lymphatic drainage, and the predetermined immune responsiveness to specific antigens. There have been descriptions of acquired agammaglobulinæmia in adult cœliac disease (Huizenga *et al.*, 1961). The tests to gluten and its fractions have been negative in cœliac patients, and peripheral eosinophilia and a personal or family history of allergy are unusual (Alvey, Anderson and Freeman, 1957).

Using the immunofluorescence method, Malik *et al.* (1964), claimed that the sera from patients with untreated cœliac disease reacts with the cytoplasm of human and monkey jejunal mucosa. This suggested that both the healthy and cœliac intestinal epithelium absorb antigen derivatives of gluten or possibly that some cœliac sera contain a humoral autoantibody to small bowel epithelial cells. Rubin *et al.*, (1965) were unable to confirm the presence of circulating autoantibodies to intestinal epithelium in cœliac disease. Nor could they demonstrate synthesis of gliadin specific immunoglobulins in small bowel immunocytes. Clearly there is much to be done on the relationship between humoral antibodies against dietary proteins, hypersensitivity states to such proteins and gastrointestinal disease.

In contrast to the concept of immunological hypersensitivity in cœliac disease, there is some evidence to suggest that immunological insufficiency may be of importance. Splenic atrophy, hypogammaglobulinæmia and lymphoma of the small intestine may occur in association with idiopathic steatorrhœa (McCarthy *et al.*, 1966). It has also been shown that patients with idiopathic steatorrhœa may be deficient in the synthesis of gamma A immunoglobulin in the alimentary tract and that gamma A immunoglobulins may be of importance in maintaining the integrity of the intestinal mucosa (Crabbé and Heremans, 1966).

CROHN'S DISEASE

While no circulating antibodies to intestinal mucosa have been found in Crohn's disease, this condition shares with ulcerative colitis a number of extra-intestinal manifestations which are of considerable interest in an immunological context.

The granulomas of Crohn's disease are similar to those found in sarcoidosis, but the gastro-intestinal tract is rarely affected in sarcoidosis and the two conditions would appear to be quite separate. They do resemble one another immunologically, however, in that both have a high incidence of negative Mantoux reactions, but the Kveim test is negative in Crohn's disease and attempts to produce a similar reaction with Crohn's tissue have not been successful (Williams, 1965). The analogy with sarcoidosis is not very close and immunology has added little to the understanding of this condition.

ULCERATIVE COLITIS

The clinical and pathological features of ulcerative colitis provide some circumstantial evidence of the possible importance of immunological factors in its characterization. The serum gammaglobulin level may be raised, there is a high frequency of extracolonic manifestations (many suspected of originating from hypersensitivity, such as arthritis, conjunctivitis, and erythema nodosum), the histology shows extensive lymphocytic infiltration in the colonic mucosa, and the response to corticosteroid therapy is well known (Broberger, 1964). There may be a slight but significant prevalence of ulcerative colitis in females (Evans and Acheson, 1965).

In ulcerative colitis abnormal immunological responses have been sought to antigens derived from three sources—the patient's own tissues, bacteria and food constituents.

Auto-antibodies. Broberger and Perlmann (1959) suggested that auto-immune reactions might be relevant to the study of ulcerative colitis and showed that hæmagglutinating antibodies to a hot phenol-water extract of human fœtal colon are present in the sera of a high proportion of children with ulcerative colitis, with a lesser incidence in adults with the disease. Some positive reactions in this test have been obtained using sera from patients with rheumatoid arthritis, systemic lupus erythematosis, some liver diseases and the nephrotic syndrome, but in a lower incidence than in ulcerative colitis (Asherson and Broberger, 1961). Immunofluorescence studies using unfixed sections of human colon have shown that the circulating antibodies react with an antigen in colonic epithelial-cell cytoplasm (Fig. 5).

There is a positive correlation between the results of the hæmagglutination and the immunofluorescence tests, the former being more sensitive (Lagercrantz *et al*, 1966). Absorption of sera with fœtal colon inhibited positive results with both techniques. 56 per cent of a group of 101 ulcerative colitis patients were found to have a hæmagglutination titre $\geq 1:16$ compared to 13 per cent of age and sex matched healthy controls or surgical cases. Of 109 patients with other gastrointestinal disorders (chronic diarrhœas of unknown ætiology, bacillary dysentery, Salmonella infection, cancer of colon and rectum, cœliac disease) only 8 had a titre $\geq 1:16$. Fluorescent antibody staining of rat colon sections confirmed these results (Lagercrantz *et al*., 1966). In this series no clear difference was noted in the incidence or titre of control of antibodies in children compared to adults.

The hæmagglutination procedure has shown that the colon antigen is also present in extracts from other parts of the gastro-intestinal tract of germ-free rats and is independent of blood group A and H antigens (Hammarström *et al*., 1965; Perlmann *et al*., 1965). Background reactivity somewhat decreases the sensitivity of the hæmagglutination test as a diagnostic tool for the comparison of different groups of sera, since only titres elevated over the low and arbitrary chosen level of the controls can be counted as positive (e.g. $\geq 1:16$).

The antigen is probably a lipopolysaccharide, but it is difficult to prepare and many preparations are inactive. The antibody will react with the patient's own colon tissue indicating that it is a true auto-antibody. The presence of colonic antibodies cannot be correlated with any clinical features, and may even persist after colectomy (Harrison, 1965a; Wright and Truelove, 1966; Lagercrantz *et al*., 1966). Using the fluorescent method Harrison (1965a) detected antibody reacting with mucosal cells of the small and large intestines in 27 out of 200 cases. All the control sera were negative. The sera of a few ulcerative colitis patients reacted with the superficial mucosa cells of the stomach. Lagercrantz *et al*. (1966) also noted a few patients with ulcerative colitis who had antibodies against the superficial mucous cells of the stomach which were distinct from those reacting with colon.

Positive sera have not been shown to be cytotoxic to colon cells, although such cells grown in culture will fix antibody (Broberger and Perlmann, 1963). The most powerful evidence so far implicating auto-immune mechanisms in ulcerative colitis is the finding that leucocytes from patients with ulcerative colitis are cytotoxic for fœtal colon cells in tissue culture (Perlmann and Broberger, 1963). Freshly obtained fœtal colon cells were labelled with ^{32}P-orthophosphate or ^{14}C-amino acids and exposed to white cells from children with ulcerative colitis or from healthy controls. Exposure of the colon cells to patients' white cells led to a rapid isotope release, significantly higher than that obtained with normal white cells. The cytotoxic action of the patients' white cells was immunologically specific, since no

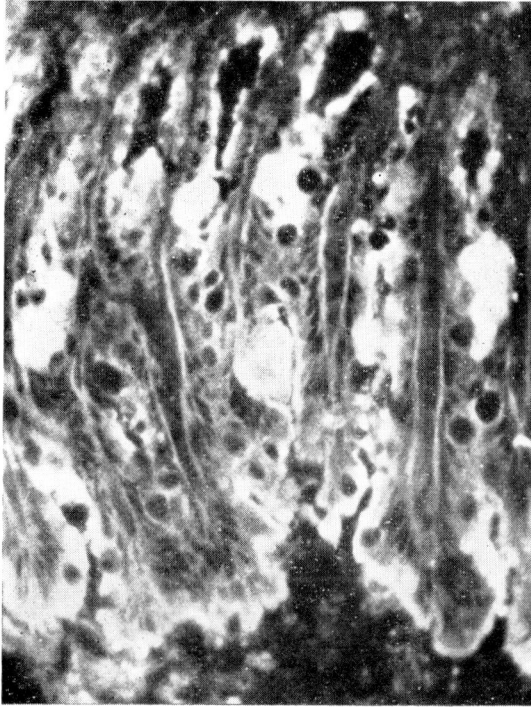

FIG. 5. Section of germ free rat colon mucosa stained by indirect fluorescence after treatment with ulcerative colitis serum (blood group A). Note specific staining of mucosal epithelial particularly of goblet cells and of inner surface of mucous membranes (mucus). Submucosal layer not stained (UV $\times$ 125).

(From Lagercrantz et al. (1966), Clin. exp. Immunol.)

difference from the controls was found in the isotope release when cells from other organs or animals were similarly treated. Complement was required in the system for a cytotoxic effect to be manifest. This observation has recently been confirmed by Watson, Quigley and Bolt (1966). It would seem that cellular antibody mediated by lymphocytes, rather than the antibody titre in the serum, may be responsible. In support of this, Watson, Styler and Bolt (1966) have shown that leucocytes from about one-third of patients with ulcerative colitis may produce autologous skin reactions. Taylor (1965) and Wright and Truelove (1966) report an increased incidence of gastric parietal cell antibody in ulcerative colitis, while Harrison (1965b) found no increase in incidence compared to controls. The presence of anti-nuclear factor in the sera of ulcerative colitis patients has been reported, but again the results are conflicting, due to lack of standardization in the detection of antinuclear factor and lack of adequate controls matched for age and sex.

Antibody to Bacteria.—The clinical observation that an intercurrent infection may provoke a relapse of ulcerative colitis raises the possibility that an immunological response against normal or non-pathogenic bacteria might trigger off an auto-immune response against related antigens in the colon. Perlmann *et al.* (1965) suggested a cross reactivity between bacterial lipopolysaccharides and colon antigen, since absorption of the sera of colitis patients with lipopolysaccharide derived from *E. coli* 014 reduced the reaction with colon antigen. A positive correlation was also found between the degree of reaction of sera with colonic and bacterial antigens. The bacterial antigen involved may be the heterogenetic antigen of Kunin (1963). Rabbits injected with various dead enteric organisms in complete Freund's adjuvant produce antibodies which react with their own colon and in some cases with ileum and stomach (Asherson and Holborow, 1966). There is yet no evidence that the production of these antibodies is associated with any pathology of the colon or elsewhere.

In testing for antibody to colon it is essential to use germ-free colon. If normal adult colon is used then 100 per cent of sera, whether from patients with ulcerative colitis or from normal controls, give positive reactions due to the bacterial contamination.

These facts are compatible with the view that ulcerative colitis is due to an auto-immune reaction against the colon mucosa perhaps caused by an antigenic similarity between certain bowel organisms and the mucosal cells of the colon. This would relate the immunological findings in ulcerative colitis to those of rheumatic heart disease and glomerulonephritis where cross-reactivity with streptococcal antigen is implicated. Alternatively, ulcerative colitis may be due to an immune response against bacteria or bacterial residues lodged in the wall of the colon, and the auto-antibodies may be an irrelevant concomitant of a strong immune response to bacteria.

Food Hypersensitivity. Taylor and Truelove (1961) reported higher serum antibody titres to the three main milk proteins (casein, lactoglobulin and lactalbumin) in patients with ulcerative colitis than in controls. Acheson and Truelove (1961) claimed that patients with ulcerative colitis had been weaned at an earlier age than control subjects. A beneficial effect of a milk-free diet in patients with a frank attack of uncomplicated ulcerative colitis has been suggested by Wright and Truelove (1965). However, the significance of antibodies to milk proteins in ulcerative colitis lacks conviction; the selective incidence and titres of milk antibodies in ulcerative colitis and the differences in the weaning habits compared to controls have not been confirmed (Dudek, Spiro and Thayer, 1965). A "milk free" diet would seem to be almost an impossibility; indeed, butter (which contains about 0·5 per cent milk protein) was allowed. Presumably this would be sufficient to perpetuate a state of hypersensitivity (Taylor, 1966). Some forms of milk intolerance may be non-immunological and due to intolerance to lactose (Jeejeebhoy, Desai and Verghese, 1964; Struthers, Singleton and Kern, 1965).

Extracolonic Manifestations. In both ulcerative colitis and Crohn's disease extra-intestinal manifestations may be prominent. Holdsworth *et al.* (1965) have presented strong clinical evidence of an association between ulcerative colitis and lupoid hepatitis or inactive cryptogenic cirrhosis. The relationship between ulcerative colitis and arthritis has been reviewed by McEwen *et al.* (1962) who state that there is no significant association with rheumatoid arthritis or rheumatoid factor, but that ulcerative colitis is clearly associated with a peripheral form of arthritis distinct from rheumatoid. In the study of 114 patients with ulcerative colitis Wright *et al.* (1965) reported that 12 per cent had evidence of past or present anterior uveitis and 17 per cent had evidence of sacroiliac involvement, whereas the incidence among controls was negligible. Wright and Watkinson (1965) described a colitic type of arthritis which usually begins as an acute arthritis, affecting a single joint of the lower limb, and then spreading predominantly in the legs in an asymmetrical manner. The improvement in the peripheral or colitic arthritis with a spontaneous or therapeutically induced remission of the ulcerative colitis would suggest that it at least is a secondary complication of the intestinal disease.The evidence that colitic arthritis, spondylitis and uveitis are related to auto-immune disease is nebulous. However, it is conceivable that these extracolonic manifestations of ulcerative colitis might result from a hypersensitivity reaction to antigens, for example, bacterial antigens released from the diseased colon, and represent true complications of the ulcerative colitis.

CONCLUSION

The alimentary diseases illustrate a wide range of immunological disorders or different forms of immunological aberration. At one end of the spectrum is the atrophic gastritis of pernicious anæmia which is one of the group of diseases (pernicious anæmia, auto-immune thyroid disease, idiopathic adrenal insufficiency and idiopathic hypoparathyroidism) that is characterised by the occurrence of organ-specific auto-antibodies and in which there is negligible incidence of antibodies reacting simultaneously with constituents of multiple tissues. In Sjögren's disease and the triad of liver diseases (primary biliary cirrhosis, active chronic hepatitis and cryptogenic cirrhosis) the majority of auto-antibodies described are non-organ-specific (e.g. antinuclear factors, antibodies to mitochondria and to smooth muscle, rheumatoid factor), but in both these groups of diseases there may be some overlap with organ-specific antibodies (e.g. thyroid and gastric) and in liver disease there may be a specific antibody to bile canaliculi or to liver cell membranes. In gluten enteropathy there is clearly an intolerance to a food constituent and this may be due to immunological hypersensitivity. The significance of food allergy in relation to ulcerative colitis is unknown; indeed, the alleged increased incidence and titre of antibodies to milk proteins in ulcerative colitis has been questioned.

Ulcerative colitis illustrates the interesting concept of immunological cross-reactivity between a bacterial antigen and an auto-antigen and places ulcerative colitis along with rheumatic fever and glomerulonephritis in this respect. The immunological aberration in relation to ulcerative colitis would therefore appear to be distinct from that occurring in pernicious anæmia and distinct again from that occurring in liver diseases although there is some overlap between hepatitis and ulcerative colitis.

Ulcerative colitis is unique in the alimentary diseases in that a cytotoxic effect of lymphocytes from a patient with the disease has been demonstrated against colon cells in tissue culture. Attempts at producing lesions of the alimentary tract by immunological techniques in animals have met with little success, except for atrophic gastritis in the monkey.

With regard to auto-antibodies as an aid to clinical or subclinical diagnosis, the presence of parietal cell antibodies in the serum may be taken to indicate some degree of atrophic gastritis while the presence of intrinsic factor antibodies in the serum shows a strong correlation with malabsorption of vitamin B_{12} due to lack of intrinsic factor secretion with advanced atrophic gastritis. The application of serological tests to the screening of subjects at risk with regard to pernicious anæmia leads to an earlier detection of the disease and should prove helpful in the elucidation of its natural history. While the detection of antibody to salivary duct tissue may prove valuable in the investigation of a suspected case of Sjögren's disease, the clinical value of mitochondrial ("M") antibodies in the differentiation between surgical and non-surgical jaundice has already been established.

Much further work requires to be done in relation to the immunological aspects of alimentary disease. In some disorders the occurrence of auto-antibodies and of hypersensitivity to exogenous antigens requires to be more clearly defined. In other disorders affecting the alimentary system where the occurrence of auto-antibodies has been defined, the reason for their development and their role in the pathogenesis of that disease remains an enigma.

References

ABELS, J., BOUMA, W., JANSZ, A., WOLDRING, M. G., BAKKER, A., NIEWEG, H. O. (1963). *J. Lab. clin. Med.*, **61**, 893.
ACHESON, E. D., TRUELOVE, S. C. (1961). *Brit. med. J.*, **ii**, 929.
ADAMS, J. F., GLEN, A. I. M., KENNEDY, E. H., MACKENZIE, I. L., MORROW, J. M., ANDERSON, J. R., GRAY, K. G., MIDDLETON, D. G. (1964). *Lancet*. **i**, 401.
ALVEY, C., ANDERSON, C. M., FREEMAN, M. (1957). *Arch. Dis. Childh.*, **32**, 434.
ANDERSON, J. R., BECK, J. S., BUCHANAN, W. W., BLOCH, K. J., BUNIM, J. J. (1965). "Autoimmunity." A Symposium of the 5th Congress of the International Academy of Pathology. Ed. R. W. Baldwin, J. H. Humphrey. Oxford: Blackwell.
ANDERSON, J. R., GRAY, K. G., BECK, J. S., KINNEAR, W. F. (1961). *Lancet*, **ii**, 456.
ANDRADA, J. A., ROSE, N. R.(1969). *Clin. exp. Immunol.*, **4**. In press.
ARDEMAN, S., CHANARIN, I. (1963). *Lancet*, **ii**, 1350.
ARDEMAN, S., CHANARIN, I. (1965a). *Brit. J. Haemat.*, **11**, 305.
ARDEMAN, S., CHANARIN, I. (1965b). *New Eng. J. Med.*, **273**, 1352.
ARDEMAN, S., CHANARIN, I., KRAFCHNIK, B., SINGER, W. (1966). *Quart. J. Med.*, **35**, 421.
ASHERSON, G. L., BROBERGER, O. (1961). *Brit. med. J.*, **i**, 1429.
ASHERSON, G. L., HOLBOROW, E. J. (1966). *Immunology*, **10**, 161.
BAUR, S., ROITT, I. M., DONIACH, D. (1965). *Immunology*, **8**, 62.
BEALL, G. N. (1963). *J. lab. clin. med.*, **61**, 67.
BECK, J. S., ANDERSON, J. R., BLOCH, K. J., BUCHANAN, W. W., BUNIM, J. J. (1965). *Ann. rheum., Dis.*, **24**, 16.
BERTRAM, U., HALBERG, P. (1964). *Acta allerg. Kbh*, **19**, 458.
BERTRAM, U., HALBERG, P. (1965). *Acta allerg. Kbh*, **20**, 472.
BLOCH, K. J., BUCHANAN, W. W., WOHL, M. J., BUNIM, J. J. (1965). *Medicine*, **44**, 187.
BLOCH, K. J., BUNIM, J. J. (1963). *J. chron. Dis.*, **16**, 915.
BOUCHIER, I. A. D., RHODES, K., SHERLOCK, S. (1964). *Brit. med. J.*, **i**, 592.
BROBERGER, O. (1964). *Gastroenterology*, **47**, 229.

BROBERGER, O., PERLMANN, P. (1959). *J. exp. Med.*, **110,** 657.
BROBERGER, O., PERLMANN, P. (1963). *J. exp. Med.*, **117,** 705.
BUNIM, J. J., BUCHANAN, W. W., WERTLAKE, P. T., SOKOLFF, L., BLOCH, K. J., BECK, J. S., ALEPA, F. P. (1964). *Ann. int. Med.*, **61,** 509.
BURCH, T. A., BUNIM, J. J., BLOCH, K. J. (1963). "The Epidemiology of Chronic Rheumatism", Vol. 1. p. 267. Ed. J. H. Kellgren, M. R. Jeffrey, J. F. A. Bell. Philadelphia: Davis.
CALLENDAR, S. T., DENBOROUGH, M. A. (1957). *Brit. J. Haemat.*, **3,** 88.
CHAN, W. C. (1964). *J. Path Bact.*, **88,** 592.
COGHILL, N. F., DONIACH, D., ROITT, I. M., MOLLIN, D. L., WILLIAMS, A. W. (1965). *Gut*, **6,** 48.
CRABBÉ, P. A., CARBONARA, A. O., HEREMANS, J. F. (1965). *Lab. Invest.*, **14,** 235.
CRABBÉ, P. A., HEREMANS, J. F. (1966). *Gut*, **7,** 119.
CROFT, D. N., POLLOCK, D. J., COGHILL, N. F. (1966). *Gut*, **7,** 333.
DAGG, J. H., GOLDBERG, A., ANDERSON, J. R., BECK, J. S., GRAY, K. G. (1964). *Brit. med. J.*, **i,** 1349.
DE BOER, W. G. R. M., NAIRN, R. C., MAXWELL, A. (1965). *J. clin. Path.*, **18,** 456.
DOIG, A., GIRDWOOD, R. H., DUTHIE, J. J. R., KNOX, J. D. E. (1957). *Lancet*, **ii,** 966.
DONIACH, D., ROITT, I. M. (1964). *Seminars in Haematology*, **1,** 313.
DONIACH, D., ROITT, I. M., TAYLOR, K. B. (1965). *Ann. N.Y. Acad. Sci.*, **124,** 605.
DONIACH, D., ROITT, I. M., WALKER, J. G., SHERLOCK, S. (1966). *Clin. exp. Immunol.*, **1,** 237.
DUDEK, B., SPIRO, H. M., THAYER, W. R. (1965). *Gastroenterology*, **49,** 544.
EVANS, J. G., ACHESON, E. D. (1965). *Gut*, **6,** 311.
FELTKAMP, T. E. W., VAN ROSSUM, A. L. (1968). *Clin. exp. Immunol.*, **3,** 1.
FISHER, J. M., REES, C., TAYLOR, K. B. (1965). *Science*, **150,** 1467.
FISHER, J. M., REES, C., TAYLOR, K. B. (1966). *Lancet*, **ii,** 88.
FONKALSRUD, E. W., LONGMIRE, W. P. (1961). *Surgery*, **50,** 134.
FROST, J. W., GOLDWEIN, M. I. (1958). *New Eng. J. Med.*, **258,** 1096.
GOLDBERG, A., LOCHHEAD, A. C., DAGG, J. H. (1963). *Lancet*, **i,** 848.
GORDIN, R. (1959). *Acta med. Scand.*, **164,** 159.
GOTTLIEB, C., LAU, K. S., WASSERMAN, L. R., HERBERT, V. (1965). *Blood*, **25,** 875.
GOUDIE, R. B., MACSWEEN, R. N. M., GOLDBERG, D. M. (1966). *J. clin. Path.*, **19,** 527.
HAMMARSTRÖM, S., LAGERCRANTZ, R., PERLMANN, P., GUSTAFSSON, B. E. (1965). *J. exp. Med.*, **122,** 1075.
HARRISON, W. J. (1965a). *Lancet*, **i,** 1346.
HARRISON, W. J. (1965b). *Lancet*, **1,** 1350.
HEINER, D. C., LAHEY, M. E., WILSON, J. F., GERRARD, J. W., SCHWACHMAN, H., KHAW, K. T. (1962). *J. Pediat.*, **61,** 813.
HOEDEMAEKER, P. J., ABELS, J., WACHTERS, J. J., ARENDS, A., NIEWEG, H. O. (1964). *Lab. Invest.*, **13,** 1394.
HOLBOROW, E. J., ASHERSON, G. L., JOHNSON, G. D., BARNES, R. D., CARMICHAEL, D. S. (1963). *Brit. med. J.*, **i,** 656.
HOLDSWORTH, C. D., HALL, E. W., DAWSON, A. M., SHERLOCK, S. (1965). *Quart. J. Med.*, **34,** 211.
HUIZENGA, K. A., WOLLAEGER, E. E., GREEN, P. A., MCKENZIE, B. F. (1961). *Amer. J. Med.*, **31,** 572.
IRONSIDE, P. N. J., DE BOER, W. G. R. M., NAIRN, R. C. (1966). *Lancet*, **i,** 1210.
IRVINE, W. J. (1963). *Quart. J. exp. Physiol.*, **48,** 427.
IRVINE, W. J. (1965a). *New Engl. J. Med.*, **273,** 432.
IRVINE, W. J. (1965b). *Lancet*, **i,** 736.
IRVINE, W. J. (1966a). *Clin. exp. Immunol.*, **1,** 341.
IRVINE, W. J. (1966b). *Clin. exp. Immunol.*, **1,** 99.
IRVINE, W. J. (1967). *Clin. exp. Immunol.*, **2,** 740.
IRVINE, W. J. (1968). *Proc. R. Soc. Med.* In press.
IRVINE, W. J., CULLEN, D. R., SCARTH, L., SIMPSON, J. (1968). *Lancet*, **2,** 184.
IRVINE, W. J., DAVIES, S. H. (1963). *Lancet*, **ii,** 538.
IRVINE, W. J., DAVIES, S. H., DELAMORE, I. W., WILLIAMS, A. W. (1962). *Brit. med. J.*, **ii,** 454.
IRVINE, W. J., DAVIES, S. H., TEITELBAUM, S., DELAMORE, I. W., WYNN WILLIAMS, A. (1965a). *Ann. N.Y. Acad. Sci.*, **124,** 657.
IRVINE, W. J., DAVIES, S. H., HAYNES, R. C., SCARTH, L. (1965b). *Lancet*, **ii,** 397.
IRVINE, W. J., STEWART, A. G., SCARTH, L. (1967). *Clin. exp. Immunol.*, **2,** 31.
JEEJEEBHOY, K. N., DESAI, H. G., VERGHESE, R. V. (1964). *Lancet*, **ii,** 666.
JEFFRIES, G. H. (1965). *Gastroenterology*, **48,** 371.
JEFFRIES, G. H., HOSKINS, D. W., SLEISENGER, M. H., (1962). *J. clin. Invest.*, **41,** 1106.
JEFFRIES, G. H., TODD, J. E., SLEISENGER, M. H. (1966). *J. clin. Invest.*, **45,** 803.

JEFFRIES, G. H., SLEISENGER, M. H. (1965). *J. clin. Invest.*, **44**, 2021.

JOHNSON, G. D., HOLBOROW, E. J., GLYNN, L. E. (1966). *Lancet*, **ii**, 416.

JOHNSON, G. D., HOLBOROW, E. J., GLYNN, L. E. (1965). *Lancet*, **ii**, 878.

KRISTENSEN, H. P., FRIIS, T. (1960). *Acta med. Scand.*, **166**, 249.

KUNIN, C. M. (1963). *J. exp. Med.*, **118**, 565.

LAWRIE, J. H., ANDERSON, N. M. (1967). *Lancet*, **1**, 68.

LEHNER, T. (1964). *Lancet*, **ii**, 1154.

LEHNER, T. (1967). *Brit. dent. J.*, **122**, 15.

LAGERCRANTZ, R. HAMMARSTRÖM, S., PERLMANN, P. and GUSTAFSSON, B. E. (1966). *Clin. exp. Immunol.*, **1**, 263.

MCCARTHY, C. F., FRASER, I. D., EVANS, K. T., READ, A. E. (1966). *Gut*, **7**, 140.

MCEWAN, C., LINGG, C., KIRSNER, J. B., SPENCER, J. A. (1962). *Amer. J. Med.*, **33**, 923.

MCFADYEN, I. J., GOLDBERG, A., DAGG, J. H., ANDERSON, J. R. (1967). *Clin. exp. Immunol.*, **2**, 737.

MCINTYRE, P. A., HAHN, R., CONLEY, C. L., GLASS, B. (1959). *Bull. Johns Hopkins Hospital*, **104**, 309.

MCINTYRE, O. R., SULLIVAN, L. W., JEFFRIES, G. H. and SILVER, R. H. (1965). *New Engl. J. Med.*, **272**, 981.

MACKAY, I. R. (1964). *Gut*, **5**, 23.

MACKAY, I. R., WEIDEN, S., HASKER, J. (1965). *Ann. N.Y. Acad. Sci.*, **124**, 767.

MACKAY, I. R., WEIDEN, S., UNGAR, B. (1964). *Lancet*, **i**, 899.

MACKAY, I. R., WOOD, I. J. (1961). "Progress in Liver Diseases", Chap. 3. Ed. H. POPPER, F. SCHOFFNER. *New York*: Grune and Stratton.

MALIK, G. B., WATSON, W. C., MURRAY, D., CRUIKSHANK, B. (1964). *Lancet*, **i**, 1127.

MILGROM, F., TUGGAC, Z. M., WITEBSKY, E. (1965). *J. Immunol.*, **94**, 157.

MOORE, J. M., NEILSON, J. McE., (1963). *Lancet*, **ii**, 645.

MORGAN, W. S., CASTLEMAN, B. (1953). *Amer. J. Path.*, **29**, 471.

PAGE, A. R., CONDIE, R. M., GOOD, R. A. (1964). *Amer. J. Med.*, **36**, 200.

PARONETTO, F., SCHAFFNER, F., POPPER, H. (1964). *New Engl. J. Med.*, **271**, 1123.

PERLMANN, P., BROBERGER, O. (1963). *J. exp. Med.*, **117**, 717.

PERLMANN, P., HAMMARSTRÖM, S., LAGERCRANTZ, R., GUSTAFSSON, B. E. (1965). *Ann. N.Y. Acad. Sci.*, **124**, 377.

PINCKARD, R. N., WEIR, D. M. (1966). *Clin. exp. Immunol.*, **1**, 33.

RØDBRO, P., DIGE-PETERSEN, H., SCHWARTZ, M., DALGAARD, O. Z. (1967). *Acta med. Scand.*, **181**, 445.

ROITT, I. M., DONIACH, D. (1967). *Clin. exp. Immunol.*, **2**, 727.

ROITT, I. M., DONIACH, D., SHAPLAND, C. (1965). *Ann. N.Y. Acad. Sci.*, **124**, 644.

RUBIN, C. E., BRANDBORG, L. L., FLICK, A. L., PHELPS, P., PARMENTIER, C., VAN NIEL, S. (1962). *Gastroenterology*, **43**, 621.

RUBIN, W., FAUCI, A. S., MARVIN, S. F., SLEISENGER, M. H., JEFFRIES, G. H. (1965). *J. clin. Invest.*, **44**, 475.

SCHADE, S. G., FEICK, P. L., IMRIE, M. H., SCHILLING, R. F. (1967). *Clin. exp. Immunol.*, **2**, 399.

SCHADE, S. G., FEICK, P., MUCKERHEIDE, M., SCHILLING, R. F. (1966). *New Engl. J. Med.*, **275**, 528.

SCHWARTZ, M. (1958). *Lancet*, **ii**, 61.

SCHWARTZ, M. (1960). *Lancet*, **ii**, 1263.

SEWELL, P., COOKE, W. T., COX, E. V., MEYNELL, M. J. (1963). *Lancet*, **ii**, 1132.

STEIN, A. A., MANLAPAS, F. C., SOIKE, K. F., PATTERSON, P. R. (1964). *J. Pediat.*, **65**, 495.

STRUTHERS, J. E., SINGLETON, J. W., KERN, F. (1965). *Ann. intern. Med.*, **63**, 221.

STURGILL, B. C., CARPENTER, R. R. (1965). *Arth. Rheum.*, **8**, 213.

TAYLOR, K. B. (1959). *Lancet*, **ii**, 106.

TAYLOR, K. B. (1965). *Fed. Proc.*, **24**, 23.

TAYLOR, K. B. (1966). *Gastroenterology*, **51**, 1058.

TAYLOR, K. B., ROITT, I. M., DONIACH, D., COUCHMAN, K. G., SHAPLAND, C. (1962). *Brit. med. J.*, **ii**, 1347.

TAYLOR, K. B., TRUELOVE, S. C. (1961). *Brit. med. J.*, **ii**, 924.

TAYLOR, K. B., TRUELOVE, S. C., WRIGHT, R. (1964). *Gastroenterology*, **46**, 99.

THAL, A. P., MURRAY, M. J., EGNER, W. (1959). *Lancet*, **i**, 1128.

TUDHOPE, G. R., WILSON, G. M. (1962). *Lancet*, **1**, 703.

VELDE, K. TE, ABELS, J., ANDERS, G. J. P. A., HOEDEMAEKER, Ph. J., NIEWEG, H. O. (1964). *J. Lab. clin. Med.*, **64**, 177.

WALKER, J. G., DONIACH, D., ROITT, I. M., SHERLOCK, S. (1965). *Lancet*, **i**, 827.

WALL, A. J., WHITTINGHAM, S., MACKAY, I. R., UNGAR, B. (1968). *Clin. exp. Immunol.*, **3**, 359.

WANGEL, A. G., CALLENDER. S. T. (1965). *Brit. med. J.*, **1**, 1409.

WARD, H. A., NAIRN, R. C. (1967). *Clin. exp. immunol.*, **2**, 565.

WATSON, D. W., QUIGLEY, A., BOLT, R. J. (1966). *Gastroenterology*, **50,** 886.
WATSON, D. W., STYLER, H. J., BOLT, R. J. (1965). *Gastroenterology*, **49,** 649.
WHITTINGHAM, S., IRWIN, J., MACKAY, I. R., SMALLEY, M. (1966). *Gastroenterology*, **51,** 499.
WIEDERMANN, G., MIESCHER, P. A. (1965). *Ann. N.Y. Acad. Sci.*, **124,** 807.
WILLIAMS, W. J. (1965). *Gut*, **6,** 503.
WRIGHT, R., LUMSDEN, K., LUNTZ, M. H., SEVEL, D., TRUELOVE, S. C. (1965). *Quart. J. Med.*, **34,** 229.
WRIGHT, R., TRUELOVE, S. C. (1965). *Brit. med. J.*, **ii,** 138.
WRIGHT, R., TRUELOVE, S. C. (1966). *Gut*, **7,** 32.
WRIGHT, R., WHITEHEAD, R., WANGEL, A. G., SALEM, S. N., SCHILLER, K. F. R. (1966). *Lancet*, **i,** 618.
WRIGHT, V., WATKINSON, G. (1965). *Brit. med. J.*, **ii,** 670.

INDEX